Dr Jon Newsome
With Sincere Best Wishes
The Anesthesiology Faculty

Thoracic Anesthesia

Thoracic Anesthesia

Edited by
Joel A. Kaplan, M.D.

Professor
Department of Anesthesiology
Director
Division of Cardiothoracic Anesthesia
Emory University School of Medicine
Atlanta, Georgia

CHURCHILL LIVINGSTONE

NEW YORK, EDINBURGH, LONDON, AND MELBOURNE   1983

Distributed in the United Kingdom by Churchill Livingstone, Robert Stevenson House, 1–3 Baxter's Place, Leith Walk, Edinburgh EH1 3AF and associated companies, branches and representatives throughout the world.

First published 1983
Printed in U.S.A.

ISBN 0-443-08166-2
9 8 7 6 5 4 3 2 1

Library of Congress Cataloging in Publication Data
Main entry under title:

Thoracic anesthesia.

  Bibliography; p.
  Includes index.
  1. Chest—Surgery.   2. Anesthesiology.
I. Kaplan, Joel A.   [DNLM: 1. Thoracic surgery.
2. Thorax—Drug effects.   3. Anesthesia.
WF 980 T4855]
RD536.T453   1982   617'.96754   82-12809
ISBN 0-443-08166-2

Manufactured in the United States of America

Contributors

David D. Alfery, M.D.
Staff Anesthesiologist, St. Thomas Hospital, Nashville, Tennessee

Jonathan L. Benumof, M.D.
Associate Professor, Department of Anesthesiology, University of California, San Diego, San Diego, California

James W. Bland, Jr., M.D.
Professor, Department of Anesthesiology, Professor, Department of Pediatrics, Director, Division of Pediatric Cardiovascular Anesthesia, Emory University School of Medicine; Medical Director, Intensive Care Unit, Henrietta Egleston Hospital for Children, Inc., Atlanta, Georgia

John T. Bonner, M.D.
Associate Professor, Department of Anesthesiology, Assistant Professor, Department of Surgery, Emory University School of Medicine; Co-Director, SICU, Veterans Administration Medical Center, Atlanta, Georgia

Patrick E. Curling, M.D.
Assistant Professor, Department of Anesthesiology, Emory University School of Medicine, Atlanta, Georgia

John B. Downs, MD.
Medical Director, Anesthesia and Pulmonary Medicine, Mercy Hospital, Urbana, Illinois; Associate Professor, Department of Anesthesiology, Northwestern University School of Medicine, Chicago, Illinois

James B. Eisenkraft, M.D.
Assistant Clinical Professor, Department of Anesthesiology, Mount Sinai School of Medicine, New York, New York

Adel A. El-Etr, M.D.
Professor and Chairman, Department of Anesthesiology, Loyola University Medical Center and Stritch School of Medicine, Maywood, Illinois

Brendan T. Finucane, M.D., F.F.A.R.C.S. (Eng.), F.R.C.P. (C)
Chief of Anesthesiology, Grady Memorial Hospital, Associate Professor, Department of Anesthesiology, Emory University School of Medicine, Atlanta, Georgia

T. James Gallagher, M.D.
Associate Professor, Department of Anesthesiology and Surgery, Chief, Division of Critical Care Medicine, University of Florida College of Medicine, Gainesville, Florida

James R. Hall, M.D.
Assistant Professor, Department of Anesthesiology, Emory University School of Medicine, Atlanta, Georgia

Eric G. Honig, M.D.
Assistant Professor, Department of Medicine (Pulmonary Diseases), Emory University School of Medicine, Atlanta, Georgia

Joel A. Kaplan, M.D.
Professor, Department of Anesthesiology, Director, Division of Cardiothoracic Anesthesia, Emory University School of Medicine, Atlanta, Georgia

Joseph I. Miller, M.D.
Assistant Professor, Department of Surgery, Emory University School of Medicine, Atlanta, Georgia

Christine H. Murphy, M.D.
Assistant Professor, Department of Radiology, Emory University School of Medicine, Atlanta, Georgia

Michael R. Murphy, M.D.
Assistant Professor, Department of Anesthesiology, Emory University School of Medicine, Atlanta, Georgia

Carl R. Noback, M.D.
Assistant Professor, Department of Anesthesiology, Emory University School of Medicine, Atlanta, Georgia

Tadikonda L.K. Rao, M.D.
Associate Professor, Department of Anesthesiology, Loyola University Medical Center and Stritch School of Medicine, Maywood, Illinois

John C. Reedy, M.D.
Assistant Professor, Department of Anesthesiology, Emory University School of Medicine, Atlanta, Georgia

George Silvay, M.D., Ph.D.
Clinical Professor, Department of Anesthesiology, Mount Sinai School of Medicine, New York, New York

Roger G. Spragg, M.D.
Associate Professor, Department of Medicine, Division of Pulmonary and Critical Care Medicine, University of California, San Diego, San Diego, California

Avron I. Weinreich, M.D.
Associate Clinical Professor, Department of Anesthesiology, Mount Sinai School of Medicine, New York, New York

Willis H. Williams, M.D.
Associate Professor, Department of Surgery, Emory University School of Medicine; Chief of Surgery, Egleston Hospital for Children, Inc., Atlanta, Georgia

Roger S. Wilson, M.D.
Assistant Professor of Anesthesia, Harvard Medical School at the Massachusetts General Hospital; Anesthetist, Department of Anesthesia, Massachusetts General Hospital

James R. Zaidan, M.D.
Associate Professor, Department of Anesthesiology, Emory University School of Medicine, Atlanta, Georgia

Foreword

Thoracic Anesthesia: A Historical Perspective

The objectives of surgery have always been clear but at one time certain basic physiological obstacles prevented their realization. The interior of the abdomen, the skull, and the thorax, were all at one time regarded as inviolate areas whose exposure would be inimical to life. Anesthesia made such formerly unapproachable recesses of the body accessible to surgical exploration and cure.

It was known to the ancients that disease, probably curable surgically, occurred in the viscera in these cavities and in particular in the thorax. The surgical technique of opening the thorax and performing such operations as a pneumonectomy was a fairly straightforward exercise in applied anatomy, and had already been perfected by the end of the 19th century—but only in animals and in the human cadaver. To carry out such procedures in the living and to ensure survival was another matter. The prime difficulty or the "pneumothorax problem" as it came to be known was soon recognized: how to maintain life with the thorax widely open?

Those pioneers who attempted pulmonary surgery were well aware of the problem. As soon as they opened the thorax the visible lung collapsed, the patient began to breathe vigorously, and the mediastinal contents moved violently with every breath (the so-called mediastinal flap). Hardly ideal conditions for diagnosis and operation! Within minutes, the patient became cyanosed, circulation began to fail, and, unless the chest was closed quickly, the patient more than likely died.

The pneumothorax problem baffled the foremost surgical minds of Europe at the turn of the century, and it was not finally solved until the beginning of the Second World War. Vesalius (1514–1564) had clearly demonstrated that an animal's breathing could be stopped and its chest opened while preserving its life by means of intermittent inflation of the lungs through a tracheal tube. Unfortunately, the level of pomposity and with it the closed mind of many of the leaders of European surgery, exemplified by Sauerbruch of Berlin, made them disinclined to listen to anyone other than themselves. There can be little doubt that Sauerbruch's refusal to accept the need for the development of anesthesia as a specialty, and his persistent adherence to his own (wrong) theory of the pneumothorax problem and its solution (spontaneous breathing under positive pressure), in spite of the growing evidence of some of his own colleagues and of anesthesiologists, physiologists, and surgeons in the rest of the world, held back the development of thoracic surgery for a generation, giving Great Britain and the United States the lead in surgery, in general, and in thoracic surgery, in particular, a lead they have maintained ever since. So great was the influence of Sauerbruch that the principle of his method of spontaneous positive pressure breathing, in spite of its obvious clinical failure to permit prolonged surgery, remained in widespread use until the Second World War, and indeed appeared as the recommended method in an English textbook of which he was co-author, in 1937.

The single most important factor enabling thoracic surgery to advance rapidly was the solution of the pneumothorax problem by artificial rhythmic inflation of the lungs after the patient had been rendered apneic. It is now clear to us that the whole marvelous edifice of modern thoracic surgery rests like an inverted pyramid on the point of artificial ventilation of the lungs.

The contributions of anesthesia are indeed great. Consider what lung and heart surgery would be like without intubation of the trachea and of the bronchi, without the easy attainment of apnea by curare and other muscle relaxants (so necessary for the performance of artificial ventilation), without the ability to remove secretions by suction, and without the huge range of powerful gases and drugs which are available to the anesthetist.

Once the primary hurdle of maintaining life with an open pneumothorax had been overcome, other developments outside the field of anesthesia quickly followed. The maintenance of fluid balance by means of blood and electrolytes, the control of infection by the administration of antibiotics, the invention of the pump oxygenator, the increase in the range of drugs available to the surgeon, the improvement of diagnosis by means of x-rays and electrocardiography, these and many other developments all made their important contributions, but without the specific anesthetic factors described above they would by themselves have been unable to sustain thoracic surgery.

Thoracic anesthesia is still a rapidly developing science probing in all the directions indicated by surgical problems as they arise. It is almost impossible for anyone not a specialist in this field to keep abreast of new developments. There is a continual need to set down the accumulated experience of those who work in this field so that their great skill and knowledge can be disseminated both to their colleagues and to the rising generation of anesthesiologists; Dr. Kaplan is eminently qualified to meet such a need.

The advances in thoracic anesthesia came not only from the field of medicine but from many other fields of science. It has its roots in the worlds of engineering, electronics, physics, biochemistry, pharmacology and physiology, as well as in medicine itself. Anesthesia and surgery must work in close harmony and mutual support in such a highly scientific and technical field as thoracic surgery. Each must transmit to the other its difficulties as they appear so that they can work together in finding solutions. It is a measure of Dr. Kaplan's understanding and appreciation of this need, born of long experience in thoracic anesthesia and surgery, that surgeons as well as anesthesiologists have helped him to complete this book.

Having been myself a modest author of books such as this, I admire Dr. Kaplan for setting out, with the help of so many distinguished colleagues, on what I know to be an arduous and exacting task. His reward will be the knowledge that he has contributed in no small measure to extending the boundaries of thoracic anesthesia, in making its problems and its practice more clear to less experienced doctors, and, above all, in making a positive contribution to the health of the public.

William W. Mushin, *CBE. MA., MBBS., FRCS., FFARCS., D.Sc. (hon.)*
Emeritus Professor of Anaesthetics
Welsh National School of Medicine
University of Wales
United Kingdom

Foreword

Thoracic Anesthesia: A Modern Perspective

The events immediately following the assassination attempt of President Ronald Reagan on March 30, 1981, demonstrated the need for a coordinated effort in Emergency Medicine, Surgery, Operating Room Staff, and Anesthesiology. The all-encompassing statement, "We did what we normally do," applies so well to the multidisciplined efforts at resuscitating, anesthetizing, and repairing the damage caused by an assassin's bullet.

One overriding factor was very clear that afternoon at the George Washington University Medical Center. There was a specific need for a working knowledge of thoracic anesthesia, especially as it applies to a patient with recent food intake, significant pulmonary trauma, and a sizeable blood loss. The anesthetic challenges presented by the President of the United States were widely publicized, but similar physiologic derangements occur daily on a national basis in patients undergoing anesthesia for thoracic surgery.

Frequently, the lung has incurred, in addition to the primary reason for surgery, a long-standing injury from smoking and industrial exposure. While the chest is open and ventilation is altered toward less physiologic gas exchange, there are multiple adverse influences upon tissue oxygenation. The ability to monitor and adjust therapy while all this is going on requires the most intelligent decisions in anesthesia.

There is a great need for a current, comprehensive textbook which discusses the additional problems related to anesthesia for thoracic surgical patients. A book similar to *Cardiac Anesthesia* by Dr. Kaplan will be well received by those professionals who want to read about concepts current among experienced authors in this field.

The textbook describes the development of thoracic anesthesia as it parallels the advances in thoracic surgery, pulmonary physiology, and the technical development of anesthesia and ventilator equipment. In addition, the text discusses the logic and appropriateness of preoperative evaluation and preparation of the patient scheduled for thoracic surgery.

Several chapters make the book additionally valuable in that they discuss subjects that are recurring adjunct problems of thoracic surgery. The need for endobronchial intubation, reliance on or need for pacemakers, the spectrum of physiologic aberration in thoracic trauma, and the necessity for sophisticated intraoperative monitoring head the list of these essential subjects.

The contributions of these outstanding authors will be highly beneficial to the anesthetic care given patients during thoracic surgery.

Manfred W. Lichtmann, M.D.   *Professor, Department of Anesthesiology*
Benjamin L. Aaron, M.D.   *Director, Department of Thoracic and Cardiovascular Surgery*

May Lin Chin, M.D.   *Resident, Department of Anesthesiology*
Charles S. Coakley, M.D.   *Professor and Chairman, Department of Anesthesiology*
Sol Edelstein, M.D.   *Associate Professor, Department of Health Care Service and Anesthesiology*
Judith Johnson, M.D.   *Resident, Department of Anesthesiology*
George A. Morales, M.D.   *Professor, Department of Anesthesiology*
Robert Roubik, CRNA   *Department of Anesthesiology*
Vickie Sidou, M.D.   *Assistant Professor, Department of Anesthesiology*

The above are affiliated with the George Washington University School of Medicine in Washington, D.C.

Preface

This book was written to improve anesthesia care for all patients undergoing thoracic surgery. The text reflects the experience of the Division of Cardiothoracic Anesthesia at the Emory University School of Medicine, as well as that of experts from the University of California-San Diego, Harvard University, Loyola University, Mount Sinai School of Medicine, and the University of Florida. The book presents methods, materials, philosophies, attitudes, and fundamentals whose use will provide safe, individualized anesthetic care.

The scope of this book ranges from the historical background to the modern practice of thoracic anesthesia and surgery, including new modes of postoperative ventilation and oxygenation. The book focuses on the patient undergoing a thoracotomy, beginning with the preoperative evaluation and preparation for surgery and continuing through to the intraoperative management and postoperative respiratory care. It is organized into five parts, consisting of twenty-one chapters and hundreds of illustrations and x-rays. The five major areas covered are: (1) thoracic anesthesia and surgery; (2) assessment of the patient; (3) cardiopulmonary physiology; (4) specific anesthetic considerations; and (5) postoperative intensive care. Throughout, the emphasis is on understanding respiratory physiology and how disease states and an open chest with one-lung ventilation may alter this physiology. The latest techniques and equipment are discussed in the areas of intraoperative monitoring, endobronchial intubation, pulmonary lavage, tracheostomy, pacemakers, and mechanical ventilators. All aspects of patient care are presented in the belief that preoperative and postoperative management of the patient are as important as intraoperative management.

The material in this book is an overview of the highly specialized field of thoracic anesthesia. Many medical disciplines including surgery, radiology, pediatrics and internal medicine have contributed to the development of this text and the new sub-specialty in thoracic anesthesia. Therefore, this work may serve as a source book for use by anesthesia residents and fellows, anesthesiologists interested in the field of thoracic anesthesia, intensivists, thoracic surgeons, pulmonary medicine specialists, and other physicians dealing with thoracic surgical patients.

I gratefully acknowledge the help of my fellow anesthesiologists at Emory for the expertly written chapters they have contributed to this book. In addition, I would like to thank my colleagues in surgery and medicine for their outstanding contributions, and most of all, I wish to express my deep appreciation to the expert anesthesiologists from other institutions whose contributions give this text balance.

My sincere appreciation goes, in addition, to my executive secretary Patricia Bailey, to Judy Hawkins and Cindy Lewis, and to the rest of our secretarial staff who spent many long hours preparing this manuscript for publication.

And, finally, my thanks to my wife, Norma, who again managed to edit a manuscript between tennis sets!

Joel A. Kaplan, M.D.

Contents

PART I.

THORACIC ANESTHESIA AND SURGERY

Joel A. Kaplan, M.D.

1
Development of Thoracic Anesthesia

DEVELOPMENT OF VENTILATION TECHNIQUES

As long ago as 1555, when Vesalius first demonstrated thoracic anatomy, the need for artificial respiration was recognized.[1] However, the multitude of problems associated with adequate ventilation and proper anesthetic techniques during open chest surgery has been solved only comparatively recently. After the introduction of aseptic operating techniques, abdominal surgery was commonly performed. Any attempts by these skilled surgeons to enter the chest cavity, however, were invariably hampered by problems due to pneumothorax.[2]

In the laboratory, early physiologists had demonstrated the presence of negative intrathoracic pressure. It had been shown that an animal's chest could be opened, provided adequate artificial respiration with a bellows was provided.[3] For many years, however, clinicians refused to accept these findings, preferring to pursue other methods to overcome the problems encountered when opening the chest. No really satisfactory method was found, unfortunately, until clinicians in the mid-eighteenth century returned to and enlarged upon the work of the early physiologists.

Some of the techniques now in use for thoracic anesthesia evolved from 18th and 19th century resuscitation methods, stimulated by societies which were formed at that time for the resuscitation of drowning victims. John Hunter, a British surgeon, recommended to the Royal Humane Society in 1774 the use of bellows for resuscitation. He had experimented on dogs, keeping them alive with double chambered bellows. The adoption of bellows for resuscitation led others to invent various pumps, intubating tubes and bellows to aid in further resuscitation efforts during this period in history. James Curry developed a series of endotracheal tubes in the early 1800s, but he felt that, in many cases, rigid muscles would preclude the possibility of introducing these tubes. Instead, he advocated the insertion of bellows into the nostril to provide respiratory support.[4]

After 1880, the use of bellows for resuscitation lost favor, chiefly due to their overzealous application and resultant problems.

3

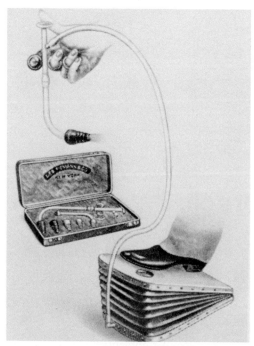

Fig. 1-1 The Fell-O'Dwyer apparatus. It incorporates Fell's bellows system and O'Dwyer's intubating cannula. The various size intubating cannulas are shown for different size patients. (Reproduced with permission from Matas R, JAMA 34:1470, Copyright, American Medical Association, 1900)

At this time, Fell, O'Dwyer and Macewen reawakened interest in intubation for lung inflation. O'Dwyer had earlier designed an intubating cannula which led to his mastery of the technique of blind oral intubation.[5] George Fell again popularized the use of bellows for resuscitation, particularly for cases of morphine poisoning, a common problem during that era.[6] Rudolph Matas, a surgeon from New Orleans, saw the advantages of Fell and O'Dwyer's ideas in thoracic surgery, and enthusiastically supported them.[7] The first successful use of the Fell-O'Dwyer apparatus, with Matas' modifications, was in 1899 for the removal of a chest-wall tumor by a colleague of Matas (Fig. 1-1).

Some thoracic surgeons at this time adopted the Fell-O'Dwyer apparatus for use in surgery. However, for the most part, they refused to try a direct-vision laryngoscope for endotracheal intubation developed by Kirstein in 1895. They preferred, instead, to use blind oral methods, not the best for hygiene or accuracy, when they used any intubation method at all.

Many European surgeons, however, still attributed the pneumothorax problem to a simple collapse of the lung. They believed they could overcome this problem by creating a differential pressure, forcing the lung up against the opening in the chest wall. They achieved this condition by enclosing the upper part of the body in a container of compressed air, avoiding intubation. Sauerbruch of Germany, assistant to von Mikulicz, became interested in a "negative pressure chamber" for use in open chest surgery (Fig. 1-2).[8] After some doubts on von Mikulicz's part of the efficacy of his assistant's developments, he was finally convinced and eventually operated in a patient's chest using Sauerbruch's chamber. The endorsement of this method from von Mikulicz's clinic gave impetus to other surgeons, most of whom used this "negative pressure" method to the exclusion of all others.

While Sauerbruch's negative pressure chambers became progressively more elaborate, Brauer (1905) and Tiegel (1909) developed smaller, positive-pressure, choroform-oxygen apparatuses, providing the same effect much more conveniently.[9] Eventually, Sauerbruch was convinced of the efficacy of the positive-pressure method and advocated its use throughout his later career (Fig. 1-3).

During this same period, in the United States, Meltzer and Auer, two physiologists, refined bellows respiration methods, using the Brauer continuous positive-pressure method.[10] Their method made use of continuous lung inflation with air-ether and rhythmical respiration only every 2 to 3 minutes. This technique, using endotracheal intubation, was accepted mostly by surgeons who had some experience with endoscopy. It also proved valuable during head and neck pro-

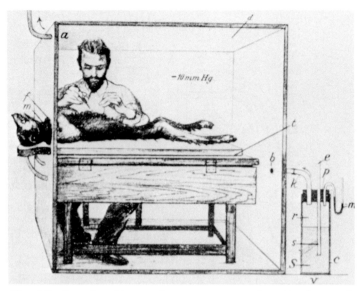

Fig. 1-2 Sauerbruch's negative pressure operating chamber used during experimental chest surgery in animals. Note that the chamber has a negative 10 mmHg pressure in it and is sealed at the animal's neck. (Reproduced with permission from Sauerbruch F: Zur Pathologie des offenen Pneumothorax und die Grundlagen meines Verbahrens zu seiner Ausschaltung. Mitt. Grenzgeb. Med. Chir. 13, 399, 1904)

cedures which endangered the patency of the patient's airway.[10]

The use of the insufflation method for thoracic surgery was developed in the United States around this time by Elsberg, who advocated intermittent ventilation to allow adequate CO_2 removal from the lungs.[11] Several apparatuses, such as that of Janeway (1913), were developed to regularly interrupt airflow, simulating spontaneous respiration. Janeway and Green, both surgeons, used rhythmic continuous ventilation with intubation in experimental surgery.[12] They advocated its use to produce artificial apnea and eliminate diaphragmatic movement. Still, at this time, the few anesthetists in practice preferred the intrapharyngeal insufflation method which was simpler and avoided endotracheal intubation. Janeway then introduced a cuffed endotracheal tube and a patient-triggered ventilator; and Chevalier Jackson invented the modern laryngoscope, but practitioners at the time rejected these as too complicated and continued to use insufflation for the next quarter of a century.

DEVELOPMENT OF VENTILATORS

The precursor of today's modern ventilators is generally considered to be the one developed by Giertz, a former assistant to Sauerbruch, around 1916. His experiments on animals showed that rhythmic inflation was more effective than either negative or continuous positive pressure ventilation.[13] In 1934, Frenckner, a Swedish ear, nose, and throat surgeon, enlarging upon Giertz's work, developed the "Spiropulsator" because he was convinced that "the rhythmic introduction of air into the trachea under favorable circumstances would be the most ideal type of positive pressure breathing" (Fig. 1-4).[14] Crafoord, working first with

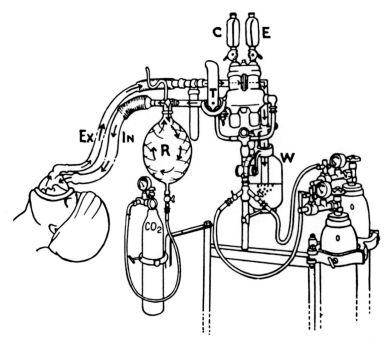

Fig. 1-3 The Tiegel-Henle positive pressure apparatus used in Sauer-bruch's clinic in 1937. This remarkably modern apparatus was used for the administration of either chloroform or ether anesthesia. (Reproduced with permission from Sauerbruch F, O'Shaughnessy L: Thoracic Surgery, Fig. 17, London, 1937, p 26)

Giertz and later with Frenckner, found with further experimentation that the "Spiropulsator" worked most effectively when the patient's own respiratory efforts were eliminated. He observed a tendency for the patient to "fight" the machine and overcame this problem by adding a bag from which the patient could draw a breath as desired. This "Spiropulsator," developed jointly by Crafoord, Frenckner and an experimental engineer, became commercially available in 1940.[15] Although Crafoord's results were enthusiastically accepted in Scandinavia, the British and American medical community, at large, continued to use the older methods of continuous positive pressure and insufflation.

In the United States, in particular, the impetus for adopting automatic ventilators was due, in large measure, to the cardiac surgeons who wanted to solve the problems associated with open heart surgery. Mautz

and Beck, in Cleveland, had developed their own version of a ventilator.[16] These surgeons, as well as other notable authorities such as Allbritten, Dennis, and Sievers, demonstrated that mechanical respiration was more efficient in removing CO_2 and greatly improved their results.[13] Their insistence upon ever-improving methods of patient ventilation led to the continued development of a series of commercially available ventilators.

The catastrophic Copenhagen polio epidemic of 1952 led to a crash production program of Engstrom volume ventilators. In 1955, Bjork and Engstrom in Sweden first described the use of their ventilator for postoperative respiratory care of poor risk thoracic surgery patients. The Jefferson ventilator was developed on John Gibbon's thoracic surgery service in Philadelphia and was introduced in 1957 as the first American ventilator for controlled ventilation.

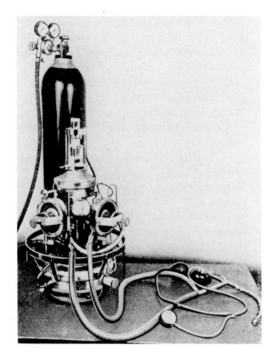

Fig. 1-4 The Frenckner spiropulsator. (Reproduced with permission from Frenckner P, Bronchial and tracheal catheterization and its clinical affability. Acta Oto-laryng, Suppl. 20:1934

DEVELOPMENT OF ANESTHETIC DRUGS AND TECHNIQUES

Prior to 1933, the agents used for continuous positive pressure and insufflation anesthesia included: (1) ether, first used by Crawford Long in 1842, and demonstrated in Massachusetts by William Morton in 1846; (2) nitrous oxide, first used for tooth extraction by Dr. Horace Wells, in 1844; and, (3) chloroform, first used by Simpson in 1848 for obstetrical delivery.[17] None of these agents induced the apnea deemed necessary by anesthetists to enable them to adequately control patient respiration during thoracic anesthesia. Therefore, during this time, many problems still existed for the surgeon desiring to perform open-chest surgery.

In 1882, Freund prepared cyclopropane, which was first used as an anesthetic agent in 1928, in experiments performed on animals by Lucas and Henderson. In 1933, Ralph

Waters and his staff at the University of Wisconsin experimented further with animals and with themselves. They published their clinical findings in 1934.[18] Cyclopropane easily induced apnea and permitted controlled respiration with good gas exchange. It became eagerly accepted and rendered most older complicated techniques obsolete.

Other clinicians, during this era, preferred "safer" anesthetic agents and techniques. Some used nitrous oxide and oxygen via a rotameter with heavy morphine-scopolamine premedications, as described by Neu in 1910.[20] This technique was adopted by many pioneer anesthesiologists and surgeons in America, such as McKesson, Gwathmey, and Crile. They popularized the use of open nitrous oxide-oxygen anesthesia with or without local field blocks for surgery.[21] The cost of the agents involved helped prompt the development of a closed circle carbon dioxide absorption apparatus to lower expense. Such a machine was invented by D. E. Jackson in 1915 and further developed by Waters and his staff.[20] Not until Waters introduced cyclopropane into widespread clinical use in 1934, did Jackson's closed circuit design gain popularity in clinical practice.

Cyclopropane had some unfortunate disadvantages inherent in its use. It was expensive, highly explosive, and precluded the use of electrocautery.[19] It also sometimes caused postoperative shock. Its use, and that of other explosive agents, was obviated in 1942 by the introduction of curare by Griffiths and Johnson.[17] Curare's advantages were induction of apnea, loss of reflexes, and unrestricted use of the cautery. Neff's meperidine-supplemented, nitrous oxide-oxygen-relaxant, controlled respiration method gained great popularity in Britain after the publication of articles by Mushin and Rendall-Baker.[20] Neff's method made use of the cautery safe, permitting wedge and segmental resections of lung for tuberculosis.

Other techniques which enjoyed limited popularity for thoracic surgery from 1935 to 1945 were spinal and epidural anesthesia.

However, these methods permitted preservation of the patient's cough reflex, making surgery more difficult.[20]

Halothane, introduced in England in 1956 by Johnstone, was the result of research begun in 1932 in the field of halogenated hydrocarbons. Its development was an answer to many needs unfilled by the other agents available. Nonflammable, it also had other characteristics eagerly sought at that time. It allowed adequate oxygen concentrations to be delivered; it was essentially inert; it had limited solubility in water and fat; it did not react with the alkali used for CO_2 absorption; it was tolerated reasonably well by the heart; and it produced a smooth induction and awakening.[22] By 1959, the use of halothane was widespread in both the United States and the rest of the world. This signalled the beginning of the era of nonflammable, inhalational anesthetics.

Since then, anesthetic drugs, techniques, and equipment for thoracic anesthesia and surgery have continued to be developed and refined. Other milestones have included neuroleptanalgesia with fentanyl-droperidol (1959); use of specialized endobronchial intubation tubes (Carlens, White, Robertshaw; 1970s); high frequency positive pressure ventilation (HFPPV; 1971–1977); and, increased invasive hemodynamic monitoring (1970s).[19]

REFERENCES

1. Vesalius A: Some observation on the dissection of living animals. DeCorporis Humanis Fabrica, Vol 7, Chapter 19, Basle, 1555
2. Murphy JB: Surgery of the lung. JAMA 31:151, 1898
3. Nissen R and Wilson RHL: Pages in the History of Chest Surgery, Charles C Thomas, Springfield, Illinois, 1960, p 6
4. Curry J: Observations in Apparent Death from Drowning. 2nd ed. London, 1815
5. O'Dwyer J: Two cases of croup treated by tubage of the glottis. NY Med J 42:605-607, 1885
6. Fell G: Fell method-forced respiration-report of cases resulting in the saving of twenty-eight human lives—history and a plea for its general use in the hospital and naval practice. Section of General Medicine, First Pan American Medical Congress, p 309, 1893
7. Matas R: On the management of acute traumatic pneumothorax. Ann Surg 29:409-434, 1899
8. Sauerbruch F: Master Surgeon, Crowell, New York, 1954, p 21
9. Tiegel M: Uberdrucknarkose, Beitr Klin Chir 64:356, 1909
10. Meltzer SJ, Auer JL: Continuous respiration without respiratory movements. J Exp Med 11:622, 1909
11. Elsberg CA: Clinical experiences with intratracheal insufflation; with remarks upon the value of the method for thoracic surgery. Ann Surg 52:23, 1910
12. Green NW: A positive pressure method of artificial respiration with a practical device for its application in thoracic surgery. Surg Gyn Obstet 2:512, 1906
13. Mushin WW, Rendell-Baker L, Thompson PW, et al: Automatic Ventilation of the Lungs. Blackwell, Oxford, pp 199-205, 1969
14. Frenckner P: Bronchial and tracheal catheterization. Acta Otolaryng Scand (Suppl.) 20:100, 1943
15. Crafoord C: Pulmonary ventilation and anesthesia in major chest surgery. J Thorac Surg 9:237, 1940
16. Mautz FR: Mechanical respiration as adjunct to closed system anesthesia. Proc Soc Exp Biol (NY) 42:190, 1939
17. Kaplan N: An American Heritage: Anesthesiology. The Anesthesia Foundation, Park Ridge, Illinois, 1976
18. Meade RH: A History of Thoracic Surgery. Charles C Thomas, Springfield, 1961, p. 758
19. Rendell-Baker L: Anesthesia for Thoracic Surgery, Anesthesiology Review. Vol. VII., No. 10, 1980
20. Mushin WW: Thoracic Anesthesia, F. A. Davis, Philadelphia, 1963
21. Crile GW and Lower WE: Anoci-Association, W. B. Saunders, Philadelphia, 1914
22. Greene NM: Halothane. F. A. Davis, Philadelphia, 1968

Joseph I. Miller, M.D.

2
Thoracic Surgery

HISTORICAL ASPECTS[1,2]

The current practice of thoracic surgery owes its development to a number of significant achievements in the fields of cardiorespiratory physiology, radiology, pharmacology, and anesthesia. The earliest problems in thoracic surgery were in controlling the airway. In 1555, Vesalius wrote of ventilating a dog through a tracheal stoma while exploring the chest. Matas, in 1899, discussed orotracheal intubation and the utilization of bellows to move the chest. The clinical application of the method of endotracheal intubation is credited to Meltzer and Auer.

Paralleling the clinical aspects of endotracheal intubation was the discovery of the x-ray by Röntgen in 1895. With this discovery, clinical knowledge of diseases of the tracheobronchial tree rapidly progressed.

At the turn of the nineteenth century, endoscopic visualization of the tracheobronchial tree was practiced by Killian and Einhern. In 1904, Chevalier Jackson combined the lighting principle of the Einhern esophagoscope with the tube of Killian. Jackson has been called the "father of bronchial endoscopy."

Physiologic studies by Graham and Bell as members of the U.S. Army Empyema Commission in 1918 established current concepts in the management of pleural empyema. These principles were drainage following the period of active pneumonia, early sterilization and obliteration of the cavity, and maintenance of the patient's nutrition.

The principles of obliteration of the pleural cavity led to the development of numerous types of thoracoplasties. Two of the most common types were the Estlander and the Schede. In 1943, Burford first performed a decortication of the lung in order to fill an empyema space.

In 1945, the discovery of penicillin completely changed the clinical course and treatment of lung abscess, bronchiectasis, and empyema.

The credit for pulmonary resection is hard to determine. Tuffer is given credit for performing the first successful partial lobectomy for a tuberculous lesion in 1892. Nissen and Sauerbruch, in 1931, are credited with performing the first pneumonectomy. This was performed in a staged manner, the hilum being encircled with rubber ligatures and the lobes allowed to slough in a patient with bronchiectasis. Haight and Alexander, in 1932, performed the first successful pneu-

9

monectomy in the western hemisphere in a patient with bronchiectasis. In 1933, Graham performed a left pneumonectomy on a physician with squamous cell carcinoma, and the individual survived 30 years.

Individual ligation technique for lobectomy was extensively used by Churchill starting in 1938. Reinhoff performed the first pneumonectomy in the late 1930s using the individual ligation technique. The work of these early pioneer surgeons in the field of thoracic surgery led to detailed anatomic studies of bronchial and hilar regions as we know them today.

The development of chemotherapy for tuberculosis, starting with streptomycin in 1944 and, subsequently, isoniazid in 1952, completely changed the therapeutic approach to pulmonary tuberculosis. Prior to this, therapy had been largely surgical, with various types of procedures such as artificial pneumothorax and various forms of collapse therapy being done. With the development of antituberculous chemotherapy, surgery became reserved for the failures of drug therapy and is now utilized predominantly in the form of pulmonary resection.

The first successful surgical resection for esophageal carcinoma was performed by Turek in 1913. When Culams and Phemister reported their success with esophagogastrectomy 25 years later, there were only 30 limited successes reported in the literature.

The present status of thoracic surgery owes its origins to the interrelationship of multiple disciplines such as bronchoesophagology, pioneering surgical efforts, developments in anesthesia, and the development of antibiotics and chemotherapy for pulmonary diseases.

SURGICAL ANATOMY

The following is a brief synopsis of surgical anatomy pertinent to the operative procedures usually performed in general thoracic surgery.

Trachea

The trachea begins at the level of the cricoid cartilage and extends into the superior mediastinum to the level of the sternal angle (lower border of fourth thoracic vertebra), where it divides into the right and left primary bronchi. The point of bifurcation is known as the *carina*. Approximately half of the trachea lies in the neck and half in the thorax.[3] The trachea ranges in length from 10 to 13 cm (mean 11.8 cm) and consists of 18 to 22 U-shaped cartilagenous rings within this length (approximately two rings per centimeter).[4]

The internal diameter of the trachea averages 2.3 cm laterally and 1.8 cm anteroposteriorly.[4] The nerve supply, both motor and sensory, to the trachea is derived from branches of the vagus; and the arterial supply is from branches of the inferior thyroid artery above and the bronchial arteries below.

Bronchial Tree

At the carina, the trachea divides into right and left main-stem bronchi. The right main bronchus deviates less from the axis of the trachea than does the left, which explains why foreign objects enter the right bronchus and its branches more often than the left.

The Right Bronchial Tree

The length of the right main bronchus is about 1.2 cm before it gives off laterally the upper lobe bronchus, which subsequently divides into three segmental bronchi. Distal to this, the primary bronchus is known as the *bronchus intermedius* and is approximately 1.7 to 2.0 cm in length. At this point, the middle lobe bronchus arises and subsequently divides into the medial and lateral branches. Just distal to this, the remaining primary bronchus divides into the superior segmental bronchus and the main basilar segmental bronchi, which subsequently divide into the four remaining basilar division bronchi.

The Left Bronchial Tree

The left main bronchus is longer than the right, and its first branch arises 4 to 6 cm distal to the carina. It subsequently divides into the lingula, anterior and apical posterior bronchus. About 0.5 cm distal to the left upper lobe bronchus, the lower lobe bronchus gives off the superior segmental branch, and subsequently the remaining basilar branches.

The Lobes and Fissures

"The right lung is composed of three lobes—upper, middle, and lower, and is the larger of the two lungs. The left lung is composed of two lobes—upper and lower."[5] Two fissures are present on the right. The oblique fissure (major fissure) separates the lower

lobe from the upper and middle lobes and the horizontal fissure separates the latter two. On the left is a single major fissure dividing the upper and lower lobes.

Bronchopulmonary Segments

The right lung is divided into 10 segments and the left into 8 segments (Fig. 2-1). Each subsegment has its own bronchus, artery, and vein.

Hilar Anatomy

From an anatomic surgical standpoint, knowledge of hilar anatomy is extremely important. On the right side, the azygous vein marks the uppermost aspect of the hilar structures. From top to bottom on the right are the right main-stem bronchus, the main pulmonary artery, and then the right superior pulmonary vein. On the left side, the aortic arch marks the superior aspect of the hilum; and from top to bottom there is first the left pulmonary artery, the left main

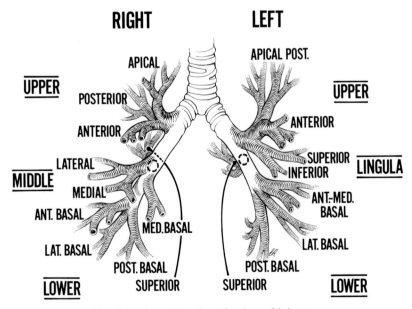

Fig. 2-1 Anatomy of tracheobronchial tree.

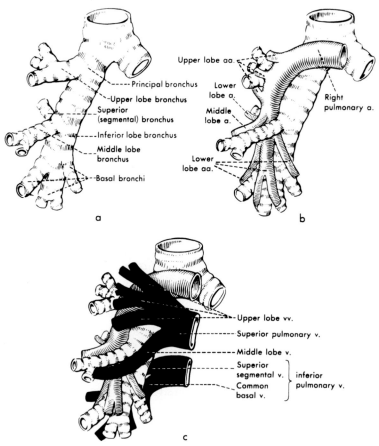

Upper lobe aa.
Principal bronchus
Lower lobe a.
Upper lobe bronchus
Superior (segmental) bronchus
Middle lobe a.
Right pulmonary a.
Inferior lobe bronchus
Middle lobe bronchus
Basal bronchi
Lower lobe aa.

a   b

Upper lobe vv.
Superior pulmonary v.
Middle lobe v.
Superior segmental v. ⎤ inferior
Common basal v. ⎦ pulmonary v.

c

Anterior view of the chief bronchi and vessels of the right lung.

Fig. 2-2 Anatomy of the right hilum. (Hollingshead WH: Anatomy for Surgeons: The Thorax, Abdomen and Pelvis, Vol II. Harper and Row, New York, 1967, p 66.)

bronchus, and then the left superior pulmonary vein. In both hilar regions, the most anterior structure is the superior pulmonary vein, behind which is the main pulmonary artery, and the most posterior structure is the main-stem bronchus (Figs. 2-2 and 2-3).

Esophagus

The esophagus is a long muscular tube approximately 40 cm in length which begins at the pharynx at the level of the sixth cervical vertebra and extends to the abdomen, passing through the esophageal hiatus at the level of the tenth thoracic vertebra. There are three important anatomic areas of narrowing within the esophagus which correspond to the points most prone to esophageal perforation. The first of these is the cricopharyngeal muscle, which is 15 cm from the incisors; the second is the aortic arch and tracheal bifurcation at 25 cm; and the third is the esophagogastric junction at the esophageal hiatus at 40 cm.

The esophagus has two layers, an inner mucosa and an outer muscular layer composed of an inner circular layer and an outer

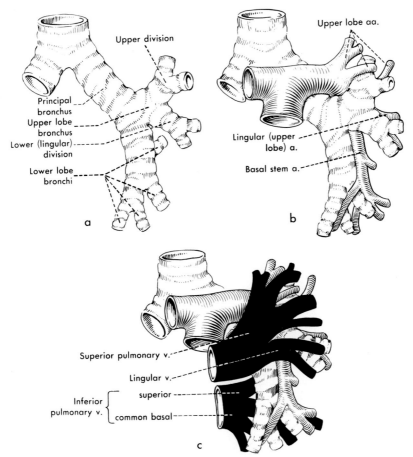

Anterior view of the chief bronchi and vessels of the left lung.

Fig. 2-3 Anatomy of the Left Hilum. (Hollingshead WH: Anatomy for Surgeons: The Thorax, Abdomen and Pelvis, Vol II. Harper and Row, New York, 1967, p 70.)

longitudinal layer without a serosa. The lack of a serosal covering best explains why esophageal anastomoses are more prone to leaks than other parts of the gastrointestinal tract.

The nerve supply to the esophagus is from the vagi; and the arterial supply is from the inferior thyroid arteries, esophageal branches from the aorta, and bronchial arteries.

Table 2-1 is a brief outline of some of the commonly encountered thoracic surgical disease entities. A brief discussion of each of these diseases entities is given.

PULMONARY INFECTIONS

Lung Abscess

According to Takaro, "A lung abscess is a localized area of suppuration and cavitation in the lung."[6] It may be a primary pyogenic lung abscess or may occur secondarily in association with other disease processes. It is seen most commonly in association with aspiration occurring secondarily to dental procedures, periods of unconsciousness from alcoholism, general anesthesia, cerebrovas-

Table 2-1
Surgical Diseases of the Thorax

I. Pulmonary infections
  1. Lung abscess and fungal disease
  2. Pleural disease and empyema
  3. Pulmonary tuberculosis
  4. Bronchiectasis
II. Tumors of the lung and bronchi
  1. Benign tumors
  2. Malignant tumors
III. Mediastinal tumors
IV. Esophageal disease
  1. Hiatal hernia and reflux esophagitis
  2. Esophageal motor disorders
    A. Achalasia
    B. Diffuse spasm
  3. Esophageal diverticuli
  4. Esophageal carcinoma
V. Pacemakers
VI. Pericardial disease

cular accidents, esophageal disease, or prolonged dependency.

The three most common sites of involvement are the superior segment of the right lower lobe, the posterior segment of the right upper lobe, and the superior segment of the left lower lobe.[7] Ninety-five percent of lung abscesses occur within these three locations. The most commonly involved organisms are *Staphylococcus aureus*, alpha *Streptococcus, Escherichia coli,* and *Klebsiella.*

The primary method of treatment is medical, with antibiotic therapy, chest physical therapy, and endobronchial drainage. Surgical treatment is reserved for failures of medical treatment, massive hemoptysis, suspected underlying malignancy, and the presence of large, thick-walled cavities greater than 6 cm in size.[8, 9] Surgery is generally resective in nature; surgical drainage is rarely performed.

Fungal Disease

The surgeon most frequently encounters fungal disease (except pulmonary tuberculosis) when he is operating for an undiag-

nosed coin lesion of the lung, and the pathologist reports this as a fungal granuloma. Histoplasmosis is the most common of the fungal infections and occurs in the Mississippi River Valley. Other fungal infections frequently seen include coccidioidomycosis, blastomycosis, cryptococcosis, aspergillosis, and actinomycosis. The primary drug treatment for all these is amphotericin B, except for actinomycosis, for which penicillin is used.

The surgeon may suspect the fungal disease by history, but generally tissue confirmation is required. The widespread use of antimetabolites and steroids for a variety of neoplastic and immunologic disease states has led to a large number of "superinfections" with these pathogenic fungi.

Pleural Empyema

Empyema is by definition a collection of purulent fluid within the pleural space. It may be loculated or free-flowing (involving the entire pleural space); and may be acute or chronic. The most common causative organisms are *Staphylococcus aureus, Pneumococcus,* and a variety of gram-negative organisms.

The goals of treatment for all stages of empyema are: (1) control of the primary infection and the empyema; (2) evacuation of the purulence of the empyema cavity and eradication of the sac to prevent chronicity; and (3) reexpansion of the underlying lung.[10]

This can generally be achieved with appropriate antibiotics and closed-chest tube thoracostomy, with later conversion to open drainage and slow removal of the chest tube over a period of several months. Occasionally, because of a poorly drained or incompletely drained cavity, open surgical drainage will be required. This is generally in the form of resection of a short segment of rib, or the creation of an Eloesser-type skin flap.[11] In some instances, decortication may be required, but only rarely is thoracoplasty required to obliterate the cavity.

The treatment of post-pneumonectomy empyema is now mostly nonsurgical after the manner described by Clagett.[12]

Pulmonary Tuberculosis

While the number of patients operated upon for pulmonary tuberculosis has declined in the past few years, there are about 30,000 new cases reported annually. In addition, approximately 3,500 patients suffer clinical relapses each year. The number of patients requiring surgery remains relatively constant at 5 to 15 percent.[13]

The predominant method of treatment of pulmonary tuberculosis is with specific chemotherapeutic agents. The most commonly employed agents are isoniazid, ethambutal, and rifampin, used in various combinations for a period of 6 months to 1½ years.

Surgery remains a valuable complement to medical therapy, and, when properly applied, is nearly 100 percent successful. "The purpose of surgery is to remove or to assist in the healing or control of destructive residuals, which would otherwise contribute to failure of medical treatment or to reactivation of the disease process."[13]

The indications for resection are well-standardized:[13]

1. An open cavity associated with positive sputum beyond 3 to 6 months after the initiation of chemotherapy
2. Persistent positive sputum cultures after adequate initial or retreatment programs in patients without demonstrable cavitation but with pathologic residuals, such as destroyed lobe or lung
3. A residual destroyed segment, lobe, or lung, blocked cavities, tuberculomas, and significant fibrocaseous disease in patients with negative sputum
4. The presence of localized infection with

one of the atypical acid-fast organisms
5. Symptomatic noncontrollable bronchiectasis of the middle and lower lobes
6. Failure of certain patients with open negative cavities to take their medication
7. Tuberculous lesions in patients with suspected malignancy
8. Recurrent, persistent, or massive hemoptysis
9. Pleural empyema together with a nonexpandable lung which may need a resection and decortication

The type of resection depends upon the extent of the disease.[13] A wedge resection is adequate for tuberculomas and for coin lesions proven to be granulomas. Lobectomy is generally the procedure of choice for destroyed lung; pneumonectomy should be reserved for those patients with a totally destroyed lung.

The most common complications of surgery are empyema and bronchopleural fistula. In a combined study of 4,126 pulmonary resections performed between 1961 and 1966 for pulmonary tuberculosis, the overall mortality was 1.7 percent.[14] The long-term results in patients undergoing resectional surgery for tuberculosis are excellent, with 90 to 96 percent of patients free of disease at 5-year follow-up.

TUMORS OF THE LUNG AND BRONCHUS

Benign Tumors

HAMARTOMA

A hamartoma is the most common benign tumor of the lung. It accounts for about 80 percent of all benign tumors of the lung and accounts for approximately 8 to 14 percent of reported solitary pulmonary nodules in large series. The majority of these are peripheral in location and present as solitary coin lesions. The peripheral lesions cannot be differentiated from carcinoma of the lung and must be removed for diagnosis.

OTHER BENIGN TUMORS

Other benign tumors of the lung occur with much less frequency. These include polyps, angiomas, hemangiopericytomas, lipomas, leiomyomas, fibromas, and chondromas.

Malignant Tumors

Table 2-2 lists the World Health Organization (WHO) Classification of Malignant Pleuropulmonary Neoplasms. A detailed discussion of each of these is not possible in the framework alloted, but a brief description of the four common types of bronchogenic carcinoma will be given.

The four common types of bronchogenic carcinoma are (1) squamous-cell carcinoma; (2) adenocarcinoma; (3) large-cell carcinoma; and (4) small-cell anaplastic carcinoma.

PATHOLOGIC TYPES

Squamous-cell carcinoma (epidermoid carcinoma) is the most common type of bronchogenic malignancy and accounts for

Table 2-2
WHO Classification of Malignant Pleuropulmonary Neoplasms

---

1. Epidermoid carcinomas (squamous cell)
2. Small-cell anaplastic carcinoma
3. Adenocarcinoma
   a. Bronchogenic
   b. Bronchioalveolar
4. Large-cell carcinoma
5. Combined epidermoid carcinoma and adenocarcinoma
6. Carcinoid tumors
7. Bronchial gland tumors
   a. Cylindromas
   b. Mucoepidermoid carcinoma
8. Papillary tumors of the surface epithelium
9. Mixed tumors and carcinosarcomas
10. Sarcomas
11. Unclassified
12. Melanoma

---

50 to 60 percent of all cases. It is generally central in location and 10 percent of these tumors may cavitate. It generally has a slow growth rate and is slow to metastasize.

Adenocarcinoma accounts for about 5 to 15 percent of bronchogenic carcinomas. It is generally a small lesion less than 3 cm in diameter, and in more than 70 percent of cases it is located peripherally. It may form in scars, has a moderate growth rate, and spreads via the bloodstream.

Large-cell carcinoma accounts for 15 percent of lung carcinomas. The diagnosis is generally made by exclusion of other cell types. It may occur in any location but is more often peripheral. It has a rapid growth rate and metastasizes early.

Small-cell carcinoma accounts for approximately 15 percent of lung cancers. The majority of these lesions occur in a central location. They spread via blood and lymphatics, have a rapid growth rate, and metastasize early. The most common sites of metastasis are bone, brain, liver, and bone marrow. At the present time, small-cell cancer is generally not considered a surgical disease.

The approach to any patient with carcinoma of the lung must consist of (1) an adequate preoperative workup; (2) appropriate preoperative staging; (3) physiologic determination of operability and evaluation of anatomic resectability; and (4) if indicated, the appropriate operation.

The standard workup used by the author in patients with suspected bronchogenic cancer is listed in Table 2-3. If symptoms or laboratory evidence of metastatic disease is present, then appropriate scans of liver, bone, and brain are indicated to confirm this and help in staging the patient. In the absence of symptoms or laboratory evidence of disease, staging scans are generally not performed. If no evidence of metastatic disease is present, then physiologic assessment of the patient and appropriate invasive procedures are performed as indicated to determine anatomic and physiologic resectability.

Table 2-3
Workup for Cancer of Lung

Symptoms and/or chest x-ray
suspicious for lung cancer

↓

History and physical examination
CBC | SMA-18 | EKG | CXR | UA
Skin test: PPD; antigen control
Sputum for cytology | C&S
Thoracoabdominal CAT scan
Pulmonary function test
Hilar oblique tomography

↙ ↘

Symptoms or laboratory evidence of metastatic disease	No evidence of metastatic disease
1. X-ray and scan of liver, bone, and brain	1. Bronchoscopy
2. Consider biopsy to confirm	2. Mediastinoscopy
3. If symptoms suggest, or another primary is suspected: IVP, BE, UGI	3. Scalene node biopsy
4. Invasive diagnostic procedures as indicated	4. Mediastinotomy
	5. Needle biopsy as indicated

The second major point to be considered is the physiologic assessment of the patient's cardiovascular and respiratory system. It must be known how much lung can safely be resected without expected mortality and whether the patient's cardiovascular system is able to tolerate the proposed surgical procedure. A full discussion of this will appear in a later portion of this chapter (see Preoperative Evaluation of the Thoracic Surgical Patient).

The third major factor to be considered before undertaking treatment is the anatomic extent of the disease. This requires appropriate preoperative staging of the patient. Staging of a lung cancer is the estimation of its anatomic extent. The staging system for classifying lung cancer adopted by the American Joint Committee for Cancer Staging and End-Results Reporting is shown in Table 2-4.[15] "This system employs the letters T (tumor), N (nodes), and M (metastasis), with appropriate suffixes to describe the extent of the tumor."[16]

Appropriate diagnostic invasive procedures such as bronchoscopy, mediastinoscopy or mediastinotomy, scalene node biopsy, needle biopsy, or thoracoscopy, as determined by the anatomic facets of the disease, are indicated to appropriately stage the disease. With appropriate staging, the incidence of unnecessary thoracotomy can be reduced to less than 20 percent.[17]

CANDIDATES FOR SURGICAL RESECTION

At the present time, definitive resection is the only approach to the treatment of non-small-cell carcinoma of the lung which holds promise for long-term survival. The criteria for selection of patients is fairly uniform for comparable medical centers. The criteria for definitive resection relate to (1) the biologic nature of the tumor; (2) the anatomic extent of disease; and (3) the physiologic status of the patient.[18]

All patients with stage I and stage II disease with squamous-cell carcinoma, adenocarcinoma, and large-cell carcinoma, and selected patients with stage III disease are considered candidates for definitive surgical resection if their physiologic status permits. At the present time, it is not felt that definitive surgery has a role in the management of small-cell cancer of the lung.

Table 2-4
Staging of Lung Cancer

Primary Tumor
T_x Malignant cell in cytology; site undetermined.
T_0 No evidence of primary tumor
T_1 Tumor $\leq$ 3 cm in size; surrounded by tissue
T_2 Tumor > 3 cm in size
T_3 Tumor of any size with extension to chest wall, parietal pleura, diaphragm, mediastinum or within 2 cm of carina

Nodal Involvement
N_0 No lymph mode metastasis
N_1 Metastasis to peribronchial or ipsilateral hilar region only
N_2 Mediastinal lymph node metastasis

Distant Metastasis
M_0 No distant metastasis
M_1 Distant metastasis present

Stage Grouping
Stage I $T_1N_0M_0$
           $T_1N_1M_0$
           $T_2N_0M_0$

Stage II $T_2N_1M_0$

Stage III T_3 with any N or M
           N_2 with any T or M
           M_1 with any T or N

According to Mountain et al "final selection of the specific operative procedure must take place at the time of exploration, but the probable extent of the resection is carefully planned preoperatively, depending on the patient's cardiovascular and pulmonary status."[18] The location of the tumor and stage of disease usually dictate the procedure of choice. The physician must also know the contraindications to surgical resection for carcinoma of the lung.

CONTRAINDICATIONS TO PULMONARY RESECTION

The absolute contraindications to resection are (1) malignant pleural effusion; (2) metastatic disease outside the thoracic cavity; (3) superior vena cava syndrome; and (4) paralysis of the recurrent laryngeal nerve. Rela-

tive contraindications include (1) general medical contraindications; (2) paralysis of the phrenic nerve; (3) oat-cell carcinoma; and (4) a positive mediastinoscopy.

TYPE OF SURGICAL PROCEDURE

Segmental Resection

Segmental resection is indicated for small peripheral lesions usually less than 3 cm in diameter for stage I ($T_1N_0M_0$) disease, and in patients with a compromised cardiopulmonary status. Relative contraindications are T_2 lesions or a lesion which crosses an intersegmental plane. Mortality for segmental resection is less than 0.5 percent.[19]

Lobectomy

At the present time, lobectomy is the operation of choice for carcinoma of the lung. It is indicated when technically feasible for stage I and II disease and some stage III lesions. It has a mortality in our series of 1.3 percent.[19]

Pneumonectomy

Pneumonectomy is indicated with more extensive disease, generally $T_2N_0M_0$ or $T_2N_1M_0$ with hilar involvement. The mortality for pneumonectomy is about 5 percent.[19]

In general, patients with stage III disease are not candidates for definitive surgical resection, with a few exceptions. These include certain patients with central lesions and hilar nodal involvement, Pancoast tumors, or certain lesions with chest wall involvement.

RESULTS OF SURGICAL THERAPY

At the present time, current reported surgical results for stage I squamous-cell carcinoma are 50 to 60 percent 5-year survival.[18] Stage I adenocarcinoma and large-cell carcinoma have a reported 35 to 50 percent 5-year survival. Survival for stage II and stage III carcinoma is markedly decreased and varies from 10 to 35 percent, depending on the cell type. Our own results are similar to the above.

BRONCHIAL ADENOMAS

The only other common malignant neoplasm is the bronchial adenoma. Pathologically, there are three types: bronchial carcinoids, 90 percent; mucoepidermoid carcinomas, 7 percent; and cylindromas, 3 percent. The majority of these occur in the proximal bronchi, and the treatment of choice is surgical resection, generally by lobectomy with or without sleeve resection.

MEDIASTINAL TUMORS

A large number of histologically different types of tumors arise from the many anatomic structures within the mediastinum. The lesion may be benign or malignant. The incidence of different types of mediastinal tumors in a collected series of 1,000 patients is given in Table 2-5.[20]

Table 2-5
Incidence of Neoplasms and Cysts of the Mediastinum in a Collected Series of 1,000 Patients

Type of tumor or cyst	Number	Percent
Neurogenic tumors	240	24
Cysts		
Pericardial	74	7.4
Bronchogenic	87	8.7
Enteric	22	2.2
Nonspecific	31	3.1
Teratodermoids	169	17
Thymomas	125	12
Lymphomas	126	13
Other	126	13
Total	1000	100

From Oldham NH, Sabiston DC: The mediastinum. pp 2153–2166. In Sabiston DC (ed): Textbook of surgery, 11th Ed. W. B. Saunders, Philadelphia, 1977.

The most common mediastinal tumors are the neurogenic tumors, followed by teratomas and lymphomas. When the mediastinum is divided into its three anatomic sections, the most common tumors are as follows: (1) *anterior mediastinum:* thymoma, teratoma, thyroid tumors and lymphoma; (2) *middle mediastinum:* pericardial cyst, bronchogenic cyst, and lymphoma; (3) *posterior mediastinum:* neurogenic tumors.

The treatment of choice is surgical resection through either a median sternotomy or a thoracotomy. The morbidity is quite low and mortality is about 1 percent.

ESOPHAGEAL DISEASE

Hiatal Hernia and Reflux Esophagitis

The surgery of hiatal hernia and its complications comprise the most common surgical disorder of the esophagus. About 5 percent of patients with hiatal hernia and reflux esophagitis will require surgical correction.

Anatomically, hiatal hernias are divided into two types: (1) sliding hernias, which comprise 95 percent of the hernias and are associated with incompetence of the lower esophageal sphincter and reflux esophagitis; and (2) paraesophageal hiatal hernias, which account for 5 percent of hiatal hernias and with which the esophagogastric junction remains below the diaphragm and competence of the lower esophageal sphincter is preserved.

Indications for surgical correction are as follows: (1) intractability of symptoms, despite adequate medical management; (2) severe reflux with ulceration; (3) stricture or bleeding; and (4) recurrent aspiration pneumonia. All patients with paraesophageal hernias should undergo surgical repair if their medical condition permits because of the high incidence of complications associated with them.

There are three currently accepted surgical methods of correcting hiatal hernias. Each has its advantages and disadvantages. All are effective in restoring esophagogastric competence and give good results when properly performed. The Nissen procedure is recognized as being the best in restoring the lower esophageal sphincter and preventing reflux, but it is also associated with a much higher morbidity than the other two procedures. Regardless of the type of procedure performed, the recurrence rate is approximately 10 percent when followed for more than 10 years.

The most important determining factor in the outcome of hiatal hernia surgery is the capability of the surgeon and his experience, regardless of the type of procedure performed.

A brief description of the three techniques is given below.

1. Belsey Mark IV. This is a transthoracic reconstruction of the cardia and repair of the hiatus. It consists of a 270-degree wrap of the cardia around the lower 3 cm of the esophagus and tightening of the crura. It is very effective in restoring competence of the lower esophageal sphincter, and its only disadvantage is that it can be performed only by the transthoracic route. It is our technique of choice for hiatal hernia repair.

2. Nissen Fundoplication. This procedure, originally reported in 1963, consists of a 360-degree wrap of the fundus of the stomach around the lower esophagus.[21] It can be performed by either the abdominal or the transthoracic route. It is very effective in restoring competence of the lower esophageal sphincter but is associated with the highest complication rate of the three procedures. The most common complication is the "gas-bloat" syndrome, which occurs in about 20 percent of cases.[22]

3. Hill Repair. This procedure is performed through an abdominal approach and is referred to as a *posterior gastropexy*. In this procedure, the crura are approximated posterior to the esophagus, and the gastroesophageal junction is sutured to the median arcuate ligament. In addition, the left border of the abdominal esophagus is sutured to the gastric fundus. The procedure is associated with few side effects.

Surgery for hiatal hernia may thus be performed through either an abdominal approach or a transthoracic approach. Indications for an abdominal approach are: (1) preference of the surgeon; and (2) associated intra-abdominal pathology, which may be repaired concomitantly (i.e., gallstones). Indications for a thoracic approach include: (1) obesity; (2) shortening and strictures of the esophagus; (3) previous surgery at the gastroesophageal junction or abdominal surgery; and (4) previous hiatal hernia repair.

Stricture of the Esophagus

Fortunately, the majority of strictures can be dilated preoperatively or intraoperatively and then one of the three standard types of antireflux procedures performed. In those patients with marked foreshortening of the esophagus in which the esophagus is dilatable but the esophagogastric junction cannot be reduced below the diaphragm, a combined Collis-Nissen procedure is the operation of choice. This consists of cutting a 5-cm segment along the lesser curvature of the stomach and then performing a Nissen fundoplication around this. This procedure has proven quite effective in these situations.

When strictures are nondilatable, a colon interposition with either right or left colon is the procedure of choice. Mansour et al recently reported our experience in 40 patients with benign strictures of the esophagus who underwent colonic interposition between 1972 and 1980.[23] The right colon was used in 28 patients, the left colon in 4, and the transverse colon in 1. In 7 patients, the stomach was employed because of vascular insufficiency of the colon. Complications developed in seven patients, and there were four deaths (10 percent mortality). This was fairly low, as the reported mortality in most series for colonic interposition procedures is 15 to 25 percent.

In general, we favor colonic interposition for benign disease of the esophagus and esophagogastrectomy for malignant disease.

ESOPHAGEAL MOTOR DISORDERS

Achalasia

According to Ellis, "achalasia of the esophagus is a disease of unknown etiology characterized by absence of peristalsis in the body of the esophagus and failure of the lower esophageal sphincter to relax in response to swallowing."[24] It is primarily thought to be caused by a loss of ganglion cells in Auerbach's plexus in the lower esophagus. Medical therapy consists of hydrostatic dilatation of the esophagus and is successful in about 80 percent of cases.

Current surgical therapy is divided into two schools of thought. Common to each is the performance of a modified Heller myotomy, which is a long esophageal myotomy just extending onto the proximal 1 cm of the stomach. Ellis feels that this is all that is required.[24] The second group feels that in addition to a modified Heller procedure, an antireflux procedure should be used because of the high reported incidence of gastroesophageal reflux (15 to 45 percent) following the Heller procedure alone.[25] We are of the latter opinion, and perform a modified Heller-Belsey procedure for routine achalasia of the esophagus.

Diffuse Spasm of the Esophagus

Diffuse spasm is a hypermotility disorder of the esophagus characterized by diffuse hyperperistaltic waves in the lower body of the esophagus. It results in marked esophageal pain. Surgical therapy consists of a long Heller myotomy carried up to the level of the aortic arch, combined with a Belsey mark IV antireflux procedure.

Esophageal Diverticuli[24]

There are three common esophageal diverticuli, classified by location, mode of development, and status as true or false diverticuli. These are (1) pharyngoesophageal; (2) midthoracic; and (3) epiphrenic diverticuli. The first and third types are generally associated with motor disorders of the esophagus and are referred to as *pulsion* diverticuli. They generally consist of an outpouching of mucosa and submucosa and are called *false* diverticuli. The midthoracic diverticulum is called a *traction* diverticulum, and is a true diverticulum, as its sac consists of all layers of the esophageal wall.

Pharyngoesophageal Diverticulum

Pharyngoesophageal diverticulum or Zenker's diverticulum is the most common of the esophageal diverticuli. It results from a weakness in the posterior fibers of the inferior pharyngeal constrictor and the cricopharyngeus muscle. The predominant symptoms are dysphagia, regurgitation, and aspiration.

Treatment is surgical and depends on the size of the diverticulum. For a small diverticulum (less than 2 cm in length), all that is required is a cricopharyngeal myotomy. This is performed through an oblique incision in the left neck and consists of a longitudinal incision through the cricopharyngeus muscle distally onto the esophagus itself. For a moderate-size diverticulum (2 to 3 cm), cricopharyngeal myotomy and diverticulo-pexy, in which the apex of the diverticulum is stitched to the prevertebral fascia, are performed. For a large diverticulum (greater than 4 cm), both a myotomy and a diverticulectomy are performed, with use of the T55 stapling instrument.

Midthoracic Diverticuli

Diverticuli in the midportion of the esophagus are rare and almost never require surgical treatment.

Epiphrenic Diverticuli

Epiphrenic diverticuli are located just above the diaphragm. The majority are associated with both a motor disorder of the esophagus and a hiatal hernia. Dysphagia and regurgitation are the most common symptoms. Surgery is indicated when symptoms become disabling and progressive. Surgery consists of diverticulectomy, a long esophagomyotomy, and an antireflux procedure.

Esophageal Carcinoma

Esophageal carcinoma is a devastating disease, and surgical therapy is generally considered palliative. There are few 5-year survivals regardless of the mode of therapy. Pathologically, the most common cell type occurring in the body of the esophagus is squamous-cell carcinoma. Malignant lesions of the esophagogastric junction are generally adenocarcinomas of gastric origin extending proximally up the body of the esophagus; these comprise approximately half the esophageal carcinomas.

Arbitrary division of the esophagus into four divisions is important prognostically and therapeutically. Gunnlaugsson et al listed the following locations and frequency of occurrence: cervical, 8 percent; upper thoracic, 25 percent; midthoracic, 17 percent; and lower thoracic and gastroesophageal, 50 percent.[26] If the lower third of the esophagus and gastroesophageal junction are considered, this anatomic area accounts for about 67 percent of all malignancies of the esophagus.

Treatment depends upon the level of involvement. The following discussion will outline the usual method of treatment in our institution, but it is not a complete discussion of the subject. There will be some individuals and institutions that differ with our approach.

Cervical and Upper Thoracic

This anatomic area includes the esophagus from the level of the pharynx to the top of the aortic arch. For this group of patients, it is felt that surgery has little to offer, and they are treated with a combination of chemotherapy and radiation therapy. Five-year survival for this level approaches 0 percent.

Midthoracic

This would include anatomic involvement from the level of the aortic arch to the inferior pulmonary ligament (or from 25 to 35 cm measured from the incisors). At this level of involvement, preoperative adjunctive treatment is favored with either chemotherapy and/or cobalt treatment to 4,000 R, followed by surgical resection with esophagogastrectomy. If the lesion is less than 5 cm in length, preoperative chemotherapy is used, followed by surgery. If the lesion is more than 5 cm in length, preoperative radiation therapy to 4,000 R is utilized, followed by esophagogastrectomy. The 5-year survival rate for lesions in this area is about 5 percent.

Lower Thoracic and Esophagogastric Junction

This includes lesions at and below the level of the inferior pulmonary ligament (35 cm). If the lesion is a squamous-cell carcinoma, preoperative adjunctive chemotherapy is used, followed by esophagogastrectomy. If the lesion is an adenocarcinoma, surgical exploration is immediately done, with resection by esophagogastrectomy, if feasible, and provided widespread metastatic disease is not present, as determined by preoperative workup. The 5-year survival for resection in this area varies from 15 to 30 percent, depending upon nodal involvement. The best prognosis is for patients with squamous-cell carcinoma of the lower third of the esophagus; while the worst prognosis is for patients with adenocarcinoma of the cardia. (See Table 2-6).

A description of esophagogastrectomy will be given in a later section.

PACEMAKERS

See Chapter 17.

PERICARDIAL DISEASE

A full discussion of surgery of the pericardium is outside the scope of this chapter. Brief indications for surgery (Table 2-7) and surgical results for pericardiectomy will be given.

The pericardium may be approached through four separate operative incisions: (1) subxiphoid; (2) bilateral anterior thoracotomy; (3) left anterior thoracotomy; and (4) median sternotomy.

Pericardiectomy is generally indicated in cases of recurrent pericardial effusion, which may occur in uremia, neoplasia, infections, and other miscellaneous conditions, and in cases of constrictive pericarditis. The pericardiectomy may be of two types: (1) pa-

Table 2-6

Five-year Survival after Resection in Carcinoma of Esophagus and Cardia*

Location of lesion	1956–1963		
	Resected	Traced	Survived
Cervical level of esoph.	7	7	1
Upper thoracic esoph.	56	52	4
Lower thoracic esoph.	44	42	12
Cardia	153	148	20
Total	260	249	37
Percent			14.9

* Reproduced in part from Gunnlaugsson GH, Wychulis AR, Roland C et al: Analysis of the records of 1,657 patients with carcinoma of the esophagus and cardia of the stomach. Surg Gynecol Obstet 130:997–1005, 1970.

Table 2-7

Surgical Indications for Pericardiectomy*

I. Congenital
   A. Congenital anomalies and defects
   B. Cysts and diverticula

II. Acute and Chronic Pericarditis
   A. Predominant effusion with or without tamponade
     1. Idiopathic recurrent
     2. Uremic
     3. Infectious
       a. Pyogenic (purulent)
       b. Tuberculous
       c. Viral
     4. Neoplastic
     5. Associated with systemic disease
     6. Traumatic
     7. Radiation
   B. Predominant constriction with or without effusion
     1. Idiopathic (nonspecific)
     2. Infectious
     3. Following cardiac surgery

* Miller, JI: Pericardiectomy. pp 147–159. In Hurst, JW, Ed: Update III, The Heart. McGraw-Hill, New York, 1980.

rietal pericardiectomy, which is the procedure done in most cases involving recurrent pericardial effusion; and (2) visceral pericardiectomy, which is required, along with parietal

Table 2-8
Indications for Pericardiectomy 1974–1978*

Condition	Pericardiectomy Number	Deaths
Uremic pericarditis	19	0
Purulent pericarditis	7	2
Constrictive pericarditis	13	0
1. Tuberculous	3	
2. Idiopathic	2	
3. After coronary artery bypass	8	
Recurrent idiopathic effusion	5	0
Radiation pericarditis	1	0
Neoplastic pericarditis	8	2
Total	53	4

* Miller, JI: Pericardiectomy. pp. 147–159. In Hurst, JW, Ed: Update III, The Heart. McGraw-Hill, New York, 1980.

pericardiectomy, in cases of constrictive pericarditis.

Our approach is to use a left anterior thoracotomy for all cases operated for predominant pericardial effusion and to use a median sternotomy with pump standby for cases of constrictive pericarditis.

Table 2-8 reflects the authors' experience with pericardiectomy at Emory University Affiliated Hospitals during the 5-year period 1974 to 1978.

PREOPERATIVE EVALUATION OF THE THORACIC SURGICAL PATIENT

The physiologic assessment of operability constitutes one of the most important aspects of the preoperative evaluation of the thoracic surgical patient. The surgeon must be able to weigh the risk involved to the patient and to calculate accurately the patient's ability to survive the surgical procedure without excessive morbidity.

The physiologic assessment requires careful evaluation of the cardiovascular and pulmonary systems, as cardiac and respiratory complications are the most common source of postoperative morbidity and mortality. It must be ascertained with accuracy whether the patient can tolerate the planned type of resection and whether the status of his cardiovascular system is satisfactory for the proposed procedure.

A more detailed description of the preoperative evaluation is given in Chapter 4, but the pertinent aspects from a surgical point of view are briefly presented here.

Physiologic Assessment of Pulmonary Function

Physiologic pulmonary function tests should be performed before any thoracic surgical procedure and are imperative if a pulmonary resection is to be performed.

Our standard approach is to perform (1) full pulmonary function tests with and without bronchodilators, (2) diffusion capacity tests, and (3) measurements of arterial blood gases.[19]

The pulmonary function criteria applied for the various types of pulmonary resection are maximum breathing capacity (MBC), forced expiratory volume in 1 second (FEV_1), and maximum midexpiratory flow rate, now known as FEV_{25-75}. Certain pulmonary ratios are also helpful. These are: (1) ratio of the forced expiratory volume in 1 second to the forced vital capacity (FEV_1/FVC) expressed as a percentage; (2)

Table 2-9
Pulmonary Function Test Criteria for Resection

Test	Unit	Normal	Pneumonectomy	Lobectomy	Biopsy or Segmental
MBC	Liters/min	>100	>70	40–70	40
MBC	Percent predicted		>55	40–70	35–40
FEV_1	Liters	>2	>2	>1	>0.6
FEV_1	Percent predicted		>55	40–70	≧40
$FEV_{25–75}$	Liters	2	>1.6	0.6–1.6	>0.6

the ratio of the residual volume to the total lung capacity (RV/TLC), expressed as a percentage; and (3) the diffusion capacity. Additional studies utilized are the Reichel pulmonary stress test and split differential perfusion lung scans.[28]

Specific criteria for various types of pulmonary resections are listed in Table 2-9. MBC and FEV_1 are expressed both in liters and percent. Ratio analysis (Table 2-10) is predominantly helpful in determining candidacy for pneumonectomy. The Reichel pulmonary stress test is also utilized mainly in determining operability with respect to pneumonectomy. Split differential perfusion scans are helpful in assessing operability for both pneumonectomy and lobectomy (Table 2-11).

These criteria were applied to 500 consecutive thoracic resections carried out under the supervision of one surgeon from 1974 to 1978.[19] The type of surgical resections were pneumonectomy, 46; lobectomy, 196; and elective wedge, segmental, or open biopsy, 248. In the pneumonectomy group, 44 patients were operated on for carcinoma and 2 for tuberculosis. Complications developed in 18 patients: 16 had significant dysrhythmias, and 2 had pulmonary emboli. There were 2 deaths in the perioperative period of 4 weeks, for a mortality of 4.4 percent. During this same interval, only five patients needing

Table 2-10
Ratio Analysis

$\dfrac{FEV_1}{FVC}$	<50%	
$\dfrac{RV}{TLC}$	>50%	Indicate that patient is not a candidate for pneumonectomy
Diffusion capacity <50% of predicted		

Table 2-11
Determining Operability for Pneumonectomy

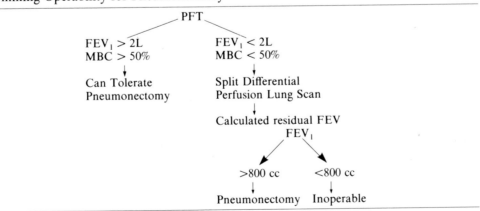

pneumonectomy were turned down solely on pulmonary function criteria. They had otherwise appeared to be operable. There were no deaths in the lobectomy group and one death in the segmental resection group. Two patients were denied elective segmental resection for carcinoma on the basis of pulmonary function tests: one with an MBC of 24 percent and one with an MBC of 30 percent.

Realizing that no one parameter is absolute, the following set of criteria is proposed as minimal values of pulmonary function for various types of pulmonary resection that result in minimum morbidity and low mortality.[19] Minimum criteria for pneumonectomy are: MBC greater than 55 percent of predicted; FEV_1 greater than 2 liters; FEV_{25-75} greater than 1.6 liters; ability to complete the Reichel stress test; and predicted residual postoperative FEV_1 greater than 0.8 liters. Minimum criteria for lobectomy are: MBC greater than 40 percent of predicted; FEV_1 greater than 1 liter; and FEV_{25-75} 0.6 liters. Minimum criteria for elective wedge or segmental resection are: MBC 35 to 45 percent of predicted; FEV_1 0.6 liters; and FEV_{25-75} 0.6 liters.

When the following values are present, the patient is inoperable for an elective thoracic resection and operation should only be performed for life-threatening necessity: MBC less than 35 percent of predicted; FEV_1 less than 0.6 liters; FEV_{25-75} less than 0.6 liters.

When these criteria have been applied, a more precise method of selecting patients as candidates for various types of pulmonary resection has resulted in lower mortality, and denial of surgery to less than 2 percent of patients who would otherwise have been candidates.

Combined xenon ventilation-perfusion lung scans are done as indicated, depending upon the patient's routine pulmonary function tests. These are extremely helpful in determining the patient's postoperative calculated pulmonary reserve. Block et al have shown that a calculated postoperative resid-

ual FEV_1 greater than 800 cc is compatible with a reasonable ventilatory reserve and the ability to function comfortably with normal activity.[29]

Physiologic Assessment of the Cardiovascular System

The heart is the organ most frequently limiting operability. According to Logue "although many cardiac risk factors can be isolated, a universally accepted set of rules governing cardiac risk is not available."[30] The easiest and most careful assessment is done by a good history of the patient. Logue has listed the important factors in determining underlying cardiac risk (Table 2-12).[30]

A careful history points to potential problems and the potential need for further studies that may be indicated. Any patient with a history of coronary artery disease, as manifested by angina pectoris or suspected angina, or any history of previous myocardial infarction should undergo cardiac exercise stress testing, including the recently developed thallium exercise cardiac nuclear scan. If the angina is stable with either a negative exercise test or negative thallium scan without exercise-induced dysrhythmias, the patient will generally tolerate pulmonary re-

Table 2-12
Determining Cardiac Risk

IS THERE

1. Evidence of heart disease?
2. History of angina or myocardial infarction?
3. Cardiac enlargement?
4. Symptoms or signs of congestive heart failure?
5. Cardiac dysrhythmias
6. Hypertension?
7. Postural hypotension?
8. History of syncope or cerebrovascular disease?
9. Phlebitis?
10. Medications: cardiac, antihypertensives, steroids?
11. Kidney or prostate disease?

Table 2-13
Lung Resection and Cardiopulmonary Risk

Group I Very low risk	Group II Very high risk (prohibitive)	Group III Moderate risk
Cardiac Normal size and cardiac function Normal blood pressure Normal ECG	*Cardiac* Intractable CHF or ventricular dysrhythmias Uncontrolled myocardial infarct	*Cardiac* *CAD* with 1. Angina 2. MI within 2 years 3. ECG abnormalities Cardiac dysrhythmias Systemic HCVD Valvular heart disease
Pulmonary Normal ABG Satisfactory overall mechanical lung function ($FEV_1 >$ 70%)	*Pulmonary* Poor mechanical lung function ($FEV_1 < 35\%$) Irreversible CO_2 retention ($PaCO_2 > 45$ mm) Pulmonary hypertension	*Pulmonary* Hypoxia with normal $PaCO_2$ Reduced overall pulmonary function FEV_1 (35–70%) predicted

section safely. If the exercise stress test is markedly positive and if the pulmonary lesion appears to be anatomically and physiologically resectable otherwise, the patient is referred for coronary arteriography to determine if the coronary disease is surgically correctable. If the coronary lesion is amenable to surgery, we have done a few combined procedures concomitantly, but our preferred approach has been to stage them, first doing the coronary artery bypass, waiting 6 weeks, and then performing the pulmonary resection. We have operated on 16 such patients in the last 2 years with no mortality by using this staged approach.

Thoracic surgery is generally not indicated if a myocardial infarction has occurred within 3 months of the proposed elective resection. In a series reported from the Mayo Clinic, 27 percent of patients operated upon within 3 months of a previous infarct had a reinfarction. If the time period was 3 to 6 months, the reinfarction rate was 11 percent, and after 6 months it was 6 percent. Of all patients having a reinfarction within 6 months of surgery, 69 percent died.[31] We believe that 3 months should pass when the patient has a history of a recent previous infarction, and then the thoracic resection of

the lesion should be done only when lung cancer is suspected.

Dysrhythmias and hypertension should be treated with proper medications prior to any thoracic surgical procedure.

Logue feels that all patients with coronary artery disease should be digitalized preoperatively before any thoracic surgical procedure because of postoperative dysrhythmias and myocardial depression.[30] However, not all authorities agree with this viewpoint. All patients with a history of angina or infarction should be treated preoperatively with nitroglycerin ointment and have intravenous nitroglycerin given during surgery as indicated to control hypertension and ischemic changes and to decrease myocardial oxygen consumption.

Ali et al from M. D. Anderson Hospital have presented a helpful table (Table 2-13) for assessing cardiopulmonary risk in the thoracic surgical patient.[32]

The combined physiologic evaluation of the pulmonary system and cardiac system allows accurate assessment of the surgical risk to the patient for the proposed procedure and discussion with the patient before surgery. The risk/benefit ratio of any surgical procedure must always be weighed.

Sound clinical judgment, combined with preoperative radiographic anatomy and endoscopic findings, and accurate assessment of the cardiopulmonary system allow the surgeon to make an accurate determination of the probabilities and risk of surgery to the patient.

THORACIC SURGICAL PROCEDURES

A brief description of a few of the common thoracic surgical procedures will be given, as well as indications and possible complications.

Invasive Diagnostic Procedures

The common invasive diagnostic thoracic surgical procedures are bronchoscopy, mediastinoscopy or mediastinotomy, scalene-node biopsy, needle biopsy, thoracoscopy, and limited thoracotomy. Their diagnostic yields are given in Table 2-14.

MEDIASTINOSCOPY

Mediastinoscopy is a useful diagnostic procedure associated with low morbidity and mortality. It is important as a diagnostic staging procedure in patients with cancer of the lung who are surgical candidates.

The indications for mediastinoscopy are (1) all central lesions; (2) small peripheral lesions with hilar enlargement; and (3) any radiologic evidence of hilar or mediastinal enlargement. It is not utilized in patients with peripheral coin lesions and a normal-appearing mediastinum on chest x-ray.

Mediastinoscopy provides access to five lymph node–bearing groups: paratracheal, subcarinal, and tracheobronchial angle nodes.

Contraindications to resection based upon mediastinal assessment are: (1) a diagnosis of undifferentiated small-cell carcinoma; (2) involvement of contralateral paratracheal lymph nodes; (3) involvement of

Table 2-14
Diagnostic Procedures

Procedure	Diagnostic yield %
Fiberoptic Bronchoscopy	
Peripheral lesion	30–50
Central lesion	70–80
With TBL biopsy	80–90
Mediastinoscopy	
Peripheral lesion	5–10
Central lesion	70
Mediastinotomy	
Left upper lobe	50–60
Scalene Node Biopsy	
Nonpalpable node	10–20
Palpable node	80
Needle Biopsy	
<3 cm	50
>3 cm	80
Thoracoscopy	95

ipsilateral paratracheal lymph nodes in the upper half of the intrathoracic trachea; (4) direct tumor invasion of mediastinal structures; and (5) lymph node involvement with large-cell carcinoma or adenocarcinoma or extracapsular nodal involvement with squamous-cell carcinoma.[33]

The morbidity and mortality are about 0.1 percent.

MEDIASTINOTOMY

Anterior mediastinotomy, or the Chamberlain procedure as it is sometimes called, is an extrapleural approach to the mediastinum through the resected bed of the second costal cartilage. It is helpful in evaluating lesions of the left upper lobe. It is indicated for predominantly left upper lobe lesions with suspected hilar involvement. If positive nodes are found, surgery is generally contraindicated. The surgical risk is low, about 0.5 percent.

THORACOSCOPY

Thoracoscopy is indicated for recurrent undiagnosed pleural effusions of undetermined etiology. After the usual modalities of thoracentesis and closed pleural biopsy have been done and if the etiology is still not known, then thoracoscopy should be considered.

The procedure is carried out in the operating room under general anesthesia. A small ½ inch incision is made and a thoracoscope or mediastinoscope is inserted into the pleural cavity. Fluid is obtained and appropriate biopsies performed. The mediastinum, diaphragm, and entire pleural space are easily examined.

Miller et al reported on 17 cases with greater than 95 percent accuracy based on use of this procedure.[34]

Thoracic Resections

LOBECTOMY

Pulmonary lobectomy is most often performed for benign and malignant neoplasms of the lung. Lobectomy may also be required for pulmonary tuberculosis, refractory lung abscess, residual bronchiectasis, pulmonary sequestration, and other infectious processes in the lung.

The preferred anesthetic technique is general anesthesia via an indwelling double-lumen endotracheal tube, such as a Carlens or Robertshaw tube. The usual position of the patient for a pulmonary resection is the lateral decubitus position with the operated side most superior. The main operative steps after the thoracotomy incision consist of control of the arterial supply and venous drainage of the respective lobe, followed by dissection of the fissures and division of the bronchus. The lobe most commonly resected is the right upper lobe, and the second most common is the left upper lobe.

The procedure is well-tolerated and does not present a major surgical stress when the patients are well-selected from the standpoint of associated medical problems and assessment of cardiopulmonary function. The perioperative 4-week mortality is about 1 to 2 percent.

Potential complications following lobectomy consist of: (1) dysrhythmias, 5 to 15 percent; (2) intrapleural air space, 10 percent; (3) prolonged air leaks, 3 to 7 percent; (4) empyema, 1 to 3 percent; (5) bronchopleural fistula, 3 percent; (6) pulmonary embolism, 1 percent; and (7) major bleeding, 1 percent.

PNEUMONECTOMY

The main indication for pulmonary pneumonectomy is the presence of a pulmonary neoplasm which involves structures such that pulmonary lobectomy is not feasible. On rare occasions, a pneumonectomy may be indicated for benign disease such as residual problems with pulmonary tuberculosis, for lung trauma, or as a result of a complication with pulmonary lobectomy.

The preferred anesthetic technique is with a double-lumen endotracheal tube. The operation is performed with the patient in the lateral decubitus position. The main operative steps consist of control of the pulmonary artery and superior and inferior pulmonary veins, and secure closure of the bronchial stump.

Pneumonectomy carries with it a high level of surgical stress and should only be performed in patients who have demonstrated sufficient cardiopulmonary reserve to tolerate such a procedure.

Potential postoperative complications consist of (1) dysrhythmias, 25 to 40 percent; (2) empyema, 2 to 10 percent; (3) bronchopleural fistula, 1 to 3 percent; (4) cardiac herniation, rare; (5) bleeding, 1 percent; and (6) tension pneumothorax, less than 1 percent.

The accepted mortality for pneumonectomy is 5 to 15 percent.

ESOPHAGOGASTRECTOMY

Esophagogastrectomy is usually indicated for carcinoma of the esophagus and carcinoma of the gastroesophageal junction. It is occasionally indicated for nondilatable esophageal strictures in patients who are not candidates for colonic interposition.

For carcinoma of the gastroesophageal junction a thoracoabdominal approach is used; and for carcinoma of the remainder of the esophagus a combined right thoracic and midline abdominal incision is used.

The abdomen is explored and assessment of resectability made. If the patient is deemed resectable, the stomach is mobilized outside the gastric-epiploic arcade. The left gastric artery is divided and the proximal stomach resected and closed. A pyloroplasty is performed and the spleen is generally resected with gastroesophageal lesions. The stomach is brought up into the chest, and a esophagogastrostomy (end to side) is performed.

The magnitude of the surgical stress is high, with a fairly high incidence of morbidity and mortality. The reported mortality in the literature is from 10 to 15 percent.

Potential complications include (1) anastomotic leak, 15 to 20 percent; (2) anastomotic stricture, 5 to 15 percent; (3) bleeding, 1 to 3 percent; (4) gastroesophageal reflux, 20 to 25 percent; and (5) empyema, 3 to 5 percent.

COLON INTERPOSITION FOR
ESOPHAGEAL SUBSTITUTE

Indications for colon replacement of the esophagus include: gastroesophageal malignancy; benign undilatable esophageal strictures; benign tumors of the esophagus which are extensive or multiple, where simpler measures are inapplicable; and congenital atresia of the esophagus, where a primary anastomosis is impossible or impractical.

The right or left colon may be used, depending upon the blood supply to the colon. A midline abdominal incision is used and the appropriate colonic segment isolated. The colon may be passed subcutaneously, retrosternally, or through the posterior mediastinum. It may be taken to the neck or left in-

trathoracically. Esophagectomy may or may not be performed. Appropriate esophageal-colonic and colonic-gastric anastomosis and/or colo-colostomy are performed.

The operation is a highly technical one and can result in significant morbidity when performed by inexperienced individuals. The mortality in reported series varies from 5 to 25 percent. The highest source of morbidity is with an esophageal-colonic leak. Leak rates of 15 to 20 percent have been reported. Other complications are similar to those listed under esophagogastrectomy.

FUTURE AREAS OF INTEREST

Lung Transplantation

Hardy and his group performed the first clinical lung transplant in 1963, with the patient surviving 3 weeks.[35] Since that time an additional 36 human lung transplants have been done. These were recently reviewed by Veith and Koerner.[36] Indications for transplant were patients with severe respiratory insufficiency due to both obstructive and restrictive diseases and to pulmonary hypertension. The majority of patients died within 1 month and the longest survival was 10 months. Death has generally been due to infection and/or rejection.

At the present time, clinical lung transplantation is not widely performed, the reason being the poor survival rate and the inability to control infection and rejection in the transplanted lung. It is felt that once the problems of infection and rejection can be controlled, lung transplants will become more successful, like renal and cardiac transplants. Recently, combined cardiac and lung transplants have been successfully performed at Stanford University. New immunosuppressive drugs may allow many more of these procedures to be performed in the future.

WHAT THE THORACIC SURGEON NEEDS FROM THE ANESTHESIOLOGIST

The successful performance of any operative procedure requires close cooperation and communication between the operating surgeon and the anesthesiologist. This begins with a preoperative discussion of the patient's problems, anticipated difficulties of the operative procedure, and potential intraoperative problems, as well as requests of the operating surgeon concerning a given case.

Pertinent aspects important to surgery are outlined below:

1. The ability to collapse the lung on the operative side increases the speed of the operative procedure, makes the technical aspects of the procedure easier, and greatly enhances all aspects of the surgical procedure. Double-lumen tubes are indicated in all thoracic and esophageal procedures for endotracheal intubation.

2. The anesthesiologist should be able to insert, maintain, and monitor central venous, pulmonary arterial, and peripheral arterial catheters.

3. The anesthesiologist must be able to adequately monitor and assess the status of the cardiopulmonary system during the operative procedure. This frees the surgeon and allows him to attend to the technical aspects of the surgery. In addition, both must have a knowledge of the pharmacology of the commonly used cardiovascular drugs.

4. At the completion of a pulmonary resection it is important that the deflated lung be allowed to inflate slowly and evenly. It should not be inflated under a great deal of pressure or too rapidly so that hypotension and production of undue tension on the bronchial and pulmonary parenchymal suture lines may be avoided. The bronchial suture lines are tested at 35 to 40 cm of water and the fissure lines and parenchymal suture lines at 15 to 20 cm of water.

5. There should be continuous communication between the anesthesiologist and the surgeon during surgery. Good postoperative care also requires close communication between both members of the operative team.

REFERENCES

1. Langston H: The development of thoracic surgery, pp 2003-2009. In Sabiston D, Ed: Textbook of surgery 11th ed. W. B. Saunders, Philadelphia, 1977
2. Meade RH: A history of thoracic surgery. Charles C Thomas, Springfield, Ill., 1961
3. Goss CM, Ed: Gray's anatomy of the human body. 28th ed., Lea and Febiger, Philadelphia, 1966
4. Grillo HC: Tracheal anatomy and surgical approaches, pp 539-554. In Shields TW, Ed: General thoracic surgery. Lea and Febiger, Philadelphia, 1972
5. Shields TW: Surgical anatomy of the lungs, pp 55-73. In Shields TW, Ed: General thoracic surgery. Lea and Febiger, Philadelphia, 1972
6. Takaro T: Lung abscess and fungal infections, pp 2074-2085. In Sabiston D, Ed: Textbook of surgery 11th ed. W. B. Saunders, Philadelphia, 1977
7. Bernard WF, Malcolm JA, Wylie RH: Lung abscess: a study of 148 cases due to aspiration. Dis Chest 43:620-630, 1963
8. Barnett TB, Herring CL: Lung abscess: Initial and late results of medical therapy. Arch Intern Med 127:217-227, 1971
9. Mattox KL, Guinn GA: Emergency resection for massive hemoptysis. Ann Thorac Surg 17:377-383, 1974
10. Takaro T: The pleura and empyema, pp 2087-2098. In Sabiston D Ed: Textbook of surgery 11th ed. W. B. Saunders, Philadelphia, 1977
11. Eloesser L: Of an operation for tuberculous empyema. Ann Thorac Surg 8:355-357, 1969
12. Clagett OT, Geraci JE: A procedure for the management of postpneumonectomy empyema. J Thorac Cardiovasc Surg 45:141-145, 1963
13. Young WG, Moor GF: The surgical treatment of pulmonary tuberculosis, pp 567-590.

In Sabiston DC, Spencer FC, Ed: Gibbon's surgery of the chest. 3rd Ed. W. B. Saunders, Philadelphia, 1976

14. Mendenhall JT: Report of thoracic surgery for pulmonary tuberculosis in VA-Armed Forces study unit hospitals. July 1, 1965-June 30, 1966. Transactions of the 26th VA-Armed Forces pulmonary diseases research conference, Cleveland, 1967

15. American Joint Committee for Cancer Staging and End-Results Reporting: system for staging of lung cancer. Chicago, 1979

16. Carr DT: Malignant lung disease. Hospital Practice, Jan. 1981, 97-115

17. Miller JI, Mansour KA, Hatcher CR: Carcinoma of the lung: five-year experience in a university hospital. Am Surgeon 46:147-150, 1980

18. Mountain CF, McMurtrey MJ, Frazier H: Current results of surgical treatment for lung cancer. The Cancer Bull 32:105-108, 1980

19. Miller JI, Grossman G, Hatcher CR: Pulmonary function test: criteria for operability and pulmonary resection. Surg Gynecol Obstet. In press, 1981

20. Oldham NH, Sabiston DC: The mediastinum, pp 2153-2166. In Sabiston DC, Ed: Textbook of Surgery 11th ed. W. B. Saunders, Philadelphia, 1977

21. Nissen R, Susetti M: Surgery of the cardia ventriculi. CIBA Symp 11:195, 1963

22. Woodard ER, Thomas HF, McAlhany JC: Comparison of crural repair and Nissen fundoplication in the treatment of esophageal hiatal hernia with peptic esophagitis. Ann Surg 173:782-792, 1971

23. Mansour KA, Miller JI, Hatcher CR et al.: Colon interposition for advanced non-malignant esophageal stricture. Ann Thorac Surg. In press, 1981

24. Ellis HF: Disorders of esophageal motility, pp

796-809. In Sabiston DC, Ed: Textbook of surgery 11th ed. W. B. Saunders, Philadelphia, 1977

25. Mansour KA, Symbas PN, Jones EL et al: A combined surgical approach in the management of achalasia of the esophagus. The Am Surg 42:192-195, 1976

26. Gunnlaugsson GH, Wychulis AR, Roland C et al: Analysis of the records of 1,657 patients with carcinoma of the esophagus and cardia of the stomach. Surg Gynecol Obstet 130:997-1005, 1970

27. Miller JI: Pericardiectomy, pp 147-159. In Hurst JW, Ed: Update III, The Heart. McGraw-Hill, New York, 1980

28. Reichel J: Assessment of operative risk of pneumonectomy. Chest 62:570-576, 1972

29. Olsen GN, Block AJ, Swenson EW et al: Pulmonary function evaluation of the lung resection candidate: a prospective study. Am Rev Respir Dis 111:379-387, 1975

30. Logue B: Personal communication

31. Steen PA, Tinker JH, Tarhan S: Myocardial reinfarction after anesthesia and surgery. JAMA 239:2566-2570, 1978

32. Ali MK, Ewer MS: Preoperative cardiopulmonary evaluation of patients undergoing surgery for lung cancer. Cancer Bull 32:100-104, 1980

33. Mountain CF, Murphy WK: Differential diagnosis and clinical evaluation of lung cancer patients. Cancer Bull 32:94-99, 1980

34. Miller JI, Hatcher CR: Thoracoscopy: a useful tool in the diagnosis of thoracic disease. Ann Thorac Surg 26:68-72, 1978

35. Hardy JD, Webb WR, Dalton ML et al: Lung homotransplantation in man: report of initial case. JAMA 186:1065-1074, 1963

36. Veith FJ, Koerner SK: The present status of lung transplantation. Arch Surg 109:734-740, 1974

PART II.

ASSESSMENT OF THE PATIENT

Christine H. Murphy, M.D.
Michael R. Murphy, M.D.

3
Radiology of the Chest

PRINCIPLES OF RADIOLOGIC INTERPRETATION

Chest radiography is a routine and essential part of the preoperative evaluation and the postoperative management of the patient undergoing thoracic surgery. Many decisions made and courses of action taken during and after surgery are the result of chest film interpretation. Even for the relatively inexperienced interpreter, a well-exposed, properly positioned PA and lateral examination on a cooperative patient can provide a wealth of information and a rather secure feeling that significant pathology may be recognized. Similarly, obtaining and interpreting the history, physical examination, and laboratory data on a cooperative patient can be relatively easy. The greatest challenges arise when one is faced with obtaining and interpreting data on acutely ill patients. Unfortunately, all too often the only obtainable radiograph on a thoracic surgery patient (especially in the acute postoperative period) is the bedside portable. Such a radiograph is often confusing and less than optimal due to the altered consciousness of the patient, the

physical alterations from surgical intervention, and the limitations of portable technique. However, it is heartening that an acquaintance with the basics of radiographic physics (why you see what you see) and a familiarity with normal "shadows" as they are altered by surgery and film technique, coupled with a disciplined, systematic approach to each film, will render significant and useful information from even the most confusing and less-than-optimal study.

X-ray is a form of electromagnetic energy, similar in many respects to visible light, radiating from its source in all directions and being absorbed in varying degrees by objects it encounters. The shorter wave length of x-ray is the medically useful property that allows it to penetrate body tissues that are opaque to light. Radiographic film allows visualization of degrees of penetration as different shades of gray. The white-gray-black value or *radiographic density* of an object is a function of its thickness, as well as its composition (physical density plus atomic number). There is a finite limit on standard radiographs to our perception of changing shades of gray. Therefore, objects of similar compo-

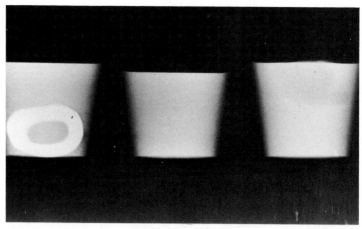

Fig. 3-1 Three cups of water, each containing a piece of body tissue, were radiographed. The cup on the left holds a piece of bone, the one in the center a piece of muscle, and the one on the right has a piece of fat floating in the water. The bone and fat are visible because they differ from water significantly in composition (radiographic density). The muscle-water interface is not visible because for radiographic purposes muscle is primarily water density. Also, notice the sharp water-air interface that is visible because of significant differences in radiographic density between air and water. (Courtesy of Basic Diagnostic Radiology Self-instructional Seminars, L. F. Squire and A. Ettinger, Programmed Seminars, Inc., N.Y., N.Y.)

sition and thickness appear the same shade of gray. The margins or *interface* between different tissues, likewise, can only be seen if they differ significantly in radiographic density. Most of the body tissues consist predominantly of water and are considered "water density." Only air, fat, and bone or calcium differ significantly in composition from the rest of the body tissues, allowing radiographic appreciation of their interfaces.[1] When two tissues of the same radiographic density abut each other, their interface is lost and they are said to "silhouette" each other.[2] Figures 3-1, 3-2, and 3-3 illustrate the concepts of radiographic density and interface. With the advent of computerized tomography, much more subtle changes in x-ray beam attenuation can be displayed on an expanded gray-scale, and many more tissue interfaces become apparent. The chest film is a static, two-dimensional image of a three-dimensional being in constant flux. The image, therefore, is a *summation* of the penetration

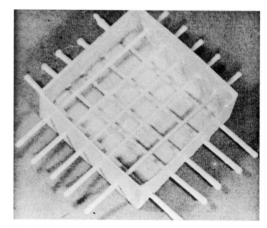

Fig. 3-2 A box was constructed with straws piercing each side in a perpendicular fashion as illustrated above. Straws running in one direction were filled with water, while those at right angles remained filled with air. Then radiographs were made of the box filled with air and then with water. See Fig. 3-3. (Courtesy of Basic Diagnostic Radiology Self-instructional Seminars, L. F. Squire and A. Ettinger, Programmed Seminars, Inc., N.Y., N.Y.)

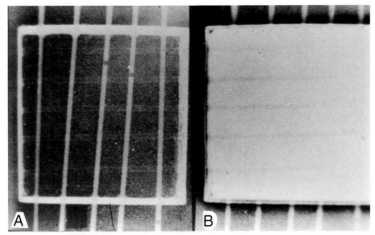

Fig. 3-3 Radiographs of the box in Figure 3-2. (A) An air-filled box with vertical straws filled with water and horizontal straws containing air. The air-filled straws are relatively invisible against the air background except for the fine lines produced by their paper walls. (B) A radiograph of the same box, now filled with water. Notice that the air-filled straws are visible, but the water filled straws being of the same radiographic density as the box are now silhouetted, and therefore, invisible. (Courtesy of Basic Diagnostic Radiology Self-instructional Seminars, L. F. Squire and A. Ettinger, Programmed Seminars, N.Y., N.Y.)

of objects superimposed in a single plane at a single instant.

Just applying the concepts of *radiographic density, interface* and *summation* will explain many shadows on a radiograph. For example, consider the paired bronchus and vessel near the hilum in Figure 3-4. In Figure 3-4A, the small vessel (water density) appears denser than the much larger descending pulmonary artery (also water density). Why is this? It is because it is seen on-end and, therefore, much thicker (effect of summation) in the frontal plane. Could this vessel be a metastatic nodule? It would be highly unlikely because metastases grow roughly as a sphere and a soft-tissue sphere of approximately 4 mm in diameter would not be that dense. However, a calcified sphere or granuloma could be (effect of composition). The bronchus on-end, being air density, is only seen normally near the hilum, where it is large enough to have a wall of such thickness that it can be resolved. Small air-filled bronchi are not normally seen because they are adjacent to air-filled alveoli and their *interface* is silhouetted. What happens to the interface or margins of these structures in various disease states? Figure 3-4B is the same patient in congestive heart failure with early interstitial edema. The vessel is now larger than its paired bronchus, partially due to vascular engorgement. Also, as fluid (water density) escapes from the capillaries into the interstitium, it appears as thickening of the wall of the vessel and the bronchus (perivascular and peribronchial cuffing). The wall or interface also becomes less distinct (perihilar haze). As the failure progresses, edema fluid fills the alveoli and obscures the vessel interface (silhouette sign) (Fig. 3-4C). Note that not only air in the major bronchus but also in smaller bronchi becomes even more apparent (the "air bronchogram") as the alveoli become fluid filled.

Total lung congestion, as in Figure 3-5, permits branching bronchi to be visualized as clearly as branching blood vessels are seen

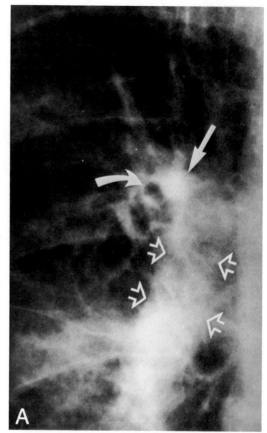

Fig. 3-4 (A) A coned-down view of the right hilum demonstrating the relative radiographic density of a small vessel on-end (*closed arrow*), the larger descending pulmonary artery (*open arrows*), and a bronchus on end (*curved arrow*) as they are affected by summation. (B) A coned-down view of the same right hilum after development of interstitial edema. The vessel on-end (*closed arrow)* is now larger due to vascular engorgement and perivascular edema. The wall of the bronchus (*curved arrow)* is also thickened by interstitial edema. (C) Development of alveolar edema obscures or silhouettes the blood vessels while making air in multiple small bronchi visible as small black circles and lines within the infiltrate.

in a normally-aerated lung. Could the lung in Figure 3-5 be totally atelectatic from proximal bronchial obstruction? No, because then the bronchi would also be airless and, therefore, as invisible as the blood vessels.

From understanding radiographic density, summation, and interface, the next step to understanding "why you see what you see" is to recognize the effects of technique, such as penetration and projection, in altering the appearance of familiar anatomy, making it appear unfamiliar or abnormal. If a film is properly exposed, then relative densities can be relied upon; but if it is underexposed, then objects that one is accustomed to seeing through become opaque. Conversely, overexposed radiographs will make some objects relatively invisible. Figure 3-6 shows a properly exposed PA and lateral study in a healthy adult. Note that the spine can be seen through the mediastinum to the degree that disc spaces can faintly be identified. By

seeing pulmonary vessels, surrounded by air, through the heart and the domes of the diaphragm, one can feel secure that there are probably no alveolar consolidations in the lower lobes, even without the aid of the lateral film.

A property of light rays that also applies to x-rays is magnification. Put your hand between a light source and the paper. As you move your hand away from the paper, the shadow of your hand is magnified. Similarly, structures in the chest that are farthest from the film are the most magnified. A PA chest film refers to the photon beam traversing the patient from the posterior chest wall to the anterior chest wall to reach the film. This projection is preferred because the heart, a relatively anterior structure, is closest to the film. It is, therefore, least magnified and its size is more truly represented. Along the same line, most lateral views are taken with the left side adjacent to the film to prevent

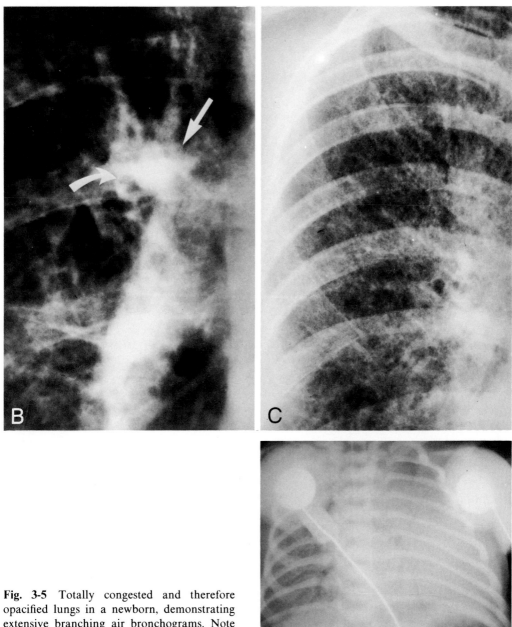

Fig. 3-5 Totally congested and therefore opacified lungs in a newborn, demonstrating extensive branching air bronchograms. Note the similarity to the air-filled straws in Figure 3-3B.

cardiac magnification. Unfortunately, portable films usually must be taken AP (anterior to posterior), and the heart appears enlarged relative to the chest wall.

Not only does the direction of the beam in the frontal plane change the appearance of the mediastinum, but degrees of rotation (obliquity) or lordosis of the patient will distort the image. Rotational distortion can be assessed by evaluation of the relationship of an anterior structure, the clavicles, to a posterior structure, the posterior spinous process

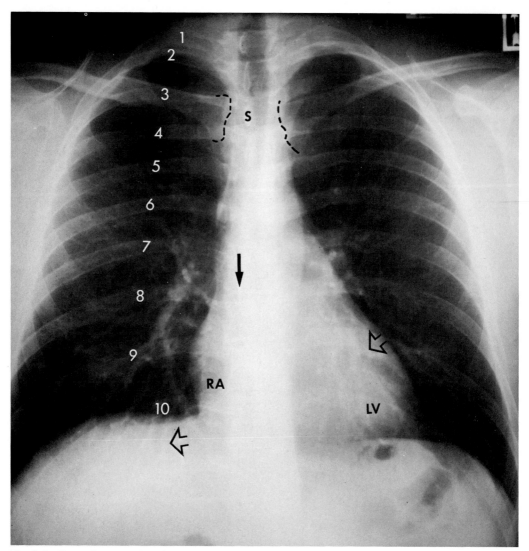

Fig. 3-6 Properly exposed and positioned PA and lateral chest films of a healthy male. The disc spaces (*closed arrow*) can be seen through the mediastinum on the PA view. The blood vessels surrounded by air (*open arrows*) are seen through the heart and diaphragm. The posterior spinous process of T-3 (S) is midway between the medial ends of the clavicles (*dotted lines*) indicating that there is no significant obliquity or rotation. The posterior ribs are numbered with the diaphragm at the 10th rib indicating a good inspiration. The cardiac chambers that are border-forming on each view are labeled. (RA) right atrium, (RV) right ventricle, (LA) left atrium, (LV) left ventricle. The approximate location of the minor fissue (*dotted line*) and major fissures (*solid line*) are illustrated on the lateral view.

of the vertebrae. On a nonrotated view, the spinous process should be seen midway between the medial ends of the clavicles. Note their position in Figure 3-6 and then in Figure 3-7. Lordosis, a common problem in semierect portable views, occurs when the

patient's chest is angled in relation to the beam as in Figure 3-8. Note that both rotation and lordosis can cause apparent mediastinal widening.

On the lateral view in Figure 3-6, it can be seen that even with good inspiration a

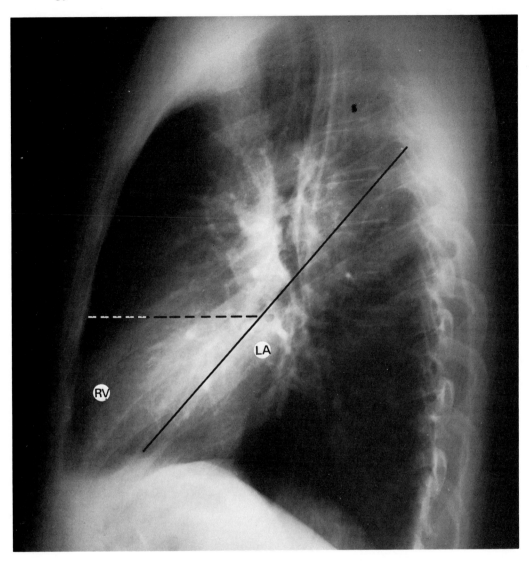

substantial portion of the lower lobes projects below the domes of the diaphragm on a frontal view. Lordosis, rotation, and AP projection can even further increase the amount of lung tissue hidden by the diaphragm. In an underexposed film, where the lung cannot be seen through the diaphragm and heart, a significant portion of the lower lobes cannot be readily assessed for infiltrate, atelectasis, or other pathology without a lateral view.

In the ideal chest film, a patient takes a deep breath for the exposure and the domes of the diaphragm will project at the 10th or 11th posterior ribs in an adult (Fig. 3-6), or the 8th to the 9th posterior ribs in a small child. However, the ability to take and hold a deep breath is, as would be expected, often inversely related to the debility of the patient. Hypoinflation can markedly change the appearance of the chest; the mediastinum widens, the heart and hila enlarge, the lungs become more opaque, and the diaphragm hides more of the lungs (Fig. 3-9). If one fails to count the ribs, then hypoinflation can easily be confused with congestive heart failure, pneumonia, mediastinal hematoma, and many other conditions. This is especially true

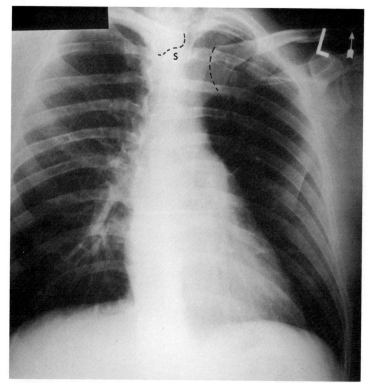

Fig. 3-7 An oblique view of the same person as in Figure 3-6. The chest is rotated to the left, distorting the apparent size and shape of the heart and other mediastinal structures. Compare the position of the medial ends of the clavicles (*dotted lines*) to the vertebral spinous process (S) here and in Figure 3-6.

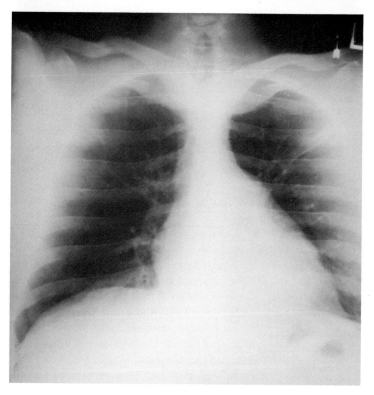

Fig. 3-8 A lordotic view of the person in Figure 3-6. Note the position and appearance of the clavicles in both views. Lordosis distorts and magnifies the cardiac shadow, and also places a greater portion of the lung bases behind the domes of the diaphragm.

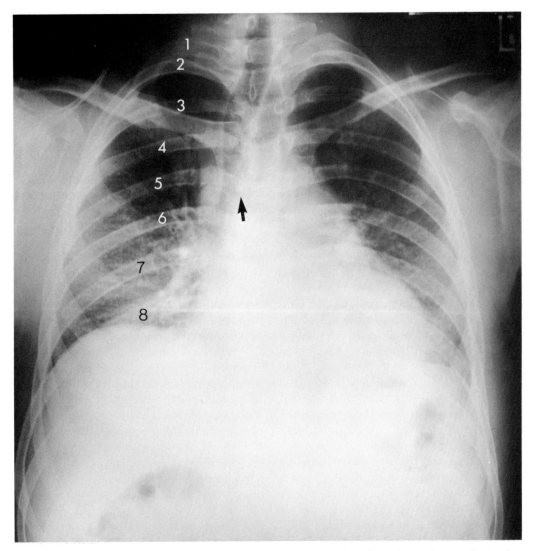

Fig. 3-9 A film of the same healthy male in Figure 3-6. The technique is unchanged except for moderate hypoinflation and an AP projection on the current study. The posterior right ribs are labeled revealing the diaphragm to now be at the level of the 8th rib. The hypoaereated lungs and widened mediastinum can mimic disease such as congestive heart failure or pneumonia. Note the position of the carina (*arrow*) on a portable examination.

in postoperative portables when the viewer glances hurriedly at the film with a high index of prejudice, wanting only to confirm clinical impressions. It has often been said in radiology that "we see only what we look for, and recognize only what we have seen before." Undoubtedly, the value and correctness of a radiologic interpretation is heightened when correlated with clinical findings.

In fact, an examination is *only* properly utilized when it is integrated with all data. Nevertheless, only when the examination is studied in a systematic fashion, and with an awareness of the technical pitfalls in interpretation mentioned above, can one hope to avoid overtreatment or mismanagement due to clinical prejudice.

The tendency when viewing a film is to

let one's eyes drift about erratically and be drawn to areas of obvious pathology. Do not fight this, but once the mass lesion in the lung has been seen, the entire film should be scanned in a set manner to avoid missing the metastasis in a rib. The easiest method is to look *at* specific structures, comparing sides for symmetry, and then look *through* them at others.[3] For example, the bony thorax and soft tissues may be scanned first, comparing sides, then looked through to assess lung parenchyma, the hila, and peripheral pulmonary vasculature. Finally the mediastinum and cardiac configuration may be examined. After the heart has been observed for size, shape should be noted and then looked through for valvular calcifications. One's own system should be developed and used every time, so that, after that film has been studied, it is certain that such things as tracheal deviation, the position of the stomach bubble, and mediastinal air have been looked for. In the postoperative study, the position of tubes and lines must be added to the list of items to scan. Remembering that the x-ray beam goes from the gown on the anterior chest wall to the gown posteriorly, and through any extraneous surgical dressings or tubing, may prevent one from coming to the wrong conclusion. Particularly on a portable examination, these artifacts may simulate pathology. In the later section on extra-alveolar air, a skin fold is shown mimicking a pneumothorax (Fig. 3-32A). Think three-dimensionally. Many shadows that at first glance appear to be pathological can be explained away by tracing their margins back to overlapping normal anatomy.

Figure 3-6 illustrates the normally appearing cardiac chambers that are border-forming in each view. Also, in Figure 3-6B, the position of the major and minor fissures is indicated. The superior extent of the lower lobe is at the level of the hila or above. Therefore, an infiltrate in the superior segment of the lower lobe, a common place for aspiration, will appear as a perihilar infiltrate in the frontal plane. Become familiar with the position of the other lobes in both planes. Knowing that an infiltrate silhouettes a certain portion of the mediastinum or diaphragm allows one to correctly identify the lobe. For example, consolidation or atelectasis of the right middle lobe will obscure the right heart border.

Abnormalities found on chest films taken in the intraoperative or postoperative period cannot always be assumed to be reflective of an acute process. Before delving into a discussion of acute pathology, we will reflect on the value of prior films. It has been said jokingly in radiologic circles that when one is faced with an unexplained finding on a film, the thing to do to avoid displaying ignorance is to ask for "another view." It is no joke, however, that the most informative, timesaving and cost-beneficial "other view" is the old film. It will often save the patient needless further workup.

When evaluating preoperative films in anticipation of surgery, or when comparing them to postoperative studies, two major assessments should be made. First, does the film reveal chronic pathology that may complicate anesthesia or postoperative recovery? This would, of course, include many types of chronic pulmonary or cardiac disease. Of particular importance in thoracic surgery patients would be recognition of any complications of the disease for which the patient is having surgery. For example, abnormalities of the esophagus such as carcinoma, stricture, or hiatal hernia, and severe motility disorders such as achalasia are usually not apparent on plain chest films—unless the esophagus becomes so obstructed and dilated that it is seen as a fluid-filled mass in the mediastinum. However, a frequent complication of these conditions is recurrent aspiration. While aspiration is often clinically apparent, it may be silent or undiagnosed. If serial preoperative films are reviewed, a pictorial history of recurrent basilar infiltrates may lead to a suspicion of chronic aspiration. The patient's lungs would likely be chronically inflamed and infected, altering his abil-

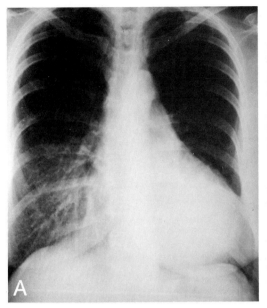
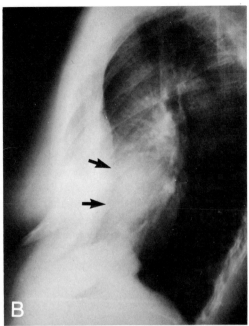

Fig. 3-10 (A) PA and (B) lateral views of a healthy female with a severe pectus excavatum simulating cardiomegaly and right lung pathology. The posterior extent of the sternum is indicated by arrows.

ity to clear secretions and increasing his chances of postoperative complications such as pneumonia and atelectasis. If lung damage is severe enough, large main pulmonary arteries reflecting pulmonary arterial hypertension and even cor pulmonale may be seen.

The second major value of a preoperative film is that pathology can be assessed that would be confusing or misleading when viewed postoperatively on a portable examination. For example, chest wall deformities such as scoliosis or pectus excavatum, by narrowing the PA diameter of the chest, change the appearance of the lung and mediastinum. Note in Figure 3-10 the accentuation of right lower lung markings and apparent cardiac enlargement, in the PA projection, in this otherwise healthy individual with severe pectus excavatum. Without a lateral view, such as on a portable examination, pneumonia or heart disease might be erroneously diagnosed. More severe thoracic cage deformities would not only present a confusing picture on a portable radiograph, but might also pose considerable problems in positioning the patient for anesthesia and surgery. Along the same line, arthritic changes such as severe cervical or thoracic spondylosis, or ankylosing spondylitis, while not necessarily confusing on portable examinations, should also be looked for preoperatively to avoid difficulty with or complications from intubation. Two other examples of diseases that tend to "muddy the water" when viewing portable examinations are chronic obstructive pulmonary disease (COPD) and mitral valvular disease. Recognition of the pulmonary parenchymal and vascular changes seen preoperatively in these conditions may help avoid misinterpretation of postoperative studies, especially when evaluating the films for signs of congestive heart failure. This is illustrated in greater detail in the section on pulmonary edema later in this chapter.

The following sections review many of the acute changes in the chest film in the intraoperative and postoperative period relating to surgical alteration or complicating disorders.

INFILTRATES

The term infiltrate is used here loosely to include all acute pulmonary parenchymal densities which may be encountered on post-operative radiographs. Unfortunately, most infiltrates seen on a single radiograph are by themselves very nonspecific. With alveolar infiltrates, the radiographic density is the same whether the alveoli are filled with edema, blood, pus or any other water density substance. Likewise, interstitial infiltrates from edema can be indistinguishable from other types of interstitial disease such as fibrosis or even lymphangitic spread of carcinoma. These limitations strengthen the argument for the importance of comparison with prior films.

When assessing an infiltrate, the clue to its nature may lie in recognition and correlation of other radiographic findings and clinical data. This will become more apparent in the following discussion of specific infiltrates.

Atelectasis

Atelectasis is by far the most common infiltrate found on postoperative radiographs, especially in the first 48 hours.[4] Multiple factors such as pain, decreased consciousness, and intubation decrease the ability to cough, clear secretions, or expand the chest. Chronic hypoinflation may produce well-defined, thin, dense lines parallel or oblique to the diaphragm. These are easily recognized as linear or "plate-like" atelectasis (Fig. 3-11). Acute hypoinflation more typically appears as patchy infiltrates that can be indistinguishable from edema or pneumonia. Occasionally, air bronchograms may be apparent as the peripheral alveoli collapse around patent bronchi. With acute hypoinflation, as in Figure 3-9, counting ribs and identifying crowded vessels should lead to a suspicion of volume loss rather than an inflammatory process or pulmonary edema. However, coexisting pneumonia or edema

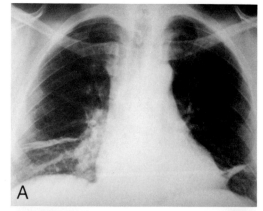

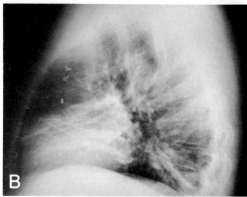

Fig. 3-11 (A) PA and (B) lateral views that demonstrate dense bands of linear or "plate-like" atelectasis produced by chronic hypoinflation.

can be difficult to exclude in the presence of marked hypoinflation. Rapid changes in configuration or location, or disappearance after physical therapy are also indications that atelectasis rather than pneumonia is present.[5]

Lobar collapse implies a proximal obstruction and produces an airless lobe so that neither blood vessels nor air bronchograms are seen. Lobar atelectasis occurs frequently after thoracic or abdominal surgery and it typically involves the lower lobes, especially the left lower lobe.[6] In a supine patient, a large heart may directly compress the left lower lobe bronchus, creating atelectasis. In open heart surgery, topical cooling of the heart is frequently employed and this has been shown to effect the left phrenic nerve producing temporary paralysis of the left leaf of the diaphragm.[7] In these cases, poor dia-

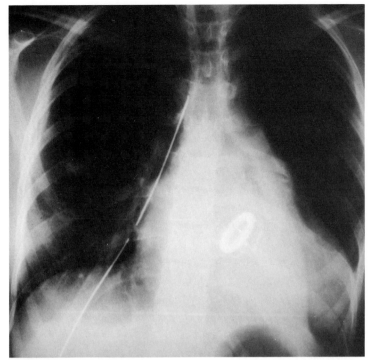

Fig. 3-12 This portable examination obtained following mitral valve surgery reveals atelectasis of the left lower lobe. The mechanism of bronchial obstruction is probably a combination of mucus plugging and direct compression by the enlarged heart. Note the abrupt cut-off of proximal air bronchograms, the changing density in the heart shadow, and the loss of definition of the medial aspect of the left hemidiaphragm as it is silhouetted by the airless lobe.

phragmatic excursion combined with increased or thickened secretions may predispose to mucus plugs, creating lobar atelectasis. The mucus plugs may be in the mainstem bronchi or in more peripheral branches. In the latter case, air bronchograms of the first and second bronchial divisions may be observed ending abruptly as in Figure 3-12. In this case of left lower lobe atelectasis, note the benefit of a well-penetrated study in identifying the collapsed lobe. A hallmark of lower lobe atelectasis or consolidation is a change in density of portions of the cardiac shadow. If the film is not sufficiently penetrated so that this differential can be appreciated, then this important finding will be missed. In lobar atelectasis, the silhouette sign plays an important role. As can be seen in Figure 3-12, the medial aspect of the diaphragm is not apparent, since it is silhouetted by the collapsed lobe. In Figure 3-13A and B, various degrees of upper lobe collapse are illustrated. Note the silhouette effect produced by adjacent atelectasis simulating mediastinal widening. Figure 3-13 also illustrates other signs of lobar atelectasis reflecting the effects of volume loss. These include elevation of the ipsilateral diaphragm and shift of the mediastinum to the involved side. The hilum will also shift toward the atelectatic lobe. However, this is often difficult to detect on a portable examination. Following wedge resection or lobectomy, the remaining lung on the ipsilateral side may not fully reexpand or may collapse secondary to a mucus plug or inadequate function of chest tubes. This is illustrated in Figure 3-14.

Total lung atelectasis, a less frequent

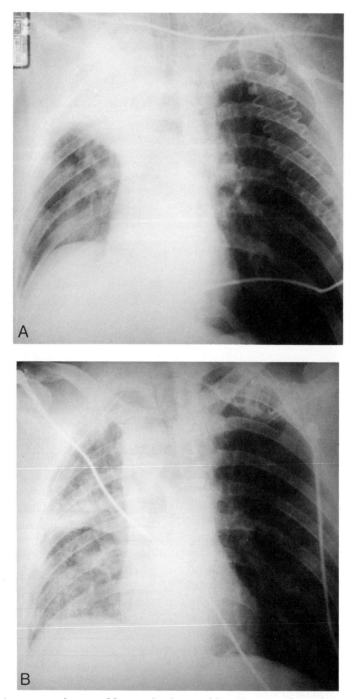

Fig. 3-13 (A) A postoperative portable examination on this patient reveals total atelectasis of the right upper lobe. The volume loss is compensated by elevation of the ipsilateral hemidiaphragm and mediastinal shift toward the atelectasis. (B) Following vigorous respiratory therapy, the right upper lobe atelectasis in (A) has partially resolved. The portion of dense atelectasis remaining medially simulated mediastinal widening.

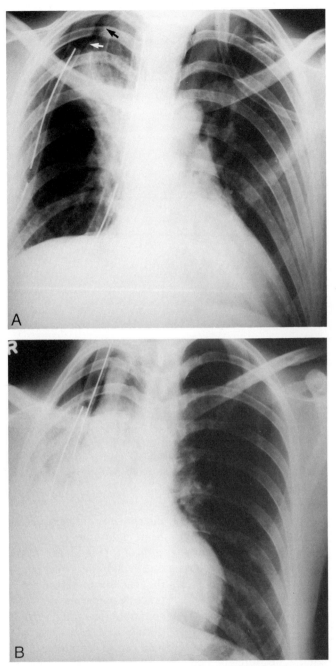

Fig. 3-14 (A) This film obtained following partial resection of the right upper lobe reveals a small residual pneumothorax (*arrows*). The infiltrate surrounding the sutures is probably a combination of atelectasis and localized hemorrhage. The remaining lung is relatively clear. (B) Several hours later a film obtained because of changing auscultatory findings reveals interval collapse of the remaining right lung with compensatory hyperexpansion of the left lung. The mediastinum also has shifted significantly to the right. This is a true shift, although it is somewhat accentuated by the great change in obliquity from one film to the other. Note the position of the clavicles.

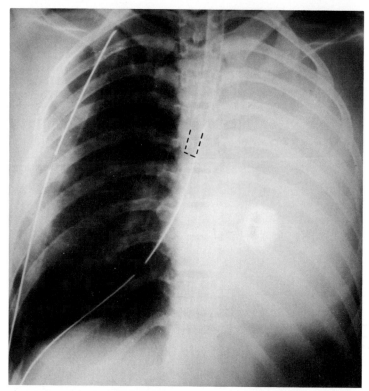

Fig. 3-15 Opacification of the left chest on this film obtained immediately after surgery is due to total atelectasis of the left lung from bronchial obstruction secondary to right mainstem bronchus intubation. There is overexpansion of the right lung and mediastinal shift to the left. The tip of the endotracheal tube (retouched) projects to the right with leftward bowing of the tube.

problem postoperatively than lobar atelectasis, also implies a mechanical obstruction to a major bronchus. In addition to formation of mucus plugs, foreign bodies such as poorly placed endotracheal tubes or aspirated teeth should be suspected with these large areas of collapse (Fig. 3-15). An adequately penetrated film is necessary for identification of the tip of the endotracheal tube and any radiopaque foreign body. Proper and improper placement of endotracheal tubes will be further discussed in a subsequent section.

Films taken immediately after extubation or removal of mechanical ventilation will often show increased density of the lungs and an apparent increase in the cardiac size due to hypoinflation. This may be mis-interpreted radiographically as congestive heart failure while the patient is improving clinically (Fig. 3-16). Conversely, infiltrates due to atelectasis may rapidly disappear after the patient is placed on ventilatory assistance. Comparing the overall degree of inspiration (counting ribs) in films obtained during and after assisted ventilation may help avoid erroneous diagnoses and mistreatment. Finally, most acute infiltrates in the lung are not entirely homogenous in etiology. Infiltrates from pulmonary edema and some pneumonias usually contain small areas of atelectasis within them. These may also appear to improve with relative hyperexpansion from ventilatory therapy while clinically the patient's condition is not improving.[6]

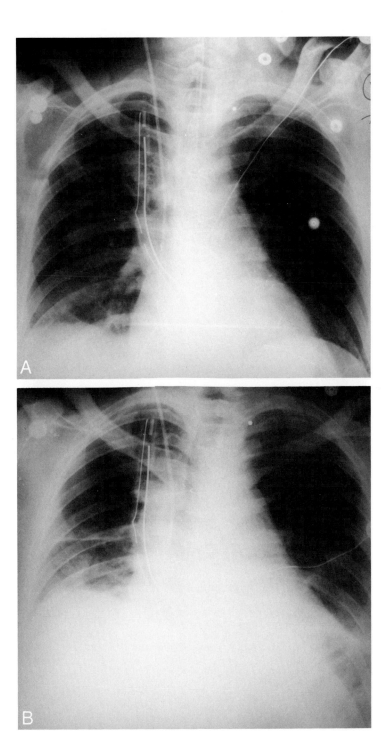

Fig. 3-16 (A) A film obtained shortly after cardiac surgery reveals relatively clear lungs and a small effusion. (B) This film taken after extubation reveals moderate hypoinflation and an accentuated pleural effusion, while the patient was making an uneventful recovery.

Pneumonia

The more common causes of nonhospital-acquired pneumonia include viruses, mycoplasma and gram-positive cocci; whereas the majority of hospital-acquired pneumonias are due to anaerobes or gram-negative bacteria, especially *Pseudomonas aeruginosa* in patients on respirators.[5,6,8] Radiographic patterns of pneumonia are often divided into three major categories, reflecting the mode of spread of the infiltrate.[9] Viral and myco-plasma pneumonias (not usually a problem in postoperative patients) tend to produce primarily bilateral interstitial infiltrates. Lobar pneumonias, classically represented by *Streptococcus pneumoniae* (formerly *Diplococcus pneumoniae*) and *Klebsiella pneumoniae,* spread contiguously in all directions within a lobe and initially present as a round or mass-like infiltrate progressing to consolidation of the entire lobe (Fig. 3-17). *Streptococcus pneumoniae,* while commonly seen in the emergency room, is not often a problem

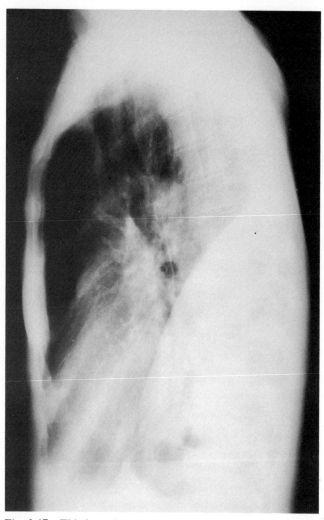

Fig. 3-17 This lateral view of a patient with Klebsiella pneumonia demonstrates total consolidation of the left lower lobe characteristic of lobar pneumonia.

postoperatively. *Klebsiella pneumoniae* is more frequently hospital-acquired than other lobar pneumonias. A characteristic feature of advanced Klebsiella infection is volume expansion of a lobe, producing bulging or convex fissures.

Most other pneumonias, and especially most hospital-acquired pneumonias, are of the bronchopneumonia pattern. They begin as a tracheobronchitis with radiographic changes of interstitial inflammation (peribronchial and perivascular fluid accumulation) that may be indistinguishable from interstitial pneumonitis or pulmonary interstitial edema. The infection spreads along the bronchial tree, producing patchy and even nodular-appearing infiltrates as alveolar involvement progresses in an acinar distribution (Fig. 3-18A,B). There is eventual coalescence into larger areas of consolidation, but they are rarely as homogenous as lobar pneumonias. Bronchopneumonia is often bilateral and may first appear as perihilar infiltrates. While peripheral air bronchograms are the hallmark of alveolar consolidation, differentiating it from atelectasis, they often are not as apparent in early bronchopneumonia as in lobar pneumonia.

Many hospital-acquired infections are also suppurative and will produce necrotic areas or abscess formation. Radiographically, these may appear as scattered lucencies within the infiltrate (microabscesses) or as large abscess cavities with fluid levels. However, air-fluid levels that simulate abscess cavities can occur in bullae in patients with COPD (Fig. 3-19). Fluid within bullae can accompany an infectious process or be seen in these patients when they are in congestive heart failure. Septic emboli, as from urinary tract infections or intravenous catheter sites, present as peripherally located nodules that then coalesce into infiltrates indistinguishable from primary pneumonic infections. These septic emboli may also cavitate.

Pseudomonas aeruginosa is the most serious pulmonary infection occurring in patients on assisted ventilation. While it is frequently found in tracheal aspirates, not all patients are clinically affected by its presence. However, when pneumonitis occurs, the mortality rate is as high as 70 percent in some series.[6,8,10,11] *Pseudomonas aeruginosa* infection is seen radiographically as a bronchopneumonia as well as septic emboli. Its early presentation can be as in Figure 3-18A,B. Later, with areas of alveolar coalescence, it is indistinguishable from any other diffuse air space infiltrate. Mottled lucencies developing within the infiltrate usually indicate necrosis with microabscess formation.

Pulmonary Edema

Pulmonary edema, the efflux of fluid from the pulmonary capillaries to the interstitium and alveoli, occurs whenever there is an imbalance between the normal hydrostatic and oncotic pressures in the lung or whenever there is an alteration in capillary permeability. Minor variations in hydrostatic or oncotic pressure, or changes in capillary permeability, are corrected by the pulmonary lymphatics which can remove up to 200 ml per minute of interstitial fluid accumulation in a normal lung. However, when the lymphatics are insufficient or overwhelmed, pulmonary edema will ensue. With slight increases in interstitial fluid, and often before most radiographic changes occur, patients may experience dyspnea due to the decreased compliance of the lungs. In patients receiving assisted ventilation, this decreased compliance may become apparent prior to changes in gas exchange or changes on the film. When interstitial fluid tension increases, some alveoli are filled while others collapse so the radiographic alveolar opacity is a combination of edema and microatelectasis. Initiation of ventilatory assistance may prevent or reverse this microatelectasis and produce a radiographic picture of improvement before it exists clinically.[12] Of the major mechanisms of pulmonary edema (Table 3-1), the one that can be differentiated from the others

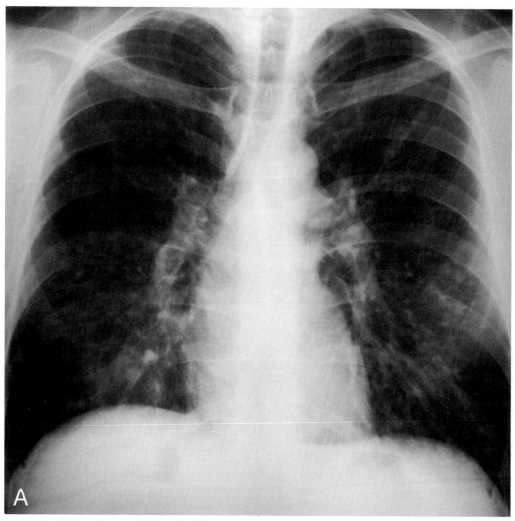

Fig. 3-18 Two early cases of bronchopneumonia. (A) The scattered bilateral small pulmonary nodules represent the early appearance of bronchopneumonia in this patient. There was subsequent coalescence into large areas of consolidation.

radiographically is increased capillary hydrostatic pressure. Pulmonary venous hypertension (PVH) produces increased capillary hydrostatic pressure. In most instances this is secondary to left heart failure or obstruction. However, in patients receiving parenteral fluids, hypertransfusion or fluid overload can also lead to PVH and then to edema, mimicking "cardiac" pulmonary edema.[13] Visualization of engorged pulmonary vasculature is the primary radiographic method of separating cardiac edema and overload from

other causes of edema and other nonedema infiltrates.[14]

What, therefore, are the radiographic findings of pulmonary venous hypertension (PVH)? In the normal erect individual, blood flow to the lungs, being influenced by gravity, is greatest in the lung bases; therefore, the diameter of lower lobe vessels is normally greater than that of upper lobe vessels. When there is an impediment to the drainage of pulmonary blood back into the heart (as in mitral valvular disease or left ventricular

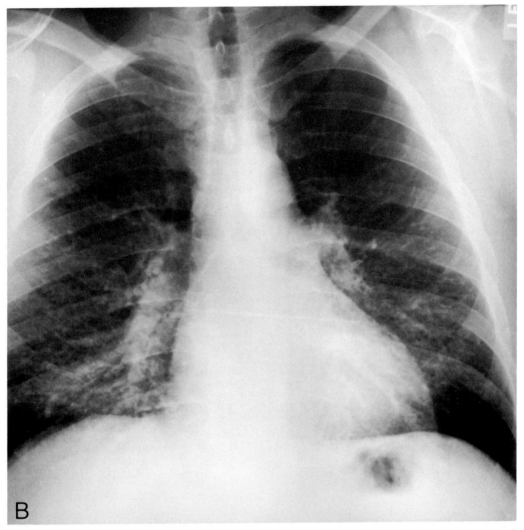

Fig. 3-18 (*continued*)   (B) This predominately perihilar and lower lobe interstitial infiltrate progressed to areas of alveolar consolidation.

dysfunction) or an overall increase in fluid in the body (as in iatrogenic fluid overload), the pressure in the pulmonary veins increases. This is observed radiographically as enlargement of the pulmonary blood vessels. Although all the pulmonary veins enlarge, this is best appreciated in the upper lobes because these vessels are not obscured by the cardiac silhouette. Also, because the capillary hydrostatic pressure is already greatest in the bases and the earliest edema occurs there, the resulting basilar lung "stiffness"

and poor gas exchange causes the pulmonary arterial blood flow to be redistributed to the upper lobes. This redistribution causes the upper lobe vasculature to appear even more prominent. To assess developing pulmonary venous hypertension and pulmonary arterial blood flow redistribution, the upper lobe vessels must be carefully evaluated for changes in size from one film to another.[15]

Since detecting pulmonary venous hypertension is of great diagnostic importance in radiographically categorizing causes of

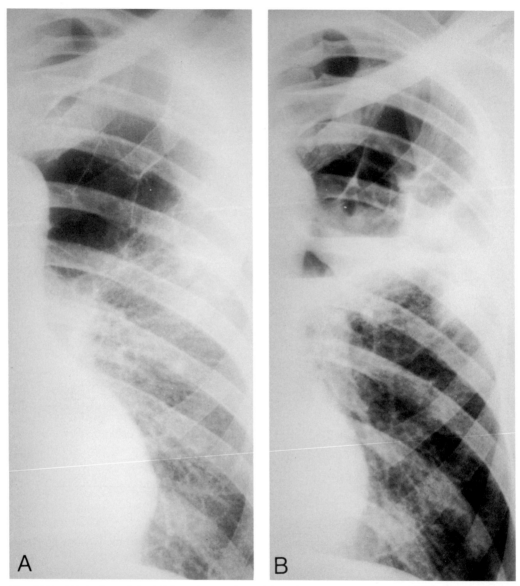

Fig. 3-19 (A) A view of the left lung in a patient with chronic lung disease reveals marked upper lobe bullous emphysema. (B) An acute infection produces fluid within these bullae as well as a surrounding infiltrate. These fluid-filled bullae could be confused with abcess cavities.

pulmonary edema, it follows that patients suspected of having edema should be radiographed in an upright position whenever humanly possible. This is often more easily said than done. Nevertheless, every effort should be made to support the patient for an upright view if the film findings are to hold any weight in clinical decisions concerning the etiology of pulmonary edema.[14]

Differentiation of heart failure from fluid overload is usually not possible radiographically. There should be clinical suspicion of the possibility of hypertransfusion any time developing pulmonary vascular engorgement, with or without edema, is found in a postoperative patient, especially if there is no known history of heart disease.[13]

Up to this point in the discussion,

Table 3-1
Mechanisms of Pulmonary Edema

I. Increased Capillary Hydrostatic Pressure
   Left ventricular failure
   Mitral valve obstruction
   Pulmonary venous obstruction
   Hypertransfusion

II. Increased Capillary Permeability
   Toxic inhalants
   Circulating toxins
   Immunological reactions
   Drug idiosyncrasy
   Infections
   Radiation injury
   Uremia
   Adult respiratory distress syndrome
   Disseminated intravascular coagulation

III. Lymphatic Insufficiency
   Chronic lung damage or disease

IV. Decreased Plasma Osmotic Pressure
   Debilitated states producing hypoalbuminemia

V. Unknown or Speculative
   High altitude
   Neurogenic
   Narcotic overdose
   Cardioversion
   Pulmonary embolism

Adapted from: CRC Critical Reviews in Clinical Radiology and Nuclear Medicine, J. H. Shapiro and U. F. Hublitz, Vol. 5, p. 389, 1974, © CRC Press, Inc., 1974. Used by permission of CRC Press, Inc.

changes in heart size have been ignored in assessing pulmonary edema. Although cardiac enlargement is a classic finding in cardiac failure, it may be absent in acute dysfunction such as myocardial infarction or dysrhythmia. Conversely, it may be present without failure. Also, because of the lack of reliability in evaluating subtle changes in heart size on portable radiographs taken in various degrees of hypoinflation, lordosis and rotation, this sign is often not helpful.[5]

Failure is often not isolated to the left heart; clinically it is the signs of right heart failure such as jugular and hepatic engorgement and pedal edema that are most obvious. In the chest film, evidence for right heart failure includes increasing size of systemic veins, specifically the superior vena cava and azygos. With iatrogenic fluid overload, the systemic as well as the pulmonary vasculature will also be engorged so that this is not a differential point between overload and failure. Assessing the size of the superior vena cava and azygos can be helpful in upright serial PA examinations as a correlative finding to PVH. However, since the mediastinum appears to widen on AP views and since changes in these vessels are not only gravity-dependent but also influenced by intrathoracic pressures, often little value can be placed on their changing appearance on portable examinations. Also, in one series evaluating the width of the azygos vein as related to central venous pressure, only about ten percent were identifiable on portable films.[16]

The typical progression from well-defined pulmonary vessels, to enlargement of these vessels, to early edema producing haziness and poor definition of vessel-air interface, and then to alveolar filling has, in part, been illustrated in Figure 3-4. The classic radiographic appearance of cardiac failure is exemplified in Figure 3-20. At the same time that the interstitial fluid is producing perivascular and peribronchial cuffing, fine but dense lines may also be seen running horizontally in the periphery of the lung base (Kerley B lines), representing fluid in the intralobular septae.[17] These can be very dramatic in upright views (Fig. 3-21), but are reportedly rarely identified on portable examination and, therefore, are of less value in assessing the postoperative patient.[18,19] Development of pleural fluid is commonly associated with pulmonary edema, but in a postoperative thoracic surgery patient where effusions are very common, this sign is not reliable.

As previously alluded to in the discussion of the value of prior films, chronic lung disease can produce confusing patterns of pulmonary edema. COPD produces areas of destruction of normal lung parenchyma with loss of vascularity to these areas. Radiographically, paucity, stretching, and attenuation of vessels are seen in the area of greatest emphysema, with increased density of the

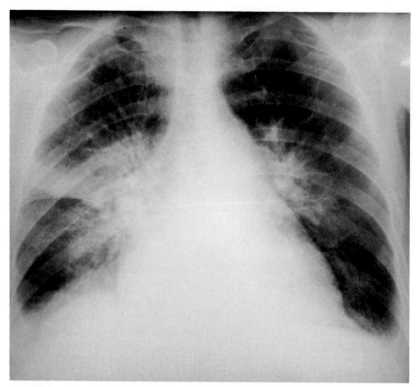

Fig. 3-20 Advanced congestive heart failure is exemplified here by cardiomegaly, prominent upper lobe vessels, bilateral small pleural effusions, and pulmonary edema, typically greatest in the perihilar and basilar areas.

remaining lung due to crowding and fibrosis. Typically, severe COPD produces an elongated mediastinum with a small cardiac silhouette due to downward displacement of the diaphragm. The central pulmonary arteries may be enlarged due to pulmonary arterial hypertension from the chronic lung disease. Congestive heart failure developing in this setting often presents a very atypical pattern. Assessment of cardiac enlargement by common criteria (transverse diameter of the heart greater than 50 percent of the transverse diameter of the chest) will not be accurate in these patients due to hyperinflation. Findings of pulmonary vascular engorgement may be altered or absent due to the chronically altered blood flow. The typical localization of pulmonary edema in the perihilar and lower lung zones in patients with otherwise normal pulmonary parenchyma cannot be expected in patients with

chronic lung disease. In general, pulmonary edema can only occur in otherwise relatively normal lung tissue. It will not occur in bullae or fibrosis or where there is absent pulmonary vasculature. Therefore, edema in chronic lung patients will be patchy, asymmetrical and can even be unilateral.[20,21] Figure 3-22 demonstrates an unusual distribution of pulmonary edema to the upper lobes due to the patient's lower lobe emphysema. As fluid fills the interstitium in these patients, it may appear as a nodular or even miliary prominence of the already chronically increased interstitial densities. A high index of suspicion and close observation of changing interstitial patterns is needed to diagnose congestive heart failure in a patient with COPD. Minor changes in compliance due to interstitial edema in these already compromised lungs may be sufficient to produce acute respiratory failure. It is not uncommon

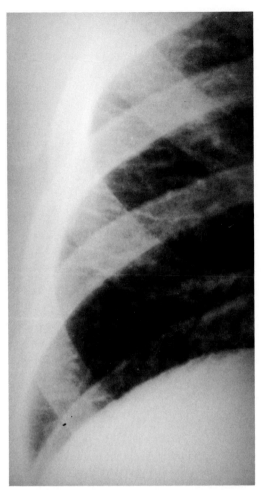

Fig. 3-21 A coned-down view of the lung periphery in a patient with interstitial edema. Thin but dense horizontal lines (Kerley B) are very apparent in this upright view, but are uncommonly appreciated on portable examinations.

to see a patient with severe COPD develop acute respiratory failure and have the chest examination show little, if any, change. It has also been postulated that, with the alteration in lymphatic drainage created in COPD, there is decreased ability to compensate for minor variations in interstitial fluid. This places the patient with COPD at a greater risk for developing edema with mild degrees of overtransfusion.[20]

Atypical patterns of pulmonary edema are also seen in other types of chronic pulmonary vascular or parenchymal derangement such as Swyer-James syndrome, or congenital and acquired heart disease with altered flow patterns.[20,21] Mitral valvular disease is the classic example. Assessing the portable film in patients with mitral valve disease poses two threats to misdiagnosis. First, the chronic changes of cardiomegaly, pulmonary vasculature redistribution, and interstitial edema and fibrosis will mimic acute failure if previous "baseline" films are not reviewed. Second, as in other patients with parenchymal disease, if acute edema does occur it may be atypical in location and distribution. With the blood flow in chronic mitral disease markedly shifted to the upper lung zones due to fibrosis and scarring of lower lobes from chronic edema, it logically follows that any blood-flow directed condition, whether it be edema, emboli from venous thrombosis, or septic emboli would selectively involve the upper lung areas.

Other causes of segmentally decreased pulmonary blood flow, such as pulmonary emboli, will present as an area devoid of infiltrate in patients with diffuse edema. In fact, this finding of a lucent area in otherwise congested lungs in a patient with no known prior chronic lung disease is a good indication that the patient may have experienced a pulmonary embolus.[5,21]

Just as areas of atelectasis have been shown to disappear, reappear and migrate with changes in mechanical ventilation or respiratory therapy, areas of pulmonary edema can also migrate or change configuration in response to changes in the patient's position. In fact, a simple test described to help differentiate edema from pneumonia is to place the patient in the lateral decubitus position for an hour or two and repeat the chest film. Edema, unlike pneumonia, should fall with gravity to the dependent lung.[22] Likewise, edema developing in a supine patient will be more uniformly distributed to both upper and lower lobes, reflecting the change in blood flow.

In all the other causes of pulmonary edema where the mechanism is other than increased capillary hydrostatic pressure

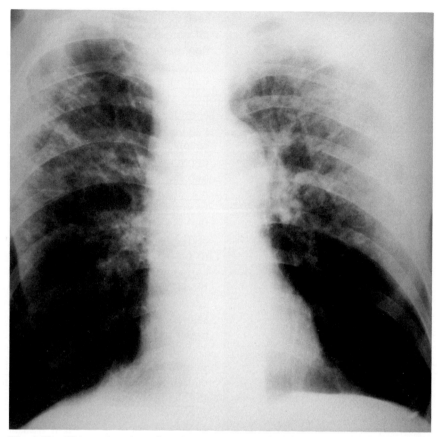

Fig. 3-22 This patient has chronic lung disease with lower lobe empnysema. Superimposed congestive heart failure has an atypical appearance due to the underlying lung disease. Here the cardiac enlargement usually associated with failure is not apparent, and the pulmonary edema is predominantly upper lobe rather than basilar.

(Table 3-1), radiographic signs of pulmonary venous hypertension and cardiomegaly are absent unless the patient has coexisting heart disease. The appearance of the infiltrate, however, is indistinguishable from edema associated with pulmonary venous hypertension. Also, as previously mentioned, evolving interstitial-to-alveolar edema can look quite similar to evolving bronchopneumonia or aspiration in some instances. Therefore, the clue to the etiology lies not in the infiltrate per se, but in the temporal sequence of its appearance, its distribution, and its associated clinical setting.

A decrease in plasma oncotic pressure (number 4, Table 3-1) is an uncommon cause

of edema. However, if patients are nutritionally debilitated by their disease, such as those with long-standing or progressive esophageal disorders, and they receive large volumes of non-colloidal fluids during surgery, decreased oncotic pressure may be a possible cause of developing pulmonary edema.[12]

Aspiration

Infiltrates from aspiration vary according to the chemical makeup of the aspirant. Aspiration of low pH fluids, typically stomach contents, classically produces hypoxia and respiratory distress (Mendelson's syndrome) within one to two hours.[23,24] Radiographs taken within 30 minutes may show little or no change, but within two to four hours there is rapid appearance of diffuse alveolar infiltrates. These may involve all lobes, but particularly the right middle lobe and superior segments of the lower lobes. The infiltrate is actually a localized pulmonary edema due to shift of fluid into the lungs secondary to chemical damage to alveoli and capillaries.[25] The pattern can be indistinguishable from other forms of pulmonary edema. However, if severe, the shift of fluid into the lungs may cause volume depletion rather than fluid overload as seen in pulmonary edema from congestive heart failure. The initial infiltrate from aspiration of gastric contents will also begin to clear rapidly, often within 24 to 36 hours. Increasing or recurrent infiltrates strongly suggest the presence of a secondary infection. Persistent areas of atelectasis may also suggest the presence of retained food particles.[5] Figure 3-23 shows a typical progression.

Adult Respiratory Distress Syndrome

In recent years, a fairly characteristic constellation of clinical, radiographic, and pathological findings has been increasingly described in patients developing respiratory insufficiency following severe trauma, major surgery, or other critical illness. Because the condition has been frequently associated with certain diseases (Table 3-2), it has been considered predisposing or causative. Various terms reflecting this association have been proposed (Table 3-3).[26-28] However, the term Adult Respiratory Distress Syndrome (ARDS) has gained the most universal acceptance, probably because its inherent vagueness encompasses these others. This would seem appropriate in that the significance of the syndrome is that, despite the multitude of associated diseases, the rather uniform pulmonary pathophysiologic re-

sponse suggests that there must be a common mechanism or that the ability of the lung to react is severely limited. ARDS is included under pulmonary edema secondary to increased capillary permeability by some investigators who feel that damage to pulmonary microvasculature represents the key event.[29]

Following the initial insult (e.g., trauma, hemorrhage, surgery, shock, sepsis) there is a latent period of variable duration, but typically 12 to 24 hours, after which clinical symptoms of tachypnea, dyspnea, cyanosis and decreased PaO_2 develop. During the next several hours of rather catastrophic clinical deterioration, the chest film typically shows no appreciable change.[29] If the chest film was clear initially, it should remain so. Immediate or concomitant development of infiltrates should suggest conditions other than ARDS such as aspiration, edema or hemorrhage. If these conditions are preexisting, they may of course be radiographically apparent, but the lack of change in light of increasing respiratory embarrassment is the hallmark of superimposed ARDS. One other condition, pulmonary embolization, may produce confusion at this stage, since it also presents with acute respiratory distress and a normal or stable chest film. Early signs of pulmonary embolization are discussed in a later section, and these, if present, may help in differentiation. Later stages of pulmonary embolization with infarction will produce focal rather than diffuse infiltrates not usually confused with ARDS.[28] Small pleural effusions common to pulmonary embolization are absent in ARDS, but in thoracic surgery patients, in whom pleural effusion is often present postoperatively, a slight increase may go unnoticed.

As clinical symptoms of increasing respiratory insufficiency (often requiring ventilatory assistance) progress, radiographic changes become apparent. The first film changes consist of patchy, ill-defined, bilateral pulmonary infiltrates. These will rapidly increase and coalesce, producing a pattern

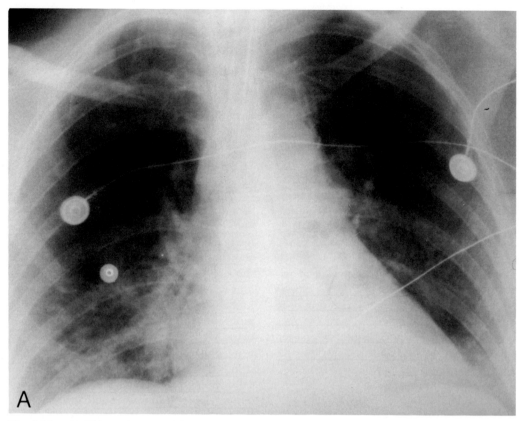

A

Fig. 3-23 (A) This patient was felt to have aspirated during intubation. This film obtained immediately afterward reveals only minimal infrahilar infiltrates although clinically there was severe respiratory embarrassment.

indistinguishable from other types of generalized alveolar pulmonary edema with diffuse air bronchograms. Unlike pulmonary edema from failure or overload, the infiltrates are unresponsive to digitalis and diuretics, and change little with changing patient position.[29]

Following the development of diffuse infiltration, the radiographic picture changes little over the next few days to weeks. After 7 to 10 days, changes in the chest film usually indicate complications.[29] Due to the decreased compliance of the lungs, complications from ventilatory assistance, especially PEEP, are common, and the films should be closely studied for signs of interstitial air or pneumomediastinum. Sudden deterioration

may mean a tension pneumothorax. Also, the congested lungs are highly susceptible to infection, especially from gram-negative organisms such as Pseudomonas. Areas of increasing consolidation, a mottled appearance suggesting microabscesses, or increasing effusion (empyema) should lead to a suspicion of superimposed pneumonia.[30]

If the patient survives and the alveolar infiltrates regress, there may be complete clearing or development of an interstitial pattern of pulmonary scarring and fibrosis. Table 3-4 summarizes the typical sequence of clinical, radiographic, and pathological findings in ARDS. In Figure 3-24 A-F, a typical radiographic progression is illustrated.

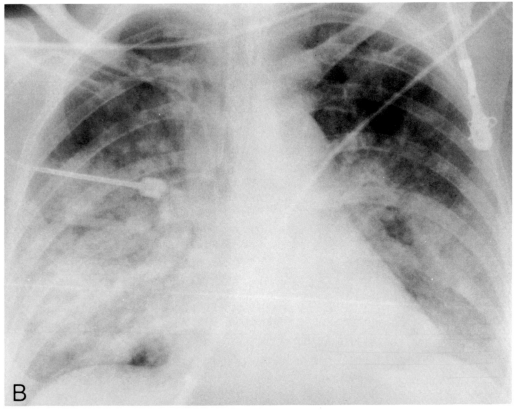

Fig. 3-23 (*continued*)   (B) A film four hours later shows interval development of extensive alveolar consolidation as pulmonary edema develops in response to the pulmonary damage. Unless secondary infection develops, or the damage is severe enough to lead to Adult Respiratory Distress Syndrome, the edema usually begins clearing within 24 to 48 hours with appropriate supportive therapy.

Pulmonary Hemorrhage

The infiltrate from intrapulmonary hemorrhage is typically a dense alveolar consolidation rapidly appearing and fairly rapidly clearing. Focal hemorrhage from contusion due to surgery or trauma can usually be suspected by its location (Fig. 3-25). Occasionally, patients receiving anticoagulant therapy or those with coagulation disorders will develop pulmonary parenchymal hemorrhages without pulmonary contusion. These typically are rapidly-progressing fluffy alveolar infiltrates. They are usually bilateral and symmetrical and can be confused with pulmonary edema.

Clinical findings such as a drop of hematocrit and occasional gross hemoptysis will be more helpful in identifying the etiology of the infiltrate than will its appearance. In a patient with clinical evidence of disseminated intravascular coagulation (DIC), the acute development of bilateral alveolar infiltrates should suggest the possibility of pulmonary hemorrhage[31] (Fig. 3-26).

Small areas of hemorrhage usually resolve completely over a few days. Massive or repetitive pulmonary hemorrhage will produce interstitial fibrosis. Delay in clearing may mean superimposed ARDS, particularly in patients with DIC.[32]

Table 3-2
Diseases Associated with or Known to Precipitate ARDS[26-28]

Trauma
Shock (hypovolemic or endotoxic)
Overhydration
Extracorporeal perfusion (cardiopulmonary bypass)
Embolism
    Fat
    Amnionic fluid
Aspiration
    Chemicals
    Low pH fluids
Viral pneumonia
Radiation pneumonitis
Burns and smoke inhalation
Carcinomatosis
Bowel infarction
Clostridial sepsis
Gram-negative sepsis
Pancreatitis
Drug abuse
Eclampsia
Oxygen toxicity
Disseminated intravascular coagulation
Transfusion of mismatched blood
Heat stroke
High-altitude pulmonary edema

Pulmonary Embolus

The typical radiographic appearance immediately following pulmonary embolus is the absence of change in the chest film.[33] This lack of change in light of a sudden deterioration in blood gases and an increase in repiratory effort is characteristic and should acutely suggest pulmonary embolization. As previously mentioned, in the appropriate clinical setting, early ARDS is also a possibility at this stage. Although the chest film may be unchanged, the radiological study that does show immediate changes of pulmonary embolization is the radionuclide lung scan. Segmental perfusion defects with a normal chest film and normal ventilation studies are considered almost pathognomonic of pulmonary embolization.[34] With preexisting pulmonary disease such as severe COPD, the scan is less specific, and angiography may be necessary for diagnosis. Plain film changes that may occur and are suggestive or supportive of the clinical diagnosis of pulmonary embolization include mild diaphragmatic elevation, small areas of atelectasis, and a small effusion. Unfortunately, these subtle findings are usually lost among the similar coexisting postoperative changes.[35] With massive or recurrent embolization, changes in the vasculature have been described including enlargement of the main pulmonary artery, vessel cutoff or lack of normal tapering, and "anemia" or decrease in caliber and number of peripheral vessels in a segment of the lung.[33] In early embolization, before the clot is lysed and blood flow is resumed, superimposed generalized pulmonary edema will be noticeably absent in the affected pulmonary segment. A segmental "clear" area in diffuse pulmonary

Table 3-3
Synonyms for Adult Respiratory Distress Syndrome[27-29]

Adult hyaline membrane disease
Adult respiratory insufficiency syndrome
Bronchopulmonary dysplasia
Congestive atelectasis
Da Nang lung
Fat embolism
Hemorrhagic lung syndrome
Oxygen toxicity
Postperfusion lung syndrome
Posttransfusion lung
Posttraumatic atelectasis
Posttraumatic pulmonary insufficiency
Progressive pulmonary consolidation
Progressive respiratory distress
Pulmonary edema
Pulmonary hyaline membrane disease
Pulmonary microembolism
Respirator lung
Shock lung
Solid lung syndrome
Stiff lung syndrome
Traumatic wet lung
Transplant lung
Wet lung
White lung syndrome

Table 3-4
Typical Sequence of Findings in Adult Respiratory Distress Syndrome[26-29]

Clinical	Radiologic	Pathologic
Primary insult and latent period (approximately 24 hr)	Normal or unchanging	Microemboli, periarteriolar hemorrhage
Onset of tachypnea, dyspnea, decreased PaO_2, decreased Pa_{CO_2} (next 6–12 hr)	Normal or unchanging	Early interstitial edema, foci of intra-alveolar edema and hemorrhage
Progression of clinical symptoms requiring assisted ventilation (occurs usually 36–48 hr after initial insult)	Perihilar haze or vague bilateral infiltrates progressing rapidly to diffuse alveolar opacification	Progression of diffuse alveolar edema and hemorrhage
Persistent arterial oxygen desaturation, respiratory and metabolic acidosis, loss of lung compliance, usually requiring PEEP therapy (36–72 hr after initial insult)	Diffuse bilateral alveolar opacification with obvious air bronchograms, but lack of pleural effusion	Solid, "beefy" or "liver-like" lungs with thickened alveolar septa, alveolar hemorrhage and edema and formation of hyaline membranes
Progressive respiratory failure requiring greater positive pressure ventilation (may last for several days or even weeks)	Persistent diffuse alveolar opacification with little change	Prominent hyaline membranes
Development of fever and increased tracheobronchial secretions	Developing focal areas of denser consolidation or areas of mottled lucency, developing effusion	Superimposed inflammatory changes with microabscesses and necrosis, empyema
Sudden deterioration in blood gases or development of soft-tissue crepitation	Interstitial air, pneumomediastinum, subcutaneous emphysema, tension pneumothorax	Extra-alveolar air from ruptured peripheral alveoli
If patient recovers, he may have symptoms of chronic pulmonary disease	Normal or varying degrees of interstitial infiltrate	Varying degrees of pulmonary fibrosis

edema should, in a patient without preexisting chronic lung disease, raise suspicion of embolization existing with or predisposing to failure.

If the embolus significantly reduces blood flow in the pulmonary circulation of a lung segment, such that systemic bronchial collaterals cannot maintain oxygenation to that segment, then it dies or infarcts. An infarcted segment of lung will develop an infiltrate due to edema and hemorrhage. The classic description of an infiltrate from pulmonary infarction is a conical or triangular alveolar consolidation with its base adjacent to a pleural surface and its apex pointing toward the hilum. Unfortunately, this classic appearance is classically rare.[33] More commonly the infiltrate is nonhomogenous or patchy and of an irregular configuration. It will be pleural based; however, this does not mean always the lateral pleural surface seen in tangent on a frontal projection. It may abut the anterior or posterior pleura, a major fissure, or even an interlobar septation, and appear to be centrally rather than peripherally located. The infiltrate will occasionally cavitate and may become secondarily infected. Radiographic resolution of a pulmo-

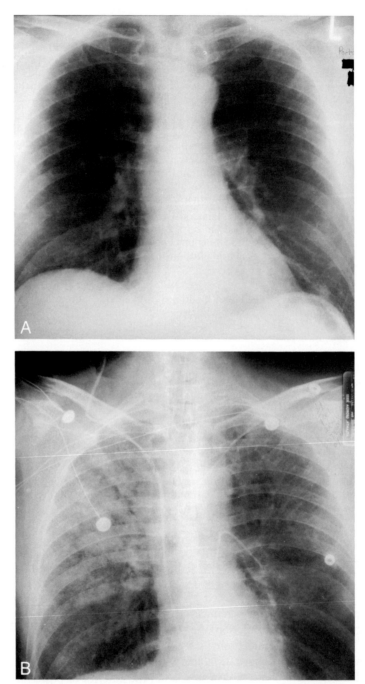

Fig. 3-24 (A) A patient with severe sepsis began experiencing increasing respiratory difficulty. The initial chest film was clear. (B) Forty-eight hours later, patchy bilateral infiltrates began to appear and respiratory failure was sufficient to necessitate intubation. Also note the Swan-Ganz (S-G) catheter tip in a slightly too peripheral location in the left lung. A left brachial venous catheter is coiled back on itself overlying the mediastinum.

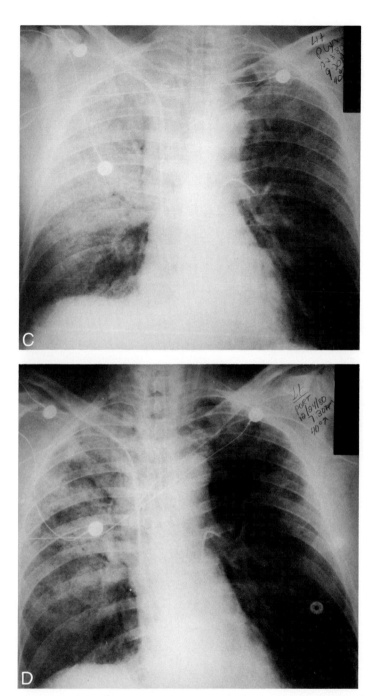

Fig. 3-24 (*continued*)   (C) The following day some of the infiltrates have further coalesced with obvious air-bronchograms. Note the now correct positions of the S-G catheter and the central venous line. (D) The next day with institution of PEEP the infiltrates appear somewhat improved, but note the development of vertical lines of subcutaneous air in the neck. This air suggests barotrauma and the patient should be closely followed radiographically and clinically for signs of mediastinal air or pneumothorax.

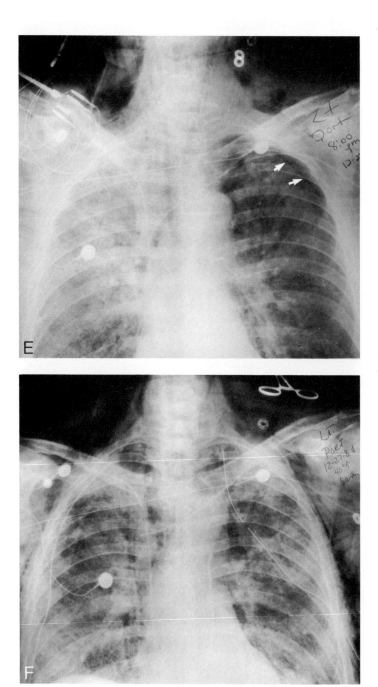

Fig. 3-24 (*continued*) (E) The following evening the subcutaneous air is more apparent bilaterally. A left pneumothorax has now developed (*arrows*), and a right pneumothorax soon followed. (F) Bilateral chest tubes have been placed because of pneumothoraces. The extra-alveolar air is now quite extensive. The diffuse infiltrates stabilized and remained until the patient's death several days later. Death was attributed to severe sepsis complicated by ARDS.

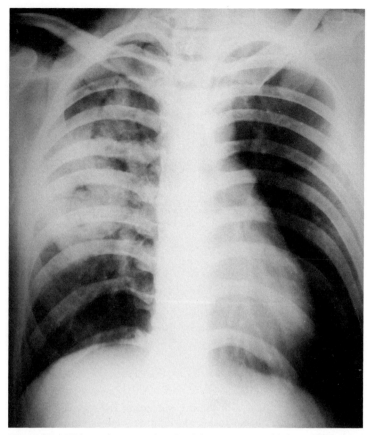

Fig. 3-25 This patient was involved in a motor vehicle accident and received blunt trauma to the right chest. This film was obtained immediately upon admission. The rounded area of consolidation represents localized pulmonary contusion with hemorrhage. Also note the subcutaneous air suggesting rupture of the lung or trachea. A pneumothorax subsequently became apparent.

nary infarction is a slow process, unlike other types of edema and hemorrhage. As it resolves, it may retract into a visible parenchymal scar.[33] Pulmonary infarction can occasionally be the result of direct occlusion of pulmonary vessels by peripherally placed pulmonary arterial catheters, illustrated in the section on Monitoring and Life Support Devices in Figure 3-50.

The incidence of venous thrombosis and subsequent pulmonary embolization in patients immobilized during surgery, and relatively immobilized in an extended recovery period, has been reported to be as high as 14 percent in one series.[12] It has been frequently stressed that a high index of suspicion must be maintained based on clinical findings, in light of the absence and nonspecificity of radiographic findings, in order to properly identify and treat pulmonary embolization. Reasonable suspicion should promptly lead to further radiologic studies such as radionuclide lung scanning or angiography. Figure 3-27 illustrates a typical sequence of films in a patient with pulmonary embolization and infarction.

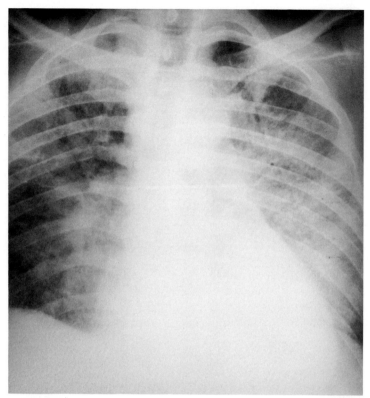

Fig. 3-26   This patient with clinical evidence of DIC developed diffuse alveolar pulmonary hemorrhage. The infiltrate itself is indistinguishable from pulmonary edema or infection.

Summary

When assessing the appearance of the lungs in the intraoperative or postoperative period, a mental checklist may lead to a proper diagnosis or at least narrow the differential.

1. What is the clinical picture and what is its temporal relationship to the developing infiltrate?

Infiltrates developing rapidly after clinical deterioration or a hypoxic event are typical in aspiration of gastric contents. Edema from fluid overload or acute cardiac decompensation often is radiographically apparent within a few hours of the onset of changing clinical symptoms; whereas abrupt clinical deterioration, respiratory distress, or hypoxia with a relatively normal radiograph would suggest ARDS or pulmonary embolization. These infiltrates often lag behind the clinical onset of symptomatology for 24 to 48 hours or more.

In contrast, a stable or improving patient who has just been extubated or removed from assisted ventilation may develop infiltrates. These are more likely areas of atelectasis. Changing areas of subsegmental or microatelectasis from hypoinflation usually do not present significant clinical symptomatology. Large areas of atelectasis, lobar or whole lung, will be symptomatic; however, their radiographic appearance is usually specific enough not to be confused

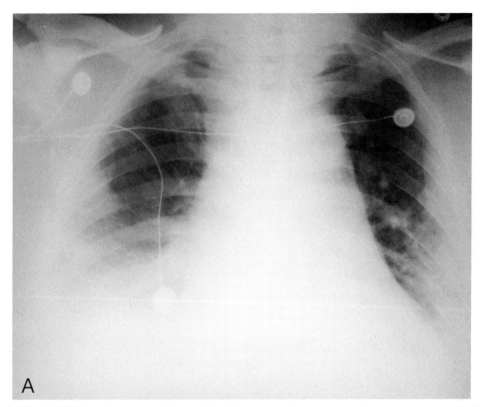

Fig. 3-27 (A) This semi-erect portable examination on a patient post-open heart surgery was obtained after extubation. The study was underexposed but demonstrated mild hypoinflation, bilateral effusions and post-surgical mediastinal widening. The patient was clinically doing well.

with other conditions such as pneumonia, ARDS, or emboli. However, it must be remembered that atelectasis may complicate or coexist with these other conditions.

2. When assessing the temporal sequence of appearance, what has been the rate of change on serial films?

Edema, once apparent, will develop rapidly within a few hours. It may also clear fairly rapidly (24 to 48 hours) following appropriate therapy such as digitalization and/or diuretics. Pneumonias show less rapid change and will often radiographically lag behind clinical resolution. ARDS, once it is radiographically apparent, may evolve quickly; however, it then stabilizes with little change over a long period of time (days to weeks).

3. What is the predominant location or distribution of the infiltrate and how does this relate to underlying lung disease, the preoperative chest film, or the patient's position?

Both aspiration and edema are gravity-dependent, and, in the supine patient, will often present in the perihilar and lower lung zones. Localized infiltrates are more typical of pneumonia, contusion, and embolus. Diffuse patterns are more characteristic of edema, massive aspiration, or ARDS. Occasionally, some pneumonias may present a diffuse pattern. In patients with underlying COPD, a normally diffuse process such as edema from congestive heart failure may appear as a patchy or segmentalized infiltrate.

4. In addition to the pulmonary paren-

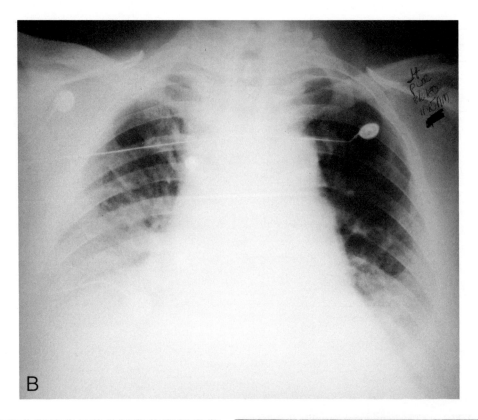

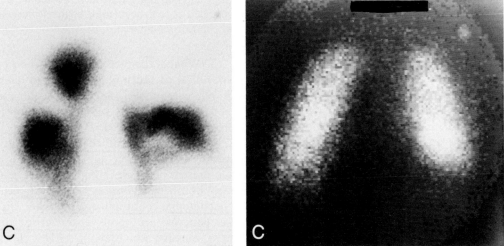

Fig. 3-27 (*continued*)   (B) The patient suddenly developed respiratory distress and hypoxia. This film was obtained immediately, and again reveals bilateral effusions and hypoinflation but essentially little change. (C) The film on the left is the PA view from a perfusion lung scan on the same patient showing large segmental perfusion defects in both lungs. The film on the right is from a normal ventilation scan obtained at the same time.

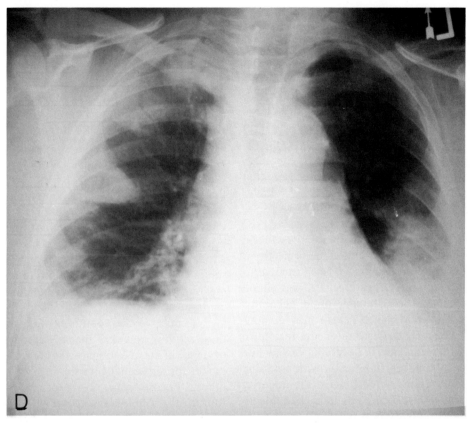

D

Fig. 3-27 (*continued*) (D) Three days after the patient began anticoagulant therapy for pulmonary embolization, the chest film demonstrated segmental areas of infarction. These slowly resolved over the next two weeks.

chymal changes, what changes have occurred in other structures such as the pulmonary vasculature, heart, or pleura that would aid in the differential diagnosis?

Accurate assessment of changing pulmonary vasculature, and occasionally of changes in heart size, is the key to differentiating types of pulmonary edema or differentiating edema from other diffuse processes. If cardiac failure or acute fluid overload are to be differentiated from other types of edema, every effort must be made to obtain an erect film. Although small effusions are difficult to assess on the portable film, they are usually present with recent thoracic surgery. Increasing effusion may indicate infection with empyema, or possibly superimposed pulmonary embolization. Effusion is noticeably absent in uncomplicated ARDS.

5. In assessing a newly apparent infiltrate, has there been recent manipulation of the patient or his support equipment?

This will be elaborated on in subsequent sections; however, placement or removal of tubing and catheters may produce various complicating pulmonary or pleural densities. Also, in assessing changing infiltrates, interval administration of physical therapy may produce significant clearing of atelectasis or change in its distribution.

Finally, to assess an infiltrate, it must first be localized. Under ideal conditions, an erect film with good inspiration and proper exposure would be expected. Unfortunately, this is not always possible. While obliquity is not desirable for assessing the mediastinum, it can be useful in assessing infiltrates. If an upright film in deep inspiration cannot be obtained, the patient can purposely be positioned obliquely to assess lower lobes that may be hidden behind the domes of the diaphragm or the cardiac silhouette. Lordosis is also often not desirable since it can hide the lower lobes; however, it can be useful in bringing out a right middle lobe infiltrate or an apical density, if one is suspected on a routine portable. When erect PA and lateral films cannot be obtained, often decubitus views can be managed. These may demonstrate changing patterns of edema related to gravity dependency. A decubitus view, while primarily used in conjunction with assessing pleural effusion, can also assess the underlying lung, often obscured by fluid. The side up on a decubitus study can expand more fully on inspiration and can be better assessed as the fluid falls toward the mediastinum.

EXTRA-ALVEOLAR AIR

Extra-alevolar air is a very common complication of various surgical manipulations, trauma, and ventilatory assistance. Its presence can be inconsequential, as in small amounts of subcutaneous emphysema, or life-threatening, as in a tension pneumothorax. The various types of extra-alveolar air include pneumothorax, pneumomediastinum, pneumopericardium, pneumoperitoneum and retroperitoneum, pulmonary subpleural and interstitial air, and subcutaneous air.

In the adult there is potential free communication between the mediastinum and the soft tissues of the neck and chest wall, and intra- or retroperitoneal spaces. Also, collections of subpleural or interstitial air from rupture of alveoli can track along vascular sheaths to the mediastinum. Mediastinal air can also rupture into the pleural space, producing a pneumothorax. In the absence of direct traumatic or surgical penetration of the pericardium in the adult, there is no communication between it and other portions of the mediastinum. In the newborn there is often no plane of communication from the mediastinum to the neck; and, therefore, a tension pneumomediastinum can occur in this age group, when it is not seen in adults. Also in newborns, pneumomediastinum can lead to pneumopericardium without implying penetrating injury to the pericardium.

Because of the communication among these various potential spaces, radiographic evidence of air in one space should raise suspicion for subsequent appearance of air in others. For instance, in barotrauma with rupture of a subpleural alveolar air space, air can dissect along the pulmonary interstitium to the mediastinum (pneumomediastinum), around the lung (pneumothorax), into the soft tissue of the neck and chest wall (subcutaneous air), and even below the diaphragm (pneumoperitoneum or pneumoretroperitoneum). Even small amounts of extra-alveolar air can be radiographically apparent due to the differences in radiographic density between air and soft tissue. As extra-alveolar air dissects tissue planes, it produces interfaces between adjacent soft tissue structures that were not previously discernible.

Extra-alveolar air in nonsurgical or nontraumatized patients is most often due to spontaneous rupture of bullae or blebs, rupture of alveoli in acute asthmatic attacks, or pleural-based cavitating processes such as necrotizing pneumonia, metastasis, or pulmonary infarct rupturing into the pleural space.[5] The incidence of tension pneumo-

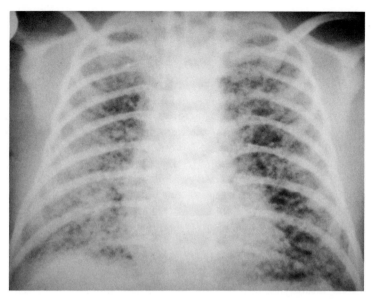

Fig. 3-28 A newborn infant on PEEP for hyaline membrane disease developed extensive interstitial air producing the "bubbly" pattern seen here.

thorax in these instances is low. In traumatic or iatrogenic causes of extra-alveolar air, however, the incidence of respiratory embarrassment due to tension pneumothorax is high.[36] Iatrogenic causes of extra-alveolar air are primarily direct surgical manipulation (including pleural tap, catheter or line placement, closed chest massage), or as a result of mechanical ventilation. The increasing use of high levels of positive end-expiratory pressure (PEEP) may produce a pneumothorax by direct rupture of the visceral pleura; however, more commonly the increased pressure produces rupture of pleural-based alveoli (barotrauma) with the subsequent dissection of extra-alveolar air as described above.[36-38]

Interstitial Air

Interstitial air, the earliest evidence of alveolar rupture due to barotrauma, is reported with some frequency in newborns on PEEP for hyaline membrane disease (Fig. 3-28), but it is often not appreciable in

adults.[37, 39] Interstitial or subpleural collection of air within normal lung tissue is relatively inapparent; however, most instances of interstitial air from barotrauma occur in diffusely consolidated lungs, and the air will be seen as a bubbly pattern within the infiltrate. It can easily be confused with air bronchograms or bullous lesions with surrounding infiltrate. However, if collections of subpleural air or peripheral interstitial air are apparent, they should be taken as an indicator of impending pneumomediastinum with a possibility of subsequent tension pneumothorax.[36, 37]

Subcutaneous Air

Subcutaneous air can be due to local disruption of tissues such as penetrating injury, surgery, tracheostomy, or chest tube insertion. Small amounts of air are inconsequential, but increasing subcutaneous air around a tube or tracheostomy site may indicate poor position of the tube or bronchopleural fistula. Subcutaneous air can dissect through the neck and produce a pneumomediastinum, or it may be the result of air dissection from a pneumomediastinum. It may be radiographically apparent before the pneumomediastinum is appreciated, especially on portable radiographs. Presence of subcutaneous air in the neck or chest without associated penetrating injury or tube placement should raise suspicions of barotrauma, and serial films should be closely scrutinized for possible developing pneumomediastinum and pneumothorax. In patients with blunt trauma, the appearance of subcutaneous air should also signal the possibility of coexistent pneumothorax (Fig. 3-25). Extensive subcutaneous air can greatly confuse or obscure changes in the underlying lung parenchyma (Fig. 3-24F).[5]

Pneumomediastinum

Pneumomediastinum may result from dissection of subcutaneous, interstitial, or pleural air. Tracheal or esophageal rupture can also produce pneumomediastinum and, if undetected, result in a life-threatening mediastinitis.

Small amounts of mediastinal air are best appreciated on a lateral projection. If this view can be obtained it should be closely scrutinized following trauma or suspected esophageal or tracheal rupture. Figure 3-29 illustrates areas where mediastinal air is most apparent on the lateral view, outlining the hila and great vessels and in the anterior mediastinum.

In postoperative portable examinations, mediastinal air is usually seen as a lucent line around the heart delineating the adjacent pleural reflection, or outlining the aortic arch (Fig. 3-30). As previously mentioned, unless there is direct penetration of the pericardium, air collections around the cardiac silhouette in the adult are most likely due to

pneumomediastinum and not pneumopericardium. Occasionally, a radiolucent halo around the mediastinum is appreciated in patients with diffuse pulmonary consolidation. This may be attributed to the MACH effect (a line perceived by the eye that is not truly present) or, as some authors feel, to the pumping action of the cardiac silhouette preventing consolidation in the adjacent lung (kinetic halo).[40, 41] This radiolucent halo, which is typically faint and indistinct, should not be confused with mediastinal air, which is usually a sharp, well-defined black line.[5] An example of the radiolucent mediastinal halo is seen in Figure 3-23B.

Pneumothorax

In a healthy lung, two forces maintain expansion: the pressure in a patent bronchial tree is atmospheric; while the intrapleural pressure is slightly less. The healthy lung, without associated pleural disease, will retract symmetrically with a pneumothorax, tending to preserve its normal configuration. This is illustrated in Figure 3-31A, which shows a spontaneous pneumothorax in a young adult due to rupture of an apical bleb. The intrathoracic, extrapulmonary air surrounds the partially collapsed lung on all sides; although on this upright view it is only seen along the superior and lateral margins. A word of caution to those who attempt to estimate a percentage of collapse: although the lung is only separated from the lateral chest wall by a few centimeters, the total volume loss, considering the three-dimensional lung, is much greater than is usually reported in percentages.

When at all possible, an upright chest film, taken in forced expiration, should be used to diagnose a pneumothorax as in Figure 3-31B. Here the absence of pulmonary markings beyond the pleural margin is easily appreciated. The difficulty in diagnosing a

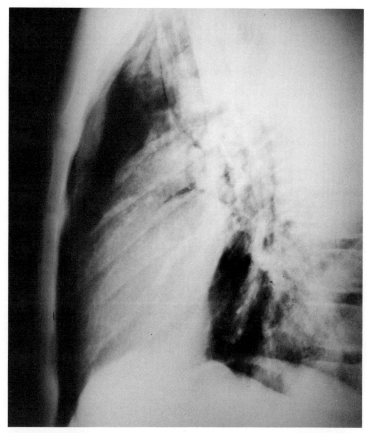

Fig. 3-29 A lateral view of a patient with extensive mediastinal air from spontaneous rupture of a bleb during an asthmatic attack. Note the thin black lines surrounding mediastinal structures and in the retrosternal area.

pneumothorax comes when the underlying lung is not normal, an upright film is difficult to obtain, or there are overlapping artifacts such as tubing or abnormal soft tissues. In patients with emphysema and bleb formation, or in patients who are hyperinflated by a ventilator, peripheral pulmonary markings may appear absent and may be mistaken for a pneumothorax. In this situation, it is important to carefully search for a pleural margin along the suspected pneumothorax. Artifacts such as overlying catheters and skin folds are very common on portable examinations. They may easily simulate a pleural margin and must be examined closely in this instance for pulmonary markings extending beyond their edge (Fig. 3-32A-C). A pneumothorax may be loculated if the underlying lung or pleura does not allow the lung to collapse symmetrically. Pneumothorax can occasionally loculate along the mediastinum and simulate a large pneumomediastinum, or it can loculate subpulmonically and mimic a pneumoperitoneum.[42] Pneumothorax with associated lobar atelectasis may preferentially loculate over the atelectatic lobe instead of around the periphery of the whole lung.[43] In a supine patient, air will rise to the

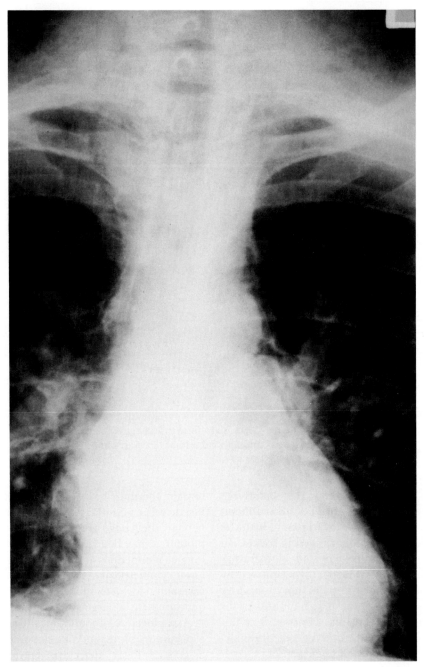

Fig. 3-30 Extensive mediastinal and some subcutaneous air in a patient with esophageal rupture. The sharp black lines of air separate mediastinal tissue planes and outline the heart and aorta.

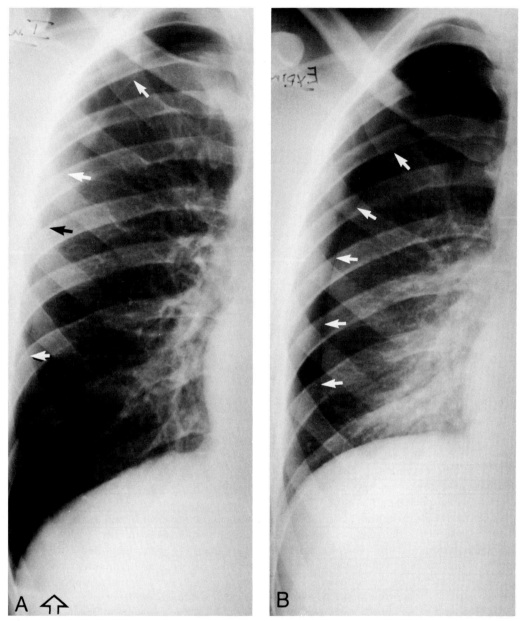

Fig. 3-31 (A) A spontaneous pneumothorax in an otherwise healthy individual. The partially collapsed lung retains its normal shape. The pleural margin (*closed arrows*) is seen as a thin white line. An air fluid level in the pleural space is indicated by the *open arrow*. (B) A film taken during forced expiration accentuates the pneumothorax in (A).

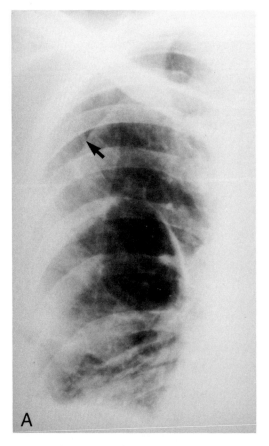

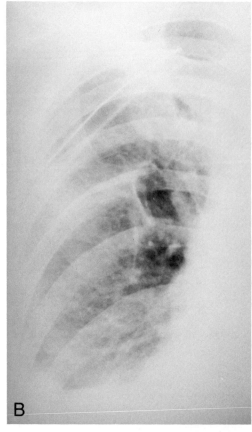

A

B

anterior surface and be relatively inapparent in the AP projection. Occasionally, the only sign of a pneumothorax on a supine view may be the development of a deep radiolucent lateral costophrenic sulcus.[44] If a pneumothorax is suspected and an upright view is difficult to obtain, a lateral decubitus view with the suspected side up may demonstrate the pneumothorax. If the patient cannot be moved, a crosstable lateral view may demonstrate air collecting in the retrosternal area. This is particularly helpful in children where there is normally no significant retrosternal air collection; however, in an adult, a large emphysematous retrosternal air space from COPD may present confusion.[5] Pleural fluid often accompanies a pneumothorax and the finding of an air-fluid level extending to the pleural surface may signal a pneumothorax that is otherwise inapparent (Fig. 3-31A).

Tension pneumothorax is an infrequent complication of pneumothorax in spontaneously breathing individuals unless there is significant trauma; but it is a very common problem in patients receiving assisted ventilation because the air leak site is kept open as more and more air is forced through it. As air pressure increases in the pleural space, overexpansion of the hemithorax with compression of adjacent structures will create serious respiratory embarrassment. Radiographic evidence of developing tension reflects this overexpansion and compression. If the lung is not significantly consolidated or "stiff," it will totally collapse into a small paramediastinal mass as tension develops. The ribs on the ipsilateral side will spread apart and the diaphragm will be depressed (Fig. 3-33A,B). If the mediastinum is not chronically immobilized, it will shift to the

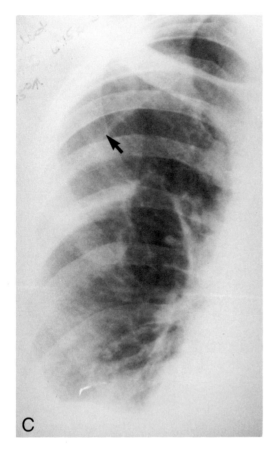

C

Fig. 3-32 (A) A curvilinear white line (*arrow*) at the periphery of the lung in this patient is produced by a skin fold. This was mistaken for a pneumothorax. (B) A chest tube was inserted as treatment for the suspected pneumothorax. (C) After removal of the tube, a white line produced by pleural reaction adjacent to the chest tube (*arrow*) is now apparent. Artifacts such as skin folds, chest tube tracts, and overlying bandages or catheters may simulate a pleural margin.

opposite side and the contralateral lung and its bronchus will be compressed. Of these findings, a depression of the ipsilateral diaphragm may be the most easily assessed and reliable finding in postsurgical patients because the ipsilateral lung or pleura is often abnormal, preventing complete collapse, and the mediastinum is fixed by surgical reaction or fibrosis, preventing appreciable shift. In fact, if the diaphragm does not appear to elevate on a film done in expiration, tension should be suspected even before the diaphragm is obviously depressed. When assessing the mediastinum for shift, it must be remembered how easily patient rotation can mimic or obscure mediastinal movement (Fig. 3-7).[5] Occasionally a tension pneumothorax may be loculated, usually in an inferior subpulmonic or paracardiac location, and the only radiographic evidence of ten-

sion may be a slight flattening of the cardiac border, or a contour change in the ipsilateral diaphragm.[45]

Occasionally, with reexpansion of a pneumothorax or rapid removal of large pleural effusions, the reexpanded lung will develop unilateral alveolar pulmonary edema. Rapid resolution of this "reexpansion pulmonary edema" differentiates it from an inflammatory process.[46]

MEDIASTINUM

Not only is *apparent* mediastinal widening from magnification, hypoinflation, and rotation to be expected when comparing a portable film to a preoperative PA projection, but *actual* mediastinal widening occurs when surgical manipulation involving the

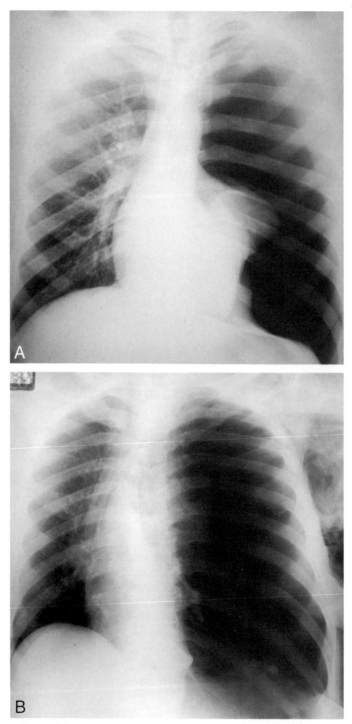

Fig. 3-33 Two patients with tension pneumothorax. Note the total collapse of the lung with spreading of the ribs, depression of the diaphragm and mediastinal shift. In (B) the changes are most marked and there is associated subcutaneous air.

heart or mediastinum creates minor degrees of hemorrhage and tissue edema. However, significant widening usually indicates gross hemorrhage and should be immediately correlated with clinical evidence of a decreasing hematocrit or increasing difficulty in ventilation or cardiovascular instability. Postoperative mediastinal hemorrhage is most common in conditions where there are abnormally dilated vessels within the mediastinum, as is seen in pediatric cardiac surgery for correction of coarctation, and in some shunts.[47] Occasionally, misplaced catheters can infuse fluid into the mediastinum creating enlargement, but they more often drain into the pleural space, creating rapidly progressive pleural effusions. Figure 3-34A,B demonstrates postoperative mediastinal hemorrhage.

If surgery involves esophageal resection with gastric pull-through or colonic interposition, the mediastinum will, of course, be enlarged. The intrathoracic stomach or colon may present as a solid mass or be filled with multiple air spaces which on an upright film will present as multiple air-fluid levels. These typically project to the right side and on a lateral view the colon interposition is usually in the retrosternal area, while the gastric pull-through is in the mid-mediastinum. Note in Figure 3-35 the nasogastric tube outlining the course of the interposition on this postoperative film. As previously mentioned, atelectasis of medial lung segments can also simulate mediastinal widening (Fig. 3-13).

PLEURAL FLUID

Small amounts of pleural fluid accumulation are common following most types of thoracic surgery; unless an embolus or empyema is suspected, usually no workup is required. Rapid or significant accumulation of fluid should, however, lead one to suspect postoperative complications such as hemorrhage. If a thoracentesis confirms hemorrhage and the hematocrit after the initial tap

appears to stabilize, a further modest increase in fluid may not necessarily mean further bleeding. Blood is a pleural irritant and will induce an effusion following intrapleural hemorrhage.[48] Occasionally misplaced catheters, especially subclavian lines, may infuse large quantities of fluid into the pleural space over a short period of time (Fig. 3-36A,B).

Pleural effusions associated with heart failure or pulmonary embolus are usually small and on a portable projection may be missed. Also, their additive effect on already existent small postoperative effusions is usually not detectable.

On an upright study the earliest evidence of effusion is blunting of the posterior sulcus on the lateral view and, as the effusion increases slightly, blunting of the lateral angles on a PA projection. The typical appearance is a meniscus (Figs. 3-20, 3-41B). On well-penetrated portable erect or semierect studies, small effusions can also be seen blunting the lateral angles or opacifying the lung base due to layering in the posterior sulcus.

In relatively supine views, the typical meniscus is lost and fluid layering along the posterior gutters produces a density to the lower hemithorax that fades out imperceptibly on its upper margin and produces indistinctness of the hemidiaphragms along its lower margin (Figs. 3-37, 3-41A). Decubitus views, when feasible, will confirm these effusions. Obtaining both decubitus views is helpful in that the dependent side shows layering of fluid laterally while the nondependent side shows layering of fluid against the mediastinum allowing for better visualization of any underlying lung pathology.

On an upright view, more than approximately a centimeter of space between the top of the stomach bubble and the hemidiaphragm on the left is considered abnormal. Widening may indicate a subphrenic process, but more commonly represents a subpulmonic collection of pleural fluid. The distance between the projected diaphragm and stomach bubble on a supine view is

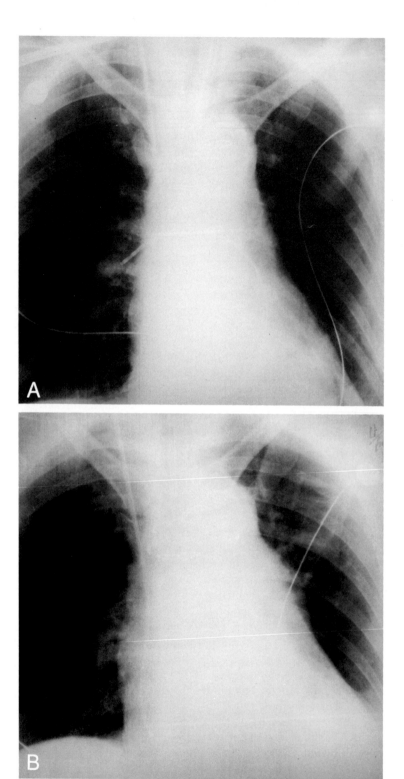

Fig. 3-34 (A) This film obtained shortly after open heart surgery reveals a normal-appearing mediastinum for an AP portable projection (note the proper position of the Swan-Ganz catheter). (B) A film the following day, also a portable AP projection without significant change in magnification or rotation shows significant enlargement of the mediastinum secondary to hemorrhage.

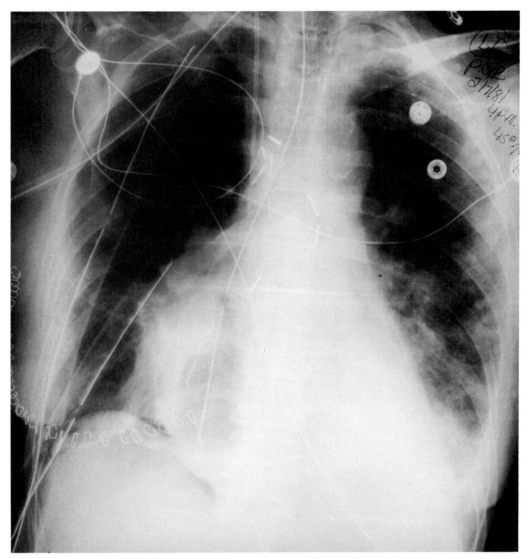

Fig. 3-35   This portable examination following distal esophageal resection for carcinoma reveals a nasogastric tube coursing to the right in a widened mediastinum. It identifies the location of the intrathoracic stomach. The mottled density of the mediastinum is due to gas within the stomach, and should not be mistaken for other postoperative pathology.

variable and does not carry the same significance. Subpulmonic fluid on the right may be more difficult to assess and quantitate as illustrated in Figure 3-38A,B.

Total opacification of a hemithorax can be caused by a number of conditions, including massive effusion. Decubitus views are of course not helpful in evaluating fluid in a total "whiteout." Typically, massive fluid accumulations cause volume expansion of the hemithorax and mediastinal shift to the contralateral side (Fig. 3-36B), while total atelectasis produces mediastinal shift to the ipsilateral side (Fig. 3-15). Unfortunately, many times when one is faced with total or near total opacification of one side of the chest in

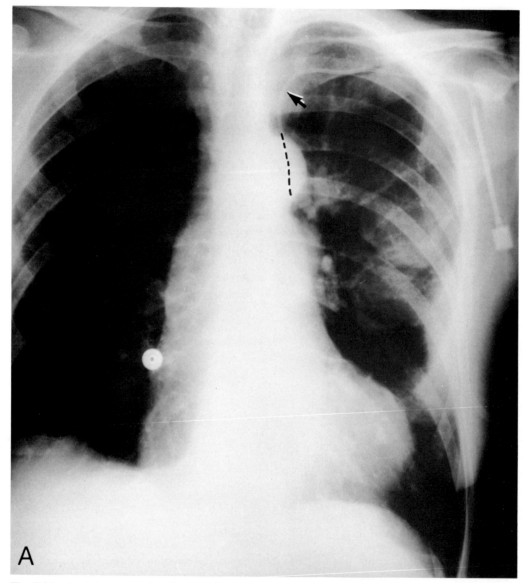

Fig. 3-36 An improperly placed subclavian catheter (retouched in A) produced hemorrhage and infused large quantities of fluid into the left pleural space (B) producing mediastinal shift and severe respiratory embarrassment.

the acute postoperative period, there is probably a mixture of fluid, atelectasis and even consolidation present at the same time. Consequently, even after a diligent search for blood vessels, air bronchograms, and mediastinal shift, they may still be absent. The very absence of mediastinal shift (assuming the mediastinum is not immobilized by fibrosis or surgery), however, should lead to a suspicion of more than one underlying process.

For completeness, other possible causes of opacification of an entire hemithorax should be mentioned. Occasionally overlying

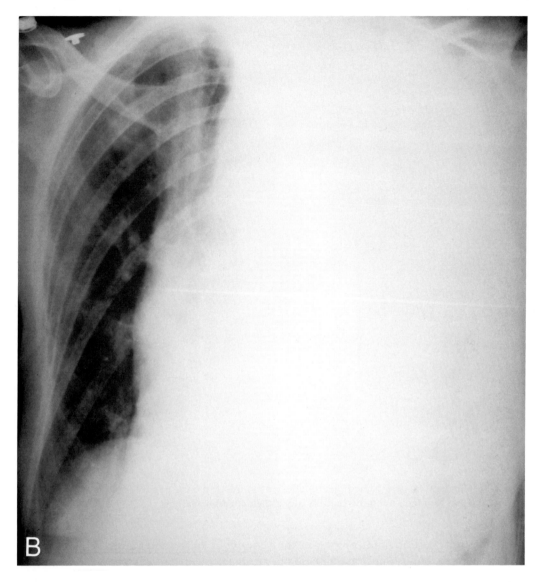

B

bandages or chest wall pathology may be sufficiently dense to produce unilateral opacification. Also, occasionally on portable projections there is a technical problem known as "grid cutoff" producing opacification of one side of the film. In both of these instances, however, the "whiteout" is not limited to the lung but should be seen extending outside into the surrounding soft tissues, suggesting the true etiology (Fig. 3-39).

Fluid accumulations may be loculated due to preexisting pulmonary scarring or to recent surgical alteration. Peripheral loculations will appear as pleural-based soft tissue masses when seen in tangent. These same collections seen en face may also appear mass-like. Fluid in the minor fissure will thicken the fissure and, if copious enough, will also present as a well-defined mass (pseudotumor) on frontal views (Fig. 3-40). Fluid layering in a major fissure on the frontal projection will be seen as a vague in-

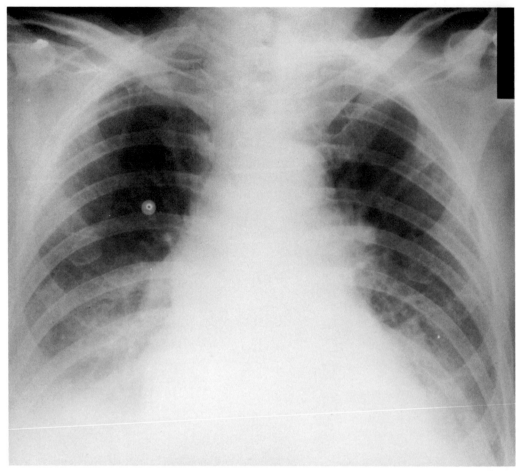

Fig. 3-37 Bilateral moderate sized pleural effusions in this semierect portable study are seen to blur the diaphragms and fade out imperceptibly along their superior margins.

creased density just as fluid layering in the posterior sulcus, but its upper margin will be demarcated as a curvilinear line overlying the fifth to sixth posterior ribs. Occasionally fluid in the major fissure will also loculate as a pseudotumor (Fig. 3-40). Fluid accumulating along the medial aspects of the lung will widen the paraspinal stripe.

It must be remembered that the presence of air within the pleural space will change the typical pleural meniscus to a sharp, straight line or air-fluid level on upright views (Fig. 3-31A). Air-fluid levels in the pleural space in a single plane may be confused with air-fluid levels in lung ab-

scesses or bullae, and a lateral view is usually recommended for differentiation. However, when this is not possible, a distinction can usually be made in that the pleural fluid line is typically longer than an abscess cavity fluid level and extends to the lateral pleural surface.[49,50] Once again, decubitus views in place of an erect lateral may distinguish pleural from parenchymal disease.

When simple maneuvers such as decubitus views are unsuccessful in evaluating pleural densities, ultrasound has been repeatedly shown to be of benefit in assessing loculated fluid accumulations. Also, recent literature on thoracic CT scanning in ICU patients suggests that in selected cases of problematic pleural, mediastinal, or chest wall postoperative complications this new modality may be definitive.[51]

PERICARDIAL EFFUSION

Progressive enlargement of the cardiac silhouette in a globular configuration is the hallmark of pericardial effusion (Fig. 3-41A,B). However, in portable examinations, assessment of changes in cardiac size and contour are limited by technique. Likewise, in the face of rapidly developing effusions or pericardial disease, restrictive pericarditis and tamponade can occur with very little change on the plain film.[52] Evidence of both systemic and pulmonary vascular engorgement from constrictive pericardiopathy should, of course, be assessed on the plain film; but if there is clinical suspicion of pericardial disease, a much more sensitive study is obtained with echocardiography. This procedure is noninvasive and can often be performed rapidly and easily at the bedside.

SPECIFIC POSTOPERATIVE CHANGES FROM THORACOTOMY FOR LOBECTOMY AND PNEUMONECTOMY

There are specific sequential radiographic findings that can be expected following lung resection, relating to compensatory changes in the diaphragm, pleura, mediastinum, and remaining lung. Local resection or enucleation of a small parenchymal nodule will result in hemorrhage in and around the site, occasionally simulating a remaining or recurring mass.[53] This "pseudotumor" slowly regresses over several days to a few weeks (Fig. 3-42A,B). Similarly, any surgical manipulation of hilar structures produces perihilar infiltrate or mass from localized edema and hemorrhage. This fuzzy and slightly full hilum should not be confused with early signs of pulmonary edema or aspiration pneumonia. Occasionally, pleural and

parenchymal densities resulting from chest tube placement may appear as "pseudotumors." This will be further exemplified in the section on Monitoring Devices.

Resection of a large pulmonary segment, lobe, or entire lung will, of course, produce significant volume loss; but this is not always apparent in the immediate postoperative studies, due to the pressure of the remaining air in the pleural space. As air is reabsorbed or aspirated through chest tubes, pleural fluid forming in response to surgery replaces the air, so volume loss again initially is often not dramatic. The resultant air-fluid level within the pleural space is best appreciated on upright views and may be a single large fluid level or multiple loculated air-fluid levels. As fluid is reabsorbed or aspirated through chest tubes, volume loss becomes apparent. Slowly, the mediastinum shifts to the ipsilateral side, the hemidiaphragm elevates, and the remaining ipsilateral lung reexpands. Eventually, the ipsilateral and contralateral remaining lung develops compensatory hyperexpansion or emphysema to fill the void. The remaining ipsilateral lobes following lobectomy may at first show diffuse opacification due to edema and residual microatelectasis. Lobar atelectasis of the remaining segments, as previously described, may simulate mediastinal widening (Fig. 3-13, 3-14).

If there is a sudden increase in the amount of intrapleural air with mediastinal shift to the contralateral side, an air leak from the bronchial stump or bronchopleural fistula should be suspected. Minor variations in the air-fluid level from film to film, however, should not cause alarm, as they are usually due to variations in patient position and variations in the daily rate of pleural absorption or chest tube aspiration of fluid versus air in the postoperative period.[53] Figure 3-43A-D represents postoperative changes acutely with later development of a bronchopleural fistula.

Elevation of a hemidiaphragm following pneumonectomy or lower lobectomy may reflect diaphragmatic or phrenic nerve

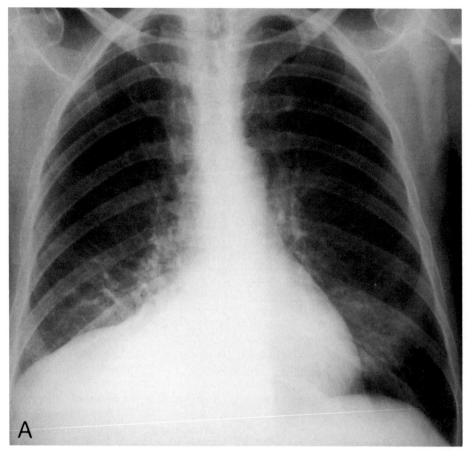

Fig. 3-38 (A) A large subpulmonic effusion on the right can mimic a high diaphragm, especially without a lateral film.

damage or simply acute volume loss in the thorax. On the left, acute gastric air distention may then result. Assessment of the degree of gastric dilatation on serial chest films is important so that a nasogastric tube may be appropriately placed to avoid the possible complication of gastric ischemia or rupture due to massive dilatation.

MONITORING AND LIFE-SUPPORT DEVICES

In the intraoperative period, the determination of proper placement of monitoring and life-support devices is usually achieved through clinical assessment of their location by physical examination or appropriate monitor readings. Only occasionally will confusing or suspicious findings suggesting malplacement or its complications lead to a call for a radiograph in the operating room. It would be inappropriately time-consuming to have radiographic confirmation of the position of every tube placed during anesthesia and surgery.

In the postoperative intensive care setting, however, radiographic monitoring of catheters and tubes becomes more appropriate, as patients and their equipment are constantly being moved and manipulated. Therefore, in a "systematic approach" to each radiograph in the postoperative period, there should be a mental "subsection" for

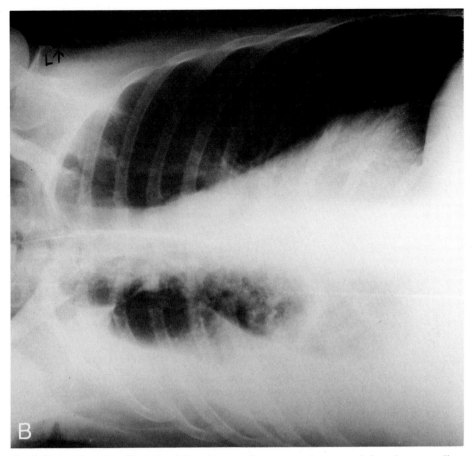

Fig. 3-38 (*continued*)   (B) A decubitus view on the same patient reveals how large a collection of fluid can be loculated in the subpulmonic space. Also note how well the lung is expanded on the non-dependent side. When assessing a lung base obscured by fluid or hypoinflation, a portable decubitus view will often show it to greatest advantage in a bedridden patient.

lines and tubes, and their possible complications.

The following sections deal with the common types of monitoring and life-support equipment, their radiographic appearance, proper and improper placement, and possible complications.

Endotracheal Tubes

Studies of the effect of flexion and extension of the neck on the position of the endotracheal tube tip indicate that it can move as much as 4–5 cm with vigorous head movement.[54] Therefore, the ideal position of the tip would be midway between the carina and the vocal cords with the head in the neutral position, to allow for maximal flexibility. In an adult, this is typically 5 to 7 cm above the carina. For localization purposes, there is a radiopaque stripe along the entire length, or at least at the distal tip, of most currently manufactured endotracheal tubes. (Refer to Fig. 3-16, 3-23, 3-24 for proper placement.)

Finding the carina in a well-penetrated mediastinum is relatively easily done by following the mainstem bronchi to their juncture (Fig. 3-9). With slight underpenetration, one aid to localization is to tilt the film, so as

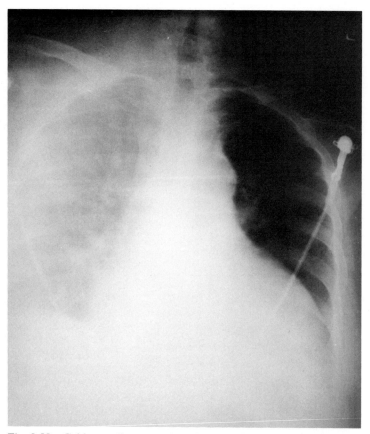

Fig. 3-39 Grid cut-off occurs when the x-ray beam is not centered to the grid and a substantial portion of the x-ray photons do not reach areas of the film. This produces, as illustrated here, underexposed portions of the film. This should not be confused with true intrathoracic pathology, as the "white-out" involves the soft tissues as well.

to look obliquely up the mediastinum. The air, soft-tissue interface between the trachea and mediastinum will become more apparent. If this is not rewarding, an approximation of carinal position can be obtained by counting vertebrae or posterior ribs. On portable radiographs, in 95 percent of patients, the carina projects over T5, T6, or T7.[55] The vocal cords overlie approximately C5 or C6. When assessing tube position, evaluation of the position of the patient's head in flexion or extension is also necessary, since a tip that appears in "good" position 2 or 3 cm from the carina with the head extended could slip into the right mainstem

bronchus on flexion. On many portable chest films, a portion of the mandible can be seen. In neutral position, it overlies the lower cervical spine; with flexion it moves over the upper thoracic spine; and with extension it moves above C4 or off of the film.[55]

If the distal portion or tip of the tube should appear to bow or bend toward the right mainstem bronchus, this may also indicate a low position in patients where the carina cannot be easily visualized (Fig. 3-15). Bowing may also create an increase in the lateral wall pressure, leading to wall erosion. Erosion into the innominate artery with massive hemorrhage and exsanguination is a

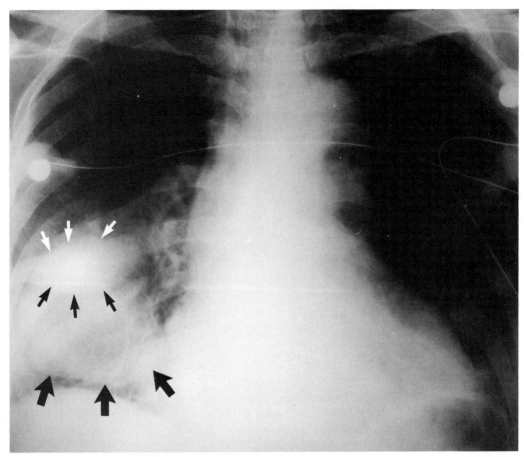

Fig. 3-40 The well-defined masses, both elliptical (*small arrows*) and round (*larger arrows*), in the right lung represent "pseudotumors" of loculated fluid in the minor and major fissures respectively. These can be confirmed with a lateral view; however, the appearance of such sharply outlined homogenous masses in a patient with chronic or recent effusion should lead one to suspect pleural fluid pseudotumor on the frontal view only.

real possibility with long-term intubation or with tracheostomy.[56]

Ideally, the diameter of the tube should be one-half to two-thirds the width of the trachea. Wider tubes increase the incidence of laryngeal injury and smaller tubes have an increased airway resistance.[57] Overinflation of the balloon cuff, which may be seen radiographically as a widening or bulging of the tracheal air column near the tube tip, will likewise lead to erosion or later tracheal stenosis due to mucosal ischemia (Fig. 3-44, 3-48).

Overinsertion of an endotracheal tube usually results in right mainstem bronchus intubation, since the angle of takeoff of the right bronchus is more in continuity with the trachea, while the left is at a more acute angle. The radiographic findings depend upon the degree of overinsertion, the duration of the misplacement, and the concentration of the inspired oxygen. Typically, varying degrees of left lung atelectasis are seen (Fig. 3-15). If the tube is low enough, the right upper lobe bronchus will also be occluded, producing right upper lobe as well as entire left lung collapse. There will be compensatory overinflation of the right middle

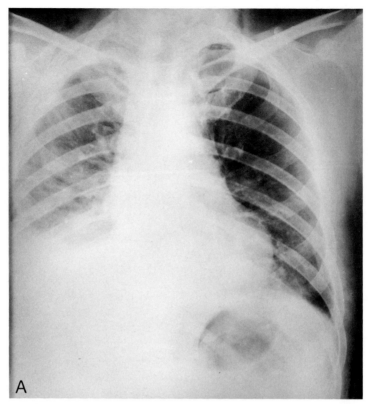

Fig. 3-41 (A) This patient sustained severe blunt trauma to the chest. This film obtained acutely demonstrates a large right effusion surrounding the lateral and apical margins of the lung as well as layering in the posterior gutter. With the subcutaneous and mediastinal air seen here, the patient should be suspected of having a pneumothorax as was proven on subsequent films. Note the normal cardiac size immediately after trauma.

and the right lower lobes. The higher the oxygen content of the inspired gas, the more rapid the collapse of the bypassed lobe due to absorption atelectasis.[58] Following repositioning of an overinserted endotracheal tube, atelectatic segments should slowly reexpand. There may, however, be some continued opacity to the reexpanding lobe or lung for several hours to a few days. A complication of long-term lobar or total lung atelectasis or collapse would, of course, be superimposed infection. If the bypassed bronchi are only partially occluded, a ball-valve-type effect may produce an obstructive emphysema picture in the bypassed lobes. In right mainstem

or bronchus intermedius intubation, because the entire tidal volume is directed at only two or three lobes, the chances of barotrauma with resulting tension pneumothorax are significantly increased, and the film should be carefully searched for signs of extra-alveolar air.[59]

A tube that is not placed deeply enough will predispose to accidental extubation. Also, if the cuff is inflated at the level of the cords (Fig. 3-44), there may be subsequent complications of ulceration and scarring. If the tube is high enough, it may be entirely excluded on the chest film and, to the unsuspecting radiologist, this will be dismissed

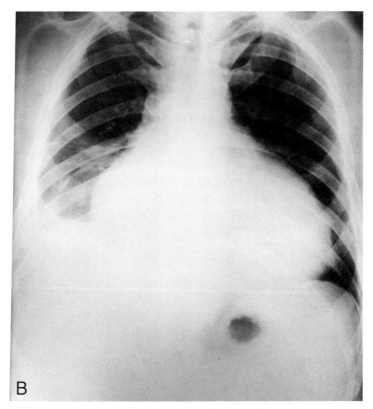

Fig. 3-41 (*continued*)   (B) A few days later serial films demonstrated progressive enlargement of the cardiac silhouette as shown here. This rapid change as well as the typically "globular" configuration is characteristic of pericardial fluid, in this case, hemorrhage.

simply as interval intentional extubation. Therefore, those who know the supposed clinical status of life-supportive devices have a special obligation to check their placement on every film reviewed.

Complications associated with intubation include aspiration or ingestion of dislodged teeth. If aspirated, they may produce atelectasis or even a ball-valve-type emphysema. Overpenetrated films are helpful in identifying their location for later removal. Unintentional esophageal intubation may produce sufficient gastric distention that decompression with a nasogastric tube is usually advisable to prevent possible spontaneous rupture and to improve diaphragmatic movement.[60] If traumatic tracheal or esophageal intubation is suspected, close observa-

tion for developing subcutaneous or mediastinal air is imperative. Undiagnosed esophageal rupture may lead to severe and often fatal mediastinitis.

Double-Lumen Endotracheal Tubes

Double-lumen endotracheal tubes greatly facilitate anesthesia when it is necessary to achieve independent control of the ventilation of each lung. Several tube designs exist. Figure 3-45 illustrates proper placement of a Robertshaw tube. The double-lumen is radiographically visible through the tracheal air column. Radiopaque markers define the terminal extent of each lumen. When correctly placed, the tip of the tracheal

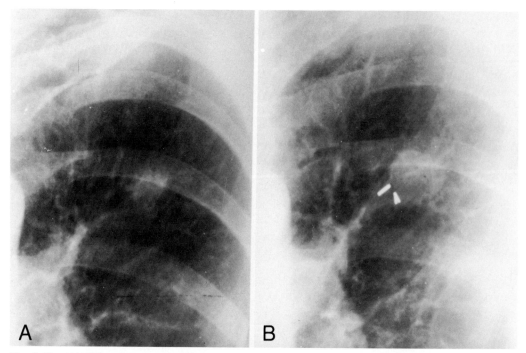

Fig. 3-42 (A) This pulmonary nodule was suspected preoperatively to represent a primary pulmonary malignancy. However, following ennucleation, frozen section pathology revealed benign chronic inflammation and further excision was not needed. (B) Postoperatively the pseudotumor of hemorrhage mimics a remaining nodule. This cleared slowly over several days.

portion lies 1–2 cm above the carina, and the tip of the bronchial portion is inserted sufficiently far into the "appropriate" main bronchus for the endotracheal cuff to seal that bronchus without projecting unduly across the carinal region or occluding the orifice of the upper lobe bronchus on that side.[61]

Complications of malplacement are primarily related to inadvertent bronchial blockage (atelectasis of a lobe) or focal overexpansion (emphysema of a lobe). When evaluating placement of a double-lumen tube on an intraoperative portable film, it is important to compare the relative radiolucency of the upper to the lower lobes. If a discrepancy exists, this may indicate poor placement. Inadvertent over-ventilation of a lung segment can lead to barotrauma with complications of extraalveolar air, as discussed previously.

Tracheostomy

Tracheostomy tubes are usually opaque enough to allow fairly easy localization. The tip should ideally be one-half to two-thirds the distance between the stoma and the carina, usually around T3 or T4. Again, the tube width should be approximately two-thirds the tracheal diameter and the cuff should not bulge the lateral tracheal walls.[62] If a lateral view is obtainable, the tip should be pointing inferiorly and not posteriorly touching the posterior tracheal wall, which can lead to erosion and subsequent tracheoesophageal fistula, or anteriorly leading to tracheo-innominate artery fistula.[55,63] Small amounts of subcutaneous air are common immediately following insertion. If the stoma is tightly sutured or packed, this air may, with positive pressure ventilation, dissect into the mediastinum. Severe air leakage may indicate an improperly placed tube in the paratracheal soft tissues. Pneumothorax after tracheostomy can result from direct puncture of the lung apex at the time of insertion, from stomal air leak with pneumomediastinum or from respirator-induced pulmonary barotrauma. Mediastinal widening after tracheostomy is usually secondary to hemorrhage and should be followed closely until it stabilizes. Late complications of intubation or tracheostomy are secondary tracheal stenosis or tracheal malacia (Fig. 3-46), usually at the cuff or stomal site.[64]

Nasogastric (NG) Tubes

Large-caliber nasogastric tubes typically have a radiopaque marker running the length of the tubing. Small-caliber feeding tubes without markers may be almost invisible through the mediastinum. Newer models have a dense, five cm marker only at their distal tip.

Proper placement is usually clinically apparent; however, when gastric contents cannot be aspirated, tip localization can best be assessed on an overpenetrated chest or thoracoabdominal view. The gastric air bubble should be analyzed on each chest film, particularly after intubation or left lung resection, so that marked or progressive gastric dilatation can be promptly treated with nasogastric tube placement to avoid gastric ischemia and rupture.

Pleural Drainage Tubes

Most chest tubes have a radiopaque stripe along their length. The side hole is marked by a discontinuity in the stripe and this should be within the chest wall for proper drainage. Subcutaneous air is common immediately after placement, but increasing air may indicate poor position of the side hole. In the supine or semierect patient, intrapleural air collects anteriorly and superiorly, while fluid layers in the posterior gutters. Therefore, the optimal position for drainage of a hydrothorax is posterior and inferior, and for a pneumothorax is anterior and superior. For true localization of these tubes, a lateral film is needed, especially if it is suspected that the tubing may be tracking along the anterior or posterior chest wall outside of the pleural space. If the patient is bedridden, a crosstable lateral film can be obtained when an erect lateral is not possible.

Unsuccessful pleural drainage by a chest tube may indicate loculation of fluid or air. Portable ultrasound examination may be exceedingly helpful in determining whether a pleural-based density represents a fluid loculation and can also identify the best approach for a successful thoracentesis.

Minor pleural or parenchymal contusion along tube tracts is common. Occasionally, curvilinear pleural tube tracts may simulate a pneumothorax after tube removal (Fig. 3-32C). Identifying pulmonary markings peripheral to the tube tract will avoid this confusion. If these cannot be identified, a film in forced expiration may be necessary to differentiate pneumothorax from pleural reaction. A wide tube tract may fill with fluid and appear as a band of density (Fig. 3-47A,B). Enlarging tracts may indicate secondary infection or empyema.[62] A rare complication of chest tubes is suction entrapment of a portion of the lung with resulting pulmonary infarction. This should be suspected if a significant infiltrate develops around a chest tube. Immediate repositioning is advisable.[65]

Central Venous Pressure (CVP) Catheters

To accurately reflect central venous or right heart pressures, a catheter should ideally be positioned in the superior vena cava or right atrium so that it is proximal to any

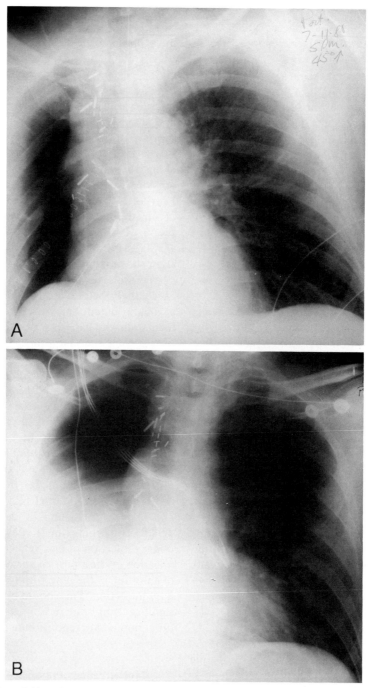

Fig. 3-43 Selected films from a series of examinations on a patient's status after recent pneumonectomy demonstrate the variations in quantity and appearance of fluid and air within the hemithorax. (A) This film obtained immediately following the right pneumonectomy reveals mild mediastinal shift toward the right, and primarily air without fluid in the right chest. (B) Two days later fluid is seen accumulating in the right chest. The lack of an air-fluid level reflects the supine position of the patient.

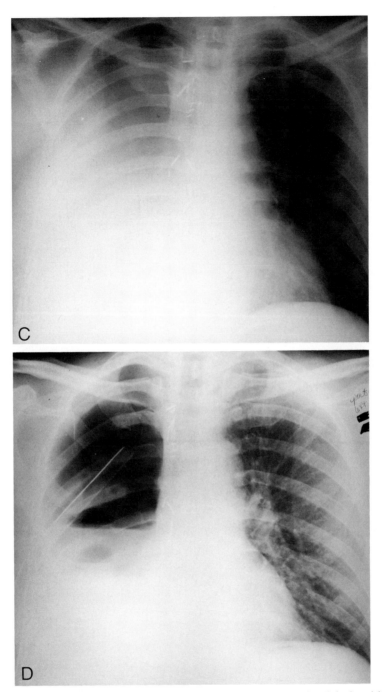

Fig. 3-43 (*continued*) (C) A day later further fluid has accumulated in the right hemithorax and the mediastinum is relatively midline. An upright film at this time would show a large air-fluid level in the apex of the hemithorax. Slowly, as air and fluid are completely reabsorbed from the pleural space over the next few weeks, there will be total opacity from fibrosis and a marked mediastinal shift into the right chest. (D) However, in this patient, now one week postoperative, a significant increase in air suggested a bronchopleural fistula and a chest tube was placed.

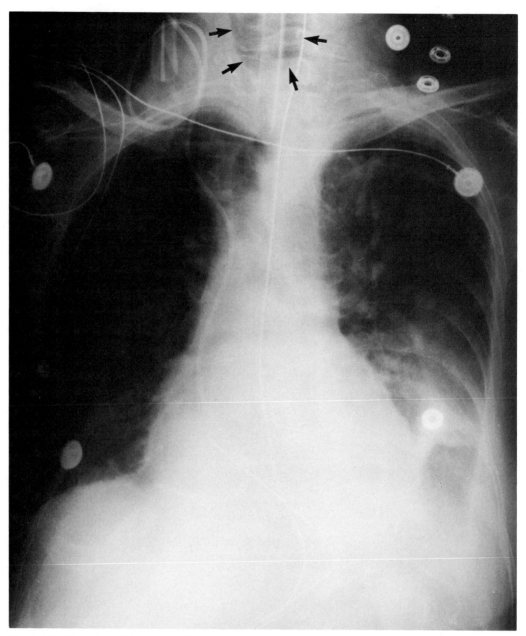

Fig. 3-44 There is malplacement of several monitoring and life-support devices on this study. The endotracheal tube is somewhat high (tip at T-2) with marked overinflation of the cuff (*arrows*) in the neck. Also note the redundant Swan-Ganz catheter in the right atrium, and the redundant N-G tube in a previously known esophageal diverticulum.

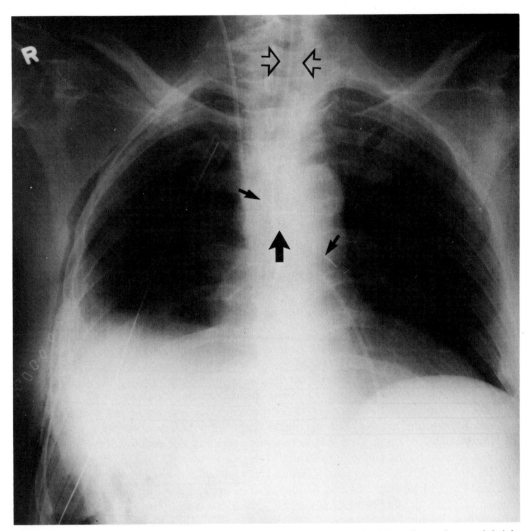

Fig. 3-45 The Robertshaw double-lumen tube is properly positioned in this patient, after partial right lung resection. Note the double-lumen seen through the upper trachea (*open arrows*), and the position of the carina (*large arrow*). The inferior tip of each lumen is defined by a radiopaque marker (*small arrows*). Both lungs are being adequately ventilated.

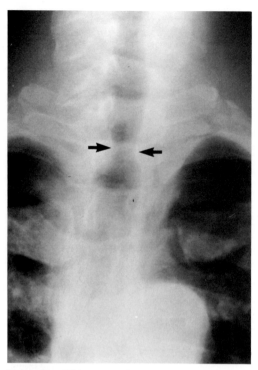

Fig. 3-46. This coned-down view of the tracheal air shadow reveals a stenosis (*arrows*) at the site of a previous tracheostomy stoma.

peripheral valves. Insertion of a central venous pressure catheter directly into the internal jugular vein should accurately reflect central pressures, since there are no valves between the internal jugular vein and right heart. Although some estimation of location can be suggested by the length of tubing advanced from a certain cutaneous insertion site, kinking and misdirection are frequent enough that radiographic evaluation may be advisable whenever these lines are placed. This is particularly advisable whenever there are unsatisfactory readings, a lack of good blood return, or suspected complications. However, fluctuations of the fluid column and ability to freely aspirate blood are not always reliable signs of proper placement, as has been frequently reported. In fact, in one prospective study, it was shown that approximately one-third of CVP catheters are incor-

rectly placed at the time of original insertion.[66]

The major complication from aberrant placement is mismanagement of the patient's fluids on the basis of erroneous CVP readings. This happens commonly when the tip advances into other peripheral veins, rather than into the central venous system. Typical aberrant locations include (1) a brachial or subclavian line going to the contralateral side or into the jugular veins (Fig. 3-48); (2) a jugular line going into the ipsilateral or contralateral subclavian; or (3) overinsertion into the inferior vena cava and even the hepatic veins. Besides problems with erroneous measurements, overinsertion may lead to right heart catheterization. Intracardiac positioning can lead to myocardial irritation producing dysrhythmias and even perforation. Central venous pressure catheters have been reported extending into peripheral pulmonary artery branches. Infusion of significant amounts of fluid through these catheters can result in unilateral pulmonary edema.[67]

The percutaneous subclavian approach, because of its close proximity to the lung apex, has the added potential complication of iatrogenic pneumothorax. If this is suspected, an immediate chest film, preferably erect and in expiration, is recommended; it is imperative before attempting puncture on the opposite side because of the possibility of creating bilateral pneumothoraces. Also, a not infrequent complication of the subclavian approach is infusion of fluid into the pleural space or mediastinum (Fig. 3-36). This will mimic intrathoracic hemorrhage. When faced with a rapidly increasing effusion or mediastinal widening in a patient with a central venous line, particularly a subclavian line, malposition can easily be confirmed by injecting water-soluble contrast material through the catheter during chest film exposure.[68] This will avoid further unnecessary angiographic or surgical procedures.

Pulmonary Arterial Catheters

Pulmonary arterial catheters are radiographically distinguishable from other venous catheters by a radiopaque stripe down the center. Ideally, the catheter should traverse the right atrium and right ventricle without redundancy or slack. The tip should lie in the right or left main pulmonary artery or their major descending branches, except when wedge pressure readings are being obtained (Fig. 3-34). Misdirection during insertion is less frequent than with other venous catheters, due to the flow-directed balloon. Redundancy within cardiac chambers will increase the incidence of myocardial irritation and dysrhythmias (Fig. 3-49). Also, with slack, the catheter tends to drift "downstream" and wedge unnecessarily.

The most significant complication is pulmonary infarction as a result of clot formation on the catheter with pulmonary embolization, or with occlusion of a pulmonary artery by the catheter itself.[69] This will happen when the tip remains in a peripheral vessel for an extended length of time or if the balloon, seen as a one cm radiolucency at the tip of the catheter, remains inadvertently inflated. If the catheter tip is seen projecting more than a few centimeters lateral to the cardiac silhouette when wedge pressure readings are not being taken, it is too peripheral and arterial occlusion may more likely occur. Although a tip projecting in or near the hilum would seem, at first glance, to be in a large-enough vessel that infarction would be unlikely, the catheter may be radiographically "foreshortened" in the AP projection with the tip actually in a small arterial branch. Development of an infiltrate around a peripherally located tip is indicative of an infarction (Fig. 3-50), although infarction has been reported at autopsy without previously recognized infiltrate. Other complications, such as pulmonary artery perforation with hemorrhage, or intracardiac knotting have been reported.[70] Rarely, the pulmonary arterial catheter may become tethered in the heart, preventing easy removal (Fig. 3-51A,B).

Transvenous Pacemakers

Proper placement of a transvenous pacemaker is best accomplished under fluoroscopic guidance. If this is not feasible, then follow-up films are recommended to assure proper placement. While clinical assessment of proper pacing usually assures a good location of the electrode in the right ventricular apex, radiographs can best evaluate the course of the lead. Sharp angulation of the lead should be avoided as this predisposes to breakage (Fig. 3-52).[71] Breakage is most common at a flexion point adjacent to a location where the lead is firmly stabilized.[72] A break may be obvious on x-ray examination, but failure to demonstrate a break radiographically does not exclude its presence, as the insulating sheath may hold the broken ends together.[71] As with central venous and pulmonary arterial catheters, excess slack increases myocardial irritation and predisposes to migration (Fig. 3-53).

If clinical evidence suggests that the electrode is in an aberrant location, both frontal and lateral films may be needed to localize it. On AP or PA projection the tip may appear to be in the right ventricular apex, while on a lateral view it is seen in the posterior portion of the heart as in Figure 3-54. This posterior location usually implies placement within the coronary venous system.[71]

When ventricular pacing alone is not producing sufficient cardiac output, A-V sequential pacing may be appropriate, as discussed in Chapter 17. Figure 3-55 illustrates proper placement of both atrial and ventricular leads.

Besides lead breakage and aberrant electrode placement within the heart and vessels, radiographic evidence of complications includes perforation of vessels or the myocardium. Figure 3-56 illustrates fluoroscopic confirmation of myocardial perfora-

(*Text continues on p. 117*)

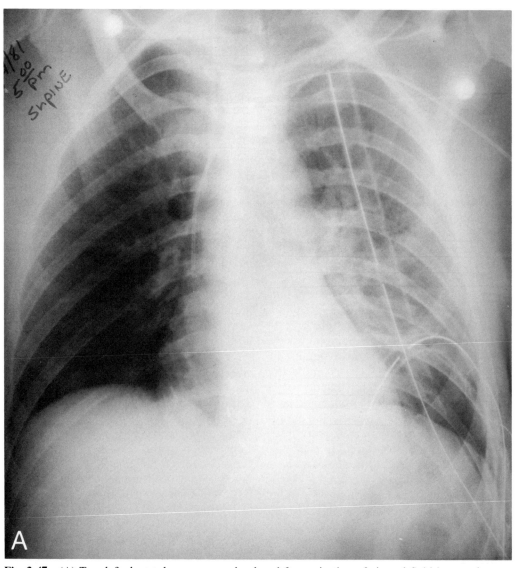

Fig. 3-47 (A) Two left chest tubes are properly placed for aspiration of air and fluid in a supine patient.

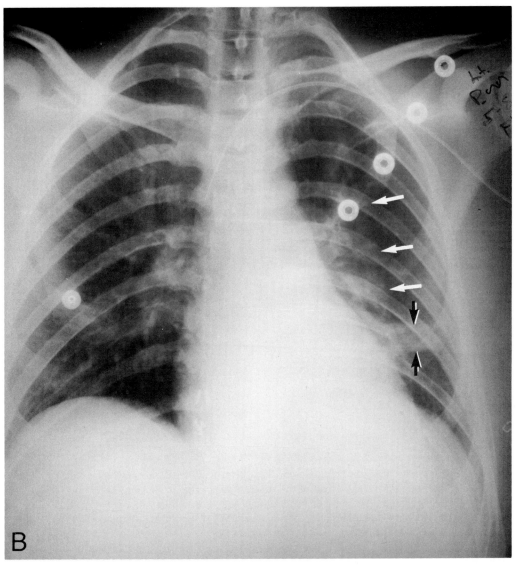

Fig. 3-47 (*continued*)   (B) After the chest tubes were removed, pleural reaction along the tube tracts produced bands of density (*arrows*) that could be confused for a pleural margin in a pneumothorax or an infiltrate. Note also the proper CVP placement in this patient.

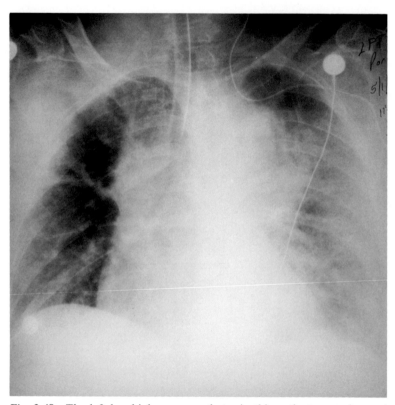

Fig. 3-48 The left brachial venous catheter in this patient was advanced into the neck veins instead of the superior vena cava, producing inaccurate CVP readings. Also note the oval radiolucency surrounding the distal end of the endotracheal tube. This represents a slightly overinflated cuff bulging the lateral tracheal walls.

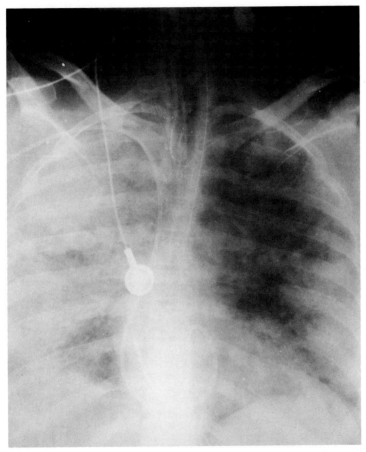

Fig. 3-49 The Swan-Ganz catheter is coiled in the right heart, increasing the chances of myocardial irritation and dysrhythmias.

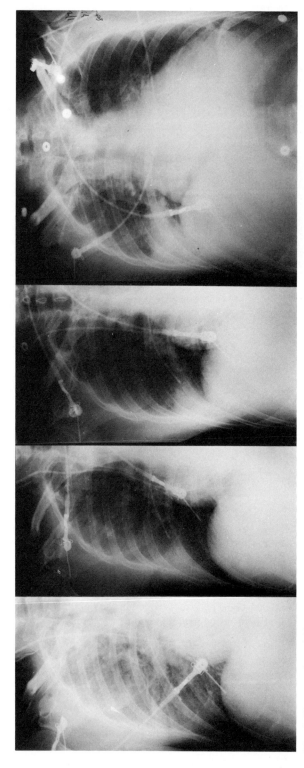

Fig. 3-50 A series of films over a two-day period demonstrates a peripherally placed Swan-Ganz catheter within the right lung. The developing wedge-shaped, pleural-based infiltrate represents pulmonary infarction secondary to direct arterial occlusion by the catheter tip. (Courtesy of Kaplan JA, Ed: Cardiac Anesthesia. By permission, Grune and Stratton, Inc., N.Y., 1979, p 94)

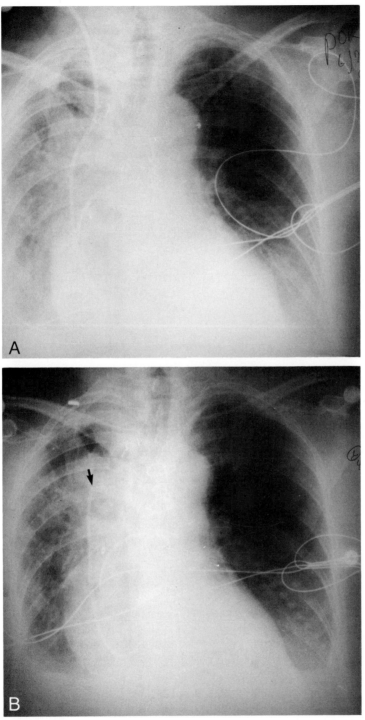

Fig. 3-51 (A) The Swan-Ganz catheter in this patient became tethered in the heart and could not be pulled free for removal. (B) It was, therefore, transected at the skin and allowed to retract inside the patient. The arrow marks the free proximal end in the SVC. It did not migrate because of its firm attachment. Except in unusual circumstances, such as this, catheter fragments loose in the veins or heart are, of course, to be strictly avoided as they will embolize to the lungs. Retrieval of loose fragments can often be accomplished by experienced angiographers using catheters, thereby avoiding further surgery.

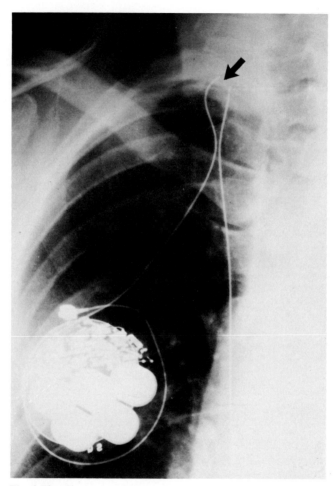

Fig. 3-52 Sharp angulation of the pacemaker lead predisposes to breakage, usually adjacent to a site of firm attachment as shown here. (From Mansour K: Complications of cardiac pacemakers. Am Surg 43:132, 1977. Reproduced with permission of publisher and author.)

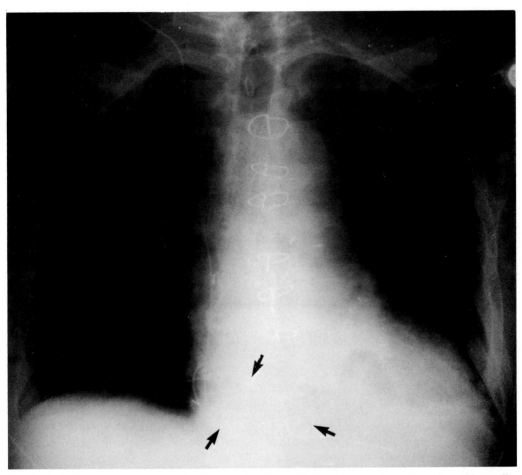

Fig. 3-53 This transvenous pacer lead is coiled in the right heart (*arrows*). Slack such as this predisposes to myocardial irritation and migration.

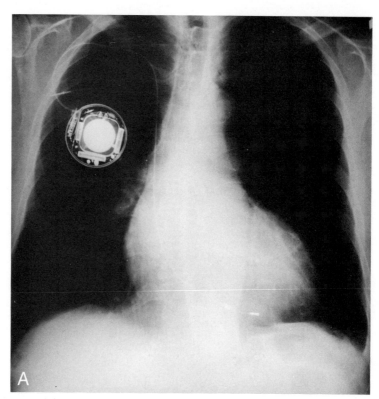

Fig. 3-54 (A) Radiographically this pacer electrode appears to be in the right ventricular apex on this PA projection. Clinically the electrode was not pacing adequately.

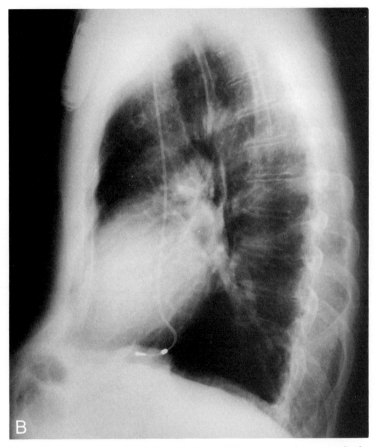

Fig. 3-54 (*continued*) (B) A lateral view of the same patient reveals the posterior location of the electrode within the cardiac silhouette. It is, therefore not within the right ventricle but probably within the coronary venous system.

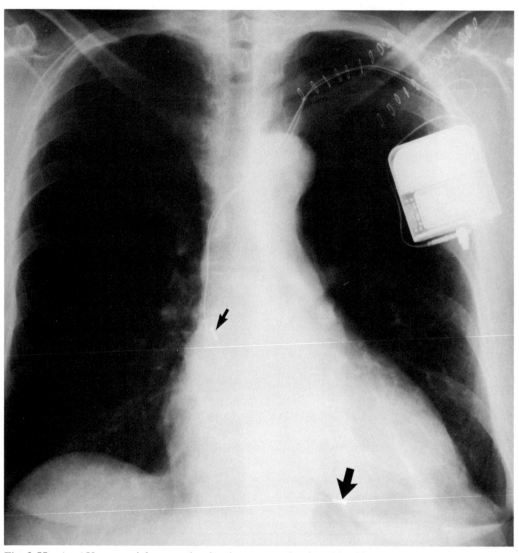

Fig. 3-55 An AV sequential pacemaker has been properly placed in this patient. The atrial electrode location is indicated by the small arrow, and the ventricular electrode is seen in the right ventricular apex (*large arrow*).

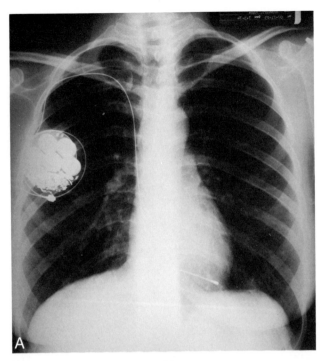

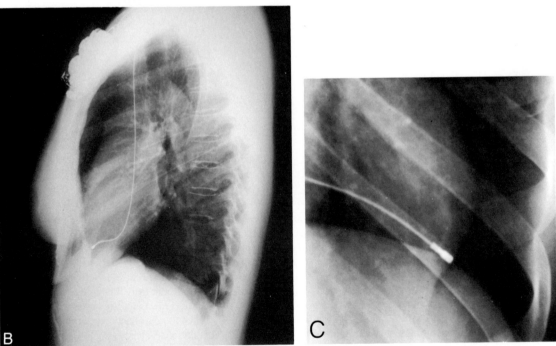

Fig. 3-56 The right ventricular electrode in this patient was felt to be too laterally positioned on the PA view (A) and possibly too anteriorly positioned on the lateral view (B). (C) Fluoroscopy with spot films made in various obliquities confirmed the suspicion of myocardial perforation. Note the tip of the electrode at the surface of the cardiac silhouette.

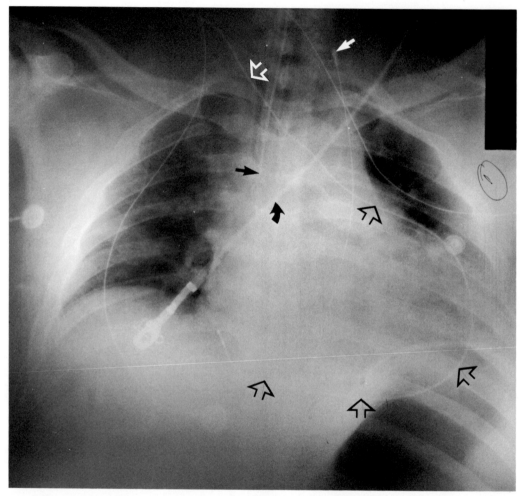

Fig. 3-57 This portable radiograph was obtained immediately after attempted placement of multiple monitoring and life-support devices in a seriously ill patient who had just suffered a massive myocardial infarction. The endotracheal tube tip (*small black arrow*) is low, just above the carina (*curved black arrow*). The transvenous pacemaker lead (*open arrows*) apparently perforated a vessel in the superior mediastinum and is seen coursing in an unusual configuration around the cardiac silhouette. A lateral view (not shown) confirmed the intrathoracic but extracardiac location of the lead. The aortic counter-pulsation balloon catheter is also improperly positioned. Its tip (*white arrow*) is quite superior to the normal location, the proximal descending aorta, and may be in either the carotid or vertebral artery. Also note the moderate gastric dilitation, post-resuscitation, in this patient.

tion, and Figure 3-57 demonstrates vessel perforation with subsequent intrathoracic but extracardiac electrode placement. With perforation or suspected injury to vessels, the radiograph should be assessed for mediastinal enlargement from hemorrhage. Superior vena caval syndrome has been reported following pacer insertion.[73] Finally, when managing patients with preexisting pacemakers, radiographs can identify the generator model and type of electrode.[74]

SUMMARY

The successful approach to chest radiology lies (1) in understanding "why you see what you see" in terms of radiographic density; (2) in understanding the limitations imposed on visualizing and assessing pathology due to altered techniques (the bedside portable) and the ways to circumvent these limitations in using serial films to develop a temporal sequence of a disease; and (3) in systematically scanning each part of the chest, each tube and line on every film.

Finally, cooperation and communication among the various clinicians (anesthesiologist, surgeon, intensivist) and the radiologist is important. Expert interpretation without history is certainly by definition objective, but isolation of radiographic findings from other data is not in the best interest of the patient. Conversely, review of a film in light of clinical bias may produce "tunnel vision" resulting in mismanagement or overtreatment (remember the skin fold?). A seemingly insignificant objective finding may take on real value within a certain clinical setting, just as a worrisome density in prejudiced eyes may dissolve into normal overlapping structures when viewed with objectivity.

The optimal approach to a film is, therefore, to view it once with objectivity and once with clinical correlation. Individually, of course, this takes discipline and strict adherence to a systematic approach. Two pairs of eyes and two points of view are often more enlightening than one. Although it is usually not routinely possible to have a team approach or joint reading of all films, when faced with a difficult or confusing clinical or radiological picture, direct consultation can be immensely profitable.

REFERENCES

1. Squire LF: Introduction and basic concepts, pp 1-13. In Squire LF, Ed: Fundamentals of Roentgenology. Cambridge, Harvard University Press, 1971
2. Felson B: Localization of intrathoracic lesions, pp 22-70. In Felson B, Ed: Chest Roentgenology. Philadelphia, W. B. Saunders, 1973
3. Squire LF: How to study a chest film, pp 30-45. In Squire LF, Ed: Fundamentals of Roentgenology. Cambridge, Harvard University Press, 1971
4. Hamilton WK: Atelectasis, pneumothorax, and aspiration as postoperative complications. Anesthesiology 22:708-722, 1961
5. Goodman LR: Cardiopulmonary disorders, pp 93-147. In Goodman LR, Putman CE, Eds: Intensive Care Radiology: Imaging of the Critically Ill. Saint Louis, C. V. Mosby, 1978
6. McCauley RGK: Radiology in respiratory intensive care unit. Int Anesthesiol Clin 14:1-29, 1976
7. Benjamin JJ, Cascade PN, Rubenfire M, Wajszczak W, Kerin NZ: Left lower lobe atelectasis and consolidation following cardiac surgery: the effect of topical cooling on the phrenic nerve. Radiology 142:11-14, 1982
8. Stevens RM, Teres D, Skillman JJ, Feingold DS: Pneumonia in an intensive care unit. Arch Intern Med 134:106-111, 1974
9. Fraser RG, Paré JAP: Diagnosis of Diseases of the Chest: An Integrated Study Based on the Abnormal Roentgenogram. Philadelphia, W. B. Saunders, 1970, pp 590-605
10. Renner RR, Coccaro AP, Heitzman ER, et al: Pseudomonas pneumonia: a prototype of hospital based infection. Radiology 105:555-562, 1972
11. Joffe N: Roentgenologic aspects of primary pseudomonas aeruginosa pneumonia in me-

chanically ventilated patients. Am J Roentgenol 107:305-312, 1969

12. De Weese JA, Stewart S III: Pulmonary complications of nonpulmonary intrathoracic
surgery, pp 215-234. In Cordell AR, Ellison
RG, Eds: Complications of Intrathoracic Surgery. Boston Little, Brown and Company,
1979

13. Westcott JL, Rudick MG: Cardiopulmonary
effects of intravenous fluid overload: radiologic manifestations. Radiology 129:577-585,
1978

14. Chait A, Cohen HE, Meltzer LE, et al: The
bedside chest radiograph in the evaluation of
incipient heart failure. Radiology 105:563-
566, 1972

15. Logue RB, Rogers JV, Gay BB Jr: Subtle
roentgenographic signs of left heart failure.
Amer Heart J 65:464-473, 1963

16. Preger L, Hooper TI, Steinbach HL, et al:
Width of azygos vein related to central venous pressure. Radiology 93:521-523, 1969

17. Grainger RG: Interstitial edema and its radiological diagnosis: a sign of pulmonary venous and capillary hypertension. Br J Radiol
31:201-217, 1958

18. Harrison MO, Conte PJ, Heitzman ER: Radiological detection of clinically occult cardiac failure following myocardial infarction.
Br J Radiol 44:265-272, 1971

19. McHugh TJ, Forrester JS, Adler L, et al: Pulmonary vascular congestion in acute myocardial infarction: hemodynamic and radiologic
correlations. Ann Int Med 76:29-33, 1972

20. Huglitz UF, Shapiro JH: Atypical pulmonary
patterns of congestive failure in chronic lung
disease. Radiology 93:995-1006, 1969

21. Calenoff L, Kruglik GD, Woodruff A: Unilateral pulmonary edema. Radiology 126:19-24,
1978

22. Leeming BWA: Gravitational edema of the
lungs observed during assisted respiration.
Chest 64:719-722, 1973

23. Mendelson CL: Aspiration of stomach contents into the lungs during obstetric anesthesia. Amer J Obstet Gynec 52:191-205, 1946

24. Gynum LJ, Pierce AK: Pulmonary aspiration
of gastric contents. Am Rev Respir Dis
114:1129-1136, 1976

25. Wilkins RA, DeLacey GJ, Flor R, et al: Radiology in Mendelson's syndrome. Clin Radiol
27:81-85, 1976

26. Tomashefski JF, Mahajan V: Managing respiratory distress syndrome in adults. Postgrad Med 59:77-82, 1976

27. Blaisdell RW, Schlobohm RM: The respiratory distress syndrome: a review. Surgery
74:251-262, 1973

28. Putman CE, Ravin CE: Adult respiratory distress syndrome, Intensive Care Radiology:
Imaging of the Critically Ill. Goodman LR,
Putman CE, Eds. Saint Louis, C. V. Mosby,
1978, pp 148-162

29. Joffe N: The adult respiratory distress syndrome. Am J Roentgenol 122:719-732, 1974

30. Petty TL, Asbaugh DG: The adult respiratory
distress syndrome: clinical features, factors
influencing prognosis and principles of management. Chest 60:233-239, 1971

31. Putman CE, Minagi H, Blaisdel FW: The
roentgen appearance of disseminated
intravascular coagulation (DIC). Radiology
109:13-18, 1973

32. Robboy SJ, Minna JD, Colman RW, et al:
Pulmonary hemorrhage syndrome as a manifestation of disseminated intravascular coagulation: analysis of ten cases. Chest 63:718-721,
1973

33. Fraser RG, Paré JAP: Embolic and thrombotic diseases of the lungs, pp 804-831. In
Fraser RG, Paré JAP, Eds: Diagnosis of Diseases of the Chest: An Integrated Study Based
on the Abnormal Roentgenogram. Philadelphia, W. B. Sanders, 1970

34. Neumann RD, Sostman HD, Gottschalk A:
Current status of ventilation-perfusion imaging. Seminars in Nuclear Medicine 10:198-
217, 1980

35. Figley MM, Gerdes AJ, Ricketts HJ: Radiographic aspects of pulmonary embolism.
Semin Roentgenol 2:389-405, 1967

36. Rohlfing BM, Webb WR, Schlobohm RM:
Ventilator-related extra-alveolar air in adults.
Radiology 121:25-31, 1976

37. Westcott JL, Cole SR: Interstitial pulmonary
emphysema in children and adults: roentgenographic features. Radiology 111:367-378,
1974

38. Zimmerman JE: Goodman LR, Shahvari
MBG: Effect of mechanical ventilation and
positive end-expiratory pressure (PEEP) on
the chest radiograph. Am J Roentgenol
133:811-816, 1979

39. Leeming BWA: Radiological aspects of the

pulmonary complications resulting from intermittent positive pressure ventilation (IPPV). Aust Radiol 12:361-374, 1968

40. Swischuk LE: Two lesser known but useful signs of neonatal pneumothorax. Am J Roentgenol 127:623-627, 1976

41. Steckel RJ: The radiolucent kinetic borderline in acute pulmonary edema and pneumonia. Clin Radiol 25:391-395, 1974

42. Kurlander GJ, Helmen CH: Subpulmonary pneumothorax. Am J Roentgenol 96:1019-1021, 1966

43. Lams PM, Jolles H: The effect of lobar collapse on the distribution of free intrapleural air. Radiology 142:309–312, 1982

44. Gordon R: The deep sulcus sign. Radiology 136:25–27, 1980

45. Gobien RP, Reines HD, Schabel SI: Localized tension pneumothorax: unrecognized form of barotrauma in adult respiratory distress syndrome. Radiology 142:15–19, 1982

46. Humphreys RL, Berne AS: Rapid re-expansion of pneumothorax: a cause of unilateral pulmonary edema. Radiology 96:509-512, 1970

47. Hipona FA, Paredes S, Lerona PT: Roetgenologic analysis of common postoperative problems in congenital heart disease. Radiol Clin N Am 9(2):229-251, 1971

48. Melamed M, Hipona FA, Reynes CJ, et al: The Adult Postoperative Chest. Springfield, Charles C. Thomas, 1977, p 307

49. Friedman PJ, Hellekant ACG: Diagnosis of air-fluid levels in the thorax: radiologic recognition of bronchopleural fistula. Am Rev Respir Dis 113 part 2:159-160, 1976

50. Schachter EN, Kreisman H, Putman CE: Diagnostic problems in suppurative lung disease. Arch Intern Med 136:167-171, 1976

51. Roddy LH, Unger KM, Miller WC: Thoracic computed tomography in the critically ill patient. Crit Care Med 9:515-518, 1981

52. Ellis K, Malm JR, Bowman FO, et al: Roentgenographic findings after pericardial surgery. Radiol Clin N Am 9(2):327-341, 1971

53. Melamed M, Hipona FA, Reynes CJ, et al: Air-fluid in the pleural space, pp 33-208. In Melamed M, Hipona FA, Reynes CJ, et al., Eds: The Adult Postoperative Chest. Springfield, Charles C Thomas, 1977

54. Conrardy PA, Goodman LR, Laing F, et al: Alterations of endotracheal tube position—flexion and extension of the neck. Crit Care Med 4:8-12, 1976

55. Goodman LR, Conrardy PA, Laing F, et al: Radiographic evaluation of endotracheal tube position. Am J Roentgenol 127:433-434, 1976

56. Lane EE, Temes GD, Anderson WH: Tracheal-innominate artery fistula due to tracheostomy. Chest 68:678-683, 1975

57. Pontoppidan H, Geffin B, Lowenstein E: Acute respiratory failure in the adult. N Engl J Med 287:690-698, 1972

58. Coryllos PN, Birnbaum GL: Studies in pulmonary gas absorption in bronchial obstruction. Amer J Med Sci 183:317-359, 1932

59. Zwillich CW, Pierson DJ, Creagh CE, et al: Complications of assisted ventilation. Am J Med 57:161-170, 1974

60. Sellery GR: Airway problems in the intensive care unit. Int Anesthesiol Clin 10:173-213, 1972

61. Black AMS, Harrison GA: Difficulties with positioning Robertshaw double-lumen tubes. Anaesth Intens Care 3:299-311, 1975

62. Goodman LR: Pulmonary support and monitoring apparatus, pp 29-63. In Goodman LR, Putman CE, Eds: Intensive Care Radiology: Imaging of the Critically Ill. Saint Louis, C. V. Mosby, 1978

63. Harley HRS: Ulcerative tracheo-oesophageal fistula during treatment by tracheostomy and intermittent positive pressure ventilation. Thorax 27:338-352, 1972

64. Mulder DS, Rubush JL: Complications of tracheostomy: relationship to long term ventilatory assistance. J. Trauma 9:389-401, 1969

65. Stahly TL, Tench WD: Lung entrapment and infarction by chest tube suction. Radiology 122:307-309, 1977

66. Langston CS: The aberrant central venous catheter and its complications. Radiology 100:55-59, 1971

67. Royal HD, Shields JB, Donati RM: Misplacement of central venous pressure catheters and unilateral pulmonary edema. Arch Intern Med 135:1502-1505, 1975

68. Ravin CE, Putman CE, McLoud TC: Hazards of the ICU. Am J Roentgenol 126:423-431, 1976

69. Roote GA, Schabel SI, Hodges M: Pulmonary complications of the flow-directed bal-

loon tipped catheter. N Engl J Med 290:927-931, 1974

70. Kaplan JA; Cardiac Anesthesia. New York, Grune and Stratton, 1979, pp 85-93

71. Hall WM, Rosenbaum HD: The radiology of cardiac pacemakers. Radiol Clin N Am 9(2):343-353, 1971

72. Rosenbaum HD: Roentgen demonstration of broken cardiac pacemaker wires. Radiology 84:933-936, 1965

73. Chamorro H, Rao G, Wholey MH: Superior vena cava syndrome: A complication of transvenous pacemaker implantation. Radiology 126:377-378, 1978

74. Chun PKC: Characteristics of commonly utilized permanent endocardial and epicardial pacemaker electrode systems: Method of radiologic identification. Am Heart J 102:404-414, 1981

Eric G. Honig, M.D.

4
Preoperative Evaluation

COMPLICATIONS OF THORACIC SURGERY

Thoracic surgery unquestionably represents a major stress on the cardiorespiratory system. Considering that the patient is paralyzed, under general anesthesia for several hours, dependent on the anesthesiologist for gas exchange as well as the bellows function of respiration, and wakes up with a painful incision in his chest wall, it is perhaps more remarkable that most thoracotomy patients escape without complication rather than that a large number do encounter difficulties. Not only does a thoracotomy pose perioperative hazards, but when the operation undertaken resects functioning lung tissue, ventilatory insufficiency and cor pulmonale become long-term risks.

Forty to sixty percent of thoracotomies are associated with respiratory complications, and overall mortality can run as high as 15 percent, although recent experience may be somewhat better as a result of careful selection of patients and improved postoperative care.[1-7]

The respiratory complications of general surgery can be basically divided into infectious and non-infectious categories. The former is represented chiefly by postoperative pneumonia and the latter by atelectasis, macro or micro. In a series of abdominal operations, pneumonia accounted for 56 percent of the observed complications and atelectasis for 42 percent.[8]

Pneumonias may result from the violation of the tracheobronchial tree by the endotracheal tube, from contamination by respiratory therapy equipment, from decreased mucociliary clearance due to drugs, oxygen, or anesthetic gases, or from any combination of these mechanisms.[1]

Atelectasis follows from the immediate intra- and postoperative changes observed in pulmonary mechanics.[9] Lung volumes tend to drop by 45 percent in the first two postoperative days. Tidal volume falls and frequency rises. Spontaneous sigh breaths are reduced in depth and frequency. As a result, surfactant production is compromised, secretions build up, and the lung loses volume and compliance. Reduction of the ventilation-perfusion ratio in such alveolar units renders them prone to collapse.[10] The tendency towards hypoventilation is accentuated by pain-induced splinting, and by sedatives and analgesic medications.

Atelectasis can be subdivided into macroatelectasis, roentgenographically-visible reduction in lung or lobar volume; and microatelectasis, which may manifest itself only as cough, lowgrade fever or a widened alveolar-arterial gradient. Both forms of atelectasis contribute to postoperative hypoxemia by promoting airway closure in the range of tidal breathing. Atelectasis may, as well, cause hypercapnia and ventilatory failure in patients with underlying lung disease. These respiratory complications have been found to occur in 3 to 10 percent of all operations.[1,11,12] The higher the incision, the higher the rate of complication, with thoracotomy presenting the highest rate of all. Curiously, however, chest wall surgery, which does not enter the pleural space, as for example, mastectomy, does not have a particularly high risk.[12]

When thoracotomy involves resection of lung tissue, the risk increases for respiratory failure. If a significant portion of the pulmonary vascular bed is resected, the possibility exists for the development of iatrogenic pulmonary hypertension and cor pulmonale.

Since the advent of effective chemotherapeutic agents for the control of tuberculosis about 25 years ago, there has been a shift in the incidence of pulmonary resections towards the management of bronchogenic carcinoma. Because this disease involves an older age population than TB, and because of the unfortunate co-existence of significant obstructive lung disease secondary to cigarette consumption, a larger number of patients present for pulmonary resection with poorer baseline respiratory function, and the incidence of postoperative respiratory insufficiency has become troubling.[13]

PREOPERATIVE ASSESSMENT OF PULMONARY FUNCTION

The concomitant application of basic respiratory physiology to the bedside led to the development of preoperative pulmonary function testing and its use in an attempt to predict the risk of cardiopulmonary morbidity and mortality from thoracotomy and other major surgery.

An extensive literature has arisen dealing with various diagnostic strategies in the evaluation of the risk of morbidity and mortality in the thoracotomy candidate. Certain difficulties arise, however, in attempting to draw general conclusions from the many sources of information available. Analysis of the literature is hampered by the variety of surgical populations involved, both general and thoracic. The thoracic surgery literature deals almost exclusively with two conditions, bronchogenic carcinoma and tuberculosis, and with two operations, pneumonectomy and lobectomy. Conclusions regarding other thoracotomies must be extrapolated from these data. Early studies, in particular, deal with different end-points, morbidity or mortality, but often lump them together or treat them interchangeably. Data about long-term outcome such as functional status or incidence of cor pulmonale are often missing.

The modifying effect of preoperative care on pulmonary function is seldom, if ever, dealt with; and the built-in bias of the sickest patients receiving the most intense care is not taken into consideration. Many studies attempt to retrospectively demonstrate a difference in pulmonary function between survivors and non-survivors, or complicated vs. uncomplicated thoracotomies. Unfortunately, this approach provides no prospective help in predicting which patients will and which patients will not develop iatrogenic problems owing to their thoracotomies.

Several studies do provide enough information to generate predictions from pulmonary function data. In general, it is found that results above a particular cut-off value give about a 90 percent likelihood of a benign course; performance below the cut-off carries a 25 to 35 percent incidence of adverse outcome (reducing the likelihood of a good outcome to 65–75 percent). Preoperative assessment of pulmonary function, then, cannot identify the patient who absolutely will suffer from his surgery any more than it can provide an ironclad assurance of a good outcome.

Applied intelligently, preoperative assessment of pulmonary function can identify patients who are at *increased risk* of complication and provide a rough numeric guess as to the likelihood of complication. Whether that risk is acceptable or precludes surgery should ultimately be up to the surgeon and his patient. Where surgery is elected, poor pulmonary function is an indication for aggressive preoperative attention to respiratory care and reassessment following that care, since the likelihood of difficulty can be substantially modified by treatment.[14]

As anywhere else in medicine, preoperative assessment of pulmonary function should begin with a complete history and physical examination.

CLINICAL EVALUATION

Medical History

A complete history and physical examination should be performed on any candidate for major surgery, but several risk factors for complications demand particular attention. The major contributing risk factors to morbidity and mortality in thoracic surgery are age, obesity, and underlying heart and lung disease. Congestive heart failure and chronic obstructive pulmonary disease (COPD) are the most important entities to identify.[1,15]

Historical investigation of the thoracotomy candidate should seek to determine the presence and severity of possible lung disease and heart disease. The following factors are important in the assessment of lung disease.

DYSPNEA

Dyspnea is a subjective sensation arising from a ventilatory output that is inappropriate for the input of muscular effort.[16]

While roughly paralleling the course of disease, it may be modified by psychologic factors. Dyspnea may be a sign of heart or lung disease and be caused either by obstructive or restrictive disease. Obesity, as a form of extra pulmonary restriction, may also cause dyspnea. Dyspnea should always be quantitated as to the degree of effort required to produce it. Patients are best asked how far they can walk on level ground, how well they can manage hills, stairs, and the activities of daily living. Are they able to continue at a normal pace or must they slow down? In general, severe exertional dyspnea implies a significantly diminished ventilatory reserve with an FEV_1 of 1500 cc or less.

A history of orthopnea should be sought. Orthopnea can be cardiac in origin, due to a shift of blood volume from the periphery to the central circulation, and is often delayed in onset by minutes to hours after assuming recumbancy. It may be respiratory in origin, due to the uncoupling of chest wall and abdominal muscles of respiration, leading to almost immediate dyspnea.[17,18] Respiratory orthopnea carries a respiratory risk, but no increased cardiac risk; while cardiac orthopnea carries a significant risk of cardiac mortality.[15]

CIGARETTE SMOKING

A tobacco history is one of the most important predictors of postoperative pulmonary difficulty.[1,2,8] Cigarettes are the most important risk factors unless pipes or cigars are inhaled. Inhalation should be inquired about. It is helpful to quantitate smoking on the basis of pack-years, that is, the number of packs smoked per day multiplied by the number of years smoked. Because patients often spontaneously cut back on smoking when they feel unwell due to intrathoracic disease, it is wise to inquire as to whether the current smoking levels reflects their usual habit over a period of years. Increasing pack years increases the risk for chronic lung disease as well as malignancy.[19]

COUGH

Cough is an extremely nonspecific symptom and may have thoracic as well as extrathoracic origins. It may indicate postnasal drip, asthma, bronchitis, or be an early manifestation of bronchogenic carcinoma.[20] The presence and frequency of cough should be established, as well as the presence and character of sputum production. The presence of a "recurrent productive cough" on most days for at least three months a year for at least two years makes a clinical diagnosis of chronic bronchitis when other causes for a productive cough have been ruled out.[21] The amount and character of the sputum should be described. The presence of hemoptysis, however, has little or no bearing on ultimate resectibility for lung cancer but may alert the clinician to a hitherto unsuspected condition.[22]

ASTHMA AND WHEEZING

A history of asthma and wheezing and/or allergies should be sought. The presence of airway obstruction in itself is a risk, but when largely reversible, as in asthma, the risk takes on somewhat lesser importance.

Cardiac factors found to be of prognostic significance include congestive heart failure with pulmonary edema, and myocardial infarction within the last six months. Angina pectoris, hypertension, remote infarction, or claudication do not appear to contribute to the risk of cardiac mortality.[15,23]

Physical Examination

Physical examination is directed towards the identification of obstructive airway disease (and its consequences) and the presence of congestive heart failure.

Peripheral edema should be looked for as a sign of possible right ventricular failure. Clubbing is not characteristic of uncomplicated COPD, and its presence should arouse

suspicion for interstitial fibrosis, or a chronic inflammatory process such as bronchiectasis, or malignancy. Cyanosis is an unreliable physical finding and more misleading than valuable.[24]

During determination of blood pressure, the presence or absence of a paradoxical pulse greater than 10 mmHg should be noted. A large inspiratory fall in blood pressure shows a fair correlation with the degree of airway obstruction and reflects afterloading of the left heart by a negative pleural pressure.[25]

Respiratory Signs

Respiratory rate and pattern should be observed and recorded with attention to the use of accessory muscles. Indications of accessory muscle use such as tracheal descent and a superior sternal vector should be noted. A prolonged expiratory time relative to inspiration may suggest airflow obstruction.[26] A forced expiratory time should be recorded by having the patient maximally inspire then exhale forcefully and completely, emptying his lungs as rapidly as possible. The diaphragm of the examiner's stethoscope should be placed over the trachea and the amount of time required for all breath sounds to cease should be noted. Prolongation beyond 5 seconds is indicative of airflow obstruction.

Elevation, collapse, and the pulse waves of the internal jugular vein should be noted. Distention more than 4 cm above the Angle of Louis at 30 to 60 degrees elevation reflects an elevated central venous pressure. The presence of jugular venous distention as a reflection of congestive heart failure carried a 22 percent cardiac mortality in a general surgery population in one large series.[15,23] A large "A" wave accompanying right atrial contraction may reflect pulmonary hypertension.

The trachea should be in the midline. Displacement to either side should prompt evaluation of the mediastinum and reassessment of the advisability of surgery.

The pattern of respiration should be noted as to its regularity and as to whether the abdomen moves out along with the chest in inspiration. Inspiratory paradox, with the abdomen moving in while the chest moves out, suggests diaphragmatic fatigue with severe respiratory dysfunction and carries ominous prognostic implications.[27-28]

Suprasternal and supraclavicular excavation on inspiration and rib retraction reflect negative intrathoracic pressure and have the same significance as pulsus paradoxus.[26,29]

Expansion of the chest should be evaluated by palpation as to extent and symmetry. Particular attention should be paid to the end-inspiratory motion of the lower ribs anteriorly. Paradoxical retraction (Hoover's sign) strongly suggests hyperinflation.[30] Motion of the diaphragm should be assessed by percussion. Less than 2 cm descent between expiration and inspiration suggests hyperinflation, particularly when associated with a hyper-resonant percussion note. Failure of a hemidiaphragm to descend in the setting of cancer may imply mediastinal metastasis involving the phrenic nerve and suggest surgical inoperability. Diminished motion of one hemithorax, or a lag in motion, suggests pleural disease and may also reflect inoperability.

A dull percussion note may be due to pleural disease, to atelectasis, or to consolidation.

The spine should be observed for evidence of kyphoscoliosis which, if severe, can lead on its own to significant pulmonary dysfunction and surgical risk.[31]

Breath sounds should be auscultated over upper, mid, and lower lung fields bilaterally, anteriorly, and posteriorly; and assessed for the quality and quantity of breath sounds, as well as for the presence of adventitious breath sounds. Diminished sounds may be due to areas of emphysema or, when accompanied by increased transmission of spoken sounds and percussive dullness, may suggest bronchial obstruction.

Inspiratory crackles are caused by opening of peripheral lung units. Early crackles may be due to atelectasis or congestive heart failure, while late crackles tend to be suggestive of interstitial pulmonary fibrosis.[32,33] Wheezes are suggestive of airflow obstruction. A localized wheeze recurring in the same area of the thorax should suggest a fixed bronchial obstruction such as a tumor. Inspiratory wheezing, as well, when intrathoracic in origin, should suggest an endobronchial tumor.

Cardiovascular Signs

Heart sounds may be distant due to hyperinflation or may be obscured by breath sounds. Signs of pulmonary hypertension should be carefully sought. These include a widened or fixed split of the second heart sound, an increased intensity of the pulmonic component of the second heart sound, or gallop sounds heard along the left sternal border that accentuate upon inspiration, suggesting a right-sided origin.

Heart rhythm should be assessed for irregularities and, if any are noted, evaluated further. An electrocardiogram should always be obtained as part of a comprehensive initial assessment.

Careful auscultation with the stethoscope bell should be performed seeking the presence of gallops, since the presence of a left-sided S_3 gallop rhythm is a major risk factor for cardiac mortality. A systolic murmur at the base suggesting aortic stenosis should be further evaluated as a potential risk factor.[15,23]

Electrocardiogram (Fig. 4-1)[34]

All surgical candidates should have an electrocardiogram prior to surgery. Signs of significant pulmonary dysfunction include

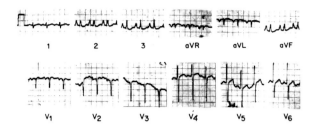

| 1 | 2 | 3 | aVR | aVL | aVF |

| V₁ | V₂ | V₃ | V₄ | V₅ | V₆ |

Pwave

ISOELECTRIC P in LEAD I or
RIGHT AXIS DEVIATION of P VECTOR

P-PULMONALE (P > 2.5mm in II, II AVF)

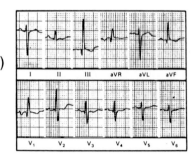

QRS COMPLEX

1 – RIGHT AXIS DEVIATION

2 – R/S V₆ < 1

3 – LOW VOLTAGE QRS IN FRONTAL LEADS - S₁Q₃ or S₁S₂S₃

4 – RIGHT BUNDLE BRANCH BLOCK USUALLY INCOMPLETE

5 – R/S V₁ > 1

6 – CLOCKWISE ROTATION OF ELECTRICAL AXIS

7 – Q or QS in INFERIOR LEADS SIMULATING
    OLD MYOCARDIAL INFARCTION

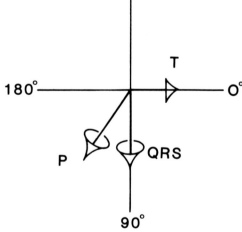

Fig. 4-1 Electrocardiographic abnormalities in COPD. Clockwise from upper right: COPD patient with cor pulmonale. Note right axis deviation, P pulmonale, poor initial anterior forces in V1-V3. Below, S1Q3 pattern and incomplete right bundle branch block. (From Holford FD: The electrocardiogram in lung disease, ch 10 In Fishman AP, Ed: Pulmonary diseases and disorders. Copyright © 1980 McGraw-Hill, New York. Used with the permission of the McGraw-Hill Book Company.) Vector depiction of ECG in COPD shows small QRS voltage with clockwise axis, large P vector with posterior and clockwise direction. T vector is nonspecific. Electrocardiographic criteria for right ventricular hypertrophy or strain in the setting of COPD.

low voltage due to hyperinflation, a vertical axis, or poor R-wave progression across the anterior precordial leads. Pulmonary hypertension will be manifested by signs of right-sided pressure overload including right axis deviation, P pulmonale (P-waves greater than 2.5 mm in height), right ventricular hypertrophy, or complete or incomplete right bundle branch block

Left bundle branch block or old dead zones are not significant cardiac risk factors, but a fresh myocardial infarction increases risk.[15] Strain patterns or subendocardial ischemia do carry a small but increased risk.[23] Any rhythm other than normal sinus or premature atrial contractions is associated with significant cardiac risk, and more than five ventricular ectopics per minute are particularly malignant.[15,23]

Laboratory Examination

Two features of the routine laboratory examination deserve particular attention. An elevated hematocrit in the absence of dehydration may be indicative of significant hypoxemia, in itself a factor suggesting increased surgical risk, and may suggest the possibility of pulmonary hypertension. Since carbon monoxide due to smoking may contribute as much to an elevated hematocrit as hypoxemia, blood gases and carboxyhemoglobin concentration should be obtained whenever the hematocrit is elevated.[35] The serum bicarbonate concentration may yield a clue as to whether the patient has a tendency towards hypercapnia.

The Henderson-Hasselbalch equation can be manipulated to solve for PCO_2 when pH is 7.40, yielding an approximation of the PCO_2 for which the patient has compensated.

Since

$$PCO_2 \text{ (mmHg)} = \frac{[H^+ \text{ (nanomol)}] [HCO_3^- \text{ (mEq)}]}{24}$$

if (H^+) is set equal to 40 (the negative antilog of 7.40), the PCO_2 for which renal compensation has evolved over the last 48 to 72 hours results.[36] Suggestion of hypercapnia makes direct measurement of arterial blood gases advisable.

Chest Roentgenogram (Fig. 4-2)

A PA and lateral chest roentgenogram should be part of the routine clinical preoperative evaluation. Chronic obstructive lung disease tends to present in two ways—hyperinflation or vascular changes.

Abnormalities in the chest film are fairly reliable. The roentgenogram is more specific than sensitive in COPD. A normal film does not exclude significant disease, but disease is usually present when the film is abnormal.

Signs of hyperinflation include a retrosternal air space greater than 2 cm, a sternal-diaphragm angle greater than 90°, flat diaphragms on PA and lateral projections, a small vertical heart, and the dome of the right hemidiaphragm appearing at the 8th anterior interspace or the 11th posterior interspace.[37] Vascular alterations include signs of decreased perfusion as in emphysema or increased vascular markings as in chronic bronchitis with cor pulmonale. Signs of vascular attenuation include sharp taper of the main pulmonary artery segments or peripheral vascular attenuation. In chronic bronchitis, bronchovascular markings may be increased in prominence particularly in the lower lobes, leading to the classic "dirty lung" pattern.

Bullae, curvilinear line shadows surrounding air density, are characteristic of emphysema.[37–39]

Because thoracotomy itself is a significant risk factor, all patients undergoing thoracotomy should go on to physiologic assessment of cardiopulmonary function; and patients exhibiting any of the abnormalities discussed should receive particularly close attention.

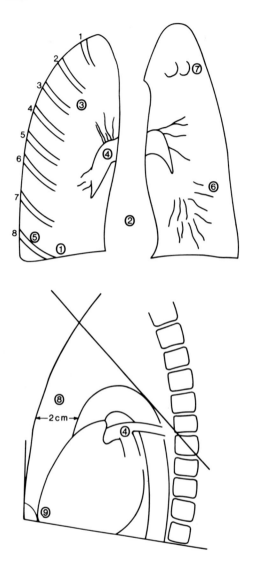

**PULMONARY FUNCTION
TESTS—INTERPRETATION**

CHARACTERISTICS OF TESTS

Epidemiologic information indicates that patients with obstructive or restrictive lung diseases are at increased risk for perioperative complications. Therefore, patients are tested preoperatively to identify those with disease who are at a particularly high risk for these complications. The ideal test would be one which perfectly separates out patients with diseases from those without the diseases of concern. Unfortunately, within any population, there is a considerable overlap in test results between those individuals who are in fact diseased and those who do not have the disease in question. Because of this overlap, any choice of limits of normal or abnormal must generate false positive or false negative as well as accurate results. The choice of normal limits for pulmonary function studies, like any others, must be guided by an understanding of what we want a test to tell us. Do we want to identify *all* individuals with abnormality at the cost of labelling some normal subjects as diseased? If so, we have a test of high *sensitivity* but low *specificity* and have a large number of false positive results. Or, do we wish to exclude *all* normal individuals and identify only those patients who certainly have disease? If so, we have a study of high specificity but low sensitivity and we may fail to identify some individuals with disease, that is, have too many false negative results. Finally, we can ask for the maximum accuracy in a test, minimizing the total number of false results irrespective of which we affect more by our choice, sensitivity, or specificity. This can be done by plotting a receiver operating characteristic curve (ROC) for the study in question: true positives or sensitivity vs. false positives, (1 - specificity) (Fig. 4-3C). A hyperbolic curve results, the elbow of which identifies the sensitivity be-

Fig. 4-2 Roentgenographic features of COPD. (Top) PA film: (1) flattened diaphragms; (2) small vertical heart due to descent of diaphragms; (3) attenuation of peripheral vascular markings; (4) enlarged main pulmonary artery segment (> 16mm) with sharp abrupt taper; (5) dome of right hemidiaphragm at 8th rib anteriorly; (6) increased vascular markings at bases (chronic bronchitis); and (7) bullae. (Bottom) Lateral Film: (8) enlarged retrosternal airspace (> 2cm); and (9) sternal-diaphragmatic angle greater than 90°

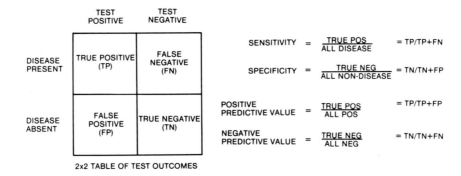

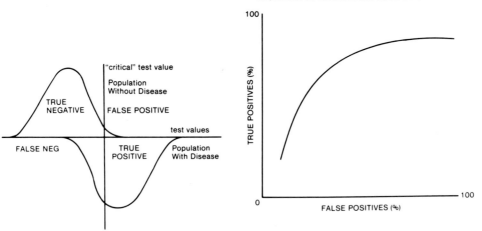

Fig. 4-3 Information content of diagnostic tests. (top) 2 × 2 table outlining possible results of tests. (bottom-left) Distribution of test results in populations with and without disease. Increasing or decreasing the critical cutoff value will change the specificity and sensitivity of a test. The amount of change will depend on how far the cutoff value is adjusted and the exact distribution of test results in a diseased or non-diseased population. (bottom-right) Receiver-operating characteristic curve (ROC) obtained by plotting the percentage of true positives versus the percentage of false positives for any cutoff value of a test given the distributions shown on the left. The "optimal" position of the ROC curve will depend on just what kind of information is desired from the test, the relative cost of testing errors, and the prevalence of the disease in question.

yond which the number of false positives increases at an excessive rate. The "best" point on a ROC curve, if one such point can be said to exist, is determined by the perception of the relative costs of false positives and false negatives, and the prevalence of the disease in the population tested.[40,41]

Specificity and sensitivity are intrinsic characteristics of a test based on the limits of normal chosen and by the distribution of test results in the population of interest (Fig. 4-3B). But specificity and sensitivity are *a posteriori* values; that is, they are calculable only when the number of normal and abnormal subjects in a population is already known.

Predictive value, which is of greater importance in a clinical situation, is influenced as much by the proportion of abnormal subjects in the population tested, as by intrinsic characteristics of the test. Sensitivity indicates how many of a population of abnormal subjects the test was able to identify; positive predictive value indicates how many individuals with an abnormal test result actually abnormal. Conversely, specificity indicates how many of a population of normal subjects the test correctly identified as normal; negative predictive value tells how many individuals with a normal test result are truly normal (Fig. 4-3A). The distinction between specificity and sensitivity on one hand, and predictive values on the other, is key to the intelligent application of any test in clinical medicine.

LIMITS OF NORMAL

Because of its influence on specificity and sensitivity, the limits of normal must be defined for any test. These limits will depend on the population studied as well as location of the study, equipment used, and technician factors. A drawback of many early normal standards for pulmonary function was that smokers were included in the so-called healthy population. This inappropriately widened the acceptable range for each age group and test.[42] Another problem was the failure of most studies to account for and deal with ethnic variability in test performance. Large-scale surveys suggest that healthy subjects of African or Asian extraction tend to have 10 to 20 percent smaller lung volumes than healthy subjects of European extraction of the same age, sex, and body habitus. The reasons for these differences are not clearly understood, but failure to adjust for them can result in false positive results in testing of these individuals.[43]

The expression of pulmonary function results as a percentage of predicted can result in further inaccuracy and error. To say that the lower limits of normal represent a fixed percentage of predicted implies that the limits of confidence for a given test are dependent on the absolute value of the test,

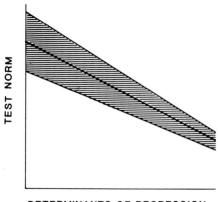

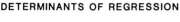

DETERMINANTS OF REGRESSION

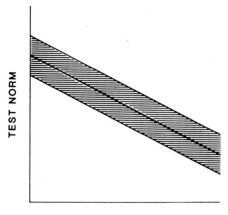

DETERMINANTS OF REGRESSION

Fig. 4-4 Limits of normal. (Top) Limits of normal set as a percentage of predicted. Note a wider confidence interval for higher predicted values. Data where the confidence limits are dependent on the absolute value of measurement are termed *heteroschedastic*. (Bottom) Limits of normal as absolute confidence limits of measurement, independent of test value. Confidence limits parallel regression. Data of this type are termed *homoschedastic*.

that is, *heteroschedastic*. In fact, the standard error of the estimate for common tests of pulmonary function has been found to be independent of the actual value of the test, that is, *homoschedastic* (Fig 4-4). This characteristic of pulmonary function data biases interpretation of studies against the smaller, older patient whose predicted values would be smaller and thus show a narrower range of normal. A sounder statistical approach would be to define the 95 percent confidence limits for a test, and not consider a test as abnormal unless the result falls outside the confidence limits (1.64 SD for a one-tailed 5% exclusion or 2 SD, ± 2½% at either end).[44] While this approach is sounder in principle, it has not been demonstrated whether this would reduce inaccuracy or uncertainty in pulmonary function testing.

Any review of the literature challenging the utility of pulmonary function testing in preoperative assessment must take these statistical problems into consideration.[45]

Two key questions need to be asked in attempting to define the limits of normal for any clinical laboratory test.

1. Are the published normal limits applicable to your patient population?

Is the makeup of the study population comparable to the population you deal with? Was the underlying disease reliably excluded in the "normal" population? Were the studies performed using equipment and techniques comparable to those used in your pulmonary function laboratory? Is adequate information provided to allow you to determine the confidence limits for the normal predictions? If not, it may become necessary to define those limits within your own local population.

2. How do you plan to use the test information?

If the test is to be used to identify individuals at risk for complications so that prophylactic measures may be employed, it is appropriate to take a bias of high sensitivity and low specificity. The limits of normal should be somewhat constricted. If the test is to be used to include or exclude the feasibility of a treatment felt to be the procedure of choice for a particular disease, the limits of normal should be made as broad as possible, high specificity and low sensitivity, so as to exclude as few patients as is absolutely necessary.

By using an appropriate reference population and selecting a cutoff value consistent with the purpose of the test, test results can more reliably yield the kinds of information for which they are intended.

The combined use of screening studies of high sensitivity to identify a population at risk, and studies of higher specificity as a basis for treatment decision, is at the root of preoperative assessment of pulmonary function.

Spirometry

In terms of simplicity, reliability, and the information yield for a given effort, no pulmonary function study offers more information than simple spirometry. Provided adequate equipment is available and the patient's effort is reasonable, obstructive lung disease can be reliably identified and quantitated, and a good estimate can be made as to the presence and degree of pulmonary restriction.

Spirometry measures the volume of air that can be inhaled or exhaled by a patient as a function of time, and is recorded as a volume-time trace. Since volume divided by time is flow, information about flow rates can also be gleaned from a spirographic tracing. Because flow is the time derivative of volume, a simple electronic differentiator permits the simultaneous generation of a flow-volume loop from the spirogram. Since volume is the timed integral of flow, the flow signal from a flow-volume loop can be integrated and plotted against time as a spirogram. Both traces, in fact, contain the same information; but for most purposes, the simplicity of the spirogram makes it the test of choice for basic pulmonary function.

PHYSIOLOGIC BASIS OF FORCED
EXPIRATORY FLOW

The information content of the spirogram derives from two basic factors: the determinants of maximal airflow, and the de-

$$\frac{V}{T} = Flow$$

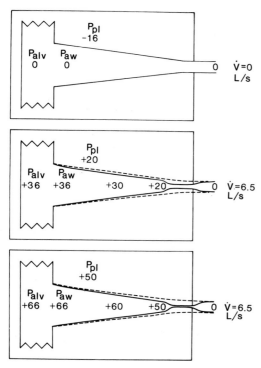

Fig. 4-5 Equal pressure point concept of maximum expiratory airflow. Upper panel: At FRC, no airflow. Driving pressure $P_{alv} = 0$. Resting pleural pressure negative, $P_{pl} = -16$. Middle panel: Expiration, $P_{pl} = +20$. Elastic recoil pressure, $P_{el} = +16$. P_{alv} equals sum of P_{pl} and P_{el} $= +36$. Airflow is initiated with P_{alv} translated to airway pressure, P_{aw}. P_{aw} drops along tube to point at which pressure inside ($+20$) equals pressure outside ($+20$). At this point in an infinitely compressible tube, narrowing and flow limitation occurs. Botton panel: Increasing expiratory effort fails to increase flow further: equal pressure point is still established, narrowing of airway and flow limitation still occurs, irrespective of effort applied (reproduced with permission from Rodarte JR, Hyatt RE: Respiratory mechanics. Basics of RD 4(4)1-6, 1976).

terminants of lung volumes. In 1960, Fry and Hyatt found that at lung volumes below 60 percent of vital capacity, maximum expiratory airflow was independent of effort. Blowing harder did not produce any futher augmentation of flow.[46] Their findings were later explained by Macklem, Mead, Permutt, and Pride in terms of the *equal pressure point concept*.[47-49]

The lung can be modelled as a balloon with a long tube representing the alveoli and airways, mounted inside a box, representing the thorax. The driving pressure to expiratory flow, alveolar pressure (Palv), is a combination of the elastic spring of the balloon (Pel), and the compressing pressure in the box, pleural pressure (Ppl). Palv drives air out of the balloon and the box into the surrounding air where it has the same pressure as the atmosphere (arbitrarily defined as 0). Therefore, Palv dissipates to zero as air flows downstream from alveoli to the mouth through the airway. Using Ohm's law as an analogy (Δ pressure = flow $\times$ resistance), the higher the air flow and the higher the resistance in the tube, the greater the pressure drop along the airway (Fig. 4-5).

The model calls for a positive pressure in the box, during expiration, Ppl. At some point in the tube, then, as pressure falls from Palv to 0, the pressure inside the tube will equal the pressure outside the tube. At this *equal pressure point*, the tube, if infinitely flexible, will collapse and limit air flow, since any further increase in Ppl will only compress the tube further.[47-49] In fact, the real bronchial tree is not infinitely compressible, and the actual choke point forms somewhere downstream from the equal pressure point and is governed by a number of factors; but the model suffices as a basic illustration of the mechanism of expiratory flow limitation.[48]

Airway resistance is one of the determinants of the maximum expiratory flow rate. The other prime determinant is the driving pressure itself, Palv. Palv, in turn, is governed by Ppl, which is a reflection of muscular effort, and Pel, a measure of the recoil of lung tissue when it is stretched.

Pel is a reflection of the *compliance* of the lung, defined as $C = \Delta V / \Delta P$, change in volume for a given pressure change, which is in fact, Pel. Pel can be expressed as $\Delta V/C$. A

$\Delta P = F \times R$ $\quad P_{el} = \dfrac{\Delta V}{C}$

$F = \dfrac{\Delta P}{R}$

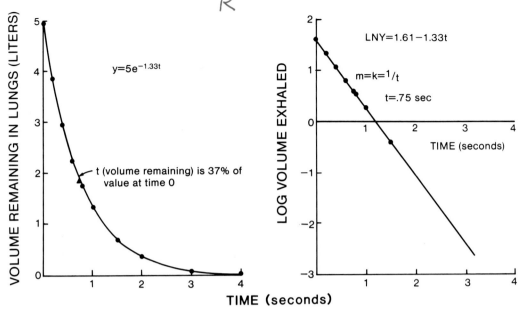

Fig. 4-6 Exponential process. Rate of change is proportional to amount of material present at any time ($Y = Y_{oe}kt$). Left: Volume vs. time trace of a single exponential. Note resemblance to normal spirogram. Right: Log volume vs time plot becomes a straight line for a single exponential. Slope is 1/time constant.

highly compliant lung will generate a small Pel, and a stiffer non-compliant lung a higher Pel for the same volume change. Pulmonary emphysema is characterized by an excessively high compliance and a decrease in elastic recoil pressure for a given inspired volume.

Therefore, alveolar driving pressure will be reduced and maximum expiratory airflow limited in emphysema, in part because of the abnormally high compliance.

If the logarithm of expired volume vs. time in a normal individual is plotted, a straight line plot results. This is a characteristic of an exponential process; that is, one in which the rate of change of some quantity is dependent on the absolute quantity at any particular time. Applied to the lung in forced expiration, it can be stated that the rate of airflow, Δ volume/Δ time, is related to the amount of volume left in the lung at that particular time.

An exponential process can be described

mathematically by its time constant τ (tau). τ is the time it takes the amount of any quantity to fall to 37 percent of its initial value, and a straight line semilog plot suggests that the normal lung operates as if it has a single time constant of about ¾ of a second (Fig. 4-6).

Returning to an electrical analogy, τ can be defined as $\tau = R \times C$, the product of resistance and capacitance. Capacitance is the equivalent of respiratory compliance. Therefore, emphysema can increase the time constant of the diseased lung by increased compliance. Asthma or chronic bronchitis can increase τ by increasing resistance. A combination of pathologic emphysema and chronic bronchitis, which is what is most often encountered in clinical COPD, will increase both resistance and compliance and produce particularly long time constants.[50-52]

What time-constant theory means to spirometry is that the normal lung with a single short time constant exhales most of its

$MEFR \simeq R \cdot P_{ALV} (P_{pL} \cdot P_{eL})$

$\tau = R \times C$

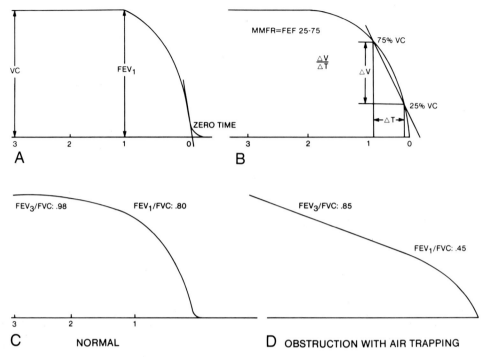

Fig. 4-7 Spirogram traces volume versus time. (A) Zero time is determined by tangent drawn to steepest portion of initial curve down to zero volume. Vital capacity is distance from zero volume to maximum volume deflection at end of trace. FEV_1 is distance from zero volume at one second from time zero. (B) MMFR or FEF_{25-27} is determined by marking flow rate ($\Delta V/\Delta T$) over middle of vital capacity. (C) Normal spirogram. Note rapid upstroke of initial flow and flattening (plateau) of terminal portion of spirogram. (D) Spirogram in obstructive lung disease. Initial flows reduced, volume is still being exhaled at the end of the trace, causing artifactual underestimation of vital capacity.

volume in a short period of time with relatively little further airflow after three seconds (Fig. 4-7C). In the abnormal lung, short time-constant airways coexist with airways with longer time-constants This means that volume continues to be exhaled by the abnormal lung well beyond three seconds of forced expiration. Time-constant theory accounts for two key features of the obstructed spirogram and helps explain at least one potentially confusing aspect of routine spirometry. In the obstructed lung, initial flow rates are abnormally low, but air flow continues for an abnormally long time. If measurement of expiration is not carried on long enough, the total volume expired will be underestimated (Fig. 4-7D).

DETERMINANTS OF LUNG VOLUMES
(FIG. 4-8)

Expiratory air flow is chiefly determined by airway resistance and the compliance of lung parenchyma. Lung volumes, in turn, are determined by the compliance of the lung and chest wall, and the forces applied to it. Each major subdivision of lung volume is a consequence of a balance of forces tending to increase lung volume and forces tending to decrease that volume.[53]

Total lung capacity (TLC) is the maximum amount of air that can be contained in the lung. TLC is determined by the strength of inspiratory muscles operating against the recoil of the lung and chest wall. A patient

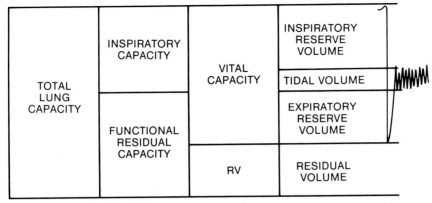

TOTAL LUNG CAPACITY	INSPIRATORY CAPACITY	VITAL CAPACITY	INSPIRATORY RESERVE VOLUME
			TIDAL VOLUME
	FUNCTIONAL RESIDUAL CAPACITY		EXPIRATORY RESERVE VOLUME
		RV	RESIDUAL VOLUME

Fig. 4-8 Static lung volumes. Data obtained from tidal breaths followed by maximum expiration to residual volume and full inspiration to TLC. VC, ERV, IC, and IRV can be determined directly from spirographic trace. RV, FRC and TLC require lung volume determinations by gas dilution, plethysmography, or estimation by chest roentgenogram. TLC = Total lung capacity; VC = Vital Capacity; ERV = Expiratory Reserve Volume; IC = Inspiratory Capacity; IRV = Inspiratory Reserve Volume; RV = Residual Volume; and FRC = Functional Residual Capacity.

with emphysema and a loss of elastic recoil would be expected to have a high TLC; a patient with pulmonary fibrosis or with kyphoscoliosis would have a reduced TLC because of increased recoil. A weakened patient may have a reduced TLC in the presence of a completely normal lung and chest wall.

Residual volume (RV) is the minimum amount of air left in the lungs after a full expiration. In young individuals, under 35-40, residual volume is determined by the strength of expiratory muscles working against the recoil of the lung and chest wall. In older individuals, residual volume is limited by airway closure.[54] The obstructed patient often has airway closure at abnormally high lung volumes. As a result, residual volume is abnormally increased. This is referred to as air-trapping.

Vital capacity (VC) is the difference between TLC and RV. It may be reduced either by a decreased total lung capacity or by an increased residual volume due to obstruction and air-trapping.

Functional residual capacity (FRC) is the resting end-expiratory lung volume. FRC is the one volume that is not dependent on

muscle activity, but rather on the balance between elastic recoil of the lung opposed by the elastic recoil of the chest wall.

Thus, the major features of the spirogram are chiefly determined by expiratory flow limitation, airway resistance, and lung and chest wall compliance.

SPIROMETRIC MEASUREMENTS

Several types of spirometers are available to record the spirographic tracing. Primary volume-recording instruments include water seal, dry rolling seal, and bellows or wedge spirometers. An acceptable instrument must be capable of recording a volume signal for at least 10 seconds, should have a volume capacity of 7 liters, and have a resistance of less than 1.5 cm/H_2O/L/sec at a 12 L/sec flow. The hard copy tracing should have at least 10 mm chart displacement per liter of lung volume, and a paper speed at least 1 cm/sec. Volume measurements must be reproducible to ± 50 ml or ± 3 percent, whichever is larger.

The actual test is performed with the patient as relaxed as possible, instructed as to the procedure and free of encumbering clothing. Dentures, if worn, should be removed. It is immaterial whether the test be performed sitting or standing. Nose clips should be worn.

The patient is instructed to take in as deep a breath as possible and then exhale forcibly as rapidly and completely as possible. Emphatic coaching is usually necessary to assure a maximum effort. In general, maximum efforts are reproducible; suboptimal efforts are not.

At least three acceptable efforts should be recorded, acceptability to be determined by the technician. Grounds for rejection of a test include (1) coughing, (2) glottic closure, (3) an effort of less than 5 seconds' duration in an obstructed patient, (4) air leak, (5) an obstructed mouthpiece (e.g., tongue, false teeth), (6) a false start or excessive hesitation at the start, or (7) excessive variability. The best 2 of 3 acceptable curves should not vary by more than $\pm$ 10 percent or $\pm$ 100 ml, whichever is greater.[55-58]

The spirographic trace takes the form of a hyperbola. The primary measurements taken from the spirogram are the forced vital capacity and timed expiratory volumes (Fig. 4-7).

The forced vital capacity is defined as the volume exhaled by the end of the trace. In the normal individual, the FVC will have reached a plateau by 4 seconds; but in an obstructed patient, long time-constant airways may still be emptying, and the spirographic trace fails to plateau. A rising terminal portion of the spirogram is evidence for airway obstruction and implies that the recorded vital capacity may be an underestimate of the "true" vital capacity due to air-trapping. A reduced vital capacity may be due to a restrictive ventilatory defect, in which case the terminal spirogram may plateau normally, rise as an artifact of obstruction, or show a combination of both characteristics. Where doubt about the significance of a reduced vital capacity exists, lung volumes should be separately determined.

The beginning of the forced expiration is determined by extrapolating the steepest initial slope back to zero volume. So long as the extrapolated volume is less than 10 percent FVC, the effort is acceptable.[56-58]

The volumes expired at one and three seconds from time zero are then measured. All volumes are converted from ATPS (ambient temperature, pressure, saturated), the conditions of measurement, to BTPS (body temperature, pressure, saturated) and reported.*

The "best curve" may be taken as the maximum sum of FEV_1 and FVC, or a "best" effort may be constructed from the best features of all three curves.[55,59] FEV_1 and FEV_3 may be compared to standard normals as absolute values, as well as a proportion of forced vital capacity so that FEV_1/FVC and FEV_3/FVC are relatively normal in restriction. In obstruction, however, they will be reduced out of proportion to vital capacity, decreasing FEV_1/FVC and FEV_3/FVC. FEV_3/FVC is extremely sensitive to even mild peripheral obstruction, and a value less than 93 percent may be taken as evidence of abnormality.[57] FEV_1/FVC is less sensitive but more specific.[40] Because FEV_1 declines with age, normality or degree of abnormality should be determined from the 95 percent confidence limits of the regression rather than some fixed value.[42,44]

It has been suggested that the maximum mid-expiratory flow rate (MMFR or

---

*Conversion factor: Volume (BTPS) =

$$\text{Volume (ATPS)} \left(\frac{273 + \text{Body } T\,°C}{273 + \text{Room } T\,°C}\right) \times \left(\frac{P_{Barom} - P_{H_2O} \text{ room } T}{P_{Barom} - P_{H_2O} \text{ body } T}\right)$$

or table of factors available.[57,95]

FEF_{25-75}) is an extremely sensitive indicator of early airway obstruction.[60] MMFR is determined by marking off 25 percent and 75 percent vital capacity on the spirographic tracing and measuring the distance between those points on the volume and time axes. The resulting straight line $\Delta V/\Delta T$ expresses the flow rate over the middle of lung volume and can reflect early obstruction (Fig. 4-7B). The usefulness of the MMFR, however, is limited by the amount of scatter inherent in the measurement.

Instantaneous flow rates can be picked off as tangents to the volume-time plot, but are much more easily assessed by a flow-volume plot. The peak expiratory flow rate can be read off a flow-volume loop or determined independently with a small hand-held peak flow meter. While peak expiratory flow is affected by airway obstruction, it is also highly dependent on patient effort.[61] Again, reproducibility is a good indication of adequate patient effort (Fig. 4-9).

Maximum voluntary ventilation (MVV), or maximum breathing capacity, is another spirometric test that is extremely effort-dependent. The MVV is a measure of the maximum amount of air that a patient could be expected to move in one minute by voluntary effort. The test is actually performed with the patient standing, in a manner similar to simple spirometry, but the patient is instructed to breathe as rapidly and as deeply as possible and effort is sustained for 12 to 15 seconds; the results are multiplied by 4 or 5 to give a minute value. The spirometer used should have an integrating pen or be capable of electronically summing exhaled volume for the test period. The spirometer should have a volume response that is constant within ± 10 percent at frequencies up to 8 Hz at flow rates up to 12 L/sec over the volume range. Volume should be accurate to ± 3 percent.[55] While a crude estimate of MVV can be obtained by multiplying the FEV_1 by 30, it is preferable to directly measure MVV as part of the patient evaluation because factors such as sustainable muscle strength and

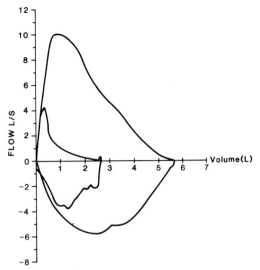

Fig. 4-9 Flow-volume loop displays essentially same information as spirogram, but is more convenient for measurement of specific flow rates. Outside: normal loop; note relative linearity of expiratory flow over lower ⅔ of lung volume. Slope corresponds to time constant of forced expiration. Inspiratory flow should at least equal expiratory flow at 50% vital capacity. Inside: loop in obstructive disease. Note reductions in peak flow, vital capacity, and flow at specific lung volumes. Compare concavity of expiratory loop with linear normal curve.

motivation may have a bearing on clinical outcome. MVV will be reduced by either obstructive or restrictive lung disease or by weakness or suboptimal effort.[62]

SPIROMETRY RESULTS AND THE
OUTCOME OF THORACOTOMY

Spirometric variables chiefly measure airflow obstruction. Since patients with obstructive airway disease are known to have a higher rate of postoperative complications than non-obstructed patients, the results of spirometric examinations have been used to predict respiratory complications of surgery. Since the natural history of chronic obstructive lung disease can be a function of spirometric variables, the assumption is further made that if the expected decline in pulmonary function due to thoracotomy or pulmonary resection is of sufficient severity, the patient is in danger of perioperative respiratory insufficiency or has a significant risk of developing cor pulmonale in the more remote future.

Clearly, retrospective studies show that patients who develop these complications have poorer preoperative function on the average than patients who escape these complications. There is general agreement that the poorer a patient's spirometric performance, the more likely respiratory complications will be.[1-5] It is more difficult to define cut-off values of pulmonary function, however, beyond which the patient is certain to encounter or escape morbidity or mortality.

Published studies tend to report the numbers of patients encountering complications with function above or below a certain level, and from these numbers some approximation of their predictive value can be derived.

VITAL CAPACITY

Vital capacity is determined by inspiratory muscle strength, pulmonary elastic recoil, and the degree of obstructive air-trapping. The predictive value of the vital capacity is based on its dependence on obstruction and on the observation that a vital capacity three times tidal volume appears necessary for an effective cough.[63] Vital capacity has been examined more as a predictor of mortality due to cardiopulmonary insufficiency rather than a predictor of complications.

Standards proposed for vital capacity as indicative of increased risk include vital capacity less than 50 percent predicted or a vital capacity less than 1.75 to 2 liters.[4,64-66] When these criteria are applied, a 33 percent incidence of respiratory failure postoperatively was found in patients with a vital capacity less than 50 percent predicted.[67] Using a vital capacity less than 70 percent predicted, Mittman was able to identify 39 percent of cardiopulmonary deaths following thoracotomy; while patients having this level of pulmonary function had a 28 percent death rate (11/39).[4] van Nostrand's data showed a 12 percent mortality with vital capacity below 2 liters; yet this criterion identified only 2/27 deaths.[68] Didolkar et al reported on 258 resections for lung cancer done at Roswell Park. They found a mean vital capacity of 65 percent predicted in their whole population. FVC in survivors, 65.6 percent, did not differ significantly from that of patients succumbing to postoperative respiratory insufficiency, 59.8 percent.[69] Gaensler likewise found the FVC to be misleading as a predictor of postoperative pulmonary function.[13] At best, an abnormal vital capacity can identify 30 to 40 percent of postoperative deaths. A patient with an abnormal vital capacity has one chance in three of complications, and a 12 to 30 percent chance of death. Mortality with a vital capacity above these cutoffs appears to run 10 to 15 percent.

FEV$_1$

FEV$_1$ is a more direct indicator of the severity of airflow obstruction. Longitudinal studies of chronic obstructive lung disease have, in general, related prognosis in terms of functional capacity and survival to the level of FEV$_1$ or its rate of decline in patients over the age of 65; and to the FEV$_1$ and the presence of cor pulmonale in patients below that age.[70,71] Since chronic obstructive lung disease often appears hand-in-hand with bronchogenic carcinoma, several authors have used an epidemiologically derived FEV$_1$ as absolute exclusions to thoracotomy or pulmonary resection for cancer on the grounds of precipitating acute or chronic respiratory failure, or cor pulmonale.

Kristersson excluded all patients with an FEV$_1$ below 1 liter, and Olsen made an FEV$_1$ less than 800 cc an absolute contraindication to pulmonary resection.[5,72] Lockwood cited an FEV$_1$ less than 1.2 liters or FEV$_1$ less than

35 percent FVC as indicative of extreme risk.[66]

When applied to patients, these limits do not appear sufficiently sensitive or specific to be absolute criteria. In van Nostrand's series, the use of these stringent criteria identified only 5 percent of deaths, and patients with this severe level of dysfunction had only a 7 percent mortality (1/15). Somewhat looser criteria appear to be more useful. Using an FEV_1 below 2 liters, 75 to 80 percent of postoperative deaths can be identified. Mortality in a group with this FEV_1 is 20 to 45 percent; while mortality with an FEV_1 above this level runs about 10 percent.[69,73]

While there is a theoretical basis for withholding thoracotomy in the face of extreme reductions in FEV_1, experience would suggest that the majority of patients operated upon in the face of this increased risk will still tolerate surgery. FEV_1, then, cannot be used as a sole criterion for determination of medical operability.

MAXIMUM VOLUNTARY VENTILATION

Maximum voluntary ventilation (MVV) is nonspecific. It is a function of restriction, obstruction, and effort on the part of the patient. Mittman suggests that the non-specificity of the MVV makes it a suitable test in preoperative pulmonary function assessment, since the outcome of surgery is as multifactorial as the MVV test.[4]

Gaensler reviewed the results of thoracotomies for tuberculosis in 460 patients. Fourteen patients died of respiratory failure, 8 within 30 days of surgery, and the rest 30 days to 6 years postoperatively. No early respiratory deaths in the series occurred in patients who had a maximum voluntary ventilation greater than 50 percent predicted, and 5 of 6 late deaths occurred in patients whose postoperative MVV was below 50 percent predicted. Postoperative dyspnea and exertional limitation were linearly related to the preoperative MVV; the poorer the initial function, the greater the ultimate compromise. He suggested that the MVV might be the best test for assessing preoperative pulmonary function.[13]

MVV has not been systematically examined as a predictor for morbidity, but four series provide information on its value as a predictor of mortality due to cardiopulmonary insufficiency. Using an MVV of less than 60 percent predicted as a cutoff, Didolkar identified 57 percent of his postoperative deaths.[69] MVV below 60 percent predicted carried a 32 percent mortality, while 90 percent of patients with a better level survived. Mittman reported on 196 thoracotomies, excluding operations involving cardiopulmonary bypass. Twenty-eight deaths occurred within six months of surgery and 24 of these were classified as cardiorespiratory.[4] An MVV below 50 percent predicted identified 46 percent of these deaths. Among patients with an MVV below 50 percent predicted, 45 percent died while 91 percent of patients with a better MVV survived. Larsen and Clifton, however, used the same cutoff for morbidity and mortality prediction and found a much poorer predictive value from the MVV. Only 27 percent of complicated cases were identified, with an 11 percent mortality among patients with an MVV below 50 percent predicted, compared with 15 percent among patients above this cutoff.[67] Boushy, using an absolute cutoff of 70 L/min, obtained more definitive results with a mortality of 25 percent for patients below 70 L/min and 8 percent for those above. He was able to identify 66 percent of the deaths with an abnormal MVV.[73]

The MVV appears to possess relatively good specificity and sensitivity when compared with other spirometric parameters. A normal MVV suggests a 10 percent risk of death or loss, and aside from Larsen and Clifton's data, an abnormal MVV suggests a risk of mortality between 25 percent and 45 percent.

MIDFLOW MEASUREMENTS

The maximum midexpiratory flow rate has been used as a test of small airways obstruction.[60] It is the only test of small airways function for which applicability to preoperative assessment has been evaluated, although one might expect that the obstruction and hypoxemia resulting from disease in small airways might have a bearing on postoperative problems such as pneumonia, atelectasis, and hypoxemia.

Gracey observed that an FEF_{25-75} less than 50 percent predicted carried an increased risk for patients undergoing a variety of surgical procedures.[14] Boushy found that the FEF_{25-75} was among the better predictors of postoperative dyspnea in his population.[73] Among the 18 of Karliner's patients for whom data is available, no patient with an FEF_{25-75} greater than 50 percent predicted had postoperative difficulty; however, only 2 of 14 with an abnormal study did, suggesting that FEF_{25-75} is highly sensitive, but rather nonspecific.[74]

PEAK FLOW

Peak flow rate is multifactorial, but primarily relates to the degree of airflow obstruction and patient effort.

Stein twice reported that the peak expiratory flow rate (PEFR) successfully discriminated between patients with postoperative respiratory complications and those who did well following a variety of surgical procedures. Sixty-six percent of patients (20/30) with an abnormal PEFR had postoperative respiratory difficulty, while only 1 of 30 with a normal PEFR had any such problems.[75,76]

MULTIPLE INDICES

In an attempt to increase the resolving power of single spirometric indices, several authors have proposed multiple test indices. In 1956, Miller et al suggested that neither the FEV_1 nor the FVC alone were sufficient

discriminators of the likelihood of postoperative respiratory insufficiency. They proposed a "single breath test" based on plotting the $FEV_{0.5}/FVC$ as a function of FVC. By so doing, they defined a four-quadrant scheme which described patients as restricted, obstructed, combined, or normal. They then prospectively studied 24 patients who underwent a series of unspecified surgical procedures. The incidence of postoperative respiratory failure defined a hyperbolic curve of function above which complications were rarely seen and defined this as a line of prohibitive function.[77] The $FEV_{0.5}$, however, reflects effort dependence at least as much as intrinsic mechanical properties of the lung and is not routinely used as a measure of pulmonary obstruction.[57] Redding and Yakaitis modified Miller's four-quadrant approach by plotting FEV_1 on the ordinate (Fig. 4-10).[78]

Meneely and Ferguson further refined the test by grading degrees of risk.[79] The four-quadrant diagram does yield a clear picture of the nature and degree of dysfunction observed in preoperative spirometric as-

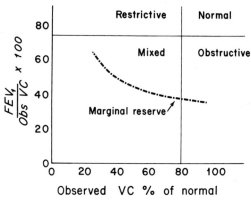

Fig. 4-10 Miller quadrant system for categorizing pulmonary function, as modified by Redding and Yakaitis.[78] Marginal reserve line denotes the combination of restrictive and obstructive defects that place patients at increased risk for postthoracotomy complications. Dot indicates values for a patient with obstructive lung disease with apparently adequate respiratory reserve. Hodgkin JE, Dines DE, Didier EP: Mayo Clinic Proceedings 48:114–118,1973. Reproduced with permission of publisher.

sessment, but it is an imperfect predictor of respiratory distress. Hodgkin reported a case of postoperative respiratory failure in a patient who clearly had "good' preoperative pulmonary function, and Williams and Brenowitz reported the results of 16 procedures in patients with "prohibitive" pulmonary function.[80,81] Among 7 patients undergoing thoracotomy, 6 had lobectomies. Postoperative respiratory failure was encountered in 3 of the 6, but all 3 survived to leave the hospital despite a preoperative FEV_1 as low as 390 ml.[81]

Bronchodilators

Recent studies have pointed out that the overall prognosis of chronic obstructive lung disease is better related to the level of spirometric function *after* bronchodilator therapy rather than the baseline function.[70,71] The larger the reversible component of airway obstruction and the smaller the irreversible component, the better the patient's outlook for survival and function.

Reversibility of airway obstruction is usually assessed in the pulmonary function laboratory by having the patient inhale an aerosolized bronchodilator and repeating spirometric tests. Commonly used bronchodilators include 0.04 to 0.3 mg isoproterenol; 1.3 to 2 mg metaproterenol; 350 μg isoetharine; racemic epinephrine; or 200 mg salbutamol.[82]

Properly done, bronchodilation begins as the patient is instructed to breathe down to residual volume and then begin a slow inspiration. At FRC the patient is told to place the mouthpiece in his mouth and actuate two puffs from the inhaler, continue the inhalation to TLC, then hold the breath for 2 or 3 seconds before exhaling.[57,83]

Post-bronchodilator spirometries are usually performed 15 to 30 minutes after bronchodilator inhalation.[57,84] Interpreting bronchodilator response is complicated by a number of factors. Because a certain amount of coordination is necessary, poor compliance, performance, or timing on the part of the patient may result in the delivery of a smaller dose of bronchodilator than thought. Each bronchodilator possesses different potencies, sites of action, duration of action, and time of peak action. Patients may have had a recent dose of bronchodilator medication prior to testing. If the patient is fully bronchodilated due to medication, no further response to bronchodilator will be seen.[85]

It has been customary to regard a 15 percent improvement in spirometric parameters as a significant response to bronchodilators. However, statistical analysis suggests that "significance" should be expressed as the absolute value of the change divided by the standard deviation of the pre-bronchodilator trials—when the change exceeds the 95 percent confidence interval ($\pm$ 1.64SD) it is regarded as significant. Using this approach it was found that tests such as airway conductance and MMFR showed the greatest post-bronchodilator change, but when compared with their standard deviations, FEV_1 and FVC were the most valuable indices of bronchodilator response.[86] Ramsdell and Tisi, however, noted that 46 of 241 patients showed a significant response to bronchodilators, consisting of a reduction in FRC, suggesting less air-trapping, or a fall in airway resistance, even when flow parameters did not change.[87]

Rather than relying on the response to a single administration of a bronchodilator, prognostic information as well as therapy may be gained from a program of respiratory therapy and bronchodilator treatment preoperatively. Gracey et al treated 157 chronic lung patients with a program of chest physiotherapy, smoking cessation, and bronchodilators, assessed pulmonary function before and after the program, and compared the response to therapy with the incidence of postoperative pulmonary complications following a variety of surgical procedures. They reported that FEF_{25-75} and MVV failed to show a significant increase in patients with an adverse outcome from surgery, while improving significantly in patients with a benign course. Arterial PCO_2 fell only in patients who went on to have a successful outcome, while dead space and alveolar-arterial oxygen gradient showed no significant change in either group.[14]

Lung Volumes

It is not possible to directly measure total lung capacity, functional residual capacity, or residual volume from the spirogram. Several methods are available for determining these volumes.

PLETHYSMOGRAPHY

Body plethysmography is considered the approach of choice for measuring functional residual capacity.[56] Determination of thoracic gas volume is determined by Boyle's law which states that in a closed system the product of pressure and volume is a constant. The patient is placed in a box of known volume and breathes through a mouthpiece. Pressure in the box and pressure at the patient's mouth are measured. In order to minimize the effects of airway resistance the patient is asked to pant at a high frequency (1/sec) and small tidal volume.

When the larynx is open, and air flow is minimal, pressure at the mouth is equal to pressure in the lungs. When the mouthpiece is temporarily occluded, the subject alternately compresses and expands the gas volume in his thorax. That small volume change results in a change in the pressure in the box. If box pressure and mouth pressure are displayed on the X and Y axes of an oscilloscope, a straight line results with a slope of

$$\frac{\Delta \text{ box pressure}}{\Delta \text{ mouth pressure}}.$$

Since the pressure-volume characteristics of the box are known, the slope becomes

$$\frac{\Delta \text{ volume}}{\Delta \text{ pressure}}.$$

Boyle's law, $PV=K$, can be differentiated with respect to pressure to yield $V = -P \, dV/dP$. P is atmospheric pressure, and dV/dP is the slope of the volume-pressure trace on the oscilloscope. V is the volume of gas in the thorax at the time of measurement. If the operator is able to consistently occlude the mouthpiece at end-expiration, an accurate determination of functional residual capacity results.[88,89] More recent evidence, however, suggests that besides being prone to artifact due to intestinal gas, plethysmographic lung volume measurements may be artifactually biased by airway closure or uneven ventilation, and yield overestimates of lung volume.[90,91]

GAS DILUTION LUNG VOLUME

Two methods for determining FRC by gas dilution are available. In the closed system method, the subject breathes a 12 percent helium–20 percent oxygen mixture in air of known volume until the measured concentration of helium reaches a stable equilibrium. According to the laws of conservation of matter:

V initial $\times$ F$_{\text{He}}$ initial = V final $\times$ F$_{\text{He}}$ final.

The final volume includes both the volume of gas in the patient's lungs plus the initial volume of the system which contained the helium. Subtracting the initial from the final volume yields the patient's lung volume. If the patient is carefully turned in and out of the measuring system at end-expiration, lung volume will be FRC. A normal subject will equilibrate with helium in 2 to 3 minutes, but an obstructed patient may not reach equilibrium for 8 minutes or more. If equilibrium is not reached, the final helium concentration will be overestimated and the resulting FRC determination biased low. Helium dilution lung volumes will also fail to measure gas in the lung hat is not communicating with patent airways; for example, large bullae in emphysema, or in the event of airway closure. For this reason, there is an increasing discrepancy between plethysmographic and helium lung volumes as the severity of airflow obstruction increases.[56,57,92-94,97]

In the open system method, the subject is asked to breathe 100 percent O_2 for several minutes. Oxygen breathing will displace the air in the lungs, which has a known concentration of 79.6 percent N_2. Exhaled N_2 concentration is monitored and all expired gas is collected until the concentration of exhaled nitrogen reaches zero or an asymptote. The volume of expired gas and its nitrogen concentration are measured. According to the conservation of matter, all expired nitrogen collected came originally from the lungs, which are now nitrogen-free. Therefore, by analogy with the helium dilution method, 79.6 percent nitrogen in air × lung volume = volume exhaled × fractional concentration exhaled nitrogen.

When the expired N_2 concentration asymptotes at a concentration greater than zero, that value should be subtracted from the room air concentration of N_2 on the left hand side of the equation.

The open circuit nitrogen method is subject to the same errors as the helium dilution method and suffers from serious methodologic as well as physiologic drawbacks. Nitrogen is a difficult gas to measure accurately because it is present in high concentration in room air, and is not well suited for mass spectrometry because it has the same molecular weight as carbon dioxide. Washing out residual nitrogen with 100 percent O_2 may cause alveolar collapse and airway closure, artifactually increasing the underestimate of lung volume.[10,94,95]

All three methods, plethysmography, helium dilution, and nitrogen washout measure resting end-tidal lung volume, FRC. When the spirometric volume between FRC and minimum end-respiratory volume, the expiratory reserve volume (ERV), is subtracted from FRC, residual volume (RV) is defined. Adding vital capacity (VC) to RV defines total lung capacity or TLC (Fig. 4-8).

RADIOGRAPHIC MEASUREMENT OF TOTAL LUNG CAPACITY

An acceptable alternative is to measure TLC directly from a standard 6-foot PA and lateral chest radiograph. The lung can be modelled as an elliptical cone and its dimensions at several heights measured. Multiplying heights of these slices by their area and adding them together yields the total volume of the thoracic cage. Subtracting corrections for the heart, diaphragm, lung tissue, and pulmonary blood volume yields the gas volume of the lung at TLC. As long as the magnification factor of the film is standardized the method is accurate, although not quite as reproducible as the physiologic methods.[55,96,97] The reliability of the radiographic TLC is limited, as well, by patient effort in taking a maximum inspiration.

From a radiographic TLC, subtracting VC yields RV, and the addition of ERV yields FRC.

LUNG VOLUMES AS PROGNOSTIC INDICES

Since residual volumes and total lung capacity in turn determine vital capacity, which in turn has an influence on FEV_1; and the ratio of residual volume to total lung capacity is an index of air-trapping and therefore of obstruction, RV and RV/TLC have been examined as predictors of postoperative difficulty. Boushy found a statistically significant difference in RV between complicated and uncomplicated resections.[73] In Mittman's series an RV/TLC over 40 percent identified 84 percent of his deaths. An abnormal ratio at this level carried a 30 percent mortality compared with 7 percent when the RV/TLC was below this level. If RV/TLC was greater than 50 percent, he found a 36 percent mortality.[4] Stein, by contrast, found no significant difference in RV/TLC between surgical patients encountering respiratory complications and those who did not.[75,76]

Lockwood attempted to improve selective resolution by using RV and RV/TLC as indices of airflow obstruction and combining them with FEV_1. By setting criteria of FEV_1 at less than 65.5 percent vital capacity, RV greater than 1.5 liters, and RV/TLC greater than 29.5 percent, he was able to generate a fairly sensitive index for predicting respiratory complications to thoracotomy. He was able to identify 41/81 (54 percent) of patients with complications. Because he matched his 81 complicated patients with an equal number of uncomplicated cases, he was able to demonstrate a 76 percent complication rate when these indices were abnormal.[65,66] If, however, tests of this specificity and sensitivity are applied to a population with a 30 percent rate of complication such as other series report, we find an expected complication rate of 42 percent when abnormal and 22 percent when normal. While sensitive, Lockwood's triple index may not be sufficiently specific for routine clinical use. The additional resolution gained by combining these measurements appears too small to justify the additional effort involved to use a multifactorial index.

Gas Exchange: Blood Gases

OXYGEN

Arterial blood gas measurements consist of the partial pressures of oxygen and carbon dioxide as well as the pH. The composition of arterial PO_2 is a consequence of three key factors: inspired PO_2, mixed venous PO_2, and the distribution of ventilation-perfusion ratios throughout the lung. Mixed venous PO_2 is chiefly determined by oxygen uptake ($\dot{V}O_2$), and modified by cardiac output, arterial oxygen content, and the shape of the oxyhemoglobin dissociation curve. Ventilation-perfusion distributions are determined by the matching of alveolar ventilation to pulmonary capillary blood flow and can be thought of as consisting of populations of alveoli

which are perfused but not ventilated (shunt, $\dot{V}/\dot{Q} = 0$); alveoli which are under-ventilated with respect to their blood flow ($1 > \dot{V}/\dot{Q} > 0$); alveoli whose ventilation is matched to their blood flow ($\dot{V}/\dot{Q} = 1$); alveoli which are ventilated in excess of their blood flow ($\infty > \dot{V}/\dot{Q} > 1$); and alveoli which are ventilated but not perfused ($\dot{V}/\dot{Q} = \infty$, dead space). The arterial PO_2 results from the average oxygen content of blood, leaving each of these alveoli weighted by their perfusion. The final mixed arterial oxygen content will be most influenced by those alveoli with the highest blood flow. Because of the sigmoid shape of the oxyhemoglobin dissociation curve, alveoli with low ventilation-perfusion ratios have a greater effect on lowering arterial PO_2 than alveoli with a higher PaO_2 have in raising it.[98]

The normal PaO_2 declines as a function of age and posture because of increasing airway closure. In a patient aged 70, a normal PaO_2 may be as low as 63 mmHg.[99]

Mechanisms contributing to clinical hypoxemia at rest include shunt, $\dot{V}/\dot{Q}$ maldistribution, or hypoventilation. Diffusion impairment, once thought to produce resting hypoxemia in lung disease via "alveolar capillary block," is not a significant factor at rest. Alveolar capillary block has been shown to be largely a consequence of $\dot{V}/\dot{Q}$ maldistribution or a low cardiac output.[98,100] Nonetheless, diffusion impairment may produce hypoxemia during exercise when the shortened transit time of erythrocytes through the pulmonary capillary bed is insufficient to permit partial pressure equilibration between alveolus and pulmonary capillary.

Shunt hypoxemia is minimally, or totally, unresponsive to an increased FIO_2. Conditions producing intrapulmonary right-to-left shunting are exemplified by acute pneumonia, adult respiratory distress syndrome, and pulmonary alveolar proteinosis; all conditions characterized by the filling of alveoli by water, pus, or proteinaceous material. $\dot{V}/\dot{Q}$ hypoxemia arises when the ventilation to well-perfused alveoli is reduced. Arterial PO_2 in $\dot{V}/\dot{Q}$ hypoxemia is responsive to an increased, inspired oxygen tension (FIO_2) in a fairly predictable manner.[101] The majority of clinical hypoxemia, particularly in obstructive lung disease, is due to ventilation-perfusion maldistribution.

Although most organ systems are affected, the primary adverse effect of clinical hypoxemia is on the heart, and particularly on the right ventricle via a hypoxia-mediated increase in pulmonary vascular resistance. Subject to modifiers such as acidosis, restriction of the pulmonary vascular bed by disease processes, and the swings of intrathoracic pressure, appreciable reduction in PaO_2 below 50 to 60 mmHg provokes active constriction of vascular smooth muscle in the pulmonary arterial bed. In order to maintain cardiac output against increased pulmonary vascular resistance, right-sided pressures must increase. The increase in right ventricular pressures and consequent elevation in stroke work is compensated by right ventricular hypertrophy. The adaptive capacity of the right ventricle is limited, and ultimately right ventricular strain or failure ensues. The syndrome of right ventricular dysfunction in the setting of pulmonary hypertension due to respiratory disease is termed cor pulmonale.[102, 103]

The presence of cor pulmonale is an extremely adverse factor in the prognosis of chronic obstructive lung disease. In patients under 65 years of age with severe obstruction, the median survival time is reduced from 5–9 years to 2–3 years in the presence of cor pulmonale.[70,71] Under these circumstances, the patients' life expectancy may be shortened more from underlying medical disease than from the disease for which surgery is contemplated.

Where directly examined, preoperative PaO_2 at rest was found to be a relatively minor predictor of postoperative outcome. In Mittman's series, abnormal oxygen saturation carried a 36 percent mortality rate as compared to a 17 percent mortality rate in patients with a normal saturation; the cutoff level is not specified.[4] Milledge and Nunn studied 12 consecutive patients with chronic obstructive lung disease presenting to a general surgery service. In the face of simple hypoxemia, they noted no increased complications after surgery. Oxygen therapy was all that was required.[104] Boushy found no difference in mean PaO_2 between complicated and uncomplicated resections for lung cancer; and Gracey reported no significant difference in the rate of postoperative pulmonary complications based on baseline PaO_2, or on the response of PaO_2 to a program of preoperative preparation.[14, 73]

CARBON DIOXIDE

Arterial PCO_2 is a function of CO_2 output ($\dot{V}_{CO_2}$) and alveolar ventilation. Alveolar ventilation is determined by minute ventilation and by dead space ventilation; which, in turn, is governed by $\dot{V}/\dot{Q}$ relationships. Any condition tending to reduce pulmonary capillary blood flow more than ventilation will produce an increase in dead space, and force either an increase in minute ventilation to defend alveolar ventilation or a rise in $PaCO_2$ and consequent respiratory acidosis.[98]

The degree to which minute ventilation can be increased is limited by the work of breathing. The work of breathing is a function of the compliance of the lung and airway resistance as well as the rate and depth of breathing. Normally, the pattern of breathing adopted is that which involves the least work of breathing. Since restrictive lung disease involves compliance more than resistance and is influenced by tidal volume, the restricted patient tends to breathe rapidly at small tidal volumes. Conversely, the obstructive picture is dominated by airway resistance, so the obstructed patient breathes at slower rates with deeper breaths.[105] Despite compensatory adjustments, however, the patient is unable to sustain any more than 55 percent of his maximal effort for any length of time. When the demands of $\dot{V}_{CO_2}$ or dead space require a work of breathing greater than 55 percent maximum, muscular fatigue and respiratory muscle pump failure may ensue.[106] The consequence of respiratory muscle pump failure is hypercapnia and respiratory acidosis.

Another determinant of alveolar ventilation is respiratory drive. The ventilatory control of $PaCO_2$ is governed by chemoreceptor neurons in the medulla which respond to CSF pH. Primary diseases of the CNS or secondary influences may blunt the CO_2 response and cause the medullary CO_2 receptor to reset for a higher level $PaCO_2$. Modifiers of ventilatory drive include increased work of breathing, hypothyroidism, metabolic alkalosis, sedative drugs, and starvation.[107,108]

Individuals can compensate for hypercapnia by increasing renal retention of bicarbonate. Metabolic compensation can allow a patient to tolerate levels of $PaCO_2$ which would otherwise cause lethal respiratory acidosis.[36] Even with compensation, however, the presence of hypercapnia suggests that the demands placed on the lung by disease are more than the respiratory apparatus can handle.

It has been suggested that CO_2 retention becomes manifest in COPD when FEV_1 falls below 800cc to 1 liter.[109] For this reason, that lower limit of FEV_1 has been used as an arbitrary criteria for exclusion for resectional surgery. Likewise, the presence of CO_2 retention, defined as a $PaCO_2 > 45$ mmHg, has been used as an exclusion for resection or as a warning of postoperative respiratory difficulty.[1,5] In view of the fact that thoracic or upper abdominal surgery will further impair an already compromised respiratory system, and pain killers may further blunt a defective drive, hypercapnia should pose a significant risk factor in thoracic surgery.

Among Stein's 100 consecutive general surgery patients, 5 were found to have clinically significant hypercapnia ($PaCO_2 > 45$). All 5 had a complicated course postoperatively, leading him to conclude that CO_2 re-

tention should be a contraindication "to all but life-saving operations."[75,76] In Milledge and Nunn's series, patients with hypoxemia and airflow obstruction postoperatively did well, but 2 of 4 with hypercapnia as well required prolonged mechanical ventilation postoperatively. They felt that arterial blood gases, particularly $PaCO_2$, were the most important preoperative determinants of prognosis.[104] Other authors note no difference in preoperative $PaCO_2$ between complicated and uncomplicated thoracotomies, but fail to state the levels involved or whether patients were excluded from surgery on the basis of their $PaCO_2$.[73,110]

Diffusing Capacity

The diffusing capacity for carbon monoxide (CO) has been used as an indicator of suitability for pulmonary resection and as a predictor of postoperative pulmonary hypertension and cor pulmonale.

The diffusing capacity for carbon monoxide (D_LCO) has been divided into membrane (D_M) and pulmonary vascular components (Vc).[111]

$$1/D_L = 1/D_M + 1/\Theta V_C$$

Membrane diffusing capacity is a function of alveolar surface area and thickness of the distance between the alveolar epithelium and red cells within an alveolar capillary. Θ is the uptake of CO by a single red cell. Multiplication by capillary blood volume, Vc, gives the red cell uptake of CO for the entire pulmonary capillary bed. Normally, the resistance to CO uptake is about equally divided between the membrane and vascular components, but disease processes can alter either component or both. By determining D_LCO at different alveolar PO_2, it is possible to separate out Dm from Vc as the cause of a reduced D_LCO, but only when the disease processes are truly isolated (Fig. 4-11).

It has been suggested that a reduction of

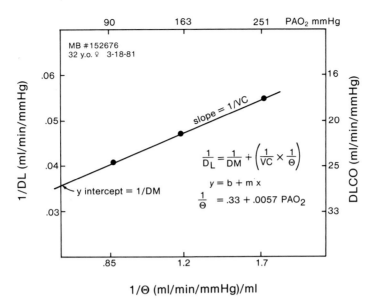

Fig. 4-11 Roughton-Forster plot separating diffusing capacity into membrane and pulmonary capillary components. DLCO measured at three different PaO$_2$. Inverse of DL plotted against $1/\theta$, yields straight-line plot with y-intercept equal to inverse of membrane diffusing capacity and slope equal to inverse of pulmonary capillary blood volume. Example is from patient with recurrent pulmonary emboli. Membrane diffusing capacity is normal, capillary volume reduced by 50 percent.

diffusing capacity to less than 50 percent of predicted normal has an adverse prognostic significance in pulmonary resection.[112] It is assumed that this reduction results from a significant diminution of the pulmonary vascular bed and that any further reduction would represent a significant risk for pulmonary hypertension and for cor pulmonale; but unless the reduction can be clearly attributed to a decreased Vc, the assumption is weak.

All measurements of D$_L$CO depend on delivering a small concentration of CO to alveoli, allowing time for CO uptake, and then measuring exhaled CO. Any such measurements are biased by the ability of the lung to ventilate and to deliver CO to alveoli. Inequalities of ventilation will reduce the measured D$_L$CO but are seen as reductions in Dm rather than V$_C$ when a Roughton-Forster plot is drawn.[113]

SINGLE BREATH D$_L$CO

Two methods for determining CO diffusing capacity are commonly available, single breath and steady state. The single breath or breath-holding method is considered the approach of choice for measuring D$_L$CO because it is somewhat less sensitive to inhomogeneities in ventilation than the steady state method.[55,93] The single breath D$_L$CO assumes that the rate of CO uptake is proportional to the alveolar concentration of CO when inhaled. If a small concentration of CO is inhaled along with a nonabsorbed gas such as helium, the volume of distribution can be calculated from the dilution of helium and the amount of CO taken up calculated.[56,57] The single breath diffusing capacity cannot be performed in patients who are too dyspneic to hold their breath for 10 seconds, or have a vital capacity too small to allow for a sufficient expirate to clear the patient's and apparatus dead space and allow collection of a sample of sufficient size to measure.[114,115]

STEADY STATE D$_L$CO

The steady state diffusing capacity is suitable for patients who are unable to perform the single breath test. CO uptake in the steady state test is defined as the product of minute ventilation and the inspired-expired CO difference. CO uptake divided by alveolar PCO defines the diffusing capacity. There is difficulty in identifying alveolar PCO in patients with uneven ventilation.[114] Two approaches have developed to estimate alveolar PCO. The Filley method uses a determination of dead space based on carbon dioxide.[116] This method carries the disadvantage of requiring arterial puncture, and it is likely that the dead spaces for carbon dioxide and carbon monoxide are not equal.[117] The Bates method is based on the assumption that end-tidal gas is a reliable estimate of alveolar gas.[118] The Bates method will be reliable only to the extent to which that assumption is correct. Both methods will be biased by uneven ventilation in lung disease and lead to underestimates of diffusing capacity.[93]

CLINICAL EXPERIENCE

In Mittman's series, a diffusing capacity (method unspecified) below 15 ml/min/mmHg carried an 18 percent mortality; while a D$_L$CO above this level was associated with only a 7 percent mortality.[4] Boushy found a significant difference in D$_L$CO patients tolerating and not tolerating thoracotomy.[73] Levels were not specified. Karliner, however, observed that patients with D$_L$CO as low as 28 percent of predicted underwent uncomplicated resections and were doing well up to 6 months postoperatively.[74] The predictive value of diffusing capacity measurements appears limited, therefore.

Exercise

A person who has marginal but compensated cardiopulmonary function at rest may be thrown into a decompensated state when stressed. Because surgery itself is a stress state and because pulmonary resection can be expected to diminish ventilatory reserve, the idea of testing a patient's ventilatory reserve by exercise arose. Most such assessments were informal and consisted of having patients walk up one or two flights of stairs while observed by the surgeon. If the patient was able to walk up two flights of stairs without severe dyspnea, he was considered a good surgical risk. Less than two flights or severe dyspnea suggested an appreciable element of risk, and a patient who could not manage one flight of stairs was deemed an unacceptable risk.[68,119]

Semb et al utilized a more formal exercise protocol in which they exercised patients on a cycle ergometer at a level of 500 kg (about 51 watts) over one minute, measuring $\dot{V}_{CO_2}$, $\dot{V}_{O_2}$, tidal volume and minute ventilation before, during, and after exercise. The authors noted that normal subjects returned to their resting CO_2 output in 2 to 5 minutes, and post-pneumonectomy patients took 8 to 10 minutes to return to baseline. Patients with a recovery time of 15 minutes or more were found not to tolerate further reduction of cardiopulmonary function.[120]

The most formal analysis of the predictive value of exercise for pneumonectomy was done by Reichel.[110] After excluding patients with known angina or abnormal electrocardiograms, he placed pneumonectomy candidates on a treadmill and had them walk 2 minutes each at staged levels of speed and elevation. The entire test lasted 14 minutes and reached a work output of approximately 185 watts for a 70 kg man.* Data are pre-

---

* Work = speed (m/sec) × wt (kg) × (1 + [9.80665 sin (arc tan % Grade)]).

sented for 25 patients; eleven completed the entire protocol. Among 12 patients completing a minimum of 12 minutes and 163 watts, there were no deaths and no cardiopulmonary complications. Seven patients were unable to complete more than 4 minutes and 63 watts, a level comparable to Semb's protocol. In this group there were 3 cardiopulmonary deaths; 3 survivors after complications; and one patient with a benign course. Four of six patients with intermediate levels of performance escaped complications, and there were no deaths.[110] Despite the small population recorded, the separation and prediction was striking enough that the Reichel test has gained wide popularity for preoperative assessment and is the only protocol published to exceed 90 percent sensitivity.

Once again, failure to pass an exercise study denoted only an increased risk rather than an absolute contraindication to intervention. van Nostrand emphasized that point in reporting the outcome of the stair-climbing test in 91 patients about to undergo pneumonectomy. Looking at patients who were able to tolerate climbing two flights of stairs with "minimal" dyspnea, 7 of 63 died (11%); while among patients failing to reach this level 4 of 28 died (14%). The added 3 percent mortality is not significantly different from that of patients successfully completing the protocol. But, if patients unable to climb two flights of stairs are noted, it is found that 2 of 4 (50%) died; only 9 of 87 (10%) patients managing two flights died, giving this test a specificity of 98 percent.[68] The close agreement between Reichel's formal study and van Nostrand's more traditional approach is consistent with a recent British study which measured work output on stair climbing in a normal population and a group of chronic bronchitics. They found an average work output for the patient group of 66 watts and correlated that output linearly with FEV_1 [work (watts) = 26.6 FEV − 1 (L) + 19.28]. Using this regression, the critical level in Reichel's study corresponded to a post-bronchodilator FEV_1 of about 1700cc.[122]

More rigorous exercise protocols have been designed which allow noninvasive quantitation of maximum work output, the cardiopulmonary response to work and a statement as to whether cardiac, pulmonary, or general fitness factors limit cardiopulmonary reserve.[121,123] The addition of arterial blood gas sampling allows a determination of dead space with exercise and the ability to follow arterial oxygenation (the latter can be done noninvasively with an ear oximeter or transcutaneous oxygen sensor; also, a transcutaneous $PaCO_2$ electrode has become available). An increase in dead space is a good, although not necessarily sensitive, indicator of pulmonary vascular compromise.[124,125] Exercise desaturation can be due to diffusion limitation, worsening ventilation-perfusion relationships, or to a limited cardiac reserve. Finally, a pulmonary artery catheter can be inserted and a patient exercised under hemodynamic monitoring allowing the physician to identify the patient who develops pulmonary hypertension under minimal stress. Like Mittman's assessment of the MVV, exercise testing may owe its utility in preoperative assessment to its attention to the *integrated* output of cardiopulmonary function, but offering the additional advantage of separate assessment of cardiac and pulmonary function.[4]

Circulation

If pneumonia and respiratory failure represent the largest group of postoperative complications in thoracic surgery, the second most common group of problems involves the circulatory system. Twenty to forty percent of postoperative deaths can be ascribed to myocardial infarction, dysrhythmia, pulmonary edema, pulmonary embolism, or progressive congestive heart failure.[126] The ASA physical status scale is somewhat vague, but the graded classifications correlate fairly well with overall surgical mortality. Goldman et al., however, noted that the ASA criteria were better predictors of non-cardiac rather than cardiac mortality.[127] In order to better define the cardiac risk of surgery, they prospectively studied 1001 patients over 40 years of age undergoing a major surgical procedure requiring general anesthesia. There were 19 cardiac fatalities, and 39 life-threatening but non-fatal cardiac complications including myocardial infarction, pulmonary edema, and ventricular tachycardia. Cardiac deaths represented 32 percent (10 of 59) of all mortality.

Nine factors were identified as significant predictors of cardiac outcome. By assigning point values to these factors, a cardiac risk index was generated. They identified a "moderate risk" group with 13 to 25 points in whom they recommended further medical evaluation and a "high risk" group with more than 26 points (Table 4-1). Ten of 18 patients identified as Class IV by the Goldman index suffered cardiac deaths, while 974 of 983 patients in Classes I to III (99%) survived. The 53 percent sensitivity and 99 percent specificity for cardiac death represented a substantial predictive improvement over the ASA criteria's 35 percent sensitivity and 89 percent specificity as a cardiac mortality predictor.

The most important risk factors in Goldman's system were found to be an S3 gallop or jugular venous distention, and a history of myocardial infarction in the previous six months. Somewhat less important but still significant risks were electrocardiographic rhythms other than sinus or premature atrial contractions, or more than 5 ventricular ectopic beats per minute. Other risks included age over 70 years, aortic stenosis, thoracic or abdominal surgery, poor hepatic, respiratory, or renal function, or an emergency operation. Insignificant variables for cardiac mortality included hypertension, diabetes, smoking, peripheral atherosclerosis, stable angina, old myocardial infarction (> 6

Table 4-1
Computation of the Cardiac Risk Index.

Criteria*	"Points"
1. History	
(a) Age > 70 yr	5
(b) MI in previous 6 mo	10
2. Physical examination:	
(a) S_3 gallop or JVD	11
(b) Important VAS	3
3. Electrocardiogram:	
(a) Rhythm other than sinus or PAC's on last preoperative ECG	7
(b) > 5 PVC's/min documented at any time before operation	7
4. General status:	
PO_2 < 60 or PCO_2 > 50 mm Hg, K < 3.0 or HCO_3 < 20 meq/liter, BUN > 50 or C_R > 3.0 mg/dl, abnormal SGOT, signs of chronic liver disease or patient bed ridden from noncardiac causes	3
5. Operation:	
(a) Intraperitoneal, intrathoracic or aortic operation	3
(b) Emergency operation	4
Total possible	53 points

* MI denotes myocardial infarction, JVD jugular-vein distention, VAS valvular aortic stenosis. PAC's premature atrial contractions, ECG electrocardiogram, PVC's premature ventricular contractions, PO_2 partial pressure of oxygen, PCO_2 partial pressure of carbon dioxide, K potassium, HCO_3 bicarbonate, BUN blood urea nitrogen, C_R creatinine, & SGOT serum glutamic oxalacetic transaminase.

Golden L, Caldera DL, Nussbaum SR et al: Multifactorial index of cardiac risk in noncardiac surgical procedures. Reprinted by permission of the New England Journal of Medicine. 297:848, 1977.

months remote), mitral valve disease, bundle branch blocks, and congestive heart failure in the absence of physical findings (determined in their series by an elevated CVP). ST and T-wave abnormalities were likewise found to be insignificant.

Since congestive heart failure is treatable and ventricular dysrhythmias are to some degree preventable, Goldman et al strongly advised dealing directly with the risk factors before attempting surgery and delaying all but the most pressing operations.[15,127]

van Nostrand similarly found that electrocardiographic (ECG) abnormalities were able to identify 53 percent of his postoperative deaths from all causes with a 10 percent death rate among patients with a normal ECG. Among patients with nonspecific ST and T-wave changes, conduction defects, old ischemia or infarct, or a strain pattern, 15 of 69 or 22 percent died. Noteworthy is a 50 percent mortality (2/4) in the face of a right ventricular strain pattern.[68] Among Karliner's pneumonectomies for bronchogenic carcinoma, an abnormal ECG carried a 44 percent mortality (4/9), while patients with a normal ECG had an 11 percent death rate. Abnormalities included nonspecific ST and T-wave changes, P wave abnormalities, axis deviation, atrial fibrillation, left ventricular hypertrophy and bundle branch block.[74] Mittman attributed great importance to an abnormal electrocardiogram. He was able to identify 21 of 28 deaths (sensitivity 75%) by electrocardiographic abnormalities. Mortality among patients with an abnormal ECG was 26 percent (24/80) while only 6 percent of patients with a normal ECG died. He found the highest mortality among patients with nonspecific abnormalities; 12 of 26 (46%). Mittman stated that together with an MVV less than 50 percent predicted, an abnormal ECG identified 64 percent (18/28) of all cardiorespiratory deaths in his entire series; a sensitivity comparable to that of Goldman, van Nostrand, and Didolkar who identified 66 percent of their operative deaths among patients undergoing resections for bronchogenic carcinoma.[4,15,68,69] Among patients with an abnormal electrocardiogram 22 percent (25/114) died while only 9 percent (13/130) of patients with a normal electrocardiogram died.[69] Several authors, however, report no significant differences in the electrocardiogram between patients surviving or failing to survive thoracotomy.[67,73,110]

These data together suggest that the Goldman index is a moderately sensitive indicator of cardiac risk. A Class IV rating carries a better than even chance of cardiac death, while a lower rating suggests an overall 1 percent mortality. For thoracic operations, electrocardiographic abnormality is a more sensitive but less specific indicator of overall prognosis. Electrocardiographic abnormalities suggest a 20 to 25 percent mortality, while a 5 to 10 percent mortality can be expected in the presence of a normal electrocardiogram.

PULMONARY ARTERY PRESSURE

As the medical management of chest diseases improves and more prolonged survivals from pulmonary resections are noted, iatrogenic cor pulmonale has become a serious problem. In one autopsy series 71 of 95 tuberculosis patients showed evidence of cor pulmonale manifested by right ventricular hypertrophy and dilatation.[64]

It is understood that the cor pulmonale resulted from elevated pulmonary artery pressures and that pulmonary artery pressures were in turn determined by pulmonary vascular resistance. Riley et al demonstrated pulmonary hypertension on exercise in patients with emphysema and suggested that the elevated pressure and resistance arose from a reduction in the pulmonary vascular bed.[128]

The pulmonary circulation has been found to act as a low pressure, high capacitance circuit which is capable of handling increased blood flow by recruitment of vessels that are normally unperfused. The ability to recruit allows the lung to defend against hypertension due to increasing blood flow by reducing overall resistance. Capillary recruitment allows a considerable circulatory reserve before increased flow causes pulmonary hypertension. This reserve is eroded in chronic lung disease by primary destruction of pulmonary capillaries as in emphysema or vasculitis; by obstruction of pulmonary capillaries as in recurrent pulmonary emboli; or by increased pulmonary vascular tone or medial hypertrophy as might result from hypoxemic lung diseases or from chronic left ventricular failure. The resting circulation assumes an increasing state of recruitment.

When the recruitable capillary reserve is limited, the patient may or may not show elevated pulmonary artery pressures at rest, depending on resting pulmonary vascular resistance. During exercise, however, cardiac output increases and, since the patient is no longer able to reduce pulmonary vascular resistance by further recruitment, pulmonary arterial pressure rises. With progressive disease, the remaining circulation becomes sufficiently distended so that resting pulmonary hypertension becomes evident. With prolonged pulmonary hypertension, right ventricular hypertrophy and dilatation, failure and cor pulmonale follow.

If reduction of the pulmonary vascular bed by disease produces pulmonary hypertension, it is clear that further reductions imposed by pulmonary resectional surgery can represent a serious contraindication to surgery. Animal experiments and theoretical considerations suggest that, in the normal individual, 50 to 60 percent of the total lung volume can be removed before pulmonary hypertension results.[129]

These theoretical concerns are borne out by the development of pulmonary hypertension and cor pulmonale perioperatively or at some time remote from the initial resection in a number of operated patients.[130,131] With the development of clinical cardiac catheterization, surgeons have begun to study the pulmonary circulation in operative patients.

Semb noted three categories of pulmonary artery (PA) pressure among his tuberculosis patients. "Normals" had a pulmonary artery pressure less than 30 mmHg at rest and less than 50 mmHg on exercise. By contrast, healthy controls had a pulmonary artery pressure below 19 mmHg at rest and below 26 mmHg on exercise. A population designated as "latent" hypertensives had a

resting PA pressure below 30 mmHg but greater than 50 mmHg during exercise; and a population with resting PA pressure greater than 30 mmHg and exercise pressure greater than 50 mmHg was identified as "overt" pulmonary hypertensives. Pneumonectomy patients were found to move from the normal to the latent hypertensive group or from the latent to the frankly hypertensive group. Semb recommended avoiding resection in the frankly or latent hypertensive groups.[120] Harrison correlated pulmonary artery pressure at rest and exercise in post-pneumonectomy patients with New York Heart Association functional state criteria. He found a mean PA pressure of 26 mmHg at rest, and 46 mmHg on mild exercise in asymptomatic (Class I) subjects contrasted with 33 mmHg and 53 mmHg in Class III and 48 mmHg and 73 mmHg in patients crippled at rest (Class IV).[131] Uggla studied 109 tuberculosis patients at the Söderby Hospital in 1956. These patients underwent a variety of thoracic procedures with an overall mortality rate of 22 percent (23/109). Fourteen patients were autopsied and all showed evidence of cor pulmonale. Preoperatively, Uggla measured pulmonary artery pressure (Ppa) at rest and at 15 watts of exercise. In addition, he measured pulmonary artery pressure resulting from balloon occlusion of the pulmonary artery (TUPAO) of the lung to be operated upon at rest and at a similar level of exercise. He then reevaluated the survivors three to four years postoperatively and classified them as fit or cardiorespiratory "cripples" based on their work capacity.[64]

There was no significant difference in pulmonary artery pressure under any conditions between the "fit" patients and "cripples," nor was there any difference in Ppa during exercise between survivors and nonsurvivors. There was, however, a significant elevation in pulmonary artery pressure on TUPAO both at rest and on exercise in nonsurvivors; Ppa averaging 35 mmHg and 53 mmHg respectively.[64]

Laros and Swierenga reported another

large series of resections for bronchogenic carcinoma. They had 10 early cardiopulmonary deaths among 110 resections (9%). Six of the ten were identified by elevated pulmonary artery pressures, two at rest, two during TUPAO, and an additional two on exercise during TUPAO. Among their survivors, however, 23 had an elevated PA pressure yielding a mortality rate of 21 percent in patients with an elevated PA pressure and a 95 percent survival rate when pressures were normal.[132]

Two series studying intraoperative TUPAO in resections for bronchogenic carcinoma came to differing conclusions regarding the value of resting TUPAO measurements in predicting surgical mortality. Rams reported a 54 percent cardiothoracic death rate (13/24) among patients with a resting Ppa greater than or equal to 25 mmHg. Sensitivity of this criterion was 68 percent with 13 of 19 deaths predicted. Among patients with a lower pulmonary artery pressure, 82 percent (28/34) survived.[133] By contrast, van Nostrand's figures were 14 percent mortality (3/21), 9 percent sensitivity (3/23), and 80 percent survival (79/99). Using pulmonary artery pressure greater than 33 mmHg upon intraoperative TUPAO, however, van Nostrand reported a 50 percent mortality (4/8) with 16 percent sensitivity, 92 percent specificity and 80 percent survival (89/109) in patients with a lower pressure.[68]

Based on these figures and the observation in other pulmonary vascular disorders that PA pressures of 30 to 40 mmHg are associated with elevated right ventricular pressures, Olsen et al concluded that an exercise PA pressure after TUPAO greater than 35 mmHg was a relative contraindication to pulmonary resection. The authors used this along with a PaO_2 following exercise and TUPAO < 45 mmHg, and a predicted post-pneumonectomy FEV_1 < 800 cc as potential exclusions for resection, but withheld surgery only when a patient met all three criteria for exclusion. Thirty high-risk patients were operated on with four car-

diorespiratory deaths (13%). Information, however, is not provided as to the function of the patients who died. Among 23 survivors, seven had pulmonary artery pressures greater than 25 mmHg during exercise, and seven more had pressures greater than 33 mmHg during exercise and TUPAO.[5]

While a 50 percent or greater reduction in the pulmonary vascular bed may be expected to produce resting pulmonary hypertension, and sustained pulmonary hypertension may lead to cor pulmonale, the reported experience in pulmonary resection suggests that inferences about the size of the pulmonary vascular bed or its pressure-volume characteristics may be neither particularly sensitive nor sufficiently specific to reliably identify patients who are extremely likely to die nor exclude the risk of cardiopulmonary death to a probability any less than 20 percent.[134] Even if it is assumed that all of Olsen's cardiopulmonary deaths had abnormal PA pressures, a mortality of 19 percent (4/21) is seen when either of Uggla's criteria are met.

Two series attempted to correlate pulmonary hemodynamics with spirometric function. The failure of either study to detect a significant correlation suggests that the two aspects of function are separable.[64,132]

Ventilatory function primarily relates to the likelihood of postoperative ventilatory failure, hypercapnia, and respiratory acidosis, but not to cardiac dysfunction. Pulmonary hemodynamics and cardiac evaluation describe the likelihood of cor pulmonale or cardiac insufficiency but do not predict ventilatory failure.

Regional Function

Thus far the discussion of preoperative evaluation for thoracotomy has centered on global cardiopulmonary function with criteria based on total organ values. If it is accepted that it is desirable to maintain an MVV above 50 percent of predicted and an

FEV_1 above 800 cc to avoid ventilatory failure following pulmonary resection, and a pulmonary vascular bed at least 50 percent of normal to avoid pulmonary hypertension and cor pulmonale, then it is clear that the amount of pulmonary tissue that is ultimately resectable is limited. The amount of tissue that can be resected can be expressed as that percent of overall function that can be lost and still preserve function above the marginal limits.

At its most simplistic level, it can be assumed that the five lobes of the lung contribute equally to overall function. Therefore, lobectomy will reduce overall ventilation and blood flow by 20 percent per lobe. A left pneumonectomy will leave the patient with 60 percent of preoperative capacity and a right pneumonectomy with 40 percent. Ventilation and perfusion are not distributed evenly throughout the lung, but rather follow a gradient from apex to base of increasing ventilation and blood flow, and function is usually greater in the right lung than the left.[98] Normally, 50 to 65 percent of ventilation and blood flow are distributed to the right lung. Therefore, a more accurate estimate might be obtained by subtracting the "true" percent function of the affected lobes from the preoperative figures.

Localized pulmonary disease, however, will cause alterations in the distribution of ventilation and blood flow, making predictions based on normal function unreliable. Several studies in the 1950s and 1960s pointed to the fact that pulmonary function was disproportionately reduced in a cancer-containing lung or lobe.[135,136] Therefore, predictions based on subtraction of a normally functioning lobe or lung from preoperative totals would overestimate the degree of postoperative impairment. A larger resection than initially expected might then be possible if the affected segment or lobe could be shown to have subnormal function. In certain conditions, such as bullous emphysema, *improved* function might even be expected on the basis of removing non-functioning tissue

that was compressing more normal parenchyma.[137]

Attention became focused on the predicted pulmonary function post-resection (which can be expressed as: preoperative function − % function of tissue to be resected) and on methods of determining regional lung function. Three basic approaches have evolved in the determination of regional lung function: bronchospirometry, the lateral position test, and scintigraphic determinations of regional ventilation and blood flow.

BRONCHOSPIROMETRY

Bronchospirometry measures the separate ventilation and gas-exchanging function of either lung by physically separating the right and left mainstem bronchi with a Carlens double-lumen endotracheal tube. The separate lumens are each connected to either simultaneous recording spirometers, or each lumen can be evaluated sequentially. Vital capacity, oxygen consumption ($\dot{V}E \times [FIO_2 - FEO_2]$) and CO_2 output ($\dot{V}E \times FECO_2$) can then be determined for each lung. Because of the resistance imposed by the narrow Carlens tube lumen, flow-dependent measurements and direct determination of regional MVV are not possible. Further localization can be achieved by placing the patient in the right or left decubitus position, head up or head down. Svanberg noticed that in patients with apical lesions, oxygen uptake was greater in the upright position than the supine, and, with basal lesions, it was greater in the supine. He further reported that oxygen uptake was impaired to a greater degree in a cancerous lung than might be predicted on the basis of regional ventilation alone, and suggested that this was indicative of vascular invasion by tumor. He suggested that marked reductions in oxygen uptake indicated surgical inoperability.[136] He extended these predictions in a retrospective study of 180 bronchogenic carcinomas and confirmed his initial impression. Increased functional loss predicted by bronchospirometry correlated with decreased resectability. He reported that early functional impairment due to cancer was primarily ventilatory; but in more advanced cases, circulation was more impaired than ventilation.[138]

Neuhaus and Cherniack attempted to indirectly predict postoperative MVV using the bronchospirometric vital capacity as their basis. They expressed the predicted MVV as the percentage of total vital capacity accounted for by the lung not to be removed, multiplied by the preoperative MVV. They successfully predicted postoperative vital capacity within $0.2 \pm 8.0\%$ and postoperative MVV to within $1.1 \pm 8.7\%$ ($r = 0.67$) in patients undergoing resections for tuberculosis.[139]

Vital capacity, MVV, and minute ventilation can then be separately assessed for each lung by bronchospirometry and a reasonably accurate prediction of postoperative function made. Measurement of oxygen uptake by bronchospirometry and comparisons with the distributions of ventilation may lead to impressions of the integrity of circulation and of operability. It is suggested that the greater the impairment of oxygen uptake, the less likely resectability. Bronchospirometry has the disadvantage of being invasive, often requiring anesthesia, and imposes an artifical external resistance on breathing.[140]

Armitage and Taylor suggested an alternative approach obviating the need for a Carlens tube. They passed polyethylene catheters through a Jackson bronchoscope and sampled expired air from the right and left mainstem bronchi for CO_2 and O_2. They then calculated the respiratory exchange ratio (R) for each lung. Since

$$R = \frac{\dot{V}_{CO2}}{\dot{V}_{O2}} = \frac{\dot{V}(F_{ECO_2})}{\dot{V}(F_{IO_2} - F_{EO_2})},$$

the measurement becomes independent of the relative ventilation of either lung. The contribution of the right lung to total oxygen uptake is expressed as

$$\text{Fractional } \dot{V}_{O_2} \text{ right lung} = \frac{R \text{ left} - R \text{ total}}{R \text{ left} - R \text{ right}}$$

Small differences in $\dot{V}_{O_2}$ were found between normal lungs. In ten diseased patients, however, no difference in R was found between the two lungs. This was interpreted as essential non-function of the diseased lung, with the healthy lung contributing the entire measured $\dot{V}_{CO_2}$ and $\dot{V}_{O_2}$. The interpretations were confirmed by bronchospirometry and pathology of the resected specimens. The affected lung was noted to have a higher RQ in patients with emphysema and lower in tuberculosis or bronchiectasis. No consistent difference was observed in patients with bronchogenic carcinoma.[135]

While this approach could be applied under local rather than general anesthesia, it still was rather invasive and depended on careful measurements of expired gas concentrations.

The subsequent development of the mass spectrometer and fine gas sampling probes has made the measurement of expired gas concentrations more elegant and simple. Under fluoroscopic guidance or with a fiberoptic bronchoscope, fine sampling catheters may be advanced into lobar or even segmental bronchi allowing an even finer definition of regional lung function than thought possible by Armitage.[141] The addition of an inert gas bronchial flowmeter by West et al allowed the measurement of bronchial flow rates giving most of the information derived from a Carlens tube without necessitating placement of any special tubes.[142,143]

LATERAL POSITION TEST

Both bronchospirometry and lobar sampling require special knowledge and competence. The lateral position test offers an assessment of relative whole lung function that can be performed with standard spirometry equipment and a minimum of training. The distribution of pleural pressure in the thorax is in part dependent on gravity so that the uppermost zone of the lung has a more negative pleural pressure than more dependent zones of the lung. Because of these differences in pleural pressure, non-dependent lung regions are more expanded at resting lung volume (FRC) than those of the dependent lung. This gravity-dependent difference is seen both in the upright lung and in lateral decubitus positions, so long as the total height of the lung is sufficient to create top-to-bottom pleural pressure differences.[144]

Bergan exploited gravity-dependent variations in lung volume to assess the relative function of either lung.[145] FRC tends to increase on the assumption of the lateral decubitus position due to the creation of a gravity-dependent pleural pressure gradient. If ventilatory function were equally distributed between the right and left lungs, then the change in FRC should be the same in either the right or left decubitus positions. If, however, a lung has reduced ventilatory function, FRC will increase less when it is placed in a nondependent position then it would were the lung normal.

In the lateral position test the supine FRC is determined and then compared with FRC in the left and right lateral decubitus positions. The changes in FRC in either decubitus are summed and the proportional contribution from right and left lateral decubitus positions determined. Each decubitus reflects the ventilatory performance of the nondependent lung so that the right lateral decubitus reflects the mechanics of the left lung and left lateral decubitus the right lung.[145,146] The test depends for its validity on the free motion of the chest wall and mediastinum and will be inaccurate if there is significant pleural disease or mediastinal fixation.[147,148]

To perform the test, the patient is connected via mouthpiece to a 9 to 13 liter spirometer equipped with a CO_2 scrubber and filled with 100 percent O_2. The mouthpiece is taped in place to prevent momentary disconnection from the circuit during position change. Nose clips should be worn. In the supine position, the patient rebreathes into the closed circuit. The end-expiratory baseline on the kymograph trace will steadily rise, reflecting a falling volume in the system due to oxygen uptake. When a stable baseline is established, the patient is turned to the right lateral decubitus position and a new FRC baseline recorded. The patient is then returned to the supine position and the original FRC is re-established. The process is then repeated in the left lateral decubitus position. A valid test requires the establishment of a reproducible FRC baseline in the supine posture and stable FRCs in either decubitus. Normally, ventilatory function is about equal in either lung (Fig. 4-12).

The lateral position test was found to correlate well with bronchospirometric determination of ventilation and was successfully used to predict post-pneumonectomy FEV_1 and FVC to a standard deviation of 400cc.[145-147]

Besides only being able to measure whole lung function, the lateral position test has other limitations. Patients with severe pain or dyspnea may be unable to complete the test, and a fixed mediastinum or pleural space may lead to inaccurate results.[147,148] This latter weakness of the lateral position test has been exploited for use as an indicator of surgical resectibility. Large differences ($\geq$ 13%) in predicted function of the involved lung based on perfusion lung scan and lateral position test successfully separated seven patients with mediastinal metastases from seven without.[149]

While the lateral position test appears to correlate well with ventilation, when disease is moderately advanced in the affected lung it tends to overestimate gas exchange function.[148] Since oxygen uptake is a function of blood flow as well as ventilation, impairment of perfusion will reduce oxygen uptake below that predicted on the basis of ventilation. DeMeester made a particular point of the failure of the lateral position test to cor-

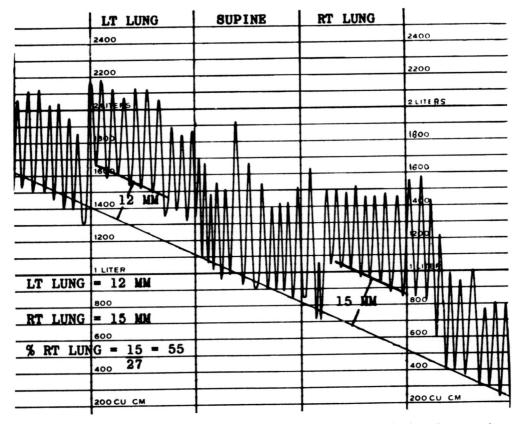

Fig. 4-12 Lateral position test. Rising trace of spirograph reflects reduction of volume in system due to oxygen uptake. Reduction of end-expiratory volume (FRC) in decubitus positions causes elevation of FRC from supine baseline. Deflections in both decubiti are summed, and proportions of ventilatory function of lung calculated as percent baseline deflection of contralateral decubitus position. In example, 12 mm deflection for L lung obtained in R lateral decubitus and 15 mm deflection for R lung obtained in L lateral decubitus (reproduced with permission from Marion JM, Alderson PO, Lefrak SS, et al: Unilateral lung function: comparison of the lateral position test with radionuclide ventilation-perfusion studies. Chest 69:5-9, 1976).

relate with a bronchospirometrically-determined oxygen uptake.[150] Since circulatory impairment appears to develop later in bronchogenic carcinoma than ventilatory impairment, the lateral position test will be less accurate in advanced disease.[136]

Overestimating the function of the involved lung will not lead to a larger resection than can be safely accomplished, but if predicted FEV$_1$ is being used strictly, some patients may be inappropriately denied surgery. Nonetheless, where bronchospirometry or scanning is not available, split whole lung function may be reasonably and simply estimated by use of the lateral position test.

NUCLEAR MEDICINE TECHNIQUES

Assessment of regional lung function by nuclear techniques has been used since 1955 when Knipping et al introduced ^{131}I and [131]Xe inhalation techniques.[151] Since that time a number of isotopes and approaches have evolved in the study of regional lung function.

All have in common the introduction of

a small dose of a radioactive isotope either by inhalation or by intravenous injection. After subtracting the number of atmospheric background counts and adjusting for uptake of isotope by the chest wall, the radioactivity of the lung fields is sensed and measured; the amount of radioactivity reflecting pulmonary ventilation or blood flow. Regional counts can be measured by fixed counters, scanners, or by the Anger gamma camera. Fixed counters have the advantage of accuracy and reliability but are difficult to handle because of their large size. A moving scanner avoids the problem of coordinating multiple inputs as from the fixed sensors, but has the disadvantage of smaller counts because of motion and a consequent decrease in statistical accuracy. The gamma camera has permitted a combination of the advantages of both devices.

The most frequently used isotope for pulmonary studies is ^{133}Xe. ^{133}Xe is a byproduct from nuclear reactors and has a half-life of 5 to 6 days. It is poorly soluble in blood (β = .21 ml gas STPD/ml blood/mmHg), so is not taken up by blood to any great extent during ventilation studies. The gas can be breathed from a spirometer, allowing for assessment of ventilation, or can be dissolved in saline, permitting assessment of blood flow. In a steady state infusion, ^{133}Xe may be used to determine regional ventilation/perfusion ($\dot{V}/\dot{Q}$) ratio.

Ventilation can be measured by wash-in kinetics, wash-out kinetics, single breath distribution, or rebreathing equilibration. The latter permits measurement of regional ventilation, volume, and ventilation-to-volume ratios. Since, if ventilation were uniform, distribution of a single inspiration should be the same as at equilibrium, a comparison technique allows an index of ventilatory unevenness.

Ventilation studies are performed by adding ^{133}Xe to a CO_2 scrubber-equipped spirometer circuit of known volume, to a concentration of 0.5 − 3 mCi/ml. The subject takes in 1 to 3 vital capacity breaths

of gas and distribution of radioactivity throughout the lung is constant. The initial breath measures ventilation, and equilibrium determines regional lung volume.

To measure the distribution of blood flow, ^{133}Xe is dissolved in saline at a concentration of .25 − 2 cmCi/ml. An IV catheter is placed as close to the superior vena cava as practicable. The subject is asked to hold his breath at FRC and the xenon is rapidly injected. After approximately another seven seconds, the subject inhales to TLC. The xenon exchanges rapidly with alveolar air because of its low solubility, allowing for counting of radioactivity over the lung fields. Counting is carried out over 10 to 30 seconds. By this method, regional blood flow can be measured to within ± 5 percent in normals and ± 10 percent in patients with lung disease.[152,153]

^{133}Xe studies involve a radiation dose less than 300 to 400 mRads as compared with about 100 mRads for a standard PA and lateral chest radiograph. These studies, while permitting a measurement of regional function, do not correspond to strictly lobar or segmental readings since there is considerable overlap of anatomic segments in any one plane of reading. Strictly anatomic estimates are available only with computerized analysis of raw count data.[152,153]

A more convenient measure of perfusion can be accomplished with isotopically-tagged macroaggregates. Ninety to ninety-five percent of particles in the 10 to 50 mm range become trapped in the pulmonary microvasculature when injected intravenously. Isotopically-tagged particles will then give a steady state index of pulmonary perfusion. ^{99}Technetium-tagged iron hydroxide or albumin particles have a half life of 4 to 8 hours and are most commonly used in the clinical setting.[5,154] The average radiation dose for a 3 mCi dose of ^{99}Tc is about 150 mRad. Because of the larger counting time, particulate ^{99}Tc offers somewhat better resolution than gas methods (Fig. 4-13).

Scans

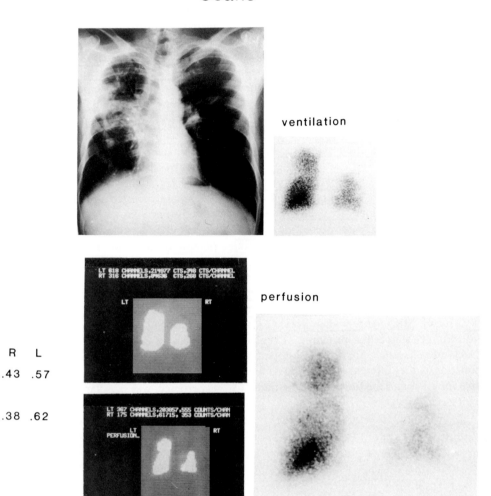

R   L

$\dot{V}$ .43   .57

$\dot{Q}$ .38   .62

Fig. 4-13   Regional lung function determined by radionuclide scanning. Patient is a 37-year-old male with tuberculosis in the right upper lobe and major hemoptysis. ^{133}Xe ventilation scan upper right, ^{99}Tc aggregate perfusion scan lower right. Scans are posterior views; therefore, right and left are opposite from roentgenogram. Computer analysis of ventilation and perfusion scans (lower left) indicate right lung receives 43 percent of total ventilation, 38 percent total blood flow. Finer anatomic resolution is possible if necessary.

CLINICAL UTILITY

Isotope scanning has been used in the assessment of surgical operability, particularly ^{67}Gallium.[155] The suggestion has been made that ^{133}Xenon or ^{99}Tc perfusion scanning may identify inoperability by indicating substantially reduced perfusion to the involved lung. A correlation was observed between decreased local perfusion and hilar vascular metastases in lung cancer; and the suggestion has been advanced that, when the involved lung received less than one-third of the total perfusion, resection was not possi-

ble.[72,156] This contention has not been sub-
stantiated. Wernly reported 15 successful
pneumonectomies in patients with less than
33 percent of the total blood flow to the involved lung, and 14 of 33 of Boysen's cases
had less than 33 percent blood flow to the involved lung.[6,157] All fourteen survived pneumonectomy.[157] Marked differences between
unilateral function as predicted by the lateral
position test and by ^{99}Tc aggregate perfusion
scan may indicate inoperable mediastinal
metastasis.[149]

Radioisotope scanning is more commonly used to assess the contribution of the
diseased lung or lobe to total pulmonary
function in order to better predict postoperative function when that tissue has been resected. Decisions involving medical operability are made on the basis of predicted
function. Pulmonary functions commonly
used as predictions in regional studies are
VC, FEV_1, MVV, and oxygen uptake.

Simply stated, the principle of regional
assessment is that predicted postoperative
function is the difference between preoperative function and the function of the tissue to
be resected.

REGIONAL LUNG FUNCTION IN
PNEUMONECTOMY

For pneumonectomy, postoperative
function can be expressed as:

1. Preoperative function × % perfusion to
   contralateral lung;
2. Preoperative function × % ventilation to
   contralateral lung; or,
3. Preoperative function × % matched
   $\dot{V}/\dot{Q}$.

In the latter case, Wernly pointed out that,
when total gas exchanging function is looked
at, both ventilation and perfusion must be
considered and that the more severely affected parameter will be the limiting factor.
Total function is expressed as the sum of the
least ventilation and perfusion percentages of
either lung. The function of the lung to be

resected is expressed as the lower percentage,
ventilation or blood flow divided by the adjusted total function.[6]

Kristersson and Miörner introduced a
combined Xenon ventilation and perfusion
protocol which they called radiospirometry,
and noted that the technique predicted postoperative vital capacity better than postoperative FEV_1.[158,159] Accuracy was comparable
to bronchospirometry. Olsen used ^{99}Tc perfusion scanning to estimate postoperative
function. He found good correlations for
FEV_1, FVC and D_LCO, although in each
case, postoperative function was underestimated somewhat.[154] Subsequently, the same
group reported assessment of 33 patients for
pneumonectomy all with preoperative FEV_1
less than 2 liters. They encountered a perioperative mortality of 15 percent and reported no incidence of postoperative respiratory insufficiency after two years' follow-up.
Despite their stated intent of prognosticating
on the basis of predicted postoperative FEV_1,
none of the deaths occurred in patients
with an FEV_1 less than 1 liter.[5,157] Wernly's
experience was similar, with three deaths
among 45 pneumonectomy patients, one respiratory. None of the deaths occurred in a
patient with a preoperative FEV_1 less than
2 liters. Comparing predicted FEV_1 with
actual post-pneumonectomy FEV_1, Wernly
found no statistically significant difference
among predictions based on perfusion, ventilation, or $\dot{V}/\dot{Q}$ ratio. Although a single
breath ventilation scan appeared to correlate best with FEV_1, all methods came
within 11 to 14.6 percent of actual postoperative function.[6]

REGIONAL LUNG FUNCTION IN
LOBECTOMY

Since lobectomy removes less tissue
than pneumonectomy, the postoperative results tend to be somewhat better.[159] Regional
function for lobectomy, though, is somewhat
more difficult to interpret.[7] Difficulty arises
because anatomic lobes and segments are

difficult to isolate without multiple projections and computer analysis. Prediction of postoperative function is further confused by the improvement of postoperative function over time.

Ali used a ^{133}Xe radiospirometry approach to study predicted vs. actual function in 44 lobectomies, and found that postoperative function tended to be better than preoperative predictions, particularly in late (> 6 months) studies.[7] He suggested introducing a correction factor into the equations to account for this. Other authors also noted this discrepancy and dismissed it as being a clinically safe error, although surgery might be denied on the basis of such an error.[5,6]

In the early (2–3 months) postoperative period, pulmonary function is considerably more impaired than in later postoperative phases. Often, predictions can be confounded because the patient receives close attention and airway obstruction is better managed postoperatively than at the time of preoperative testing. Pulmonary hypertension may not occur despite resection because the resected tissue contained areas with low ventilation-perfusion ratios or frank shunts. Consequent postoperative improvement in $\dot{V}/\dot{Q}$ relationships may improve PaO_2 and relieve pulmonary hypertension when hypoxic vasoconstriction was a contributing factor.[72]

Functional loss from lobectomy has been expressed in terms of the number of segments removed. Miörner divided the lung into 19 functional segments, 10 in the right lung (RUL 3, RML 2, RLL 5), and nine on the left (LUL 5, LLL 4).[158] Several mathematical expressions have been presented to summarize functional loss in lobectomy:[6,7,159]

$$(1) \ \text{PREOP FEV}_1 \times \left(\frac{\text{Number of segments in lobe resected}}{\text{Total segments in both lungs} \times \% \text{ function in resected lobe}} \right)$$

$$(2) \ \text{PREOP FEV}_1 \times \left(\frac{\text{Segments in lobe resected}}{\text{Segments in that lung} \times \% \text{ function in affected lung}} \right)$$

$$(3) \ \text{PREOP FEV}_1 \times \left(\frac{\text{Functional segments in lobe resected}}{\text{Total number of segments both lungs}} \right)$$

Wernly et al studied 40 lobectomies using ^{133}Xe ventilation scanning, single breath, equilibrium and washout, and ^{99}Tc for perfusion. As with the pneumonectomy group, they reported no difference in the accuracy of prediction using any scan technique, nor any difference among methods of calculation. They concluded that since ^{99}Tc perfusion scanning was cheaper and simpler, it should be considered the approach of choice.[6] Kristersson, using ^{133}Xe radiospirometry, had earlier concluded that local function was best reflected by perfusion, that regional function was more reproducibly measured by perfusion scanning, and that a $\dot{Q}$ scan would predict postoperative MVV as well as a ventilation scan. Error of prediction was small, about 10 percent.[159]

Studies of regional lung function have been employed for assessment of operability when preoperative FEV_1 is less than 2 liters for pneumonectomy or less than 1.5 liters for lobectomy.[5] An attempt is made to predict postoperative function on the basis of preoperative function and the expected loss of function upon resection, which, in turn, is determined by the function of that segment, lobe, or lung. If the whole-lung criteria of postoperative $FEV_1 > 800$ to 1000cc and/or MVV greater than 50 percent predicted are employed, the cardiopulmonary mortality of pneumonectomy can be held to 15 percent in high-risk patients and the risk of lobectomy brought to approach that of the normal population.

Among available techniques, bronchospirometry, lobar sampling, the lateral position test, and isotope scanning, are all capable of providing estimates within 10 to 15 percent of actual postoperative function.

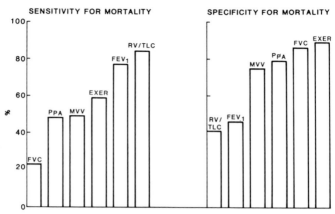

Fig. 4-14 Relative sensitivity and specificity of pulmonary function tests in predicting mortality from thoracotomy. Note that FEV_1 and RV/TLC are relatively sensitive, but have poor specificity as predictors. This makes them better suited as screening tests. Highest specificity comes from exercise tolerance testing, pulmonary artery pressure measurements, and vital capacity. These are best suited as followup studies when a initial screen indicates a patient at risk.[4,66-69,73,75-76,110,132-133]

Since the gas exchanging function of the lung is ultimately determined by blood flow, and ventilation usually correlates well with blood flow, perfusion-based studies should represent the approach of choice.[157] Based on simplicity and reproducibility, the ^{99}Tc perfusion scan is probably the procedure of first choice for pneumonectomy evaluation as well as for lobectomy. Where nuclear medicine support is not available, the lateral position test provides a satisfactory alternative. Since lobectomy is usually performed for peripheral lesions in which ventilation and blood flow are relatively well preserved, subtraction of the number of functional segments to be removed is a sufficient prediction of function in lobectomy when scanning is not available.[6]

It must be borne in mind, however, that failure to meet predicted whole-lung postoperative parameters is still associated with a 65 to 75 percent survival rate, and that among the reported series utilizing studies of regional function, deaths occurred among patients with less, rather than more, severe pul-

monary dysfunction. The predictive value of studies of regional lung function, therefore, is no greater than that of the whole lung function they were designed to modify.

CONCLUSIONS

A significant risk for cardiorespiratory failure or death is associated with thoracotomy. Patients with pre-existing cardiopulmonary disease, obesity, advanced age, or those undergoing pulmonary resections have been repeatedly shown to be at particular risk. When these factors are identified and treated, the risk of complications or death can be minimized.

All patients undergoing thoracotomy and all patients facing general anesthesia who have histories, physical examinations, or routine laboratory abnormalities suggesting cardiopulmonary disease should undergo physiologic assessment of pulmonary function and have surgery delayed, when possible, to treat the abnormalities.

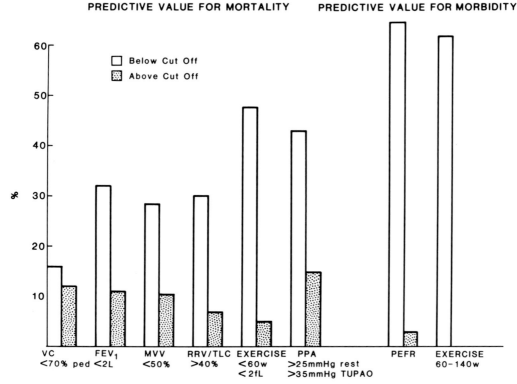

PREDICTIVE VALUE FOR MORTALITY   **PREDICTIVE VALUE FOR MORBIDITY**

Fig. 4-15 Predictive value of pulmonary function studies for morbidity and mortality in thoracotomy. Note excellent separation of high-risk from low-risk groups with exercise protocol and pulmonary artery pressure measurement. Predictive values for morbidity, while impressive, require further corroboration.[4,66-69,73,75-76,110,132-133]

In principle, when screening for potentially dangerous abnormalities, a highly sensitive test should be used first, with specificity of only secondary concern. Once an at-risk population is identified, more specific tests should then be applied, particularly where the treatment, dangerous though it be, may be life-saving. In this way, high risk patients are identified, but as few patients as possible are denied therapy (Fig. 4-14, 4-15, 4-16).

Routine spirometry, particularly FEV_1 and lung volumes with RV/TLC, are fairly sensitive indicators of the likelihood of perioperative difficulty and can identify prospectively up to 80 percent of potential complications. Patients with an FEV_1 below 2 liters or RV/TLC greater than 40 percent

should have their pulmonary function optimized by smoking cessation and bronchodilator therapy for at least 48 to 72 hours and then be retested.

Persistent abnormality indicates the need for a more specific evaluation. The MVV and exercise studies appear to offer sufficient specificity to reduce the operative risk to about 10 percent when these studies are normal.

If, however, the MVV is less than 50 percent of predicted or the patient is unable to complete a 60 watt exercise protocol, split function studies and pulmonary artery pressures may be employed to better define the risk of surgery.

It must be recognized that no one abnormality or constellation of pulmonary func-

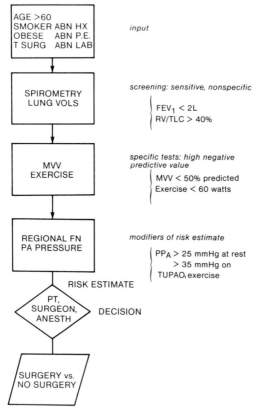

Fig. 4-16 <u>Suggested sequence for preoperative pulmonary assessment.</u> Once a population at risk is identified, sensitive screening tests should be used to define particular subjects at risk. Individuals thus identified should be evaluated with more specific tests and reclassified as high or moderate risk. High-risk patients may still be considered for surgery if highly specific predictors show acceptable results. The end result of assessment should be a rough numeric estimate of risk, and the ultimate decision for surgery should be shared among the patient, the anesthesiologist, and the surgeon given the risk of surgery weighed against the desirability of treatment.

tion abnormalities can identify a patient who *will* have a complicated course or a patient who will have an uncomplicated course with anything greater than 90 percent probability. <u>Failure to meet any of the most commonly stated criteria: postoperative</u> $FEV_1 > 800cc$, <u>MVV>50 percent predicted, or pulmonary artery pressure < 45 mmHg on temporary</u>

balloon <u>occlusion of the PA during exercise is associated with no more than a 35 percent morbidity or mortality</u> as compared with published rates of 10 to 20 percent when such patients are carefully excluded.

Given a chance at a cure of an otherwise lethal disease, a 25 percent risk of death or disability may be acceptable to the patient; or, a 15 percent risk, which is perfectly acceptable to the surgeon, may not be to the patient. As a group, patients are more risk-aversive than their physicians and may, when informed of the relative probabilities of death by disease, death in surgery, or cure, choose the natural course of their disease.[160]

Besides alerting the medical care team to the existence of abnormalities requiring correction, preoperative pulmonary assessment allows a rough quantitation of the risk of surgery which should be presented to the patient as part of the informed consent to surgery.

While the concept of "prohibitive pulmonary function" may be a fiction insofar as the literature is concerned, it may represent a reality for the individual patient and his physicians.

That any more elegant or involved a work-up can provide any further predictive information is not supported by the literature. The incidence of post-thoracotomy morbidity and mortality is multifactorial, and any predictions based on cardiopulmonary function alone must, of necessity, be incomplete. Until all such factors are identified and evaluated, preoperative assessment can do no better than educate our guess about the likelihood of morbidity and mortality and identify those patients who require vigorous preoperative and vigilant postoperative care.

REFERENCES

1. Tisi GM: Preoperative evaluation of pulmonary function: validity, indications, and benefits. Am Rev Respir Dis 119:293–310, 1979

2. Garibaldi RA, Britt MR, Coleman ML, et al: Risk factors for postoperative pneumonia. Am J Med 70:627-80, 1981

3. Latimer RG, Dickman M, Day WC, et al: Ventilatory patterns and pulmonary complications after upper abdominal surgery determined by preoperative-postoperative computerized spirometry and blood gas analysis. Am J Surg 122:622-32, 1971

4. Mittman C: Assessment of operative risk in thoracic surgery. Am Rev Respir Dis 84:197-207, 1961

5. Olsen GN, Block AJ, Swenson EW, et al: Pulmonary function evaluation of the lung resection candidate: a prospective study. Am Rev Respir Dis 111:379-87, 1975

6. Wernly JA, DeMeester TR, Kirchner PT, et al: Clinical value of quantitative ventilation-perfusion lung scans in the surgical management of bronchogenic carcinoma. J Thorac Cardiovasc Surg 80:535-43, 1980

7. Ali MK, Mountain CF, Ewer MS, et al: Predicting loss of pulmonary function after pulmonary resection for bronchogenic carcinoma. Chest 77:337-42, 1980

8. Wightman JAK: A prospective survey of the incidence of postoperative pulmonary complications. Br J Surg 55:85-91, 1968

9. Rehder K, Sessler AD, Marsh HM: General anesthesia and the lung. Am Rev Respir Dis 112:541-564, 1975

10. Dantzker DR, Wagner PD, West JB: Instability of lung units with low $\dot{V}_A/\dot{Q}$ ratios during O_2 breathing. J Appl Physiol 38:886-895, 1975

11. Harman E, Lillington G: Pulmonary risk factors in surgery. Med Clin North Am 63:1289-1298, 1979

12. Pierce AK, Robertson J: Pulmonary complications of general surgery. Ann Rev Med 28:211-21, 1977

13. Gaensler EA, Cugell DW, Lindgren I, et al: The role of pulmonary insufficiency in mortality and invalidism following surgery for pulmonary tuberculosis. J Thor Surg 29:163-67, 1955

14. Gracey DR, Divertie MB, Didier EP: Preoperative pulmonary preparation of patients with chronic obstructive pulmonary disease: a prospective study. Chest 76:123-129, 1979

15. Goldman L, Caldera DL, Nussbaum SR et al: Multifactorial index of cardiac risk in noncardiac surgical procedures. New Engl J Med 297:845-850, 1977

16. Campbell EJM, Howell JBL: The sensation of breathlessness. Brit Med Bull 19:36-40, 1963

17. Richards DW: The nature of cardiac and pulmonary dyspnea. Circulation 7:15-29, 1953

18. Derenne J-Ph, Macklem PT, Roussos C: The respiratory muscles, mechanics, control and pathophysiology. Am Rev Respir Dis 118:119-134, 373-90, 581-602, 1978

19. Ayres SM: Cigarette smoking and lung diseases: an update. Basics of RD 3(5):1-6, 1975

20. Irwin RS, Rosen MJ, Braman SS: Cough: a comprehensive review. Arch Intern Med 137:1186-1191, 1977

21. Meneely GR, Renzetti AD, Jr, Steele JD, et al: Chronic bronchitis, asthma and emphysema: a statement by the Committee on Diagnostic Standards for Nontuberculous Respiratory Diseases. Am Rev Respir Dis 85:762-68, 1962

22. Cohen MH: Signs and symptoms of bronchogenic carcinoma. Semin Onc 1:183-189, 1974

23. Goldman L, Caldera DL, Southwick FS et al: Cardiac risk factors and complications in noncardiac surgery. Medicine 57:357-70, 1978

24. Comroe JHJr, Botelho S: The unreliability of cyanosis in the recognition of arterial anoxemia. Am J Med Sci 214:1-6, 1947

25. Robotham J: Cardiovascular disturbances in chronic respiratory insufficiency. Am J Cardiol 47:941-949, 1981

26. Campbell EJM: Physical signs of diffuse airways obstruction and lung distention. Thorax 24:1-3, 1969

27. Ashutosh K, Gilbert R, Auchincloss JH, Jr, et al: Asynchronous breathing movements in patients with chronic obstructive pulmonary disease. Chest 67:553-557, 1975

28. Sharp JT, Goldberg NB, Druz WS, et al: Thoracoabdominal motion in chronic obstructive pulmonary disease. Am Rev Respir Dis 115:47-56, 1977

29. Permutt S: Physiologic changes in the acute asthma attack, Ch 2, pp 15-24. In Austin KF, Lichtenstein LM, Eds: Asthma: physiology, immunopharmacology and treatment. Academic Press, New York, 1973

30. Hoover CF: Definitive percussion and inspection in estimating size and contour of the heart. JAMA 75:1626-1630, 1920

31. Bergofsky EH: Respiratory failure in disorders of the thoracic cage. Am Rev Respir Dis 119:643-670, 1979

32. Forgacs P: The functional basis of pulmonary sounds. Chest 73:399-405, 1978

33. Nath AR, Capel LH: Inspiratory crackles—early and late. Thorax 29:223-227, 1974

34. Holford FD: The electrocardiogram in lung disease, Ch 10, pp 139-145. In Fishman AP, Ed: Pulmonary diseases and disorders. McGraw-Hill, New York, 1980

35. Calverly PMA, McElderry L, Leggett RJE, et al: Secondary polycythemia and carboxyhemoglobin from smoking in hypoxic cor pulmonale (abstract). Am Rev Respir Dis 119 suppl: 118, 1980

36. Goldring RM, Turino GM, Heinemann HO: Respiratory-renal adjustments in chronic hypercapnia in man. Am J Med 51:772-784, 1971

37. Burki NK, Krumpelman JL: Correlation of pulmonary function with chest roentgenogram in chronic airway obstruction. Am Rev Respir Dis 121:217-223, 1980

38. Thurlbeck W, Simon G: Radiographic appearance of the chest in emphysema. Amer J Roentgen 130:429-440, 1978

39. Fraser RG: The radiologist and obstructive airway disease. Caldwell lecture 1973. Amer J Roentgen 120:737-775, 1974

40. Griner PF, Mayewski RJ, Mushlin AI, et al: Selection and interpretation of diagnostic tests and procedures. Principles and applications. Ann Intern Med 94 (suppl) 553-600, 1981

41. McNeil BJ, Adelstein SJ: Determining the value of diagnostic and screening tests. J Nucl Med 17:439-448, 1976

42. Morris JF, Koski A, Johnson LC: Spirometric standards for healthy nonsmoking adults. Am Rev Respir Dis 103:57-67, 1971

43. Oscherwitz M, Edlavitch SA, Baker TR, et al: Differences in pulmonary functions in various racial groups. Am J Epidem. 96:319-27, 1972

44. Sobol BJ, Sobol PG: Percent of predicted as the limit of normal in pulmonary function testing: a statistically valid approach. Thorax 34:1-3, 1979

45. Boehlecke B, Merchant JA: The use of pulmonary function testing and questionnaires as epidemiologic tools in the study of occupational lung disease. Chest 79:114s-122s, 1981

46. Fry DL, Hyatt RE: Pulmonary mechanics: a unified analysis of the relationship between pressure, volume and gas flow in the lungs of normal and diseased human subjects. Am J Med 29:672-682, 1960

47. Mead J, Turner JM, Macklem PT, et al: Significance of the relationship between lung recoil and maximum expiratory flow. J Appl Physiol 22:95-108, 1967

48. Pride NB, Permutt S, Riley RL, et al: Determinants of maximal expiratory flow from the lungs. J Appl Physiol 23:646-662, 1967

49. Rodarte JR, Hyatt RE: Respiratory mechanics. Basics of RD 4(4)1-6, 1976

50. McIlroy MB, Tierney DF, Nadel JA: A new method for measurement of compliance and resistance of lungs and thorax. J Appl Physiol 18:424-427, 1963

51. Otis AB, McKerrow CB, Bartlett RA, et al: Mechanical factors in distribution of pulmonary ventilation. J Appl Physiol 8:427-441, 1956

52. Thurlbeck WM: Aspects of chronic airflow obstruction. Chest 72:341-9, 1977

53. Rahn HA, Otis AB, Chadwick LE, et al: The pressure-volume diagram of the thorax and lung. Am J Physiol 146:161-78, 1946

54. Leith DE, Mead J: Mechanisms determining residual volume of the lungs in normal subjects. J Appl Physiol 23:221-227, 1967

55. Gardner RM (chairman): ATS statement: Snowbird workshop on the standardization of spirometry. Am Rev Respir Dis 119:831-838, 1979

56. Ferris BT (Principal Investigator): Epidemiology standardization project: recommended standardized procedures for pulmonary function testing. Am Rev Respir Dis 118:(suppl) 1-102, 1978

57. Kanner RE, Morris AH: Clinical pulmonary function testing. Intermountain Thoracic Society, Salt Lake City, 1975

58. Smith AA, Gaensler EA: Timing of forced expiratory volume in one second. Am Rev Respir Dis 112:882-5, 1975

59. Sorensen JB, Morris AH, Crapo RO, et al: Selection of the best spirometric values for

interpretation. Am Rev Respir Dis 122:802-5, 1980

60. McFadden ER, Kiker R, Holmes B, et al: Small airway disease: an assessment of the tests of peripheral airway function. Am J Med 57:171-182, 1974

61. Hyatt RE, Black LF: The flow-volume curve: a current perspective. Am Rev Respir Dis 107:191-9, 1973

62. Shephard RJ: Some factors affecting the open-circuit determination of maximum breathing capacity. J Physiol 135:98-113, 1957

63. O'Donoghue WJ, Baker JP, Bell GM et al: Respiratory failure in neuromuscular disease: management in a respiratory intensive care unit. JAMA 235:733-5, 1976

64. Uggla LG: Indications for and results of thoracic surgery with regard to respiratory and circulatory function tests. Acta Chir Scand 111:197-212, 1956

65. Lockwood P: The principles of predicting the risk of post-thoracotomy function-related complications in bronchial carcinoma. Respiration 30:329-344, 1973

66. Lockwood P: Lung function test results and the risk of post-thoracotomy complications. Respiration 30:529-542, 1973

67. Larsen MC, Clifton EE: The prognostic value of preoperative evaluation of patients undergoing thoracic surgery. Dis Chest 47:589-594, 1965

68. van Nostrand D, Welsberg MO, Humphrey EW: Preresectional evaluation of risk from pneumonectomy. Surg Gynecol Obstet 127:306-12, 1968

69. Didolkar MS, Moore RH, Takita H: Evaluation of the risk in pulmonary resection for bronchogenic carcinoma. Am J Surg 127:700-703, 1974

70. Diener CF, Burrows B: Further observations on the course and prognosis of chronic obstructive lung disease. Am Rev Respir Dis 111:719-24, 1975

71. Traver GA, Cline MG, Burrows B: Predictors of mortality in chronic obstructive pulmonary disease: a 15 year follow-up study. Am Rev Respir Dis 119:895-901, 1979

72. Kristersson S, Lindell SE, Svanberg L: Prediction of pulmonary function loss due to pneumonectomy using ^{133}Xe-radiospirometry. Chest 62:694-698, 1972

73. Boushy SF, Billig DM, North LB, et al: Clinical course related to preoperative and postoperative pulmonary function in patients with bronchogenic carcinoma. Chest 59:383-391, 1971

74. Karliner JS, Coomaraswamy R, Williams MH Jr: Relationship between preoperative pulmonary function studies and prognosis of patients undergoing pneumonectomy for carcinoma of the lung. Dis Chest 54:32-38, 1968

75. Stein M, Koota GM, Simon M, et al: Pulmonary evaluation of surgical patients. JAMA 181:765-770, 1962

76. Stein M, Cassara EL: Preoperative pulmonary evaluation and therapy for surgery patients. JAMA 211:787-790, 1970

77. Miller WF, Wu N, Johnson RL: Convenient method of evaluating pulmonary ventilatory function with a single breath test. Anesthesiology 17:480-493, 1956

78. Redding JS, Yakaitis RW: Predicting the need for ventilatory assistance. Md State Med J 19:53-57, 1970

79. Meneely GR, Ferguson JL: Pulmonary evaluation and risk in patient preparation for anesthesia and surgery. JAMA 175:1074-1080, 1961

80. Hodgkin JE, Dines DG, Didier PE: Preoperative evaluation of the patient with pulmonary disease. Mayo Clin Proc 48:114-118, 1973

81. Williams CD, Brenowitz JB: "Prohibitive" lung function and major surgical procedures. Am J Surg 132:763-766, 1976

82. Freedman BJ, Meisner P, Hill GB: A comparison of the actions of different bronchodilators in asthma. Thorax 23:590-597, 1968

83. McFadden ER, Jr: Aerosolized bronchodilators and steroids in the treatment of airway obstruction in adults. Am Rev Resp Dis 112: (suppl) 89-96, 1980

84. Mushin GJ: Time factor in the measurement of response to bronchodilators. Thorax 22:538-42, 1967

85. Dull WJ, Alexander MR, Kasik JE: Isoproterenol challenge during placebo and oral theophylline therapy in chronic obstructive pulmonary disease. Am Rev Respir Dis 123:340-42, 1981

86. Light RW, Conrad SA, George RB: The one best test for evaluating the effects of

bronchodilator therapy. Chest 72:512-516, 1977

87. Ramsdell JW, Tisi GM: Determination of bronchodilatation in the pulmonary function laboratory: role of changes in static lung volumes. Chest 76:622-628, 1979

88. DuBois AB, Botelho SY, Bedell GN, et al: A rapid plethysmographic method for measuring thoracic gas volume in comparison with a nitrogen washout method for measuring functional residual capacity in normal subjects. J Clin Invest 35:322-326, 1956

89. Leith DE, Mead J: Principles of body plethysmography. Nat Heart and Lung Institute, Div of Lung Diseases, Bethesda, 1974

90. Brown R, Scharf S, Ingram RH Jr: Nonhomogeneous alveolar pressure swings in the presence of airway closure. J Appl Physiol Respir Env Exerc Physiol 49:398-402, 1980

91. Rodenstein D, Stanescu DC, Cauberghs M, et al: Failure of body plethysmography to accurately measure lung volume in bronchial obstruction (abstract). Am Rev Respir Dis 123: (suppl) 88, 1981

92. Hathirat S, Renzetti AD, Jr., Mitchell M: Measurement of the total lung capacity by helium dilution in a constant volume system. Am Rev. Respir Dis 102:760-770, 1970

93. Bates DV, Macklem PT, Christie RV: Respiratory function in disease. 2nd ed. WB Saunders, Philadelphia, 1971, pp 13-14

94. Comroe JH, Forster RE, DuBois AB, et al: The Lung: Clinical physiology and pulmonary function tests 2nd ed. Yearbook Medical Publishers, Chicago, 1962

95. Cotes JE: Lung function: assessment and application in medicine. 4th ed. Blackwell, Oxford, 1979

96. O'Shea J, Lapp NL, Rusakoff AD, et al: Determination of lung volumes from chest films. Thorax 25:544-9, 1970

97. Nicklaus TM, Watanabe S, Mitchell MM, et al: Roentgenologic, physiologic and structural estimations of the total lung capacity in normal and emphysematous subjects. Am J Med 42:547-553, 1967

98. West JB: Ventilation/Blood flow and gas exchange. 3rd ed. Blackwell, Oxford, 1977

99. Harris EA, Kenyon AM, Nisbet HD, et al: The normal alveolar-arterial oxygen-tension gradient in man. Clin Sci Mol Med 46:89-104, 1974

100. Wagner PD, Dantzker DR, Dueck R et al: Distribution of ventilation-perfusion ratios in patients with interstitial lung disease. Chest 69 (Suppl):256-7, 1976

101. Mithoefer JC, Keighley JF, Karetzky MS: Response of the arterial PO_2 to oxygen administration in chronic pulmonary disease: interpretation of findings in a study of 46 patients and 14 normal subjects. Ann Intern Med 74:328-335, 1971

102. Fishman AP: Chronic cor pulmonale. Am Rev Respir Dis 114:775-794, 1976

103. Fishman AP: Hypoxia on the pulmonary circulation: How and where it acts. Circ Res 38:221-231, 1976

104. Milledge JS, Nunn JF: Criteria of fitness for anesthesia in patients with chronic obstructive lung disease. Brit Med J 3:670-3, 1975

105. Otis AB: The work of breathing, Vol I Ch 17 Sec 3 (Respiration) pp 463-476. In Fenn WO, Rahn H, Eds: Handbook of Physiology. American Physiol Society, Washington, 1964

106. Macklem PT, Roussos CS: Respiratory muscle fatigue: a cause of respiratory failure? Clin Sci Mol Med 53:419-422, 1977

107. Mitchell RA, Berger AJ: Neural regulation of respiration. Am Rev Respir Dis 111:206-224, 1975

108. Pavlin EG, Hornbein TF: The control of breathing. Basics of RD 7(2):1-6, 1978

109. Segall JJ, Butterworth BA: Ventilatory capacity in chronic bronchitis in relation to carbon dioxide retention. Scand J Resp Dis 47:215-224, 1966

110. Reichel J: Assessment of operative risk of pneumonectomy. Chest 62:570-576, 1972

111. Roughton FJW, Forster RE: Relative importance of diffusion and chemical reaction rates in determining rate of exchange of gases in the human lung with special reference to true diffusing capacity of pulmonary membrane and volume of blood in the lung capillaries. J Appl Physiol 11:290-302, 1957

112. Cander L: Physiologic assessment and management of the preoperative patient with emphysema. Am J Cardiol 12:324-6, 1963

113. Forster RE: Exchange of gases between alveolar air and pulmonary capillary blood: Pulmonary diffusing capacity. Physiol Rev 37:391-452, 1957

114. Kreukniet J, Visser BF: The pulmonary CO

diffusing capacity according to Bates and according to Filley in patients with unequal ventilation. Pflügers' Archiv 281:207-211, 1964

115. Ogilvie CM, Forster RE, Blakemore NS, et al: A standardized breathholding technique for the clinical measurement of the diffusing capacity of the lung for carbon monoxide. J Clin Invest 36:1-17, 1957

116. Filley GF, MacIntosh DJ, Wright GW: Carbon monoxide uptake and pulmonary diffusing capacity in normal subjects at rest and during exercise. J Clin Invest 33:530-39, 1954

117. Hlastala MP, Robertson HT: Inert gas elimination characteristics of the normal and abnormal lung. J Appl Physiol: Resp Environ Exerc Physiol 44:258-266, 1978

118. Bates DV, Boucot NG, Dormer AE: The pulmonary diffusing capacity in normal subjects. J Physiol (London) 129:237-252, 1955

119. Souders CR: The clinical evaluation of the patient for thoracic surgery. Surg Clin North Am 41:545-556, 1961

120. Semb C, Erickson H, Bergan F, et al: Cardiorespiratory function in pulmonary surgery. Acta Chir Scand 109:235-247, 1955

121. Jones NL, Campbell EJM, Edwards RT, et al: Clinical Exercise Testing. WB Saunders, Philadelphia, 1975, pp 63-66

122. Johnson AN, Cooper DF, Edwards RHT: Exertion of stair-climbing in normal subjects and in patients with chronic obstructive bronchitis. Thorax 32:711-16, 1977

123. Wasserman K, Whipp BJ: Exercise physiology in health and disease. Am Rev Respir Dis 112:219-49, 1975

124. Nadel JA, Gold WM, Burgess JH: Early diagnosis of chronic pulmonary vascular obstruction: value of pulmonary function tests. Am J Med 44:16-25, 1968

125. Mohsenifar Z, Tashkin DP, Levy-SE et al: Lack of sensitivity of measurements of VD/VT at rest and during exercise in detection of hemodynamically significant pulmonary vascular abnormalities in collagen vascular disease. Am Rev Respir Dis 123:508-512, 1981

126. Feigal DW, Blaisdell FW: The estimation of surgical risk. Med Clin North Am 63:1131-43, 1979

127. Goldman L: Index of cardiac risk in noncardiac surgery (letter). New Engl J Med 298:340, 1978

128. Riley RL, Himmelstein A, Morey HL, et al: Studies of the pulmonary circulation at rest and during exercise in normal individuals and in patients with chronic pulmonary disease. Am J Physiol 152:372-382, 1948

129. Schilling JA: Pulmonary resection and sequelae of thoracic surgery, vol II Ch 67 Sec 3 (Respiration) pp 1531-1552. Fenn WO, Rahn H, Eds: Handbook of physiology. Amer Physiol Soc., Washington, 1965

130. Adams WE, Perkins JF Jr, Flores A, et al: The significance of pulmonary hypertension as a cause of death following pulmonary resection. J Thor Surg 26:407-418, 1953

131. Harrison RW, Adams WE, Long ET, et al: The clinical significance of cor pulmonale in the reduction of cardiopulmonary reserve following extensive pulmonary resection. J Thor Surg 36:352-68, 1958

132. Laros CD, Swierenga J: Temporary unilateral pulmonary artery occlusion in the preoperative evaluation of patients with bronchial carcinoma. Comparison of pulmonary artery pressure measurements, pulmonary function tests and early postoperative mortality. Med Thorac 24:269-283, 1967

133. Rams JJ, Harrison RW, Fry WA, et al: Operative pulmonary artery pressure measurements as a guide to postoperative management and prognosis during pneumonectomy. Dis Chest 41:85-90, 1962

134. Fishman AP: Dynamics of the pulmonary circulation, Vol 2 Sec 2 (Circulation) p 1667. In Hamilton WF, Dow P, Eds: Handbook of Physiology. Washington, Amer Physiol Society, 1963

135. Armitage GH, Taylor AB: Nonbronchospirometric measurement of differential lung function. Thorax 11:281-6, 1956

136. Svanberg L: Bronchospirometry in the study of regional lung function. Scand J Resp Dis supp 62:91-103, 1966

137. TenHolder MF, Jones PA, Matthews JI, et al: Bullous emphysema: progressive incremental exercise testing to evaluate candidates for bullectomy. Chest 77:802-5, 1980

138. Svanberg L: Regional function decrease in bronchial carcinoma. Ann Thorac Surg 13:170-180, 1972

139. Neuhaus H, Cherniack NS: A broncho-

spirometric method of estimating the effect of pneumonectomy on the maximum breathing capacity. J Thorac Cardiovasc Surg 55:144-8, 1968

140. Gaensler EA, Maloney JV, Björk VO: Bronchospirometry II: experimental observation and theoretical considerations of resistance breathing. J Lab Clin Med 39:935-53, 1952

141. Sackner MA; Bronchofiberoscopy. Am Rev Respir Dis 111:62-88, 1975

142. Hugh-Jones P, West JB: Detection of bronchial and arterial obstruction by continuous gas analysis from individual lobes and segments of the lung. Thorax 15:154-64, 1960

143. Hugh-Jones P: Localization of disordered function. Bull Physiopath Resp 3:419-29, 1967

144. Agostoni E: Mechanics of the pleural space. Physiol Rev 52:57-128, 1972

145. Bergan F: A simple method for determination of the relative function of the right and left lung. Acta Chir Scand suppl 253:58-63, 1960

146. Hazlett DR, Watson RL: Lateral position test: a simple, inexpensive yet accurate method of studying the separate function of the lungs. Chest 59:276-279, 1971

147. Walkup RH, Vossel LF, Griffin JP, et al: Prediction of postoperative pulmonary function with the lateral position test: a prospective study. Chest 77:24-27, 1980

148. Marion JM, Alderson PO, Lefrak SS, et al: Unilateral lung function: comparison of the lateral position test with radionuclide ventilation-perfusion studies. Chest 69:5-9, 1976

149. Solomon DA, Goldman AL: Use of the lateral position test and perfusion lung scan in predicting mediastinal metastases. Chest 79:406-408, 1981

150. DeMeester TR, vanHeertum RL, Karas JR, et al: Preoperative evaluation with differential pulmonary function. Ann Thorac Surg 18:61-71, 1974

151. Knipping HW, Bolt W, Venrath H et al: Eine neue Methode zur Prüfung der Herz- und Lungenfunktion. Deut Med Wochschr 80:1146-7, 1955

152. West JB: Regional Differences in the Lung, Academic Press, New York, 1977, pp 33-83

153. Hughes JMB, Glazier JB, Maloney JE, et al: Effect of lung volume on the distribution of pulmonary blood flow in man. Resp Physiol 4:58-72, 1968

154. Olsen GN, Block AJ, Tobias JA: Prediction of postpneumonectomy pulmonary function using quantitative macroaggregate lung scanning. Chest 66:13-16, 1974

155. Alazraki NP, Ramsdell JW, Taylor A, et al: Reliability of gallium scans and chest radiography compared to mediastinoscopy for evaluating mediastinal spread in lung cancer. Am Rev Respir Dis 117:415-420, 1978

156. Secker-Walker RM, Provan JL: Scintillation scanning of lungs of preoperative assessment of carcinoma of bronchus. Brit Med J 3:327-330, 1969

157. Boysen PG, Block AJ, Olsen GN, et al: Prospective evaluation for pneumonectomy using the 99^m technetium quantitative perfusion lung scan. Chest 72:422-5, 1977

158. Miörner G: ^{133}Xe-Radiospirometry: a clinical method for studying regional lung function. Scand J Resp Dis suppl 64:1-84, 1968

159. Kristersson S, Arborelius M, Jungquist G, et al: Prediction of ventilatory capacity after lobectomy. Scand J Resp Dis 54:315-25, 1973

160. McNeil BJ, Weichselbaum R, Pauker SG: Fallacy of the five-year survival in lung cancer. New Engl J Med 299:1397-1401, 1978

John T. Bonner, M.D.

5
Preoperative Preparation

BASIS FOR PREOPERATIVE PREPARATION

Contrasted to the essentially healthy patient scheduled for lower abdominal or extremity operations, thoracic surgery draws special attention to the preoperative evaluation and preparation of the patient.[1] Thoracic surgery, chronic lung disease, a heavy smoking history, obesity, and advanced age (>70 years old) are risk factors which can be altered by adequate preparation to lessen the chances for postoperative pulmonary complications. The spectrum of physiologic changes imposed upon the patient during the perioperative period carry a greater risk of resulting in morbidity or mortality when superimposed upon an acutely or chronically compromised cardiopulmonary system.[2-4] Even though patient morbidity exists as a wide spectrum of problems, it is defined as segmental lung collapse (atelectasis), a change in sputum character (pneumonitis), evidence of consolidation (pneumonia), or bronchoconstriction (wheezing) for thoracic surgical patients. The incidence of postoperative pulmonary complications varies from 3 to 70 percent, depending upon the criteria selected.

Optimal preoperative preparation can reduce this morbidity.[5] In a group of patients with abnormal tests of gas flow, distribution, and $PaCO_2$, Stein found that postoperative complications developed in 5 of 23 well-prepared patients (22%), compared to 15 of 25 patients (60%) who did not receive any preoperative preparation (Table 5-1).[6] Preoperative preparation of 190 of 357 men with chronic obstructive pulmonary disease (COPD) resulted in a decrease in pulmonary complications from 43 percent without preparation to 24 percent with preparation; however, no change in overall mortality was found.[7] A later series from the same institution supported this initial observation, with postoperative pulmonary complications occurring in only 19 percent of 134 prepared patients with COPD who underwent surgery and anesthesia.[5] In both series, the incidence of complications was highest in patients undergoing upper abdominal and thoracic surgery.

The responsibility for carrying out preoperative preparation is shared by the thoracic surgeon, pulmonary medicine specialist, and anesthesiologist-intensivist. Too often in the past an internal medicine consult was requested to "clear the patient for sur-

Table 5-1
Pulmonary Complications In Prepared (Group A) vs. Unprepared Patients (Group B)

| Operative Site | N | No. Patients with Pulmonary Complications | Severity of Complications | | | |
			1+ Least	2+	3+	4+ Worst
Group A						
Thorax	17	4	3	1	0	0
Abdomen	5	1	1	0	0	0
Other	1	0	0	0	0	0
Total	23	5	4	1	0	0
Group B						
Thorax	17	13	1	3	5	4
Abdomen	3	1	0	0	1	0
Other	5	1	0	1	0	0
Total	25	15	1	4	6	4

Stein M, Koota GM, Simon M et al: Preoperative pulmonary evaluation and therapy for surgery patients. JAMA 211:787–790, 1970

gery." The consultant's function should be to classify the stages of chronic diseases, identify acute problems, and propose or implement therapy. The consultant who serves this function contributes to the patient's data base from which other physicians and the patient can make decisions regarding the timing of surgery. The consultant who "clears" or "does not clear" the patient for surgery, or dictates the choice of anesthetic or surgical technique, often compromises the efficient functioning of the surgical-anesthetic team and usually contributes little to patient care.

In the preparation of a patient for thoracic surgery, objectives should be formulated according to the anticipated intra- and postoperative events. Within the time frame dictated by the urgency of the surgical procedure, therapeutic activities in the preoperative period should treat acute illness, return the patient to the steady state of chronic disease, and anticipate postoperative functional derangements. The obese, heavy smoker with chronic bronchorrhea and wheezing who requires a diagnostic thoracotomy for an isolated pulmonary lesion affords the surgical team time for adequate preoperative preparation, in contrast to the victim of a thoracic gunshot wound with an enlarging

hemothorax who may require immediate thoracotomy for hemostasis.

CONDITIONS AMENABLE TO PREOPERATIVE THERAPY (TABLE 5-2)

Acute Illness

INFECTION

Pneumonitis producing bronchorrhea or pneumonia with consolidation represent acute treatable illnesses in the preoperative period. Good medical practice dictates delay of elective surgery if an acute respiratory infection exists. However, chronic respiratory infections are often treated with a "broad spectrum" antibiotic, such as ampicillin or

Table 5-2
Conditions Amenable to Preoperative Therapy

Acute Illness	Chronic Illness
Infection	Wheezing (chronic)
Dehydration	Bronchorrhea
Electrolyte disturbances	Obesity
Wheezing (acute, reversible)	Smoking
	Cor pulmonale
	Malnutrition

tetracycline, and surgery is allowed to proceed. These antibiotics are also given to all COPD patients with a change in character of sputum, fever, or leucocytosis.[8,9]

Cooper's prospective series of 221 patients undergoing thoracotomy supports the preoperative, empirical use of prophylactic antibiotics.[10] Both pneumonectomy space and pulmonary infections occurred less frequently in patients treated with prophylactic antibiotics (ampicillin/flucloxacillin). Routine sputum cultures were of no predictive value in the selection of antibiotic therapy. Mortality was 9 percent in the group treated with prophylactic antibiotics, and 17 percent in the group receiving no preoperative antibiotics. Consequently, an empirical therapeutic regimen has become common practice, unless the likelihood of an unusual pathogen is suggested by the clinical setting; e.g., the immunosuppressed patient may need therapy for mycobacterial, fungal, or parasitic infestation.

A distinction should be made between the widespread bronchorrhea of tracheobronchitis and a pneumonic process producing consolidation demonstrable on a radiograph. A localized infection should be treated with antibiotic therapy combined with intermittent ultrasonic mist inhalation to promote coughing, bronchodilator therapy, and gravity drainage. Routine cultures of sputum produce a variety of bacteria representing oral flora and provide less precise information for directing antimicrobial therapy than transtracheal aspiration, bronchoscopic lavage and aspiration, or lung biopsy.[11,12]

Early antimicrobial treatment of the acutely ill patient should be directed by a Gram stain of the sputum which may indicate the predominant type of infection that can be confirmed later by sputum and blood cultures. If the history and examination indicates tuberculosis, an acid-fast stain of the sputum can provide a diagnosis weeks before information is derived from sputum cultures. Active tuberculosis is initially treated with a combination of isoniazid, ethambutal, rifampin and streptomycin. A summary of antimicrobial classification, presumed mechanism of action, common indications, and drug examples is provided in Table 5-3.[13]

Due to the efficient lung defense mechanisms, the bronchial tree is normally sterile from the first bronchial division to the alveolus.[14] These defense mechanisms protect the lung against a multitude of insults such as bacteriologic agents, air pollutants, allergenic antigens, smoke, and industrial byproducts.[15] The defense system includes (1) efficient nasal filtration during gas inhalation, with larger particles being impacted on the surface of the turbinates; (2) airway reflexes that protect against larger particulate inhalation and against liquid aspiration; (3) the alveolar macrophage system, representing an efficient immunologic defense; and (4) the mucociliary blanket, which is a transport system that moves pathogens and other particulate matter out of the lungs towards the glottis to be cleared by swallowing or coughing.

The mucociliary blanket is a continuous sheet of mucus that is in continuity with the mucous glands. It represents a large surface area held away from the epithelial surface on the numerous cilia which act as hands propelling it towards the glottis (Fig. 5-1). In normal tracheal epithelium only the tip of the cilia are in contact with the mucus blanket. In pathologic states the mucus blanket is tethered to the mucous glands and not moved by the cilia.[14,16,17] Poorly hydrated secretions behave more as a thick gel than a movable sheet.[16] Each cell has about 200 cilia that beat at a frequency of approximately 20 cycles per second. One-third of the cycle is active motion toward the glottis. The velocity of removal from the lung of a particle suspended in the mucus blanket is about 1 mm per minute from the small airways, and 20 mm per minute in larger airways such as the trachea.[14]

The mucociliary blanket can be altered by pharmacologic intervention. In cats ren-

Table 5-3 Antimicrobial Drugs

Type of Anti-microbial Agent	Mechanism	Use	Examples	Adverse Effects
penicillins	inhibit cell wall formation	non-hospital acquired pneumonias	penicillin G ampicillin (semisynthetic) methicillin, nafcillin, oxacillin (penicillinase sensitive) Carbenicillin, ticarcillin (effective against pseudomonas, often used in combination with gentamycin)	sensitivity
cephalosporin	inhibits wall formation	synergistic with aminoglycosides	cephalothin (venosclerotic) cefazolin cephalexin (oral preparation only)	cross-sensitivity in penicillin allergic individuals
tetracycline	inhibits protein synthesis: bacteriostatic	pneumonococcus, *H. influenzae*	tetracycline, oxytetracycline, doxycycline	gastrointestinal symptoms
aminoglycoside	inhibits protein syntheses: binds to intracellular ribosomes	gram negative, broad spectrum	gentamycin kanamycin (may be aerosolized) amikacin, neomycin tobramycin	auditory ototoxicity, vestibular ototoxicity, neuromuscular blockade, nephrotoxic
polymyxin	damages cell membranes	mostly topical	polymyxin E (bowel prep) B (topical opthalmic) bacitracin	nephrotoxic, neuromuscular blockade
macrolides	interferes with protein synthesis	penicillin alternate	erythromycin	estolate hypersensitivity producing jaundice
lincomycin	interferes with protein synthesis	anaerobes: lung abscess, empyema	clindomycin, lincomycin	diarrhea, cardiovascular collapse with rapid IV injection
chloramphenicol	interferes wiuth protein synthesis	Salmonella, wide spectrum	chloramphenicol	hematologic, neonatal cardiovascular ("grey-baby")
sulfonamides	antimetabolite: inhibits di-hydrofolic acid synthesis	pneumonococcus *H. influenzae* streptococcus	sulfisoxazole sulfadiazine	photosensitivity, gastrointestinal, hematologic, urinary tract crystallization

Modified from: Ziment, I. Respiratory Pharmacology and Therapeutics, Philadelphia, W. B. Saunders Co., 1978 pp 340–386.

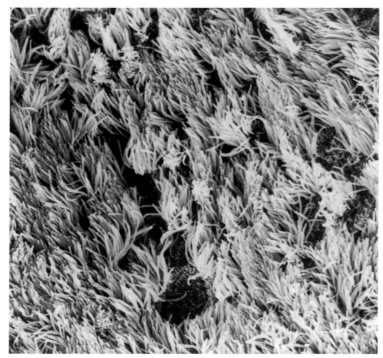

Fig. 5-1   Normal tracheal cilia as shown by a scanning electron microscope.

dered hypoxic, cardiac glycosides improved disordered ciliary beating.[18] Another study demonstrated a depression of mucus flow when it was exposed to a high concentration of oxygen. This depression was reversed by epinephrine.[19]

Atropine has been regarded as a harmful drying agent in chronic bronchitis, producing dessication and impaction of sputum. Ciliary clearance of sputum is probably impaired by atropine only in patients with excessive airway secretions. Particularly when given by the inhalation route, atropine does not impair mucus clearance in patients with scant sputum production.[20,21]

The effect of acute and chronic cigarette smoke exposure on mucociliary function is regarded to be harmful, and evidence exists that ciliary function is inhibited by smoking.[14] Immediately after cessation of chronic smoking, however, a bronchorrhea often occurs, and may last two to three days.[22,23]

DEHYDRATION AND ELECTROLYTE DISTURBANCES

Intra- and extracellular water contributes up to 50 to 60 percent of body weight.[24] Derangements of body water may be classified as water losses (dehydration), or water excesses (dilutional). Overt respiratory failure has been noted to be associated with dilutional manifestations of water retention by Sladen.[25] Similarly, sodium losses or excesses produce electrolyte derangements in clinically encountered conditions of vomiting, diarrhea, diuretic therapy, pituitary disorders, enteral fistulae, and corticosteroid therapy. Leaf classified hyponatremia as dilutional, with expanded circulatory volume; and non-dilutional, with contracted extracellular fluid volume.[26] For purposes of understanding pathophysiology and therapy, a distinction must be made between primary water loss or primary sodium loss when using the term "dehydration." Primary salt depletion produces circulatory insufficiency with tachycardia and hypotension; while primary water depletion tends to preserve extracellular water at the expense of intracellular water, leading to intense thirst and oliguria.[26]

Dehydration which results in interstitial or intracellular water loss may compromise the efficiency of the mucociliary host defense system.[14,27,28] Repletion of any water deficit represents an important aspect of preoperative preparation in these patients. Estimates of the presence and degree of dehydration should be made in any clinical setting in which water loss may occur. Examples include the patient with vomiting, diarrhea, hyperglycemia, diuretic-induced diuresis, or compromised oral intake of water from inanition or diagnostic procedures. Forehead and sternal skin turgor can be estimated by physical examination and is a useful sign of interstitial water content. In addition, serum sodium and hematocrit are elevated when significant degrees of dehydration are present.

Repletion of water should be accomplished either enterally or parenterally. Humidification of inspired gases simply prevents water loss and tracheal mucosal dessication in the intubated patient, and water repletion cannot be practically accomplished by the inhalation of vaporized or evaporated water in an adult patient.

The total body potassium stores are approximately 4,000 mEq, with only about 3 percent being extracellular. The intracellular concentration is normally 115 to 160 mEq/liter, depending on the cell type, and the extracellular concentration is about 4.5 mEq/liter. An obligate urinary loss occurs, and varies between 40 and 90 mEq/24 hours. Inadequate oral intake such as often occurs in esophageal carcinoma, or excess loss by vomiting, gastrointestinal fistula drainage, or by drug-induced diuresis may contribute to total body potassium depletion with a low extracellular concentration. Potassium depletion, reflected in low serum levels, should

be treated preoperatively to minimize the occurrence of dysrhythmias and potentiation of muscle relaxants.

In addition to disturbances in sodium and potassium, certain thoracic surgical patients may also have abnormal chloride and calcium concentrations. Patients with esophageal carcinomas and prolonged vomiting can have a hyponatremic, hypochloremic, hypokalemic metabolic alkalosis which can produce problems with weaning from mechanical ventilation. Ionized calcium levels have also been found to be markedly decreased in patients undergoing cancer operations, producing abnormalities in myocardial and neuromuscular function.

Potassium should be replaced intravenously at a maximum rate of 0.5 mEq/kg/hr and not to exceed 240 mEq/24 hrs. This therapy should be monitored by blood and urine potassium levels and constant ECG observation. The minimum time needed to replace large body deficits of potassium is 12 to 48 hours.

WHEEZING (ACUTE)

Reversible smooth muscle constriction, accumulation of secretions, and mucosal edema can each contribute to audible gas flow obstruction which is treatable with bronchodilators, mobilization of secretions, and steroids (see therapy section below). Documentation of the effectiveness of bronchodilators may be provided by measurements of air flow before and after drug therapy. The acute asthmatic attack represents a life-threatening episode which mandates therapy and resolution before elective surgical procedures. Mild asthmatic episodes may produce changes only in small airways (less than 3 mm in diameter) and result in minimal increases in flow resistance and mild wheezing. About three-fourths of the total airways' cross-sectional area is provided by these small airways (Table 5-4). In contrast, smooth muscle constriction, mucosal edema, or accumulation of mucus in large airways

Table 5-4
Airway Dynamics

Size of Airway	Flow Resistance	Cross-Sectional Area
Large (nose, trachea, bronchi)	Large	Small
Small ($<$ 3 mm diameter)	Small	Large

greatly compromises the total airway and re-sistance to air flow rises markedly with se-vere wheezing.

Acute wheezing represents a medical emergency requiring definitive therapy and postponement of all but the most emergent surgical procedures. Blood gases in the asth-matic patient usually demonstrate hypocar-bia and hypoxemia. A rising or elevated $PaCO_2$ in the acutely wheezing patient de-mands serious consideration of mechanical ventilatory support.

Chronic Illness

WHEEZING (CHRONIC)

Contrasted against the acute, reversible asthmatic episode is the presence of gas flow obstruction producing wheezing in chronic lung disease. The responsiveness of the air-ways to bronchodilators is variable and un-predictable, but adequate preoperative prep-aration should include a trial of drug therapy. Empirical preoperative preparation reduced the frequency of occurrence of post-operative pulmonary complications in Stein's and Gracey's series, where therapy consisted of aerosolized bronchodilator drugs given without regard for the degree of indi-vidual patient responsiveness.[5,6]

Rational treatment of audible air flow obstruction manifested by wheezing includes appropriate use of pharmacologic agents that relax bronchial smooth muscle, as well as other therapeutic modalities to produce hu-midification and clearing of secretions. Just as antibiotics are used in combination with methods of draining infected lung units in pneumonia or emphysema, bronchodilators

should be combined with the use of physio-therapy, humidification of inspired gases, and perhaps steroids in the treatment of chronic airflow obstruction. Constriction of smooth muscle may occur only in small air-ways, and be detectable only by sensitive tests such as the FEF_{25-75}, or may be wide-spread resulting in audible wheezing and large reductions in the FEV_1 and VC.[29] Compromise in airflow may be acute and in-tense, as in the acute asthmatic episode, or chronic and less intense in the COPD patient with profuse secretions, mucosal edema, and slight smooth muscle constriction. Cautious trials of bronchodilator therapy are appro-priate during the preoperative preparation of all patients with any evidence of airflow ob-struction, regardless of the duration or inten-sity of the bronchospasm. Inhaled steroids may provide an additional valuable mode of therapy in the chronically wheezing patient. Minimal to no adrenal suppression occurs with the newer halogenated steroids (beclo-methasone, betamethasone, triamcinolone) given by the inhalation route.[30]

BRONCHORRHEA (MUCUS PRODUCTION)

Abundant secretions present a dramatic aspect of the pathology of chronic bron-chitis.[31,32] Frequently, a stethoscope is not even needed to hear post-tussive rhonchi and wheezing if a patient's chronic bronchitis is far advanced. The assumption is frequently made that retained secretions cause atelec-tasis, but patients may develop atelectasis without having profuse secretions.[1] Resorp-tion of oxygen-rich gases by perfusion of relatively underventilated alveoli reduces the volume of those lung units, putting them at

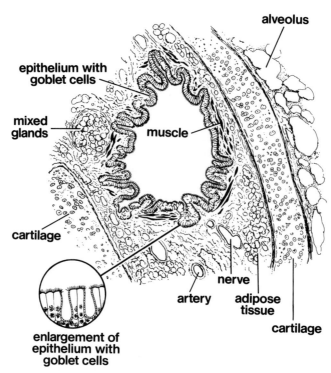

epithelium with
goblet cells

mixed
glands

muscle

cartilage

alveolus

nerve

artery

adipose
tissue

cartilage

enlargement of
epithelium with
goblet cells

Fig. 5-2 The normal respiratory histology of the trachea is demonstrated. The enlargement shows the epithelium with goblet cells.

risk for total collapse.[33] Secretions can compromise airway lumen and provide the airway obstruction necessary for resorption atelectasis to occur; but low lung volumes, in general, and decreased lung compliance with a painful incision may also compromise ventilation of lung units and allow atelectasis to develop.

Mucus is secreted by the mucous glands and goblet cells of the respiratory epithelium which primarily consist of ciliated columnar epithelium, and line the nose, paranasal sinuses, trachea, and large bronchi. Nonciliated, cuboidal epithelium is present in non-rigid portions of the airway such as the pharynx, terminal bronchioles, and respiratory bronchioles. Goblet cells are more abundant toward the proximal portion of the tracheobronchial tree and at the bifurcations of the large bronchi (Figs. 5-2, 5-3, 5-4). Mucous glands are present in clumps in the submucosa of cartilage-containing bronchi.[34]

The complex process involved in moving mucus up the respiratory tree is called mucokinesis, and drugs that result in removal of sputum or mucus are termed mucokinetics. The most commonly used mucokinetic agents are water, saline, propylene glycol, and iodine. Mucolytic drugs are capable of breaking mucoprotein molecules into smaller, less viscous residues. The important mucolytic drugs are acetylcysteine (Mucomyst) and the various inhalational enzymes (e.g., Dornase). The choice of drug therapy depends on the type of symptoms (e.g., excessive respiratory secretions versus inability to expectorate) present in each patient.[13]

OBESITY

In addition to the increased oxygen cost of breathing due to the extra work of moving the stiffer lung-thorax ventilatory apparatus, obesity produces chronic hypoxemia by re-

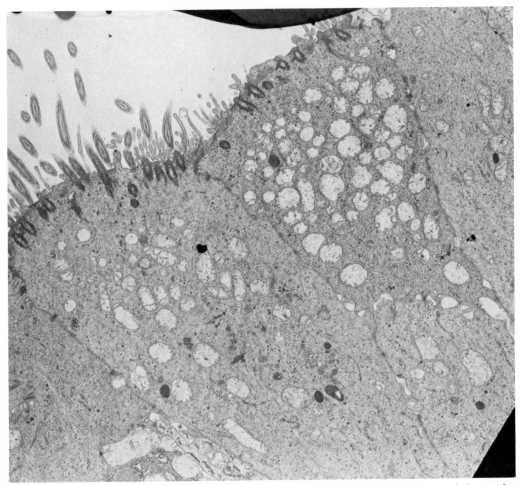

Fig. 5-3 Normal tracheal epithelium is demonstrated on a poorly preserved autopsy sample by regular electron microscopy. The microvilli and cilia can be seen in the upper left hand part of the photograph. The desmosomes clearly divide the columnar epithelial cells.

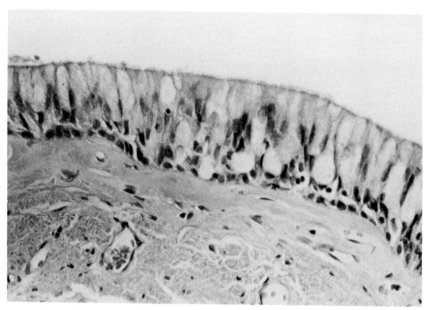

Fig. 5-4 A high-powered microscopic view of normal respiratory epithelium with goblet cells is demonstrated.

ducing functional residual capacity (FRC) towards closing volume.[35,36] The FRC is further decreased during anesthesia by as much as 10 to 25 percent.[37-39] These changes are presumed to be the etiology for the widened P (A–a) O_2 in obesity. Postoperative pulmonary complications may result from accentuation of the known pulmonary derangements.

In massive obesity, elective weight loss in a period shorter than three months is not practical. Obesity is one of the preoperative risk factors that is not easily amenable to correction over a shorter time. Caloric restriction or malabsorption resulting in weight loss may actually be detrimental to respiratory function in the early stages. In one study a reduced forced vital capacity (FVC) occurred during rapid weight loss in GI-by-passed patients who lost 27 percent of their pre-bypass weight, after which a gradual return of FVC occurred.[35]

SMOKING

Cigarette smoking is a clear example of a potentially reversible, patient-controlled

pulmonary insult that results in airway disease. The increased incidence of postoperative pulmonary complications in smokers has been recognized for decades.[40] The quantity and duration of smoking (pack-years) are directly related to the measureable changes in airflow and closing volume.[41,42] Changes in the FVC and MMEFR occur in smokers as young as 15 years of age.[43] Small airways (less than 3 mm in diameter) are affected by smoking earlier than larger airways. Therefore, in the development of airway disease related to smoking, clinical signs of airflow obstruction occur later than do derangements of tests designed to detect small airway abnormalities.

Cessation of smoking is usually encouraged as part of the preoperative preparation of the smoker being considered for thoracic surgery. Decreased symptoms of a productive cough are evident when the amount of smoking is decreased by 25 percent.[42] Reversibility of airway abnormalities is presumed to occur rapidly, but the actual slow rate of return of function toward normal is frequently not appreciated. In one study of smokers, evidence of improvement in small airways disease was detected only after eight weeks of cessation of smoking.[42] Abnormal frequency-dependent compliance, a sign of small airways disease, improved after two months of smoking abstinence in another series of smokers.[44] Improvement of mucociliary transport occurred in smokers after cessation of smoking for 3 months, while no improvement occurred in one week. Forced vital capacity and the FEV_1 have been found to decline with age, but the rate of decline is slower in nonsmokers and former smokers than in current smokers.[45] Improvement in closing volume can also occur after smoking cessation.[46]

Bode et al found that only 10 of 50 smokers stopped smoking after their physician's advice and encouragement.[46] Those 10 patients who complied demonstrated indirect evidence of improvement in small airways disease by decreased closing volume and increased $MMEFR_{25-50}$ with helium. However, these changes occurred only after 6 to 14 weeks of stopping smoking. No significant change in abnormal spirometric testing occurred in 5 volunteer smokers who stopped smoking for one week.[47] Thus, smoking abstinence would not appear to allow measureable pulmonary function improvement in any period shorter than a month, but the demonstrable improvement in function that may occur in that time represents a major step toward optimal preoperative preparation. Modification of smoking habits should decrease symptoms of cough and sputum production within one month, and should be encouraged. Considerable psychological support should be given the patient during the initial period of behavior modification. In addition to improvement in ciliary function, small airway function, and sputum production, carbon monoxide levels decrease and oxygen transport improves.

COR PULMONALE

Cor pulmonale, or pulmonary heart disease, is caused by inadequate pulmonary function. The pulmonary derangement may be intrinsic, such as emphysema, or extrinsic, such as pectus excavatum or obesity with hypoventilation.[48,49] Right ventricular enlargement and pulmonary hypertension are always present, and are necessary to make the diagnosis. The left ventricle is not primarily involved in cor pulmonale, and clinical signs of left ventricular failure are usually considered evidence for an independent cardiac problem rather than occurring secondary to pulmonary disease.[49] However, the possibility exists that severe and chronic hypoxemia may lead to left ventricular dysfunction.[50,51]

The pulmonary vasculature may be significantly obliterated by recurrent emboli independent of parenchymal lung disease. In the presence of hypoxia, pulmonary vasoconstriction contributes to an increased pulmonary arterial pressure.[52] Acidosis has long been known to potentiate hypoxic pulmonary vasoconstriction.[53] The unusually high resistance of the right-sided circulation results in increased right ventricular work and consequent right ventricular enlargement. The pulmonary circulation has a large cross-sectional area and low resistance. In order to incriminate vascular obliteration in the etiology of the pulmonary hypertension, a large proportion (as much as 75%) of the circulation would have to be involved[54,55] (see ch. 7).

Treatment of the patient with cor pulmonale who is considered for thoracic surgery assumes that there is reversibility of some element of the disease. Patients with cor pulmonale in whom the right ventricular disease is related to chronic bronchitis or emphysema are more amenable to therapy than those who have an anatomic obliterative pulmonary circulatory disorder. Hypoxic pulmonary vasoconstriction may be treated by supplemental oxygen therapy, as well as by treatment of the cause for the hypoxia, if it is an acute process such as infection or bronchorrhea. The pulmonary circulation is not practically amenable to direct pharmacologic methods of vasodilitation in the setting of hypoxia and acidosis.[52] Even though isoproterenol, acetylcholine, nitroprusside, and nitroglycerin have been shown to be pulmonary vasodilators, their use to improve right ventricular performance has not often been satisfactory.[52,56-58]

Increased lung water in cor pulmonale is usually considered a consequence of independent left ventricular disease, or of increased capillary permeability. Pulmonary edema, however slight, may be amenable to therapy, since it may contribute to increased pulmonary vascular resistance by extrinsic pressure on the pulmonary vasculature.[59] Since ischemic heart disease may contribute to overall mortality in thoracic surgery, optimal preoperative therapy should include control of angina and heart failure using vasodilators, digitalis, and diuretics.[60] Hypertension with a diastolic pressure above 110 mmHg also deserves adequate pharmacologic control before elective thoracic surgery.[61,62]

Bed rest, appropriate oxygen supplementation, and judicious diuretic therapy are useful modes of therapy in the treatment of cor pulmonale. Digitalis is often used as therapy for cor pulmonale, but the response is variable because the cause of the right ventricular dysfunction is so intimately related to the pulmonary disorder. The frequent presence of hypoxemia, acidosis, and diuretic-induced electrolyte disorders in patients with cor pulmonale suggest that digitalis therapy should be undertaken with caution in order to avoid digitalis toxicity.[52] Digitalis blood levels which are usually considered therapeutic may be toxic in the presence of hypokalemia or hypoxemia.

Clear indications for preoperative digitalis in patients without cor pulmonale undergoing thoracic surgery include congestive heart failure and supraventricular dysrhythmias with a rapid ventricular response.[63,64] If digitalization is contemplated for congestive heart failure, manifestations of left-sided failure should be sought that include ventricular (S_3) gallop, pulsus alternans, or radiographic evidence of pulmonary water accumulation. Without definite evidence of heart failure, prophylactic preoperative digitalization for pulmonary surgery is not indicated.[65]

Some cardiac patients with COPD require treatment with beta-adrenergic blocking drugs. Potentially serious respiratory dysfunction may occur when susceptible patients are given beta-blockers. Theoretically, such risk can be reduced by using (a) relatively $beta_1$ selective blockers (e.g., metoprolol, atenolol), (b) beta-blockers with partial agonist activity (e.g., oxprenolol, pindolol), or (c) a combined alpha and beta-blocker (e.g., labetalol). However, even these newer drugs should be used with caution in patients with COPD being prepared for thoracic surgery. It may be preferable in these patients to use slow channel calcium blockers instead of beta-blockers whenever possible. Verapamil can be used for control of tachyarrhythmias, and nifedipine, diltiazem or verapamil for ischemic heart disease.

MALNUTRITION

The nutritional status of the patient being considered for thoracic surgery represents a potential additional insult if malnutrition exists. In as short a period as 5 days, acute caloric restriction in healthy volunteer subjects led to a reduction of the ventilatory response to hypoxia and CO_2 production. Refeeding restored the ventilatory response to hypoxia and the intrinsic CO_2 production (Fig. 5-5).[66] Previously unrecognized malnutrition as manifested by at least one abnormality in weight history, skinfold measurements, albumin levels, transferrin levels, creatinine index or delayed sensitivity reactions was found to be present in 97 percent of a group of 64 preoperative hospitalized patients on a surgical service.[67] Postoperative morbidity and mortality were related to the degree of preoperative malnutrition. Driver found that adequate nutrition is often not provided surgical patients who cannot eat normally.[68]

The demands for oxygen are inordinately increased during exercise in patients

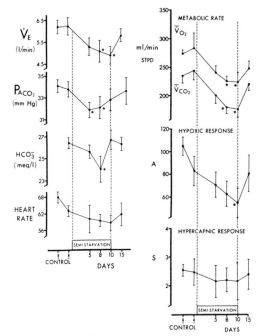

Fig. 5-5 The effects of semi-starvation on ventilation, blood gases, metabolic rate and the response to hypoxia, hypercarbia are shown. The stars indicate significant depression from the control values. Reproduced with permission from Dokel, Depression of hypoxic ventilatory response. N. Engl. J. Med. 295:358-361, 1976.

who have emphysema and bronchitis.[69] The weight loss and cachexic state often associated with chronic lung disease may be associated with increased energy substrate utilization in order to overcome the abnormally high work of breathing and oxygen cost of breathing.[70,71] Studies at Emory's Clinical Research Center have provided additional observations on the hypermetabolic state often present in emphysema and chronic bronchitis. They have shown that the increased caloric utilization is not related to the use of theophylline bronchodilators.[72] Alterations have also been noted in the lung ultrastructure of starved rats.[73] A study of patients with respiratory failure manifested by hypoxemia and respiratory acidosis demonstrated decreased concentrations of ATP and creatine phosphate in intercostal and quadriceps muscles.[74] After parenteral nutrition,

accompanied by traditional therapy for respiratory failure, levels of ATP and creatine phosphate rose, suggesting a vital role of nutritional supplementation during respiratory failure.

A significant aspect of preoperative preparation is the recognition and treatment of any degree of malnutrition. The demand for the provision of nutritional supplementation exceeds many hospitals' ability to provide such support, but hyperalimentation, whether enteral or parenteral, represents one of the more significant advances in surgery of the past decade.[75-78] Nutritional assessment has become extremely valuable and necessary for knowledgeable management of the patient undergoing thoracic surgery. Careful weight histories, skinfold measurements, creatinine-height index, albumin, lymphocyte count and transferrin levels provide a data base from which the nutritional status of the patient can be assessed. Implementation of hyperalimentation as part of the preoperative preparation offers some patients a significant advantage, when evidence exists for an inadequate caloric intake, particularly in the setting of hypermetabolism and chronic lung disease. Nutritional supplementation by parenteral hyperalimentation is indicated in many patients in whom evidence exists for malnutrition, since the ventilatory response to stimuli, immune responses, and wound healing are improved. However, supplementation in the previously caloric-depleted patient must be done with the realization that glucose loads sufficient to promote lipogenesis can increase the respiratory quotient several times over normal; the respiratory quotient (CO_2 excretion divided by oxygen consumption) associated with conversion of carbohydrate to fat can in theory increase to a value of 8 although measurements of the respiratory quotient in patients receiving glucose load indicate a value of approximately 2 to be more likely.[79] Significantly increased CO_2 loads can therefore be presented to the lung, and gross respiratory failure can result from inability to ex-

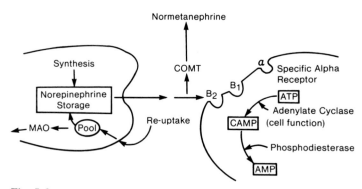

Fig. 5-6 A summary of norepinephrine storage, release, and re-uptake is shown.

crete the CO_2.[80,81] Hypophosphatemia may also occur in patients who are nutritionally depleted, and should be excluded as a possible cause of generalized weakness which could result in overt respiratory failure.[82,83]

BRONCHODILATOR THERAPY

Mediators of Bronchoconstriction

Bronchodilators may act by modifying neuroeffector events at the adrenergic nerve junction, altering release of bronchoactive substances, or influencing kinetics of intracellular messengers of cell function. Pharmacologic manipulation of bronchial smooth muscle tone involves specific intervention at various points of the complex neurohumoral mechanism controlling muscle tone.[84,85] These mechanisms involve the sympathetic and parasympathetic functions of the autonomic nervous system as well as other vasoactive substances.

Norepinephrine synthesis proceeds from tyrosine through DOPA and dopamine. Nerve stimulation releases the stored norepinephrine, which crosses the synaptic cleft, producing activation of the alpha- and beta-receptors on the cell membrane receptors (Fig. 5-6). Autonomic sympathomimetic agonists were first proposed by Ahlquist, in 1948, to be stimulators of alpha- and beta-receptors.[86] Alpha-receptors mediate vaso-

constriction, and may be involved in bronchoconstriction.[29,87] Specific beta-receptors were first proposed by Lands et al in 1967.[88] Beta$_1$ stimulation results in cardiac stimulation, while beta$_2$ stimulation results in bronchodilation. Newer drugs like terbutaline, albuterol, isoetharine, and metaproterenol have more selective beta$_2$ agonist action than the older mixed beta-bronchodilators. However, even these drugs are not totally devoid of beta$_1$ activity.

Beta-stimulation by beta-agonists such as isoproterenol results in augmentation of intracellular conversion of ATP to cyclic 3'5' AMP (C-AMP) and consequent relaxation of bronchial smooth muscle (Fig. 5-7). Adenyl cyclase promotes the conversion of ATP to C-AMP, and is increased by beta-stimulation. Phosphodiesterase catalyzes the breakdown of C-AMP, and is inhibited by the methylxanthines, causing an accumulation of C-AMP.

The actions of theophylline may also include increasing catecholamine synthesis, since it activates tyrosine hydroxylase, the rate-limiting enzyme in catecholamine synthesis. In addition, the xanthines may influence calcium kinetics. Bronchodilators, such as epinephrine, act as direct cell membrane beta$_2$-receptor stimulators; while drugs like ephedrine produce the indirect release of stored norepinephrine.

A balance exists between sympathetic and parasympathetic receptor stimulation.

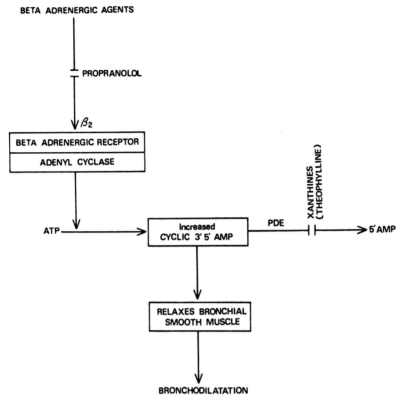

Fig. 5-7 Beta-adrenergic pathways through which C-AMP is increased in the bronchial smooth muscle cell leading to bronchodilatation. Reproduced with permission from Webb-Johnson DC, et al: Bronchodilator therapy. N. Engl. J. Med. 297:476-482, 1977.

That balance may be adversely altered by stimulation of the sympathetic autonomic nervous system with an alpha-agonist such as phenylephrine or norepinephrine resulting in decreased C-AMP and bronchoconstriction.[87] Bronchoconstriction may also result from stimulation of the parasympathetic autonomic nervous system (vagal stimulation), with a resulting increase in cyclic guanosine monophosphate (C-GMP) (Fig. 5-8).

In allergic asthmatic individuals, antibodies (IgE) bound to mast cells provoke release of histamine and eosinophil chemotaxic factor of anaphylaxis (ECF-A) when challenged by an antigen such as pollen or house dust. Synthesis of slow-reacting substances of anaphylaxis (SRS-A) may be stimulated by the antibody-antigen combination.[29] Other important chemical mediators in asthma include prostaglandins, kallikrein, bradykinin, and serotonin. Each of these appears to react through a separate receptor system. These vasoactive substances can produce bronchospasm directly and also by activation of cholinergic receptors and increased C-GMP.

**Classification of Bronchodilators
(Table 5-5)**

Drugs which promote bronchial smooth muscle dilitation may be classified as autonomic (sympathomimetics or parasympatholytics), methylxanthines, antimediators, or prostaglandins. Sympathomimetics include epinephrine, isoproterenol, and isoetharine.

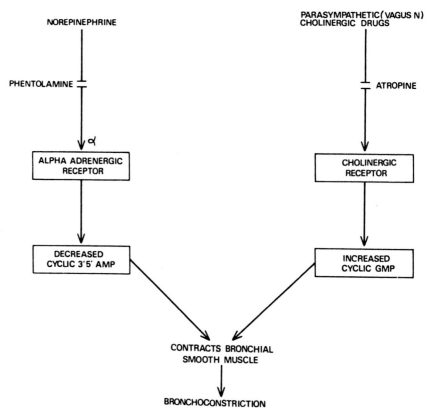

Fig. 5-8 Alpha-adrenergic and cholinergic pathways through which C-AMP is decreased, or C-GMP is increased, in the bronchial smooth muscle cell, thus causing bronchoconstriction. Reproduced with permission from Webb-Johnson DC, et al: Bronchodilator therapy. N. Engl. J. Med. 297:476-482, 1977.

Parasympatholytics include atropine and ipratroprium bromide (SCH-1000).[30,89] For years, atropine has been avoided in the wheezing patient because of concern that secretions might become more viscous and obstruct small airways. However, it has been shown that aerosolized atropine may be a clinically useful bronchodilator with only infrequently occurring side effects (Table 5-6).[89-91] The systemic absorption of inhaled atropine was studied in six patients with chronic bronchitis who received a dose of 0.05 mg/kg. Improvement of their previously reduced FEV$_1$ occurred within 15 minutes; maximal blood levels were 1.3 to 5.8 nanograms/ml, and measureable blood levels persisted for 4 hours.[92] Recently, Marini et al

examined the additive properties and the sites of action of inhaled atropine (0.05 mg/kg) and terbutaline (0.005 mg/kg) in 12 patients with COPD.[92] They found that both atropine and the combination of atropine with terbutaline improved airflow significantly more than did terbutaline by itself. The FEV$_1$ increased 85 percent with atropine and 93 percent with the combination, compared to only 56 percent with terbutaline. Atropine was shown to dilate proximal larger airways more effectively than terbutaline.

Steroids are given by aerosol, oral, and parenteral routes. They may potentiate the bronchodilation produced by sympathomimetics, but are not considered to be directly-acting bronchodilators. Steroids decrease

Table 5-5
Classification of Bronchodilators

I. Bronchoactive autonomic drugs
  A. Sympathomimetics
    1. Catecholamines
      a. Epinephrine
      b. Isoproterenol
      c. Isoetharine
      d. Ephedrine (indirect acting)
    2. Resorcinols [not metabolized by catechol-O-methyl transferase (COMT); B_2 specificity]
      a. Terbutaline
      b. Metaproterenol
    3. Saligenin
      a. Salbutamol (B_2 specificity)
    4. Others
      a. Protokylol (Ventaire)
      b. Ethylnorepinephrine (Bronkephine)
      c. Methoxyphenamine (Orthoxine)
  B. Parasympatholytic
    1. Anticholinergic
      a. Atropine
      b. Ipratroprium (SCH-1000)
II. Methylxanthines
  A. Phosphodiesterase inhibitors
    1. Theophylline ethylene diamine (aminophylline)
III. Antimediator drugs
  A. Glucocorticoids
    1. Hydrocortisone
    2. Methylprednisolone
    3. Beclomethasone
    4. Triamcinolone
    5. Betamethasone
  B. Antihistamines
  C. Bischromes
    1. Cromolyn
IV. Prostaglandins

mucosal edema, and their clinical usefulness may be attributed to improving gas flow in edematous, obstructed airways. In addition, they may prevent release of some bronchoactive substances.

Disodium cromoglycate (cromolyn-Intal) is used to prevent acute asthmatic episodes. Cromolyn stabilizes mast cells and inhibits degranulation with release of histamine and SRS-A; mediators of smooth muscle constriction. Cromolyn is useful for pre-treatment to prevent bronchospasm provoked by the classic antibody-antigen reaction.[93,94] Since cromolyn is not primarily a bronchodilator, it has no role as a first line therapeutic agent in the hospitalized patient.

Clinical Use of Theophylline

Measurements of VC and FEV_1 demonstrate that the therapeutic bronchodilation occurring after theophylline administration is directly related to the blood level of the drug. The measurement of blood levels of theophylline gives a valuable guide to therapy and is highly desirable in all cases. A loading dose of aminophylline is used to

Table 5-6 Preparations of Bronchoactive Drugs

Drug Generic-Trade	Preparation	Usual Dose	Onset	Duration	Mechanism of Action	Route	Side Effects	Comments
Sympathomimetics								
Epinephrine; Sus-phrine (Aqueous)	5 mg/cc (1:200)	0.1 to 0.3 cc (0.5 to 1.5 mg) subcutaneously test dose = 0.1 ml	Minutes	May repeat in 4–6 hours	α and β stimulation	subcu only	Anxiety, tachycardia, hypertension, injection site ischemia	For acute therapy: subcutaneous route only.
Epinephrine Injection	1 mg/cc (1:1000)	0.2 to 0.5 cc (.2 to 0.5 mg) subcutaneously	Minutes	subcutaneous dose may be repeated in 20 minutes	α and β stimulation	subcu only	Anxiety, tachycardia, hypertension, injection site ischemia	For acute therapy: subcutaneous route only
Racemic Epinephrine Micronephrine	Racemic Methamino-Ethanol Catechol Hydrochloride 2.25 gm/100ml	0.2 to 0.4 ml diluted to 5 ml	Minutes	May repeat inhalation in 2 to 4 hours	Topical vasoconstriction (α) and bronchodilation (β_2)	Inhaled aerosol	Tachycardia	Useful in glottic edema, croup
L-Epinephrine Primatine[R] Bronkaid[R]	0.2 mg/puff	1–2 puffs	Minutes	May repeat in 2–3 hours	α and β stimulation	Inhaled	Tachycardia, Dysrythmias	Non-prescription, cardiac effects prominent
Isoproterenol Isuprel-[R]	1:100 (10 mg/cc) 1:200 (5 mg/cc)	Nebulization: intermittent (undiluted) or over 10 minutes (diluted)	Minutes	May repeat in 3–4 hours	β_1 and β_2 effects	Inhaled	Tachycardia, dysrythmias	Dose determined by drops placed in nebulizer. IPPB: 0.5 ml of 1:200 diluted to 2 ml.

Drug	Preparation	Dose	Onset	Duration	Type	Route	Side effects	Comments
Isoproterenol Norisodrine[R]	Hydrocarbon propellant 0.12 mg/puff	1–2 puffs	5 minutes	May repeat in 4–6 hours	β agonist	Inhaled	Tachycardia, dysrhythmias	Significant cardiac side effects, alteration in V/Q may worsen hypoxemia.
Isoetharine Bronkosol[R]	1% 0.25% (unit dose)	1 unit dose by nebulizer O₂ drive, or IPPB	Minutes	May be repeated in 4 hours	More β₂ specificity	Inhaled	Occasionally refractory	Formerly manufactured, combined with phenylephrine
Ephedrine	Elixirs and capsules	15 to 50 mg	One hour	3–5 hours: may be given q 3–4 hours	Indirect alpha and beta (β₁ & β₂) catecholamine release	Oral	Somnolence in children, CNS stimulation	Not Metabolized by COMT or MAO. Good oral absorption. CNS stimulation. Tachyphylaxis frequent.
Resorcinols								
Terbutaline: Brethine[R]	Tabs 5 mg 2½ mg	5 mg	Hour	May be given q. 6 hours	β agonist possibly β₂ specific	oral	Tremor	Not metabolized by COMT or MAO
Terbutaline	solution 1 mg/ml	0.25 mg subcutaneously	15 minutes	90 minutes to 4 hours	Little β₂ specificity when given parenterally	subcutaneous	Tachycardia, dysrythmias, muscle tremors	Muscle tremors up to 30% of patients
Metaproterenol: Alupent[R]	10 mg tabs 20 mg 10 mg/5 ml	20 mg TID or QID	hour	q. 6 hours	Some β₂ specificity	oral	17% adverse effects: tachycardia tremor,	Not metabolized by COMT, inconsistent bronchoactive effects *(continued)*

Table 5-6 (continued) Preparations of Bronchoactive Drugs

Drug	Preparation	Usual Dose	Onset	Duration	Mechanism of Action	Route	Side Effects	Comments
Saligenin								
Albuterol Ventolin[R] Proventil[R]	inhalation	1–2 puffs q. 4–5 hrs.	minutes		β_2 agonist	inhalation		1/10 cardiac effect of isoproterenol appvd. by FDA (1981)
Others								
Protokylol Ventaire[R]								
Ethylnorepinephrine Bronkephrine[R]	2 mg/ml	0.5–1.0 ml Subcu or IM						Minimal CNS stimulating
Methoxyphenamine Orthoxine[R]								
Parasympatholytic								
Atropine	0.4 mg/cc injectable	1–2 mg diluted and aerosolized	minutes	2–4 hours	Blocking Acetylcholine muscaric receptors	inhaled	Tachycardia, CNS stimulation, mouth dryness, blurred vision	Not first line therapeutic drug for bronchodilation
SCH-1000 Ipratroprium[R]	available for experimental use in US							

Methylxanthine Aminophylline	85% theophylline, 15% ethylenediamine (250 mg/10ml)	5–6 mg/kg loading dose over 20 minutes. Maintenance dose range = 0.2 to 0.9 mg/kg/hr	minutes	continuous with maintenance dose	Phosphodiesterase inhibition, promotion cyclic 3'5' AMP		nausea, CNS stimulation, dysrythmias, inappropriate ADH	Monitor serum levels to 10–20 μg/ml, caution in CHF or liver dysfunction
Inhaled Steroids Beclomethasone Vanceril[R] Betamethasone Valisone[R]	Metered aerosol	1–2 puffs (50–200 μg) qid		Long acting	Decrease edema	Inhaled	oral candida	No adrenal suppression
Cromolyn sodium Intal[R]	aerosol	20 mg Spinhaler capsule	2–6 hrs.	days to months	Blocks release of mast cell granuales	Inhaled	Throat irritation, bronchospasm	Prophylactic use only; *not* for asthmatic attacks

Table 5-7
Guidelines for Intravenous Aminophylline

	Loading	First 12 hours Maintenance	Beyond 12 hours Maintenance
	mg/kg	mg/kg/hr	mg/kg/hr
Under 16	5 to 6	0.9	0.8
Liver disease, heart failure	5 to 6	0.3 to 0.5	0.1

(Adjusted slightly downward from FDA drug bulletin recommendations)[96]

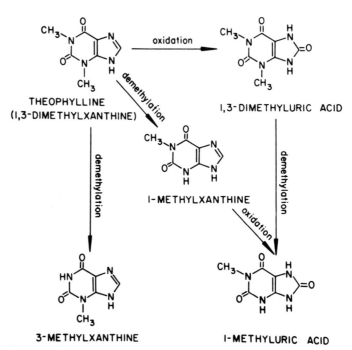

Fig. 5-9 Metabolism of theophylline in man is shown. About 87 percent of the administered dose is excreted as metabolites in the urine and 13 percent as unchanged theophylline. Reproduced with permission from Miech RP: Metabolism in Pharmacodynamics of theophylline. In Stein M, Ed: New Directions in Asthma, American College of Chest Physicians, 1975, p 377.

avoid the long time necessary to establish an equilibrium between infusion and biodegradation. The therapeutic level of theophylline of 5-20 μg/ml (mg/liter) can usually be obtained by a loading dose of 5 to 6 mg/kg of aminophylline given over 20 to 30 minutes.[95] Therapeutic blood levels are maintained by administration of a continuous infusion at a rate determined by the patient's age, smoking history, and the presence or absence of liver disease or congestive heart failure. The infusion rate needed to maintain optimum blood levels is highly variable among individuals. An empirical infusion rate of 0.9 mg/kg/hr resulted in toxic blood levels above 20 μg/ml (mg/L) in 34 percent of one group studied.[96] For young patients (under 16 years) an infusion rate of 0.9 mg/kg/hr can be given for 12 hours, decreasing to 0.8 mg/kg/hr beyond 12 hours. For patients with a smoking history, evidence of liver disease, or heart failure, the continuous infusion rate should be adjusted downward to 0.3 to 0.5 mg/kg/hr for 12 hours and 0.1 mg/kg/hr beyond 12 hours (Table 5-7). Measurement of blood levels should be done to confirm the presence of adequate but nontoxic concentrations.[97] Manifestations of toxicity are closely related to blood levels of theophylline, most likely being present if levels exceed 20 μg/ml.[98,99] However, the levels at which toxicity occurs are extremely variable. The narrow therapeutic range of this drug has led to great interest in its pharmacokinetics.

If the patient has received theophylline therapy recently, a blood level should be obtained to guide the amount of an additional loading dose; if needed, 2.5 mg/kg should increase the blood level by about 5 μg/ml.[97]

Biodegradation of theophylline occurs by oxidation and demethylation. Demethylation to 1- and 3-methylxanthine occurs in the liver. Oxidation produces 1, 3 dimethyluric acid and 1-methyluric acid. These metabolites are found in the urine (Fig. 5-9).[100] The serum half life of theophylline in man is 8 hours, with a range of 3 to 9.5 hours.

REFERENCES

1. Tisi GM: Preoperative evaluation of pulmonary function: state of the art. Am Rev Resp Dis 119:293-310, 1979
2. Bryant LR, Rams JJ, Trinkle JK et al: Present-day risk of thoracotomy in patients with compromised pulmonary function. Arch Surg 101:140-144, 1970
3. Stein M, Koota GM, Simon M et al: Pulmonary evaluation of surgical patients JAMA 181:765-770, 1962
4. Wightman JAK: A prospective survey of the incidence of postoperative pulmonary complications. Brit J Surg 55:85-91, 1968
5. Gracey DR, Divertie MB, Didier EP: Preoperative pulmonary preparation of patients with chronic obstructive pulmonary disease. Chest 76:123-129, 1979
6. Stein M, Koota GM, Simon M et al: Preoperative pulmonary evaluation and therapy for surgery patients. JAMA 211:787-790, 1970
7. Tarhan S, Moffitt EA, Sessler A et al: Risk of anesthesia and surgery in patients with chronic bronchitis and chronic obstructive pulmonary disease. Surgery 74:720-726, 1973
8. Finlayson D: Pharmacology for the anesthesiologist, 16th Annual Postgraduate Course: therapeutic problems in respiratory and intensive care of critically ill patients. Atlanta, 1980
9. Chodosh S, Enslein K: Comparison of ampicillin vs tetracycline for exacerbations of chronic bronchitis. Am Rev Resp Dis 98:134, 1968
10. Cooper DKC: The incidence of postoperative infection and the role of antibiotic prophylaxis in pulmonary surgery: a review of 221 consecutive patients undergoing thoracotomy. Brit J Dis Chest 75:154-160, 1981
11. Burrows B, Nevin W: Antibiotic mangement in patients with chronic bronchitis and emphysema. Ann Int Med 77:993-995, 1972
12. Barrett-Connor E: The non-value of sputum culture in the diagnosis of pneumococcal pneumonia. Am Rev Resp Dis 103:845-848, 1971
13. Ziment I: Respiratory pharmacology and therapeutics. W. B. Saunders, Philadelphia, 1978
14. Newhouse M, Sanchis J, Bienenstock J: Lung defense mechanisms. NEJM 295:990-998, 1045-1052, 1976
15. Green G: In defense of the lung. Am Rev Resp Dis 102:691-703, 1970
16. Denton R, Forsman W, Hwang SH et al: Viscoelasticity of mucous. Am Rev Resp Dis 98:380-391, 1968
17. Bang BA, Bang FB: Responses of the upper respiratory mucosa to dehydration and infection. Ann NY Acad Sci 106:625-630, 1963
18. Laurenzi GA, Yin S: Studies of mucous flow in the mammalian respiratory tract. I: the beneficial effects of acetylstrophantanin on respiratory tract mucous flow. Am Rev Resp Dis 103:800-807, 1971
19. Laurenzi GA, Yin S, Guameri JJ: Adverse effect of oxygen on tracheal mucous flow. NEJM 279:333-339, 1968

20. Lopez-Vidriero MT, Costello J, Clark TJH et al: Effect of atropine on sputum production. Thorax 30:543-547, 1975

21. Klock LE, Miller TD, Morris AH et al: A comparative study of atropine sulfate and isoproterenol hydochloride in chronic bronchitis. Am Rev Resp Dis 112:371-376, 1975

22. Hee J, Guillerm R: La Fonction Muco-ciliare et ses modifications sous l'influence de certaines agressions (Mucociliary function and its alteration by certain irritants). Bulletin Europeen de Physiopathologie Respiratoire 13 (1):11-25, 1977

23. Bibliography on smoking and health. U.S. Dept. of Health, Education and Welfare. U.S. Gov't Printing Office, 1978, p. 20

24. Goldberger E: A primer of water, electrolyte and acid-base syndromes. Lea and Febiger, 1975

25. Sladen A, Laver MB, Pontoppidan H: Pulmonary complications and water retention in prolonged mechanical ventilation. NEJM. 279:448-453, 1968

26. Leaf A: The clinical and physiologic significance of the serum sodium concentration. NEJM 267:24-30, 77-83, 1962

27. Johanson WG, Gould KG: Lung defense mechanism. Basics of RD, 1977

28. Bang BG, Bang FB: Responses of the upper respiratory mucosa to dehydration and infection. Ann NY Acad Sci 106:625-630, 1963

29. Webb-Johnson DC, Andrews JL, Kock-Weser EE: Bronchodilator therapy. NEJM 297:476-482, 1977

30. McFadden ER: Aerosolized bronchodilators and steroids in the treatment of airway obstruction in adults. Am Rev Resp Dis 122:89-96, 1980

31. Restrepo GL, Heard BE: Mucous gland enlargement in chronic bronchitis: extent of enlargement in the tracheobronchial tree Thorax 18:334-339, 1963

32. Reid L: Measurement of bronchial mucous gland layer: diagnostic yardstick in chronic bronchitis. Thorax 15:132-141, 1960

33. Dery R, Pelletier J, Jacques A et al: Alveolar collapse induced by denitrogenation. Can Anes Soc J 12:531-544, 1965

34. Cherniack RM, Cherniack L, Naimark A: Respiration in health and disease. 2nd ed. WB Saunders, 1972, p 167

35. Stalnecker MC, Surratt PM, Chandler JG: Changes in respiratory function following small bowel bypass for obesity. Surgery 87:645-651, 1980

36. Barrera F, Reidenberg MM, Winters WL: Pulmonary function in the obese patient. Am J Med Sci 254:785-796, 1967

37 Marshall BE, Wyche MQ, Jr: Hypoxemia during and after anesthesia. Anesthesiology 37:178-209, 1972

38. Laws AK: Effects of induction of anesthesia and muscle paralysis on functional residual capacity of the lungs. Can Anes Soc J 15:325-331, 1968

39. Couture J, Picken J, Trop D et al: Airway closure in normal, obese, and anesthetized supine subjects. Fed Proc 29:269, 1970

40. Morton HJV: Tobacco smoking and pulmonary complications after operation. Lancet, 368-370, 1944

41. Burrows B, Knudson RJ, Cline MG et al: Quantitative relationships between cigarette smoking and ventilatory function. Am Rev Resp Dis 115:195-205, 1977

42. Buist AS, Sexton GV, Nagy JM et al: The effects of smoking cessation and modification on lung function. Am J of Resp Dis 114:115-122, 1976

43. Beck GJ, Doyle CA, Schachter EN: Smoking and lung function. Am Rev Resp Dis 123:149-155, 1981

44. Martin RR, Lindsay D, Despas P et al: The early detection of airway obstruction. Am Rev Resp Dis 111:119-125, 1975

45. Bosse R, Sparrow D, Rose C et al: Longitudinal effect of age and smoking cessation on pulmonary function. Am Rev Resp Dis 123:378-381, 1981

46. Bode FR, Dosman J, Martin R et al: Reversibility of pulmonary function abnormalities in smokers. Am J Med 59:43-52, 1975

47. Chodoff P, Margand PMS, Knowles CL: Short-term abstinence from smoking: it's place in preoperative preparation. Crit Care Med 3:131-133, 1975

48. McCormack WH, Spalter HF: Muscular dystrophy, alveolar hypoventilation, and papilledema. JAMA 197:127-130, 1966

49. Burwell CS: Extreme obesity associated with alveolar hypoventilation: a Pickwickian syndrome. Am J Med 21:811-818, 1956

50. Penaloza D, Sime F: Chronic cor pulmonale

due to loss of altitude acclimatization (chronic mountain sickness). Am J Med 50:728-743, 1971

51. Steele P, Ellis JH, Jr., Van Dyke D et al: Left ventricular ejection fraction in severe chronic obstructive airways disease. Am J Med 59:21-28, 1975

52. Fishman AP: Chronic cor pulmonale: state of the art. Am Rev Resp Dis, p. 355-374, 1966-1967

53. Ferrer MT: Disturbance in the circulation in patients with cor pulmonale. Bull NY Acad Med 9:942-957, 1965

54. Dunnil MS: An assessment of the anatomical factor in cor pulmonale in emphysema. J Clin Path 14:246-258, 1961

55. Hicken P, Brewer D, Heath D: The relationship between the weight of the right ventricle of the heart and the internal surface area and number of alveoli in the human lung in emphysema. J Pathol Bacteriol 92:529-546, 1966

56. Harris P, Heath D: The human pulmonary circulation. Churchill-Livingstone, London, 1962

57. Zapol WM, Snider MT: Pulmonary hypertension in severe acute respiratory failure. NEJM 296:476-480, 1977

58. Hyman AL: The direct effects of vasoactive agents on pulmonary veins. Studies of responses to acetylcholine, serotonin, histamine, and isoproterenol in intact dogs. J Pharmacol & Exp Ther 168:96-105, 1969

59. West JB, Dollery CT, Heard BE: Increased pulmonary vascular resistance in the dependent zone of the isolated dog lung caused by perivascular edema. Cir Res 17:191-206, 1965

60. Goldman L, Caldera DC, Nussbaum SR et al: Multifactorial index of cardiac risk in noncardiac surgical procedures. NEJM 297:845-850, 1977

61. Goldman L, Caldera DC: Risks of general anesthesia and elective operation in the hypertensive patient. Anesthesiology 50:285-292, 1979

62. Owens WD, Spitznagel EL: Anesthetic side effects and complications: an overview. Int Anes Clinics 18:1-9, 1980

63. Deutsch S, Dalen JE: Indications for prophylactic digitalization. Anesthesiology 30:648-656, 1969

64. Shields TW, Ujiki CT: Digitalization for prevention of arrythmias following pulmonary surgery. Surg Gyn Obst 126:743-746, 1968

65. Meyer J: Concerning the question of pre-intra, and postoperative digitalis administration. Survey Anes, 16:9, 1972

66. Doekel RC, Zwillich CW, Scoggin CH et al: Depression of hypoxic ventilatory response. NEJM 295:358-361, 1976

67. Mullen JL, Gertner MH, Buzby GP et al: Implications of malnutrition in the surgical patient. Arch Surg 114:121-125, 1979

68. Driver AG, LeBrun M: Iatrogenic malnutrition in patients receiving ventilatory support. JAMA 244:2195-2196, 1980

69. Levison H, Cherniack RM: Ventilatory cost of exercise in chronic obstructive pulmonary disease J Appl Physiol 25:21-27, 1968

70. Margaria R, Milic-Emili A, Petit JM et al: Mechanical work of breathing during muscular exercise. J Appl Physiol 15:354-358, 1960

71. Bartlett RG, Brubach HF, Specht H: Oxygen cost of breathing. J Appl Physiol 12:413-424, 1958

72. Heymsfeld S, Rudman D: Personal communication.

73. Sahebjami H, Vessalo CL, Wirman JA: Lung mechanics and ultrastructure in prolonged starvation. Am Rev Resp Dis 117:77-83, 1978

74. Gertz I, Hedenstierna G, Hellers G et al: Muscle metabolism in patients with chronic obstructive lung disease and acute respiratory failure. Clin Sci and Mol Med 52:395-403, 1977

75. Kaminski MU: Enteral hyperalimentation. Surg Gyn and Obst 143:12-16, 1976

76. Dudrick SJ: Long-term parenteral nutrition with growth, development, and positive nitrogen balance. Surgery 64:134-142, 1968

77. VanNay CU, Meng HC, Sandstead HH: An assessment of the role of parenteral nutrition in the management of surgical patients. Ann Surg 177:103-111, 1973

78. Fisher J: Total parenteral nutrition. Little, Brown and Company, 1976

79. Askanazi J, Rosenbaum JH, Hyman AI et al: Respiratory changes induced by the large glucose loads of total parenteral nutrition. JAMA 243:1444-1447, 1980

80. Askanazi J, Elwyn DH, Silverberg PA et al: Respiratory distress secondary to the high carbohydrate load of TPN: a case report. Surgery 87:596, 1980

81. Askanazi J, Carpentier YA, Elwyn DH et al: Influence of total parenteral nutrition on fuel utilization in injury and infection. Ann Surg 191:40, 1980

82. Knochel JP: The pathophysiology and clinical characteristics of severe hypophosphatemia. Arch Int Med 137:203-220, 1977

83. Newman JH, Neff TA, Ziporin P: Acute respiratory failure associated with hypophosphatemia. NEJM 296:1101-1103, 1977

84. Said, Sami I: The lung as a metabolic organ. NEJM 279:1330-1334, 1968

85. Nadel JA: Autonomic control of airway smooth muscle and airway secretions. Am Rev Resp Dis 115:117-126, 1977

86. Ahlquist RP: A study of the adrenotropic receptors. Am J Physiol 153:586-600, 1948

87. Gaddie J, Legge JS, Petrie G et al: The effect of an alpha-adrenergic receptor blocking drug on histamine sensitivity in bronchial asthma. Br J Dis Chest 66:141-146, 1972

88. Lands AM, Arnold A, McAuliff JP et al: Differentiation of receptor systems activated by sympathomimetic amines. Nature 214:597-598, 1967

89. Deal EC Jr, McFadden ER, Jr, Ingram RJ, Jr et al. Effects of atropine on potentiation of exercise-induced bronchospasm by cold air. J Appl Physiol 45:238-243, 1978

90. Hensley MJ, O'Cain CF, McFadden ER et al: Distribution of bronchodilation in normal subjects: beta agonist versus atropine. J Appl Physiol 45:778-782, 1978

91. Kradjan WA, Lakshminarayen, Hayden PW et al: Serum atropine concentrations after inhalation of atropine sulfate. Am Rev Resp Dis 123:471-472, 1981

92. Marini JJ, Lakshminarayan S, Kradjan WA: Atropine and terbutaline aerosols in chronic bronchitis. Chest 80:285-291, 1981

93. Cox JSF: Disodium cromoglycate (Intal®). Adv Drug Res 5:115-196, 1970

94. Cox JSG: Disodium cromoglycate: mode of action and its possible relevance to the clinical use of the drug. Brit J Dis Chest 65:189-204, 1971

95. Mitkenko PA, Ogilvie RI: Rational intravenous doses of theophylline. NEJM 289:600-603, 1973

96. Kordash TR, Van Dellen RG, McCall JT: Theophylline concentrations in asthmatic patients. JAMA 238:139-141, 1977

97. FDA drug bulletin, Feb 1980

98. Jacobs MH, Senior RM, Kessler G: Clinical experience with theophylline: Relationships between dosage, serum concentration and toxicity. JAMA 235:1983-1986, 1976

99. Weinberger MW, Matthay RA, Ginchansky EJ et al: Intravenous Aminophylline dosage, use of serum theophylline measurement for guidance. JAMA 235:2110-2113, 1976

100. Miech RP, Lohman SM: Metabolism and pharmacodynamics of theophylline, p. 377. In Stein M. Ed: New Directions in Asthma, American College of Chest Physicians, 1975

Carl R. Noback, M.D.

6
Intraoperative Monitoring

Anesthesia and surgery represent major deviations from the physiologic norm, and anesthesiologists have the responsibility to monitor the effects of what both we and the surgeons do to our patient during an operation. Virtually any body function, from the mundane (urine output) to the exotic (biventricular stroke work) can presently be monitored. Which functions should be monitored in any given case is a matter of much debate and speculation. In the course of development of new monitoring devices and systems, the initial response has often been, "Why do we need this new device? We are doing fine as we are"; yet many items initially scoffed at are now included in the anesthesiologist's armamentarium. It has not been long since an intraoperative electrocardiogram (ECG) was a novel idea, yet now ECG monitoring is routine. The eminent pulmonologist Thomas L. Petty was severely chastised during his internship for doing arterial punctures on humans, but arterial blood gas analysis is presently available in virtually every hospital. Not every new idea stands the test of time, and risks may outweigh benefits. Nonetheless one must keep an open mind and keep abreast of new developments, especially in a field as young as ours. The days of "the finger on the pulse" serving as complete and adequate monitoring have faded, but it is still a useful adjunct to newer techniques.

A subtle distinction exists between *monitoring* and *measurement*. While measurement implies a single determination of a specific variable (e.g., a urine output of 45 ml from 8 to 9 A.M.), monitoring entails the continuous visualization of specific measured phenomena, which can be performed in either an analog (graphic) or digital (numerical) fashion.[1] The data monitored may be displayed on an oscilloscope, recording system, small-screen cathode-ray tube (CRT), or the anesthetist's record. Such data are subject to being interrupted, altered, or invalidated during any of the phases from acquisition to presentation. These include preprocessing, conversion, storage, retrieval, processing, and reduction.[2] The information garnered by a receptor may be disrupted by patient motion, electrical interference, inadequate handling or inappropriate usage of equipment, defective equipment, or faulty preparation.[3] The concept of monitoring also includes trend identification, one of the major values of monitoring. Isolated values, unless grossly abnormal, give information of only limited usefulness. Two of the aims of effective monitoring are: (1) to provide accurate measurement of the chosen variable at a frequency determined by the clinical situation; and (2) to provide a clear display of the trend as that variable changes over time.[4]

For maximum usefulness, a clinical monitoring system should fulfill the following conditions:[5]

1. The recorded parameters should represent "hard" data.
2. Instrument operation should be simple and safe.
3. Compact and space-saving construction is necessary.
4. Prompt repair service is mandatory.
5. The system should be reasonably priced.

For accurate recording of the data so obtained, the system must: (1) be accurate under static conditions, i.e., there should be no baseline or sensitivity drift over the measurement range and there should be linearity of response over the range regardless of changes in the external condition; (2) not interfere with the physiologic event being recorded, i.e., the catheter should not occlude the vessel in which it is placed; and (3) have dynamic accuracy in that it can accurately record rapidly changing events.[6] The requirements for acceptable monitor function are stringent, and institution of a particular monitor in a given case should not be blithely undertaken. Full and complete familiarity with the equipment, its capabilities, and limitations will avoid many of the problems associated with monitoring.

NONINVASIVE MONITORING TECHNIQUES

Electrocardiogram

The electrocardiogram (ECG) is one of the staples of noninvasive monitoring, and it is well known that intraoperative electrocardiographic monitoring can provide information on heart rate and cardiac rhythm; however, the intraoperative use of the ECG for ST-segment analysis is relatively new, having awaited the development of calibrated multichannel strip chart recorders and knowledge of proper lead selection. It is not the intent of this section to provide a complete review of electrocardiography—for that the reader is referred to any of several excellent texts—but to emphasize those aspects of electrocardiography peculiar to thoracic anesthesia.

Many of the patients presenting for thoracic surgery have concomitant coronary artery disease, and the ECG can prove invaluable in tracking myocardial ischemia. The use of the ECG to diagnose myocardial ischemia intraoperatively was not mentioned by Cannard in 1960 or Russell in 1969.[7,8] At that time the ECG was used primarily for dysrhythmia diagnosis, and lead II was used because its axis parallels the P wave vector pointing from the sinoatrial to the atrioventricular node. Monitoring lead II made identification of the P waves easier and consequently facilitated differentiation of ventricular and supraventricular dysrhythmias. For many years, cardiologists have recognized the benefits of multiple-lead ECGs in diagnosing and localizing myocardial ischemia. According to Blackburn, approximately 90 percent of the ST-segment information contained in a 12-lead exercise ECG may be found in the V_5 lead.[9] Confirmation of this was provided by Mason et al, who found that in 56 patients with ST-segment changes, leads V_4 to V_6 proved most useful and lead I the least useful.[10] Despite this knowledge and the fact that the operating room experience is stressful, it was not until 1974 that Foëx and Prys-Roberts recommended the use of precordial ECG leads in hypertensive patients to detect myocardial ischemia intraoperatively.[11] Shortly thereafter, Kaplan and King recommended the use of multiple-lead ECG monitoring, including V_5, for all patients with coronary artery disease.[12]

The placement of leads for the patient

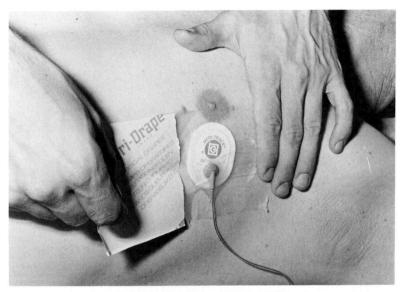

Fig. 6-1 Placement of steridrape over V_5 ECG lead. This allows surgical prep over the ECG lead, which remains in the surgical field, allowing analysis of V_5 intraoperatively.

undergoing thoracic surgery offers some problems. For a left thoracotomy, a disposable ECG pad in the V_5 position is in the midst of the surgical field. Dalton proposed a method which avoids this situation by placing a sterile spinal needle in the V_4 position after the skin preparation has been completed.[13] Although this may be efficacious intraoperatively, the postinduction placement of the precordial lead does not allow monitoring of ischemia in the distribution of the left anterior descending or circumflex coronary arteries during the stressful times of induction, laryngoscopy, and intubation. A standard disposable pad could be placed before induction and then removed before skin preparation begins and after assumption of the right lateral decubitus position, to be replaced by a needle electrode after skin preparation. For right thoracotomy and supine cases, the V_5 lead may be placed and then covered with a section of steridrape which can be prepped over by the surgical team (Fig. 6-1). The impermeable steridrape not only provides a barrier but will keep the lead from being dislodged. The newer permeable

adhesive plastic materials now being used for dressings over IV sites will not work in this regard, as prep solution may leak through causing faulty contact, and the barrier over the unprepped area is not intact. Current practice is to place the four standard limb leads and the V_5 lead (covered with steridrape) prior to induction in all patients with coronary artery disease (CAD). At this time all seven available lead configurations (I, II, III, AVR, AVL, AVF, and V_5) are observed and recorded for future reference. Patients younger than 40 years without a diagnosis of CAD generally do not have a V_5 lead placed. In all patients, two leads (II and V_5 or II and AVF) are simultaneously displayed on an oscilloscope with use of two separate ECG channels (Fig. 6-2). If only one ECG channel is available, it is necessary to intermittently check the leads not being displayed for ischemic changes, since ischemia may occur and not be apparent in the V_5 lead.[14] While the five-electrode system described, including the unipolar V_5 is preferred, not every operating room has this capability, and appropriate modifications must be made. B?

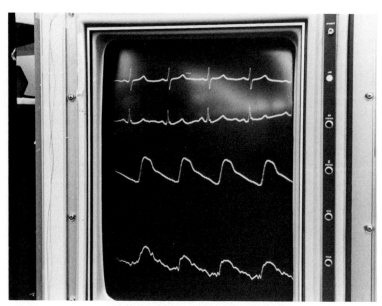

Fig. 6-2 Two-channel ECG display. Leads V_5 (Top) and II (Bottom) are continuously monitored intraoperatively.

zaral and Norfleet recently compared leads V_5 and CB_5 (a bipolar lead with a negative electrode over the right scapula and a positive electrode over the V_5 chest location) for the diagnosis of ischemia in patients undergoing coronary artery bypass grafting.[15] They theorized that CB_5 should provide ST-segment information equivalent to V_5 with better P wave definition, and this indeed proved to be the case. In patients with known disease in the distribution of the right coronary artery, a V_{4R} or V_{5R} lead (a unipolar lead in the V_4 or V_5 position but on the right side of the chest) is now being placed in order to better diagnose ischemia of the right heart.[16] Patients who have had previous inferior infarctions often have involvement of the right heart, and the right-sided V lead is useful in these patients as well.[17]

With the standard leads, including V leads, there may be difficulty distinguishing atrial dysrhythmias. For example, atrial fibrillation may be difficult to distinguish from atrial flutter with a varying block. Kistin and Copeland recognized the value of interpretation of simultaneous esophageal and standard ECG tracings to facilitate the diagnosis of such complex dysrhythmias in nonsurgical patients.[18,19] Kates recently presented data evaluating the esophageal electrode during cardiac surgery.[20] An esophageal stethoscope was modified with two external silver-silver chloride electrodes and connected to a bipolar lead II circuit. The esophageal stethoscope was then passed down the esophagus until the maximum amplitude biphasic P wave was seen on the ECG. To avoid the possibility of esophageal injury during electrosurgery, the stethoscope was attached to a high-impedance filter. In most of the 20 cases reported, the esophageal P wave was larger in amplitude than the QRS, allowing diagnosis of complex atrial dysrhythmias (Fig. 6-3). Ischemic changes of posterior origin were also observed in the esophageal lead. There are thus new, or newly used, ECG leads which may aid in the diagnosis of ischemia (V_5, V_{5R}, V_{4R}) and dysrhythmias (esophageal ECG connected to lead II) and about which anesthesiologists should be aware.

Regardless of the ECG leads chosen, it

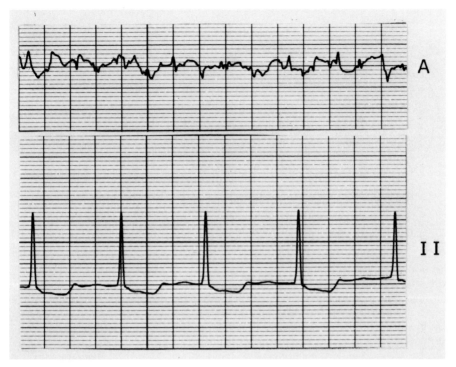

Fig. 6-3 Example of esophageal ECG tracing. The esophageal ECG (A) is compared with lead II, allowing the correct diagnosis of atrial fibrillation, which is not readily apparent from lead II.

is not enough to merely observe the complexes as they traverse the oscilloscope. The ability to freeze and hold a set of complexes is a useful adjunct, but hard-copy recordings of each lead used should be readily available. These hard copies are of minimal value, however, if the recorder is not meticulously standardized, e.g., so that 1 mV = 10 mm deflection on the ECG paper. One millimeter of ST-segment depression from the baseline is a significant sign of myocardial ischemia and may not be detected if the standardization is not appropriate.[21] ST-segment elevations greater than 1 mm are considered to represent severe ischemia. Such ST-elevations reflect transmural rather than subendocardial ischemia. J-point depression, or upsloping ST-segment depression, may represent ischemia but is nonspecific. This subtle change is easily overlooked when only observing complexes on the screen.

Blood Pressure

Interestingly, the first measurements of blood pressure were invasive rather than noninvasive. Hales, in 1733, inserted tubing ⅙-inch in diameter into a horse to measure its blood pressure.[22] Indirect blood pressure measurement was ushered in with the oscillometric method described by Étienne Jules Marey in 1876, in which a liquid-filled occluding chamber was placed around an artery, with arterial pulsations then being transferred to the fluid.[23] The maximum oscillation observed was found to be approximately the mean arterial pressure.

In the 1890s, Riva-Rocci developed the blood-pressure cuff, which allowed Von Recklinghausen to develop the oscillotonometric technique. For this, a double cuff encircles the extremity and the oscillotonometer displays the impact of arterial

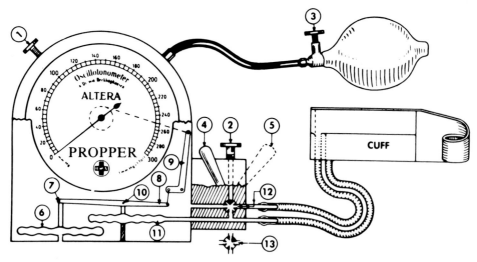

Fig. 6-4 Modified oscillotonometer: (1) zero adjust; (2) bleed valve adjustment screw; (3) bulb pressure release valve; (4) control valve lever—normal position, read pressure; (5) control valve lever—position to bleed, observer oscillometry; (6) pressure wafer; (7, 8, 10) pivot points on internal lever; (9) bell crank; (11) sensitive oscillometric wafer; (12) connection port to valve rotor shown in pressure or normal position (control lever in position 4); (13) position of valve rotor to bleed, observe oscillometry. (Bruner JMR: Handbook of Blood Pressure Monitoring. PSG Publishing Co., Inc. Littleton, MA, 1978. Reproduced with permission.)

pulsations on the lower cuff as the upper cuff is deflated (Fig. 6-4).[4] Although systolic pressure may be accurately determined with this technique, especially at lower levels of blood pressure, determination of diastolic pressure is inaccurate.[4] Additionally, a stethoscope or other means of peripheral pulse detection is not required, in contrast to auscultatory methods. Recently, automated oscillotonometric devices have been produced and marketed. An example of such a device is the Dinamap (Critikon) (Fig. 6-5), which automatically inflates the cuff at intervals of 1 to 16 minutes, depending on the user setting. As the cuff is deflated from above systolic blood pressure (on the initial inflation the cuff is filled with increasing volumes until pulsations are no longer detected), systolic pressure, diastolic pressure, mean arterial pressure, and heart rate are derived and displayed on a digital LED readout. The Dinamap also has the capability of providing a hard copy of the data in a cumu-

lative digital and graphic form. A reliable artifact detection feature is provided. The machine automatically stops deflations until the artifact has disappeared and abandons the measurement if the artifact persists. To compensate for possible increases in systolic pressure since the previous measurement, the machine is programmed to inflate the cuff to just above the previous systolic reading and verify pulse obliteration prior to initiating deflation. In clinical trials at the Mayo Clinic, the Dinamap was found to be accurate in low blood pressure and low cardiac output situations as well as in normotensive and hypertensive conditions.[24] However, with pressure determinations more frequent than every 2 minutes and bradycardia in the subject, the device would not complete its cycle prior to the time to begin the subsequent cycle, thus occluding both arterial and venous flow in the extremity. Dysrhythmias may yield either erroneous readings or no determination, owing to signal rejection.[23]

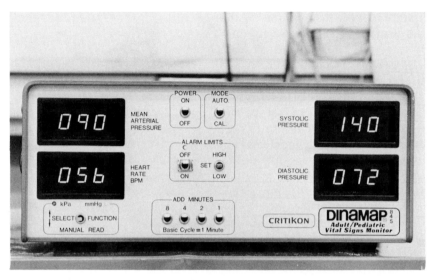

Fig. 6-5 Dinamap automated blood pressure monitor. Automated determinations may be made at intervals from 1 to 15 minutes. Systolic pressure, diastolic pressure, mean pressure, and heart rate are displayed. A printer to graphically display the results may be added.

An auscultatory method of determining blood pressure was described by Korotkoff in 1905, and this remains the "gold standard" throughout medicine. After the cuff has been inflated to obliterate the pulse pressure, it is slowly released. The systolic pressure is determined at the point at which two consecutive beats are heard, while diastolic pressure is read at the point at which the sounds are suddenly muffled.[25] Unfortunately, this technique cannot be readily automated, is least accurate with systolic pressures less than 80 mmHg, and is inapplicable during cardiopulmonary bypass.

The simplest method to determine systolic pressure is detection of resumption of flow (i.e., pulse) distal to an inflatable cuff as the cuff is deflated. The use of an ultrasonic flow detector can facilitate this method.

Principles common to both auscultation and detection of flow beyond the cuff methods are employed by the doppler ultrasound method of determining blood pressure (Fig. 6-6). A cuff over the brachial artery covers both an 8 MHz ultrasound source and a receptor. Resumption of flow as the cuff is deflated causes the vessel walls to move apart, producing the first signal (systolic pressure) for the ultrasound receptor (the turbulence created by this same situation causes the first Korotkoff sound). As the cuff pressure falls during the same pulsation (i.e., as blood pressure decreases toward diastolic), the vessel walls tend to come closer together, owing to falling blood pressure and constriction provided by the partially inflated cuff, thereby producing the second signal for the ultrasound receptor. With continued cuff deflation, the vessel is open longer during the passage of each pulse and the second signal is delayed more until it merges with the first signal of the following pulse (diastolic pressure). Below this point, the cuff causes no vessel constriction, the vessel being open throughout systole and diastole, and there is no significant vessel wall motion to produce a signal for the ultrasound receptor.

Problems exist with all these methods with the patient in the thoracotomy position. Blood pressure determined by any of the cuff methods in the "up" arm is not equal to that recorded in the "down" arm, owing to the vertical distance between the two arms. With a maximum vertical distance between arms of only 30 to 40 cm, however, this error is minimal. In general, blood pressure measurements by cuff during thoracotomy are taken in the up arm so as to: (1) underestimate the blood pressure if there is to be an error (hypotension which remains unrecognized and untreated may cause problems before similar errors in hypertension would); and (2) avoid alterations in blood pressure measurement which may be caused by kinking of the axillary artery in the down arm. However, the pressure can also be measured from the down arm, as long as the axillary artery is not compressed and the hydrostatic pressure difference is remembered.

Heart Sounds

The auscultation of heart sounds during anesthesia can provide useful information about cardiac rate and rhythm. With the ubiquitous use of intraoperative ECGs, some centers have ceased using either precordial or esophageal stethoscopes routinely, feeling that adequate information regarding rate and rhythm can be garnered from the ECG. The vast majority of the time, however, ECG signals are lost during electrocautery, and the patient's cardiac rate and rhythm are unmonitored unless a precordial or esophageal stethoscope is in use. The precordial stethoscope is not without use in thoracic anesthesia. Placement in a classical position may be difficult during a mediastinoscopy or Chamberlain procedure, but this difficulty can be overcome. In the thoracotomy position, the stethoscope may be placed over the down-lung field, thereby providing important information about breath sounds, particularly during one-lung anesthesia. During esophageal surgery, the precordial stethoscope may be the only source for intraoperative auscultation of breath sounds. When a precordial stethoscope placed over the left chest or an esophageal stethoscope is used, changes in intensity of heart sounds may be determined

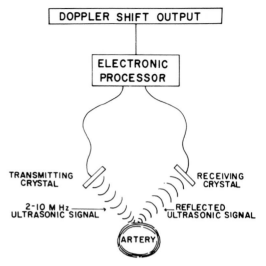

Fig. 6-6 Doppler ultrasound method of measuring blood pressure. Sudden vibrations in the arterial wall when cuff pressure falls below systolic pressure cause variation in the reflected ultrasonic signal frequency. Similarly, when diastolic pressure is reached and there is no occlusion of flow, variation in reflected ultrasonic signal frequency is eliminated. Reprinted by permission of the publisher, from Saidman/Smith: *Monitoring in Anesthesia,* New York: John Wiley and Sons, 1978; Woburn: Butterworth Publishers, 1981.

and related to contractility. Both stethoscopes serve in part as respiratory monitors allowing early detection of wheezing, rales, ronchi, etc. In case of an air embolus, a millwheel murmur may be heard early. Changes in pre-existing cardiac murmurs may also be detected. Since the introduction of the esophageal stethoscope in 1954, few hazards have been associated with its use.[26] Schwartz and Downs reported two cases in which the presence of the stethoscope in the esophagus during surgery resulted in erroneous surgical incisions into the esophagus, with subsequent complications.[27] In one case the surgeon misidentified the esophagus with stethoscope as the trachea with nasotracheal tube; while in the other the surgeon incised the esophagus thinking it was the internal jugular vein. In my personal experience surgeons have thought on several occasions that the "mass in the esophagus" was a "lesion" and had to be dissuaded from biopsying the assumed lesion. In thoracic operations involving the esophagus (colonic interposition, esophagogastrectomy) the esophageal stethoscope probably should not be used; and in other cases such as mediastinal exploration, the surgeon should be informed of its presence.

Urine Output

When a urinary catheter is in place, urine output should be monitored regularly and routinely. Urine output rather than being a specific parameter is a general indication of adequate cardiac output and sufficient peripheral and renal perfusion. The validity of urine output as an indicator is lessened in certain situations, e.g., high-output renal failure, diuretic therapy, or dopamine infusion. Renal perfusion sufficient to meet the metabolic demands of the kidney may be present despite the lack of urine output. Nonetheless, to be on the side of safety, maintenance of urine output greater than 0.5 ml/kg/per hour is recommended. Catheterization should be performed when the patient has known cardiac, major vascular, or renal disease; when lengthy procedures (over 1 to 2 hours) are anticipated; when major blood loss or fluid volume shifts are anticipated; and when the thoracic aorta will be cross-clamped.

Temperature

Monitoring of patient temperature during surgery has become virtually routine. Although such monitoring was originally proposed to facilitate early detection of malignant hyperpyrexia, it may also serve to identify cases of intraoperative hypothermia. The anesthetized human is a poikilotherm, the heat-regulating mechanism is impaired (as first noted by Simpson in 1902), and the tendency is to assume ambient temperature.[28] This results in hypothermia, not only in the operating room but in the recovery room or intensive-care unit. Deleterious effects of hypothermia include: shivering, with increased oxygen consumption, and therefore increased CO_2 production in the face of an altered CO_2 response due to anesthetics; and increased peripheral vascular tone, with increased afterload and the possibility of myocardial ischemia.

Many types of thermometers are available for intraoperative use, the most commonly used being a thermistor or thermally sensitive resistor. This is a bead made of a mixture of oxides of nickel, cobalt, and manganese heated to 95° C for three 8-hour periods.[29] Electrodes are then applied by firing on metal colloids or by fusing the material around wires. The thermistor is a semiconductor with a negative temperature coefficient; that is, the higher the temperature, the lower the resistance (Fig. 6-7).[30] Response time varies among different probes and manufacturers but averages only a few seconds. Accuracy is in general ±0.2° C. Temperature trend information may be obtained from newer devices consisting of liquid crystal material on adhesive-backed strips. These, however, have a narrow range and may not be accurate.[31]

The choice of temperature-measuring site is less crucial for thoracic anesthesia than for cardiac anesthesia, where hypothermic cardiopulmonary bypass might be employed. Monitoring rectal temperature alone is suboptimal, for there is a significant lag in rectal temperature change with acute changes in core temperature. The presence of feces may further insulate the probe from detecting either hyperthermic or hypothermic changes, and the possibility of rectal perforation with attendant sepsis exists. Holdcroft and Hal found poor correlations between rectal and esophageal or aural temperatures.[32] Tympanic membrane temperature has been touted by Benziger as a fine measure of core temperature.[33] However, two major prob-

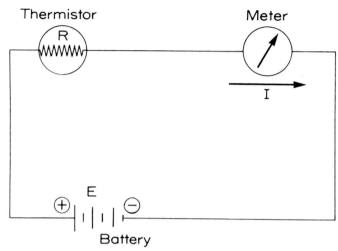

Thermistor   Meter

I

E

Battery

Fig. 6-7 Basic thermistor circuit. Different thermistor compositions provide different resistances R. The circuit is an illustration of Ohm's law, I = E/R where the current I which is measured by the meter is a function of the voltage E of the battery and the total resistance R of the circuit. (Leonard PF, Anesth Analg (Cleve) 45:249, 1966. Reproduced with permission.)

lems exist with tympanic membrane temperature: (1) it represents brain temperature, which may or may not represent "core" temperature—e.g., face fanning may decrease tympanic membrane temperature through the return of venous blood from the facial skin to the cavernous sinus, where arterial blood to the brain can be cooled; and (2) it risks possibly irreparable damage to a special sense organ while not being clearly superior to posterior nasopharyngeal or esophageal temperatures.[32–34] In the relative steady state in the operating room, without induced hypo- or hyperthermia, it matters little whether one assesses "core" or brain temperature. A temperature measured in the posterior nasopharynx, with the probe inserted through the nares a length equivalent to the distance from the tip of the nose to the earlobe, provides an accurate representation of brain temperature.[35] As this probe is easily dislodged, it should be firmly affixed to the patient. Core temperature may be assessed with an esophageal temperature probe with the thermistor at the level of midesophagus. Placement entails no more difficulty than

placement of the esophageal stethoscope, of which the thermistor is usually an integral part. During thoracic surgery surgeons often wash the chest with warm water to search for pulmonary leaks, locate bleeding points, or remove debris. This wash is quite often at a temperature (around 40°C) higher than body temperature. As the thoracic cavity is washed, spurious elevations of esophageal temperature, due to the local heating, occur. Therefore, the preference is to monitor nasopharyngeal temperature during thoracic surgery in adults. In children with uncuffed endotracheal tubes, leak of unwarmed anesthetic gases may falsely decrease nasopharyngeal temperature, and in these cases rectal, esophageal, or axillary temperatures are used.

A new development for core-temperature monitoring has been a Foley catheter which incorporates a thermocouple in the tip. A thermocouple, as opposed to a thermistor, is made of two dissimilar metals completing a circuit. When the junctions of the two metals are maintained at different temperatures, an electromotive force proportional to the temperature difference is generated (Fig. 6-8).[36] The thermocouple in the Foley tip indicates the temperature of either the bladder wall or the urine surrounding it (which in turn is in contact with the bladder wall). Clinical trials have shown that bladder temperature is close to rectal temperature ($\pm 0.2\,^{\circ}$ C) and that it accurately tracks changes in core temperature over a wide range.[37]

Another temperature should be monitored intraoperatively, namely ambient temperature. As mentioned above, anesthetized humans become poikilothermic and lose heat to the environment. Morris found that ambient temperatures less than $21\,^{\circ}$ C resulted in significantly lower patient temperatures than ambient temperatures higher than $21\,^{\circ}$ C and recommended $21\,^{\circ}$ C as a minimum ambient operating room temperature.[38,39] Recent studies by Roizen and Noback tend to dispute this, showing no effect of ambient temperatures between 17 and $23\,^{\circ}$ C on intraoperative core temperature.[40,41] It must be assumed, however, until proven otherwise, that ambient temperatures less than $17\,^{\circ}$ C may be deleterious, and elevation of ambient temperature to this minimum level should be undertaken if possible.

Despite the ability to diagnose the development of intraoperative hypothermia, there are few modalities for intraoperative rectification of the problem. As noted above, elevation of room temperature does not solve the problem in adults. Similarly, warming blankets, often touted as being effective, have not been shown to be so in adults.[42] It has recently been shown that warming blankets may delay but not eliminate core temperature decrease in patients undergoing major vascular surgery.[43] This, however, may not carry over to thoracic surgery. Warming blankets are not innocuous; burns may occur owing either to too high a blanket temperature or to prolonged pressure over a blanket with a normal pad temperature.[44,45] Such a case is illustrated in Figure 6-9. Lateral decubitus positions are very likely to cause

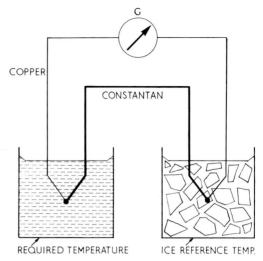

Fig. 6-8 Principle of the thermocouple. See text for explanation. Reproduced with permission from Scurr C, Feldman S: Scientific Foundations of Anaesthesia. William Heinemann Medical Books Ltd., London, 1974, 2nd ed., pp 80-86.

problems in this regard, particularly with the down shoulder, iliac crest, femoral head, and knee as the primary support points.

The use of heated, humidified inspired gases seems to be promising, but studies of the efficacy of this technique are presently lacking. Artificial "noses" such as the Brethaid are designed to trap moisture and heat which would normally be expired, thus conserving natural heat and water without the risks of respiratory heat burns and bacterial contamination associated with heated humidification. The efficacy of these new devices in thoracic surgery has yet to be established. In severe cases of inadvertent intraoperative hypothermia, washing the thoracic cavity with warm solutions until a core temperature assessment other than esophageal (i.e., nasopharyngeal or rectal) rises may be useful.

As with any monitoring device, hazards are attendant on usage. With temperature probes the hazard may be probe malfunction, with failure to indicate a rapidly rising temperature. Ben-Zvi described the failure of temperature probes soaked in Cidex for

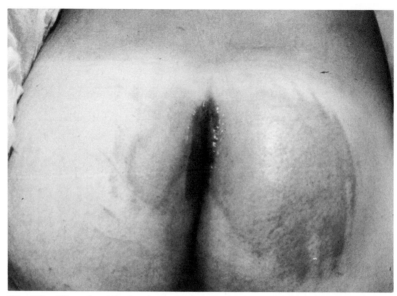

Fig. 6-9 Warming blanket burn. The burn in the intergluteal crease later required skin grafting.

cleaning and sterilization.[46] Apparently, the Cidex penetrated the plastic sheath, causing significant capacitance to build up and cause incorrect temperature readings. The solution was to wash the probes in water and Vesphene prior to gas sterilization. An axillary skin sensor probe of the button type has been reported to serve as a ground site for the electrocautery, with a faulty capacitor resulting in third-degree burns (Fig. 6-10).[47] Thus, even with devices seemingly as simple as a thermistor, appropriate maintenance must be performed and equipment inspected routinely prior to use in order to avoid situations such as those described.

Oxygen Delivery

In an effort to prevent the administration of hypoxic gas mixtures, as well as to provide a check that the desired oxygen concentration is being delivered, it is desirable to monitor the oxygen source. A well-functioning rotameter may provide an accurate estimate of oxygen concentration, but errors may occur from sticking bobbins, broken needle valves, and cracks in the tubing.[4] Such errors may be magnified at low flows. Therefore, the routine usage of oxygen analyzers is strongly recommended. Several methods of oxygen analysis have been described over the years, and these are outlined below.

VOLUMETRIC GAS ANALYZERS

In the Haldane gas analyzer (Fig. 6-11) a known volume of the gas to be analyzed is presented to a series of absorbents and the diminution in volume is noted after passage through each absorbent.[48] Because each absorbent is specific for a given component gas, the volume percent of a given gas is determined by the ratio of volume absorbed to total volume. A disadvantage of the Haldane device is that it needs relatively large volumes of gas. The micro–gas analyzer of Scholander allows determination of O_2, N_2, and CO_2 concentrations in gas samples as small as 0.5 cc.[49] In the Scholander apparatus, the gas sample is introduced into a reac-

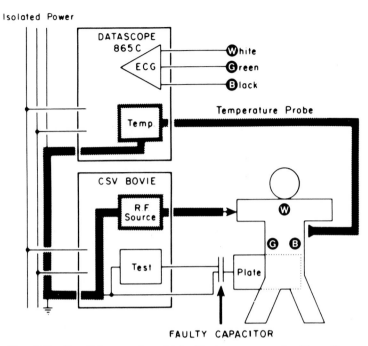

Fig. 6-10 Conditions under which skin burn occurred with axillary temperature probe. Owing to a faulty (open) capacitor, RF current passed from the bovie through the temperature probe (as well as ECG machine). Stippled line shows the assumed current pathway. (Schneider AJL, Apple HP, Braun RT: Electrosurgical burns at skin temperature probes. Anesthesiology 47:72-74, 1977. Reproduced with permission.)

tion chamber connected to a micrometer burette. Absorbents for the various gases are deposited sequentially into the reaction chamber. A side arm holds the O_2 absorber. The ratio of micrometer readings times 100 gives the percentage by volume of the components of the analyzed gas.[50]

MANOMETRIC GAS ANALYZERS

The Van Slyke manometric gas analyzer is the "gold standard" of gas analysis devices. Both precision and accuracy are greater than in volumetric devices. In the device developed by Van Slyke and Neill (Fig. 6-12), a burette has a double stopcock to which are attached a measuring cup and outlet tube.[51] The burette is attached to a manometer and to a mercury-leveling bulb and reservoir.

Changes in pressure occur within the system as "releasing agents" are introduced to liberate combined and dissolved gases.[50]

PHYSICAL METHODS

Physical methods of gas analysis offer the greatest usefulness for measurement of oxygen tension during anesthesia. These methods include (a) paramagnetic, (b) polarographic, (c) fuel cell, and (d) mass spectrometry analysis. The first three will be covered here, while mass spectrometry will be discussed in the section on Gas Exchange.

A. Pauling, Wood, and Sturdivant described the paramagnetic analysis of oxygen in 1946.[52] Oxygen, a paramagnetic gas, is attracted to the strongest part of a non-

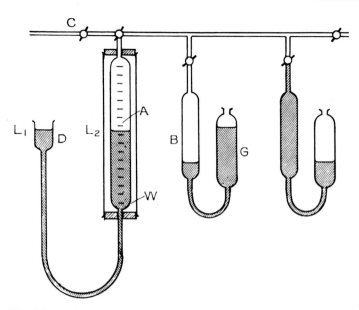

Fig. 6-11 Schematic diagram of a Haldane volumetric gas analyzer. (A) 10-ml calibrated burette into which sample is drawn through inlet (C); (D) mercury level which changes with addition of gas sample; (B) absorption pipette into which known volume of gas is forced; (G) reagent reservoir. During absorption reagent passes from G to B; (W) water jacket to stabilize burette temperature. (Reproduced with permission from Scurr C, Feldman S: Scientific Foundations of Anaesthesia. William Heinemann Medical Books Ltd., London, 1974, 2nd ed., pp 80-86.

homogenous magnetic field. The other respiratory gases are diamagnetic and locate in a weaker area of the magnetic field. The device (Fig. 6-13) consists of a glass dumbbell containing a diamagnetic gas (N_2), which is suspended by a quartz thread between the poles of a magnet. Oxygen contained in the gas to be analyzed displaces the dumbbell from the strong portion of the magnetic field. A beam of light reflected from a mirror affixed to the dumbbell onto a visual scale indicates the degree of rotation, thereby indicating the concentration of oxygen in the gas.[53] Low flow rates through the measuring cell contribute to the major disadvantage of paramagnetic analysis, namely a prolonged response time.

B. The polarographic analysis of oxygen utilizes a Clark-type electrode. The basic electrode (Fig. 6-14) consists of four components: a platinum and a silver terminal, an electrolyte solution, and a gas-permeable (polypropylene) membrane. The platinum terminal (negative terminal or cathode) is the cross-section (10 to 25 mm) of a fine wire embedded in glass through which a negative voltage is applied. The silver anode (positive terminal) is in contact with the cathode through the electrolyte (KCl) solution. The membrane separates the electrolyte and terminals from the measured phase. Oxygen molecules pass through the membrane and electrolysis occurs at the polarized platinum surface. The breakdown of O_2 alters the conductivity of the KCl solution, and current flow is proportional to the concentration of O_2 in the electrolyte solution. Modifications to the original

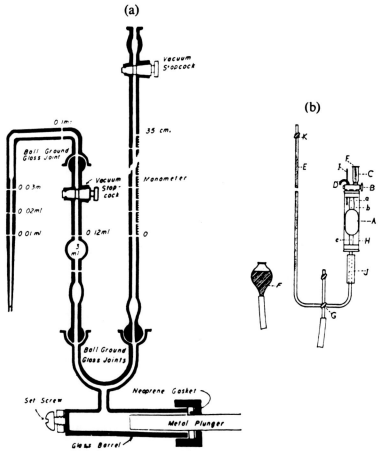

Fig. 6-12 Schematic diagram of manometric Van Slyke apparatus. (A) micro version; (B) macro version. (Reproduced with permission from Scurr C, Feldman S: Scientific Foundations of Anaesthesia. William Heinemann Medical Books Ltd., London, 1974, 2nd ed., pp 80-86.

apparatus have made breath-by-breath gas analysis possible.[53]

C. A rapid response time is also a characteristic of the solid-electrolyte fuel cell. The cell (Fig. 6-15) consists of calcium-stabilized zirconium oxide electrolyte molded into a tube. Both the internal and external surfaces are coated with porous platinum, forming two electrodes. The outside of the tube is exposed to a known O_2 concentration (ambient air) and the sample to be analyzed is drawn through the tube. The electrolyte acts as a semipermeable membrane conductive to O^{2-} ions but not electrons [when the two surfaces are exposed to differing O_2 concentrations the following reactions occur: (1) cathode $O_2 + 4e^- \rightarrow 2\ O^{2-}$; and (2) anode: $2\ O^{2-} \rightarrow O_2 + 4e^-$]. The electromotive force thus generated is related to the relative partial pressures of oxygen, and the O_2 concentration is determined.[53] Although heating the fuel cell to 800 to 1,000°C increases the conductivity of O^{2-} ions, a number of O_2 analyzers utilizing unheated fuel cells are available. Such electrochemical micro–fuel cells consume O_2 from the sample surround-

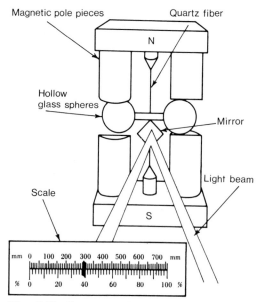

Fig. 6-13 Paramagnetic oxygen analyzer. See text for details. (Wilson RS, Laver MB: Oxygen analysis: advances in methodology. Anesthesiology 37:113, 1972. Reproduced with permission.)

ing the detector, generating an electrical current proportional to the O_2 concentration. This current then drives a microammeter whose scale is calibrated to indicate oxygen percentage.[53]

Advantages of fuel-cell O_2 analyses include ease of calibration, durability, portability, and lack of maintenance. Westenskow et al compared the function of four commercially available oxygen analyzers for use during anesthesia.[54,55] The sensors tested were: Beckman model OM 10 (Beckman Instruments Inc., Palo Alto, CA), Critikon Model 800-021 (Critikon, Irvine, CA), IL Model 402 (Instrumentation Laboratory, Andover, MA), and Teledyne Microfuel Cell Class C-1 (Harris-Lake Inc., Cleveland, OH). The first three are polarographic while the fourth is a fuel-cell type. Each sensor was calibrated by using 100 percent N_2 and 100 percent O_2 at flow rates of 5 liters/min. Performance was then assessed under conditions of room air, 3 percent halothane, 100 percent humidity, and 100 percent N_2O. During exposure to room air no drift in O_2 sensor out-

put voltage occurred—each sensor, when reexposed to 100 percent O_2 recorded the appropriate O_2 value. After exposure to 3 percent halothane for 6 hours, the Critikon sensor and Teledyne sensor showed significant variations from baseline (Table 6-1). Following exposure to 100 percent humidity only the Beckman sensor had a significant variance from baseline, reading approximately 20 percent low (Table 6-2). Nitrous oxide had little effect on any of the sensors (Table 6-3). The authors concluded that the Critikon, Teledyne, and IL sensors were appropriate for operating-room monitoring of inspired oxygen concentration. The data show that the IL Model 402 provided the most reliable across-the-board data. The failure of the Beckman sensor to function appropriately under conditions of high humidity was due to the fact that it has a small recessed membrane, which is quickly covered by condensate under high humidity conditions. Fortunately, it erred on the side of safety

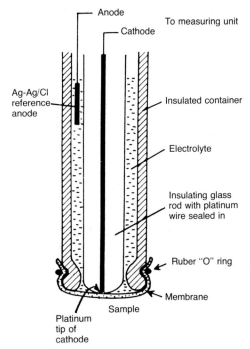

Fig. 6-14 Clark-type oxygen electrode. See text for discussion. (Wilson RS, Laver MB: Oxygen analysis: Advances in methodology. Anesthesiology 37:114, 1972. Reproduced with permission.)

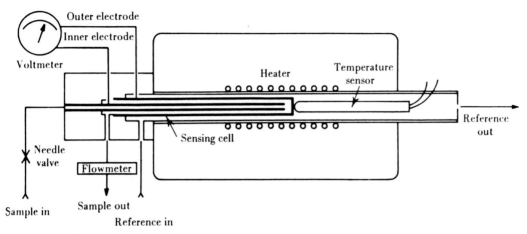

Fig. 6-15 Solid-electrolyte fuel cell. Reference gas is passed along external surface of heated electrolyte tube. Sample gas passes along internal surface. (Wilson RS, Laver MB: Oxygen analysis: Advances in methodology. Anesthesiology 37:117, 1972. Reproduced with permission.)

Table 6-1
Oxygen Sensor Reading Following Exposure to 3% halothane*

Time	Beckman	Critikon	Teledyne	IL
hr				
0	100.0	100.0	100.0	100.0
2	100.2 ±0.99	102.3† ±1.93	98.5 ±0.59	98.8 ±1.11
4	100.0 ±1.27	103.2† ±2.01	97.3† ±0.83	98.6 ±1.23
6	100.0 ±1.45	103.3† ±2.03	97.4† ±0.38	99.5 ±1.10

* Values are means ±1 SD. Oxygen sensor reading when placed in 100% O_2 following an exposure to 3% halothane in air for 2, 4, and 6 hours.
† Indicates a statistically significant difference from 100 at the $p<0.05$ level using multivariate analysis of variance.
(Westenkow DR, Jordan WS, Jordan RB, et al: Evaluation of oxygen monitors for use during anesthesia. Anesth Analg (Cleve) 60:53–56, 1981. Reproduced with permission.)

(except in the case of surgery on premature neonates) in underestimating the delivered oxygen percentage.

Conditions under which data from oxygen monitors may be deceiving include:

1. When the sensor is placed in the expiratory limb, where the O_2 reading is influenced by CO_2 and water vapor
2. When the sensor is calibrated prior to allowing sufficient warm-up time
3. When a slow response time is not considered during calibration
4. When the temperature coefficient is not considered

The temperature coefficients (i.e., percent change in reading per degree C) vary, as do the response times (Table 6-4), and familiarity with the particular device being used is mandatory.[54] Incorrect readings may occur when:

1. The cell lifetime is exceeded
2. The membrane is punctured
3. The battery supplying the sensor is low

As the battery of an oxygen sensor fails, a false high O_2 reading may be seen in the presence of N_2O.[56] An additional problem has been pointed out by Mazza.[57] The IL 402, a polarographic analyzer, has three

Table 6-2

Oxygen Sensor Reading Following Exposure to High Humidity

Time	Beckman	Critikon	Teledyne	IL
hr				
0	100.0	100.0	100.0	100.0
2	81.2†± 12.68	97.5 ± 1.92	97.3 ± 2.41	92.6†± 6.66
4	81.0†± 10.45	97.3 ± 3.58	93.2†± 1.27	96.5 ± 1.27
6	79.8†± 30.17	97.4 ± 4.41	93.8 ± 2.28	98.6 ± 1.04

Values are means ± 1 SD. Oxygen sensor reading when placed in 100% O_2 following exposure to air with 100% humidity at 34 °C for 2, 4, and 6 hours.

† Indicates a statistically significant difference from 100 at the $p < 0.05$ level using multivariate analysis of variance.

(Westenkow DR, Jordan WS, Jordan RB, et al: Evaluation of oxygen monitors for use during anesthesia. Anesth Analg 60:53–56, 1981. Reproduced with permission.)

4.05-V mercury batteries, but the battery check tests only the two circuitry batteries, not the third alarm battery. It is possible then to administer low concentrations of O_2 and have the sensor detect this but the alarm not function. The alarm needs to be tested independently and prior to, if not during, each case. Oxygen analyzers, like every other monitoring device, have hazards. Klick and du Moulen reported an oxygen analyzer as a source of *Pseudomonas* in four intensive-care-unit (ICU) patients.[58]

It is not sufficient to know only that an appropriate oxygen concentration is being administered. It is also necessary to assess the extent to which oxygen is being taken up and delivered to the tissues. To this end, digital oximeters and transcutaneous oxygen pressure (tc PO_2) sensors have been developed. The Minolta model 101 digital oximeter (Corning Medical) has recently been evaluated.[59,60] The device transilluminates a fingertip and compares the absorption of two wavelengths of light (650 and 805 nm) at a rate of five samples/per second so that sampling occurs during both systole and diastole. The results are displayed digitally. Oxygen saturation (SaO_2) readings are stable in less than 1 minute, with a variation of ± 2 percent. The readings produced correlate well with in vitro oximetry when oxygen satura-

tions are greater than 90 percent; however, overestimation of SaO_2 as saturation dropped has been reported (Fig. 6-16).[59] The deviation is linear and the instrument and/or user can be programmed to make the appropriate correction. Whitcher evaluated the device in 98 cases with 1,509 hours of recording time and concluded that the device not only was accurate but could provide early warning of hypoxemia (Fig. 6-17), hypoventilation, and esophageal or endobronchial intubation.[60] Decreased saturation occurring with bucking, suctioning, placement of abdominal packs, or air embolism could also be detected.

The use of tcPO_2 monitoring has been recommended for infants in order to avoid a

Table 6-3

Effect of Nitrous Oxide on Oxygen Sensors

	Reading with exposure to 100% N_2O
Beckman	0.17 ± 0.22*
Critikon	0.36 ± 0.81
Teledyne	−0.12 ± 0.11
IL	1.16 ± 1.84

* Values are means ± 1 SD.

(Westenkow DR, Jordan WS, Jordan RB, et al: Evaluation of oxygen monitors for use during anesthesia. Anesth Analg 60:53–56, 1981. Reproduced with permission.)

Table 6-4
Temperature Coefficient and Response Times of Oxygen Sensors

	Temperature coefficient (% $\triangle$ reading, $^{0}C^{-1}$)	Average O_2 reading in 100% N_2	Response time (seconds)
Beckman	0	0	10.1
Critikon	+0.27	+0.4	5.1
Teledyne	−1.1	−0.14	20.6
IL	−0.43	+0.1	2.9

(Westenkow DR, Jordan WS, Jordan RB, et al: Evaluation of oxygen monitors for clinical use. Anesthesiology 53:S382, 1980. Reproduced with permission.)

hyperoxic state which may be correlated with the development of retrolental fibroplasia. Under usual conditions the tcPO$_2$ at the skin surface is variable and below PaO$_2$. When the skin is made hyperemic by the application of heat, tcPO$_2$ and PaO$_2$ approach each other.[61] A specially designed Clark electrode (Fig. 6-18) with a heating coil is applied to the skin and heated to around 44° C to sense tcPO$_2$. The performance of the Roche cutaneous oxygen monitor 630, module 632 was evaluated in infants by Patel, who found good correlation with PaO$_2$ in the hypoxic and normoxic states (r=.99 and .94, respectively) but poor correlation in the hyperoxic state (r=.51 for PaO$_2$ of 105 to 439 mmHg), which one wishes to avoid in these infants.[62] Errors in oxygen analysis from the reduction of anesthetics by polarographic electrodes have been reported.[63] Patel did not find an effect of N$_2$O or halothane on the Roche sensor, but Lane found with the Radiometer

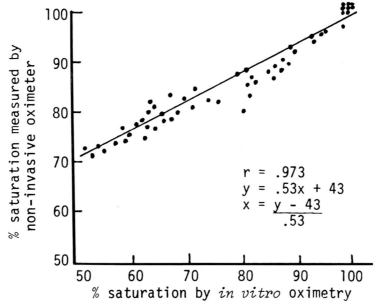

$$r = .973$$
$$y = .53x + 43$$
$$x = \frac{y - 43}{.53}$$

Fig. 6-16 Accuracy of Minolta Oximeter Model 101. A significant correlation between in vitro saturation determinations and noninvasive saturation determinations is seen. (Sarnquist FH, Todd C, Whitcher C: Accuracy of a new non-invasive oxygen saturation monitor. Anesthesiology 53:S163, 1980. Reproduced with permission.)

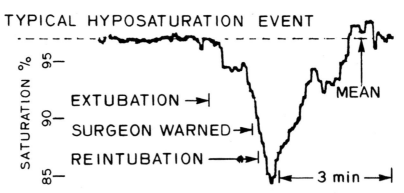

Fig. 6-17 Hyposaturation detected with digital oximeter and effect of reintubation. (Whitcher C, Flynn M: Use of a digital oximeter in resident training. Anesthesiology 53:S355. Reproduced with permission.)

tcPO$_2$ monitor that halothane increased the apparent PO$_2$ when polypropylene membranes were applied to the electrode.[64] Usage of a Teflon membrane obviated the problem, and no effect on apparent O$_2$ by N$_2$O or enflurane was observed. Whitesell evaluated the Biochem International tcPO$_2$ monitor in adults with and without vascular disease.[65] The sensor was heated to 42.5° C and the location changed every 3 hours to minimize burns. The patients with vascular disease were found to have a low tcPO$_2$ in the extremities despite high PaO$_2$ and adequate blood pressure; and in a series of 30 simultaneous determinations, no correlation was found between PaO$_2$ and tcPO$_2$. In the patients without vascular disease PaO$_2$ and tcPO$_2$ correlated, but PaO$_2$ averaged 133 mmHg while tcPO$_2$ averaged 100 mmHg. It is apparent that these devices need further refinement before finding widespread use in anesthesia.

As a corollary to monitors of oxygen delivery and uptake, disconnect alarms have been recommended. A breathing circuit disconnection was the most frequent problem in 35 percent of preventable anesthetic accidents studied by Cooper.[66] Half of those incidents resulted in hypoxia, cardiac arrest, or death. This has led to the recommendation that ventilators be used in conjunction with low-pressure or patient-disconnect alarms.[67] These devices sound an alarm when no pressure above a preset threshold is detected

in approximately 15 seconds. Examples are an Ohio Medical Products fluidic disconnect alarm with a preset pressure of 8 cm H$_2$O (if this pressure is exceeded, an audible alarm is cancelled); and a North American Drager DPM electronic pressure monitor, which has both audio and visual alarms and provides for the user to select pressure units of 5, 12.5, or 25 cm H$_2$O. McEwen found that each of these devices may not function in the face of a disconnect with low pressure thresholds (8 cm H$_2$O for the Ohio and 5 cm H$_2$O for the Drager).[68] Although the Drager sounded with higher threshold settings, neither device would detect disconnections of the gas supply at the vaporizer. Mazza noted that the Drager monitor required a higher current drain to run the alarm (11 to 19 mA) than the monitor (25 to 30 μA) and that the alarm could fail when the sensor did not.[57] As with tcPO$_2$ monitors these devices need further development. In any case, they should not replace scrutiny of the patient and anesthetic equipment by the anesthesiologist.

Gas Exchange

Noninvasive assessment of gas exchange can best be determined by use of a mass spectrometer. Most anesthesia departments do not have access to such an expensive apparatus, but an end-tidal CO$_2$ monitor in conjunction with known oxygen delivery can

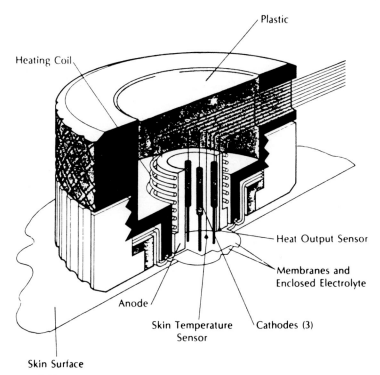

Plastic

Heating Coil

Heat Output Sensor

Membranes and
Enclosed Electrolyte

Anode

Skin Temperature
Sensor

Cathodes (3)

Skin Surface

Fig. 6-18 Transcutaneous PO$_2$ electrode in cutaway view. (Huch A, Huch R: Transcutaneous Noninvasive Monitoring of PO$_2$. Hospital Practice 11(6): 43, 1967. Art by Dan Todd. Reproduced with permission.)

provide important details with respect to gas exchange.

The first use of a mass spectrometer for measurement of respiratory gases was at the University of Pennsylvania nearly 30 years ago. Because of the possibilities of breath-to-breath analysis of gases, with implications regarding uptake and distribution, education, and development of automated anesthetic gas delivery systems, much development has taken place in adapting mass spectrometers to anesthesia usage.

There are two types of mass spectrometer, the magnetic-sector fixed collector type (Fig. 6-19) and the quadrupole type (Fig. 6-20). The magnetic-sector fixed collector functions as follows:[69]

1. A capillary inlet tube is connected to the flow-through tube attached to the endotracheal tube.
2. A mechanical pump pulls the gas sample through this tube past a gold leak.

3. A fraction of this gas is bled through the leak into an ionization chamber where a pressure of 10^{-6} mmHg is maintained.
4. The molecules are bombarded by an electron beam from a cathode.
5. Some molecules are transformed into positively charged ions, while others are fragmented.
6. The ions are accelerated, focused, and projected into an analyzer section.
7. A magnetic field at 90 degrees to the direction of exit from the ion source acts on the beam.
8. This diverts the ions into circular paths with radii proportioned to particle mass (thus the name *mass* spectrum).
9. Collectors measure the current carried by each species of ions, and this current is amplified for display.

The quadrupole mass spectrometer uses a mass filter consisting of direct current (DC) and radio frequency (RF) potentials applied

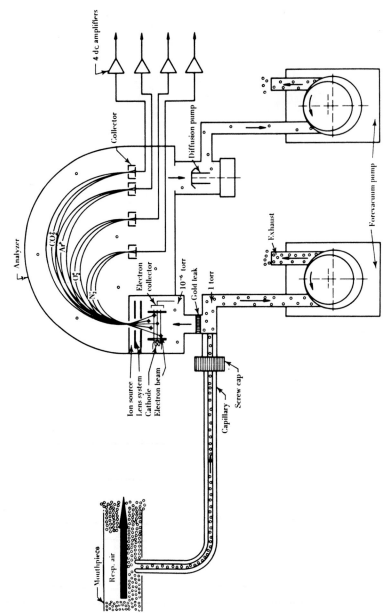

Fig. 6-19 Fixed collector mass spectrometer. (Wilson RS, Laver MB: Oxygen analysis. Anesthesiology 37:116, 1972. Reproduced with permission.)

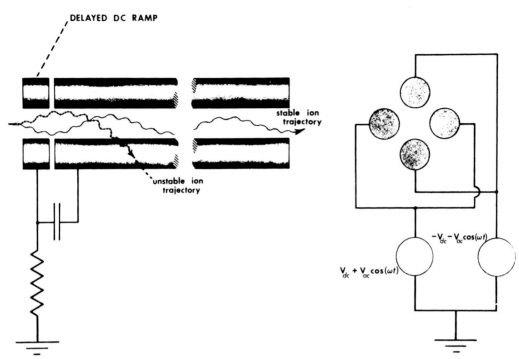

DELAYED DC RAMP

stable ion trajectory

unstable ion trajectory

$-V_{dc} - V_{ac}\cos(\omega t)$

$V_{dc} + V_{ac}\cos(\omega t)$

Fig. 6-20 Schematic representation of a quadrupole mass filter for mass spectrometry. The AC/DC potential applied to the four rods generates a rotating electromagnetic field such that charged particles with a charge-to-mass ratio matching the charge of the field will pass through the filter to be collected at the distal end. (Sodal FE, Swansen GD: Mass spectrometry: current technology and implications for anesthesia. pp. 167-182. In Aldrete JA, Lowe HJ, Virtue RW, Eds: Low Flow and Closed System Anesthesia. By permission of Grune and Stratton, New York, 1979.)

to four parallel rods (quadrupole); opposite rods are connected to the RF and DC voltage generators. Positive ions extracted from the ion source are accelerated into the quadrupole mass along the longitudinal axis of the rods. The trajectories are determined by the DC and oscillating RF fields. To reach the collector, the ions must traverse the quadrupole filter without colliding with the rods. For a particular RF/DC voltage ratio only ions of a specific mass-to-charge ratio avoid collision. The mass spectrum is scanned as voltages are swept from minimum to maximum values. Such a scan can be completed in a few milliseconds. The spectrometer is connected to a computer for analysis.

Figure 6-21 shows typical mass spectra for anesthetic gases. Expired air has peaks at the molecular weights of the components (water vapor at 18, nitrogen at 28, oxygen at 32, CO_2 at 44). The relative peak heights indicate relative composition.

Because of fragment overlap (CO_2 peak at 44, N_2O with a dominant peak at 44 and a strong fragment peak at 30) it is necessary to define an isolated peak for each fragment. Table 6-5 shows where various gases are measured in the mass spectrum. In practice, for example, CO_2 is measured at 44 and N_2O at 30.

Recently, a Perkin-Elmer Corporation quadrupole mass spectrometer has been used which can be time-shared to monitor respiratory and anesthetic gases in up to 16 patients. The system is an adaptation of earlier Perkin-Elmer systems for monitoring respiratory ICU patients. Additional requirements for operating room usage include:[70]

1. Longer sampling line lengths due to more dispersed patient locations (multiple operating rooms rather than ICU beds)
2. An increase from four to at least six gases to be analyzed
3. Remote cathode-ray-tube (CRT) data display (in each operating room rather than only at a central location)
4. Airway CO_2 waveform displayed on the CRT rather than only tabular data
5. Continuous pumping on all patient lines to speed up sequential analysis
6. Priority sampling to allow checking some patients more frequently than others

With the time-sharing system, it is not possible to continuously monitor each patient. Each monitoring location is connected via small-bore tubing to a rotary valve, which routes gas from one room at a time to the mass spectrometer. While the spectrometer is connected to one patient, the other 15 patients are connected to a second continuous pump to keep the gas sample in each line up to date. The frequency of patient sampling depends on the duration of sampling time (10 to 25 seconds), the switching time (around 3 seconds), the number of stations on line at a given time, and the number of priority sampling sites on line. In a nonpriority setting, sampling frequency ranges from 2 to 6 minutes.

Gases analyzed include O_2, N_2, CO_2, argon, N_2O, halothane, and enflurane. Although the cost of the system is not inconsequential, the cost of providing individual monitors for each of the gases would exceed the cost of the mass spectrometer system. An

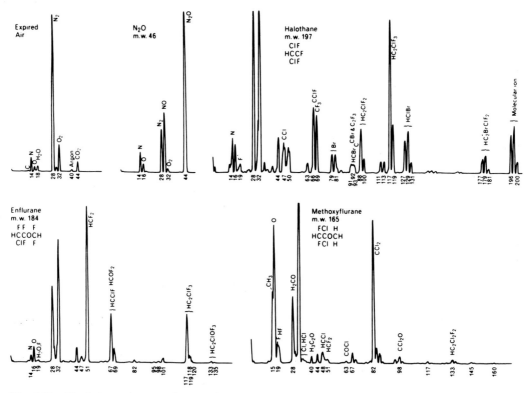

Fig. 6-21 Typical mass spectra for anesthetic gases. Analysis performed by a quadrupole mass spectrometer. (Sodal FE, Swansen GD: Mass spectrometry: current technology and inplications for anesthesia. pp 167-182. In Aldrete JA, Lowe HJ, Virtue RW, Eds: Low Flow and Closed System Anesthesia. By permission of Grune and Stratton, New York, 1979.)

Table 6-5
The Mass Number and Fractions Where Common Gases are Measured in the Mass Spectrometer

	Gas	AMU*	Measured at (AMU)
He	Helium	4	4
CH_4	Methane	16	16
H_2O	Water	18	18
Ne	Neon	20	20
C_2H_2	Acetylene	26	26
N_2	Nitrogen	28	28
$C^{18}O$	Carbon monoxide	30	30
N_2O	Nitrous oxide	44	44,30
O_2	Oxygen	32	32
Ar	Argon	40	40,20
CO_2	Carbon dioxide	44	44,12
Kr	Krypton	84	84
	Halothane	197	69,117
	Enflurane	184	51
	Methoxyflurane	165	82

* Atomic Mass Unit

advantage of the system is continuous display of the CO_2 wave form. The availability of end-tidal CO_2 measurements has decreased the required frequency of obtaining arterial blood gases for CO_2 measurements. End-tidal CO_2 measurements are approximately 2 ± 1 mmHg lower than direct measurements. This may be due to fresh gas contamination while withdrawing the required 220 cc/min from the sampling site at the endotracheal tube–system junction.

Clinical events which have been detected include:[70]

1. Partial failure of anesthetic vaporizers
2. Partial disconnection of the CO_2 absorber (high inspired CO_2 levels)
3. Cross-contamination of vaporizers (e.g., mixing halothane and enflurane)
4. Intermittent right mainstem intubation
5. Unexpected return of spontaneous ventilation
6. Unexpected high CO_2 levels in patients with high metabolic rates
7. Air embolism in sitting-position neurosurgical cases (decreased expired CO_2)

On a breath-to-breath basis, when the mass spectrometer is used, inspired concentrations of all measured gases are known, as are the expired concentrations. Gas exchange (adequacy of ventilation and O_2 uptake) is similarly monitored.

In combination with measurements of arterial and mixed venous blood gases, the following determinations can be made:[71]

1. *Quantification of dead space:* Since, by the Bohr equation,

$$\frac{V_d}{V_t} = \frac{PaCO_2 - PeCO_2}{PaCO_2}$$

V_d/V_t can be determined with a $PaCO_2$ measurement and $PeCO_2$ determination from the mass spectrometer.

2. *Quantification of shunt:*

$$\frac{\dot{Q}_s}{\dot{Q}_T} = \frac{(PAO_2 - PaO_2) \times .0031}{(a-\bar{v}DO_2) + (PAO_2 - PaO_2) \times .0031}$$

PAO_2 can be determined with the mass spectrometer, with the other values being calculated from arterial and mixed venous blood gases.

3. *Quantification of respiratory index (RI):*

$$RI = \frac{PAO_2 - PaO_2}{PaO_2}$$

Again, PAO_2 can be determined with the mass spectrometer and PaO_2 from a blood gas. Normally RI < 2. If RI > 2, O_2 is not being adequately transferred to arterial blood. If RI > 6, there is a 90 percent chance of fatality.

4. *Oxygen consumption* $(\dot{V}O_2)$

$\dot{V}O_2$ can be calculated knowing inspired and expired O_2 concentrations (FiO_2 and FEO_2, respectively). The addition of a means of collecting expired gas for a period of time and then using the mass spectrometer sampling line to sample the bag after mixing allows determination of FEO_2. Since FiO_2 is known, $\dot{V}O_2 = (FiO_2)$ (gas flow) − (FEO_2) (expired volume) can be derived.

5. *Cardiac output*

$$\dot{Q}_T = \frac{\dot{V}O_2}{(CaO_2 - C\bar{v}O_2)}$$

$\dot{V}O_2$ has been determined in (4) and CaO_2 and $C_{\bar{v}}O_2$ can be measured.

The mass spectrometer, then, is not simply a toy, for it allows noninvasive determination of several major metabolic, respiratory, and hemodynamic parameters, as well as providing information about anesthetic uptake.

In the absence of a mass spectrometer, end-tidal CO_2 monitoring can provide breath-to-breath information about ventilatory adequacy. These devices (such as the Siemens 930 CO_2 analyzer and Puritan-Bennett/Datex CO_2 monitor) generally operate on an infrared (IR) absorption principle.[72] A pump in the monitor draws the gas sample into a measuring chamber located adjacent to a reference chamber containing ambient air. Infrared rays are passed through both chambers, where the CO_2 in the sample gas absorbs some of the rays. Those IR rays passing through then go through a narrow-band IR filter, which allows only the radiation in the absorption band to reach a detector (Fig. 6-22). The ratio of the radiation through the measuring chamber to that through the reference chamber is obtained and the CO_2 content of the sample determined. The direct effect of N_2O on CO_2 measurement is negligible; however, N_2O molecules interact with CO_2 to produce the *collision broadening effect*, whereby IR absorption of CO_2 is greater with N_2O present than in ambient air. In oxygen a similar but opposite and less significant *collision narrowing effect* occurs. Devices such as the Puritan-Bennett/Datex CO_2 monitor have built-in compensation circuitry to minimize these effects. Besides monitoring expired CO_2, attempts have been made to use the output from an end-tidal CO_2 analyzer (Siemens 930 CO_2 analyzer) as part of a feedback circuit to control ventilation.[73] In addition, a device being tested by Ohio Medical Products uses IR absorption to determine end-tidal anesthetic gases (halothane, enflurane,

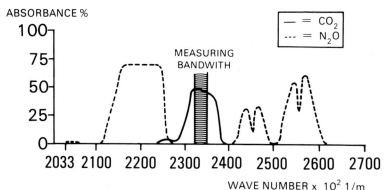

Fig. 6-22 Infrared absorbance. The electromagnetic spectrum is near the absorption peak of CO_2. (Puritan-Bennett/Datex CO_2 Monitor Operating Instructions with permission from Datex Instrumentation, Oy, Helsinki, Finland.

and isoflurane). Monitoring of inspired and expired gases offers exciting possibilities for noninvasive measurements of physiologic functions.

INVASIVE MONITORING TECHNIQUES

Despite the excellence of noninvasive monitoring techniques in areas such as detection of myocardial ischemia, intermittent determination of blood pressure, and end-tidal gas analysis, deficiencies exist in blood pressure determination on a beat-to-beat basis, measurement of acid-base status, and assessment of hemodynamic parameters (right and left atrial pressures, pulmonary artery and pulmonary capillary wedge pressures), and cardiac output and its derivatives. Invasive monitoring techniques (arterial cannulation, central venous cannulation, and pulmonary artery cannulation) allow measurement of the latter variables.

Often, not only in the literature but on a day-to-day basis, the utilization of such invasive monitoring techniques is referred to as the "placement of lines." Appropriate commentary on this usage of the language is provided by Zauder who states:[74]

> The literature abounds with references to central venous lines, pulmonary artery lines, and the insertion of arterial lines. Conventionally, a line refers to: a long, slender cord, a rope carried on a ship, a device for catching fish, a scope of activity, a horizontal row of written characters, a short note, a limit, a chronological series, a group of football players, and military officers of junior rank ... or characterization on the basis of material carried (e.g., sewer lines).

The intent of most invasive monitoring techniques is to measure pressure or to sample blood. In order to accurately measure and interpret the pressure data transduced, it is necessary to have some knowledge of the pressure-transducing system and its characteristics. The initial criteria for recording pressure waveforms with adequate fidelity

were established by Otto Frank in 1903.[75] In 1947, Lambert and Wood demonstrated the usefulness of a liquid-filled catheter and strain gauge for the measurement of arterial pressure.[76] These principles hold true for the measurement of venous and pulmonary artery pressure as well.

Once such a system of cannula–liquid-filled tubing–transducer–amplifier–oscilloscope–meter–recorder is inserted and connected, it is assumed, after calibration, to present precise information. Calibration of the system is performed to adjust the gain of the amplifier against an electrically simulated signal or a statically applied pressure against the transducer. Another major factor in determining the accuracy of such a system is in the capability of the system to respond accurately to rapidly changing pressure waveforms. This capability is not tested by the application of static pressure to the system.[77] The catheter-transducer systems generally used during anesthesia may be characterized as an "underdamped, second-order dynamic system," analogous to a bouncing tennis ball.[78] Such a second-order system can be characterized by three mechanical parameters:[78]

1. *Elasticity:* The overall stiffness of the system. Flexibility of the transducer diaphragm is a normal constituent. Elasticity may be altered by air bubbles, compliant tubing, or other elastic elements.
2. *Mass:* The fluid mass moving in the system (usually in the catheter and connecting tubing).
3. *Friction:* Friction in the catheter and tubing as the fluid moves with each pulsatile change in pressure.

These variables determine two measurable parameters, the *natural frequency,* which refers to how rapidly the system oscillates, and the *damping coefficient,* which refers to how quickly the system comes to rest.

In clinical usage, the underdamped catheter-transducer systems may result in

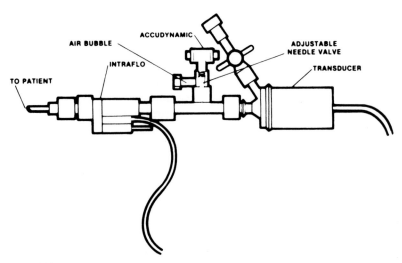

Fig. 6-23 Accudynamic damping device in typical location. The adjustable needle valve and 0.1 cc sealed air bubble are also indicated. (Gardner RM: Direct blood pressure measurement—dynamic response requirements. Anesthesiology 54:227-235, 1981. Reproduced with permission.)

two major errors in pressure measurement: overestimation of systolic pressure by 15 to 30 mmHg or as much as 30 percent above reference pressure waveforms, and amplification of artifact in the measurement system ("catheter whip" in the pulmonary artery or "ringing" at rest or with a flush).[77,78] Because most electronic pressure systems look at peak and valley pressures to determine systole and diastole, clinically relevant errors may be caused by both the above factors.[78] However, when mean pressures are electronically determined, reference and recorded pressures may not differ appreciably (calculation of mean pressure from systolic and diastolic pressures may be in error).[77]

It is clear that optimum dynamic response of the system is required for accurate determination of systolic and diastolic pressure. A device (Accudynamic, Sorenson Research Co., Salt Lake City UT) consisting of a 0.1-ml sealed air bubble and adjustable needle-valve resistor (Fig. 6-23) has been developed to optimize impedance matching of the catheter-transducer system. The inclusion of an air bubble in a monitoring system increases the damping coefficient and de-

creases the natural frequency, the effect being similar to an increase in tubing length.[77,78] The adjustable needle valve in the Accudynamic provides a method of adjusting the damping frequency of a system (natural frequency should not decrease with installation of the device, if it does the system is not properly set up and may contain air). After inclusion in the system, the Accudynamic should be adjusted to the optimum damping coefficient, which in practice is achieved when a flush results in one undershoot followed by a small overshoot which then settles into the patient's waveform (Fig. 6-24).[78] Calculations such as the rate-pressure product require an accurate determination of systolic pressure, for which an appropriately damped system is required. If only mean pressures are required, dynamic response requirements are of little importance. Characteristics of connecting tubing have been tabulated by Shinozaki and are presented in Table 6-6.[77] The combination of correct damping and knowledge of the characteristics of the components will result in more accurate determination of the relevant pressures.

Table 6-6
Weighted Sums of Percentage Differences Between Theoretical and Actual Responses Between 2 Hz and 20 Hz (WSD)

	Strain Gauge	Transducer and Length	Arterial WSD* (Per Cent)	Pulmonary WSD (Per Cent)	Resonant Frequency (Hz)	Time Delay (ms)
Standard arterial tubings and transducers	Statham P50A	—	7.2	6.8	46	<1
	Hewlett Packard	—	5.7	6.4	39	<1
	Trantek	—	9.5	8.1	54	<1
20-gauge Cathlon 1½ inch catheter and transducers	Statham P50A	—	0.1	0.2	113	—
	Hewlett Packard	—	1.1	1.3	81	—
	Trantek	—	0.4	0.5	265	—
Various lengths of connecting tubing (Cobe)		Statham P50A				
	—	3 feet	7.2	6.8	46	<1
	—	6 feet	9.2	10.7	32	<1
	—	8 feet	31.3	32.4	23	4–8
	—	7-Fr Swan-Ganz	18.0	17.0	25	4–6
		Hewlett Packard				
	—	3 feet	5.7	6.4	39	<1
	—	6 feet	16.4	16.3	26	2–4
	—	8 feet	47.2	44.4	21	5–12
	—	7-Fr Swan-Ganz	32.1	29.9	20	6–12
	—	7-Fr Swan-Ganz, 6 feet	70.2	59.1	12	20
Effect of electronic filter						
	—	Statham P50A 6-foot Cobe	6.6	6.0	—	25
	—	7-Fr Swan-Ganz	1.2	1.5	—	26–28
	—	Hewlett Packard 6-foot Cobe	2.7	2.8	—	24
	—	7-Fr Swan-Ganz	5.2	4.0	—	28–31

Reproduced from: Shinozaki T, Deane RS, Mazuzan JE: The dynamic responses of liquid-filled catheter systems for direct measurements of blood pressure. Anesthesiology 53:49–504, 1980
* WSD = weighted sum of the percentage differences

Arterial Cannulation

According to Prys-Roberts, "direct, continuous monitoring of arterial pressure should no longer be regarded as a complex esoteric measurement pertinent only to cardiac surgery, an intensive therapy unit, or the laboratory."[79] Cannulation of a peripheral artery is performed for three prime indications:

1. Desire for measurement of blood pressure on a beat-to-beat basis
2. The necessity or desire for frequent blood gas sampling
3. Prolonged surgical procedures, or those in which large fluid and volume shifts are anticipated

Although an automated oscillotonometric device such as the Dinamap presents accurate data regarding systolic, diastolic, and mean blood pressures, the maximum frequency with which pressure can be determined is once per minute. Quite often during thoracic surgery, especially during vascular procedures or those employing one-lung anesthesia, potentially lethal changes in blood pressure can occur within a 60-second period. An awareness of the pressure on a beat-

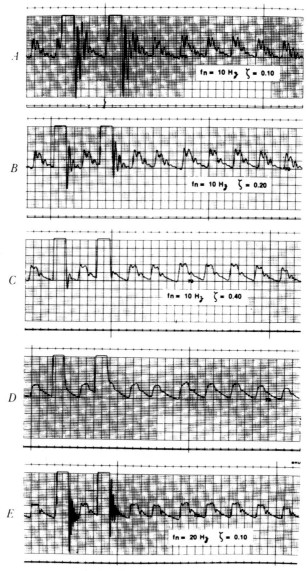

Fig. 6-24 Utilization of Accudynamic to optimize damping. Five pressure tracings show method of optimizing damping using the flush technique and Accudynamic. Each tracing has two flushes. (A) Patient waveform with two flushes, showing a low natural frequency of 10 Hz and a low damping coefficient of 0.01. Note overshoot and ringing in the patient waveform. (B) Damping coefficient increased to 0.2 by adjusting the needle valve. Natural frequency the same. Ringing after flushing decays more quickly. (C) Near optimum damping (0.4). Note that there is little ringing on the flush signals. (D) Overadjustment of damping on an overdamped system. From the flush the damping coefficient and natural frequency are not easily determined; however the flush clearly indicates overdamping because there is no ringing. (E) A waveform whose natural frequency has been increased to 20 Hz by shortening the interconnecting tubing length but with a damping coefficient of 0.1. Note that the patient waveform is much less distorted than in Figure 6-24 A. This figure also illustrates the importance of timing of the flushes to measure the damping. Tracing 24 A has two flushes which occur and are distorted by the systolic pulsation of the aortic pressure signal. On the other hand, in Figure 24 E the flushes were made during the more desirable time of the diastolic runoff when there is less artifact added to the flush signal.

to-beat basis allows prompt identification of a trend or change in pressure and a more accurate response. This may forestall wide swings in pressure due to overvigorous therapeutic responses and thereby minimize risk to the patient. During one-lung anesthesia or in those cases in which part of the lung is packed down, increased intrapulmonary shunting and subsequent arterial hypoxemia occur owing to incomplete or inadequate hypoxic pulmonary vasoconstriction (see Chs. 7 and 8). In the absence of a mass spectrometer, multiple arterial blood gas samples are required to follow the degree of shunting, level of hypoxemia, hyper- or hypocarbia, and acid-base status. The most efficacious way to obtain the necessary samples is from an indwelling arterial cannula. Where major fluid and volume shifts may occur (i.e., in repair of a thoracic aortic aneurysm), the arterial cannula will be valuable for both pressure monitoring and sampling. In addition to blood gas analysis, arterial blood may be used in the determination of electrolyte levels (Na^+, K^+, Ca^{2+}), glucose concentrations, and colloid oncotic pressures.

One of the major concerns about arterial cannulation has been the safety of the procedure. Percutaneous cannulation of the radial artery has fewer vascular complications than does cannulation of brachial or femoral arteries.[80] Several major studies now exist attesting to the safety of the procedure of cannulation of the radial artery. An early study by Bedford and Wollman of 105 percutaneous radial artery cannulations showed no major ischemic complications despite a 38 percent rate of thrombosis of the artery after cannulation.[81] With a cannulation duration of less than 2 hours, thrombosis did not occur, and the rate of thrombosis did not exceed 38 percent when cannulation persisted beyond 40 hours. Bedford followed up this work in 1978 with a study of radial artery function in 114 patients.[82] Cannulation lasting 1 to 3 days had an 11 percent incidence of occlusion, while cannulation for 4 to 10 days produced a 29 percent incidence of occlusion

($p < .05$). The conclusions were that the risk of vascular complications with 20-gauge Teflon catheters rose after 3 days of cannulation and that occluded arteries did not lead to vascular complications. Davis and Stewart reported on 333 radial artery cannulations and found that complete occlusion of the vessel occurred in 30 percent of the patients one day after decannulation, this incidence decreasing to 24 percent by the eighth day.[83] Of those arteries which were occluded, only 3 percent had been cannulated with a 20-gauge Teflon catheter. Virtually no difference was seen among occlusion rates with 18- and 20-gauge polypropylene and 18-gauge Teflon catheters, each being around 30 percent. Previous studies had documented the increased perfusion patency rate with 20-gauge cannulae.[84,85] Part of the reason for the decreased rate of vascular occlusion with 20-gauge cannulae is shown in data from Bedford (Fig. 6-25), indicating that the incidence of occlusion increases linearly as more of the vessel lumen is occupied by the cannula.[85] That is, small cannulae in large vessels rarely cause occlusions, while larger cannulae in smaller vessels increase occlusion rate.

Increased safety of arterial cannulation may be obtained by assessing the patency of ulnar arterial collateral flow to the palmar arch. Classically, this is done by performing an Allen's test, first described in 1929, although Doppler ultrasound and digital plethysmography may also be used.[86] Although the results of an Allen's test are frequently reported as "positive" or "negative," this descriptive terminology is not appropriate.[87,88] What should be reported is the time delay between release of the compressed artery and the palmar flush.[87] Further information may be obtained from reporting the "refill time" for the ulnar artery as well.[88] A short time span should elapse between radial and ulnar artery tests to avoid misinterpretation of the second test due to reactive hyperemia from the first test.[89]

If an Allen's test is used as a determinant of suitability of radial arterial can-

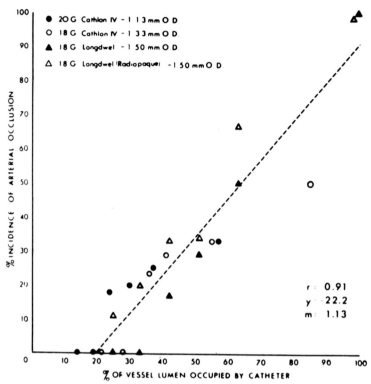

Fig. 6-25   Incidence of radial artery occlusion after 24 hours of cannulation. Incidence of occlusion increases linearly as more of the vessel lumen is occupied by the cannula. Bedford RF: Radial artery function following percutaneous cannulation with 18 and 20 gauge catheters. Anesthesiology 47:37-39, 1977. Reproduced with permission.)

nulation, an appropriate refill time must be selected. Bedford found no ischemic complications when a 5-second refill time was used, while in a prior study he found a 10 percent incidence of distal ischemia when a 15-second refill time was used.[81,85] Davis and Stewart found no complications when arteries were cannulated with use of 8- to 14-second refill times.[83] It appears that a refill time of 14 seconds is at the outer limits of acceptability, and that the adoption of a 5- to 10-second limit on refill time as a determinant of suitability for cannulation is reasonable.

As an adjunct to the Allen's test, wrist circumference may be used for predicting the likelihood of postcannulation radial artery occlusion. The incidence of postcannulation occlusion increases markedly when wrist circumference is less than 18 cm (Fig. 6-26).[90] Further decreases in the postcannulation occlusion rate may be obtained by removing any thrombus generated during cannulation at the time of decannulation.[91] When the cannula is removed in the usual fashion, by applying direct digital pressure over the arterial cannulation site while the cannula is withdrawn, any thrombus generated during cannulation which is adherent to the catheter is effectively left within the arterial lumen, thereby increasing the tendency to thrombosis. Bedford used a method shown in Figure 6-27, consisting of digital occlusion proximal and distal to the arterial cannula and application of continuous suction to the hub of the catheter with a 10-ml syringe while

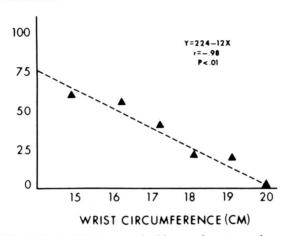

% INCIDENCE
OF OCCLUSION

WRIST CIRCUMFERENCE (CM)

Fig. 6-26   Relationship between incidence of postcannulation radial artery occlusion and wrist circumference. Patients with smaller wrists have a higher incidence of occlusion than those with larger wrists. (Bedford RG: Wrist circumference predicts the use of radial arterial occlusions after cannulations. Anesthesiology 48:377, 1978. Reproduced with permission.)

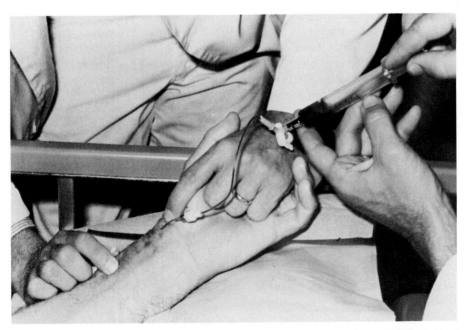

Fig. 6-27   Withdrawal of arterial thrombus. Note occlusion of vessel proximal and distal to cannulation site. From Bedford RF: Removal of radial artery thrombi following percutaneous cannulation for monitoring. Anesthesiology 46:430, 1977. Reproduced with permission.

withdrawing the catheter, to decrease arterial occlusion after decannulation.[91] Occlusion dropped from 75 to 27 percent of cases when moderate to total occlusion by thrombus existed arteriographically prior to the decannulation and from 5 to 0 percent when no thrombus or only a small thrombus was present prior to decannulation.[91]

An additional concern as far as increasing safety and patency rate has been catheter composition. The statement has been made that the heavy metals such as bismuth or barium used to make Teflon radiopaque also make the catheter more thrombogenic than nonradiopaque catheters, yet Bedford and others found almost no difference in incidence of occlusion with radiopaque (31 percent) vs. nonradiopaque (36 percent) catheters.[85,92,93]

Complications other than arterial occlusion may occur with arterial cannulation.[94] These include loss of time during insertion, laceration of the artery, hematoma formation, local pathologic changes (mycotic aneurysm, dissecting aneurysm, pseudoaneurysm, arteriovenous fistulae, atheromatous emboli), embolism of the catheter or its parts, infection, improper injections, air embolism, cerebral embolism (especially if flushing with volumes larger than 2.5 ml), and exsanguination.[95] Median nerve compression secondary to blood in the carpal tunnel has also been reported.[96] The technique is clearly not without hazard, and, as with any procedure, the risk-benefit ratio must be considered.

The various sites and methods of arterial cannulation have been described and do not need to be repeated here. A comment, however, is in order regarding the "preferred" method of arterial cannulation. Jones recently found no increased risk of vascular complications when a transfixion method of cannulation was used vs. a direct threading technique, which thus makes the former a reasonable alternative.[97]

As mentioned above, the arterial catheter may be used for blood sampling as well as for pressure determination. A comprehensive discussion of arterial blood gas analysis is beyond the scope of this text, and for that the reader is referred to standard textbooks on the subject.[98]

Central Venous Cannulation—Pulmonary Artery Catheterization

The other invasive monitoring technique commonly employed, besides arterial cannulation, is catheterization of a central vein from either a central (internal jugular, external jugular, subclavian, or femoral vein) or peripheral (basilic or cephalic vein) approach with or without passage of a pulmonary artery catheter (PAC). A comprehensive description of the techniques involved for both initial venous cannulation and placement of the PAC can be found in standard texts.[99]

In any given case, a decision must be reached as to whether to use the central venous pressure (CVP) to monitor cardiac function or to obtain more detailed information (pulmonary artery pressure, pulmonary capillary wedge pressure, cardiac output, etc.). If the latter is preferred, placement of a pulmonary artery catheter is mandated. Major questions exist, however, regarding the utility and/or accuracy of information derived from the PAC during certain thoracic cases—namely those operations performed in a lateral decubitus position or with one-lung anesthesia. Little information exists as to hemodynamic changes in the lateral position or with one-lung ventilation.

Although it appears that right atrial pressure (RAP) correlates well with pulmonary capillary wedge pressure (PCWP) in patients without heart disease in the supine position, it is unclear if this holds true in the lateral decubitus position with or without one-lung ventilation.[100]

The risks of central venous cannulation for the measurement of CVP include, but are not limited to:

1. Arterial puncture
2. Pneumothorax (especially with subclavian cannulation)
3. Local and systemic infection
4. Thromboembolism and/or thrombophlebitis
5. Infusion of fluid into the mediastinum
6. Thoracic duct laceration
7. Hematoma formation
8. Air embolism
9. Shearing of catheter parts and embolic sequelae
10. Injury to nerves adjacent to the cannulation site
11. Pericardial tamponade

To take these risks, assurance is needed that the parameter being monitored is of use and accurately represented. For the present, that assumption is made with respect to RAP. The PCWP correlates poorly with RAP in patients with heart disease, and there is no reason to assume that this relationship would improve with the lateral decubitus position or one-lung ventilation. Therefore, commonly accepted criteria are used as indications for the insertion of PACs in thoracic anesthesia (Table 6-7). The risks of insertion of the PAC are primarily those of cannulation of the central vein, with the notable exception of dysrhythmias during passage

Table 6-7
Indications for Pulmonary Artery Catheterization in Thoracic Surgery

1. Patients with known cardiac disease, vascular or valvular, with or without failure
2. Surgery in which cross-clamping of the aorta is anticipated
3. Patients in respiratory failure
4. Patients with suspected or diagnosed pulmonary emboli
5. Patients who have undergone previous cardiac surgery
6. When a pneumonectomy is anticipated
7. When large volume shifts are anticipated
8. In the presence of sepsis
9. Patients who are maintained on inotropes, vasodilators, or the intra-aortic balloon pump prior to surgery

through the right ventricle.[100-102] The additional risks of maintenance of a PAC are numerous and include:[103]

1. Rupture of the balloon
2. Pulmonary infarction
3. Pulmonary artery rupture
4. Catheter knotting
5. Infections (both local and systemic with endocarditis possible)
6. Thrombogenesis and thrombocytopenia

Again, to justify taking these risks, one would like assurance that accurate information is necessary. In the supine patient, the ability to estimate left-sided function from pulmonary artery and PCW pressures has been well established.[104, 105] The use of lateral positions and/or one-lung ventilation, however, throws a proverbial "monkey wrench" into the works.

For the PAC to present accurate information, its tip should not be in a zone 1 region of the lung (where alveolar pressure exceeds pulmonary artery and venous pressure). In such a case the PCWP recording will reflect airway pressure rather than left atrial pressure. Benumof found, in a retrospective analysis of 314 PACs placed, that the vast majority of catheter tips were located in the right middle and lower lung fields (Fig. 6-28).[106] He also found that around 5 percent of the catheter tips were 9 cm or more lateral to the midline, an area which would possibly be a zone 1 when the patient was placed in the lateral position. Kronberg et al found similar catheter tip location on anteroposterior chest roentgenograms (Fig. 6-29).[107] Clearly, if the patient is to be in the left lateral decubitus position for a right thoracotomy and the PAC has been placed supine, a question must arise regarding reliability of the data obtained.

In view of the propensity for the PAC to enter the right middle and right lower pulmonary arteries, it would be nice to be able to selectively direct the catheter. For instance, more reliable readings might be obtained during a right thoracotomy if the

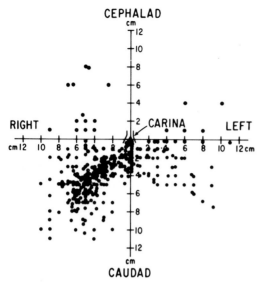

Fig. 6-28   Intrathoracic distribution of locations of pulmonary artery catheter tips. (Benumof JL, Saidman LJ, Arkin DB, et al: Where pulmonary arterial catheters go: intrathoracic distribution. Anesthesiology 48:336-338, 1977. Reproduced with permission.)

catheter tip were in the distribution of the left main pulmonary artery and therefore in close proximity to the left atrium. By utilizing a technique described by Kopman with a sterile sleeve (Fig. 6-30) whereby the catheter can be manipulated without the risk of contamination, it may be possible to place the catheter in the pulmonary artery trunk, turn to the lateral position (and deflate the up lung if one-lung ventilation is to be used), and advance the catheter to the wedge position.[108] The potential success of this technique depends in part on the effect of gravity on redistribution of blood flow to the down lung as well as on hypoxic pulmonary vasoconstriction. Early clinical trials utilizing this technique have been promising.

The position of the catheter tip is not the only variable affecting reliability of pulmonary artery pressures; positive pressure ventilation, particularly with the use of positive end-expiratory pressure (PEEP), and the time during the respiratory cycle at which pulmonary artery pressure is measured may affect the pressure obtained. PEEP may alter validity of pulmonary artery pressure readings in two ways: first by altering intrapleural pressure; and second by transmitting pressure generated by PEEP to the pulmonary microvasculature.[109] The latter condition occurs when pulmonary alveolar pressure exceeds pulmonary venous or left atrial pressure.

Lozman et al have suggested that mean wedge pressure no longer indicates left atrial

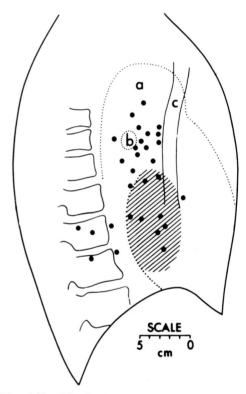

Fig. 6-29   Distribution of PAC tips on lateral roentgenograms: a = aortic arch; b = left main-stem bronchus; c = superior vena cava; shaded area = left atrium. Each dot represents a PAC tip after supine placement. Most tips are cephalad to the left atrium but do not differ markedly in vertical location in the supine position. However, changes in patient position may result in significant variation in these relationships. (Kronberg GM, Quan SF, Schlobohm RM et al: Anatomic locations of the tips of pulmonary-artery catheters in supine patients. Anesthesiology 51:467-469, 1979. Reproduced with permission.)

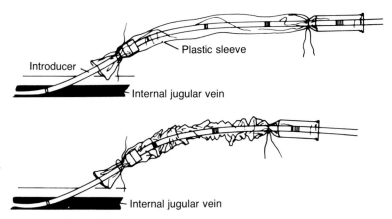

Fig. 6-30 Utilization of a plastic sleeve, either made on the spot with a sleeve from a CVP set (as illustrated) or from commercial sources, allows manipulation of the PAC without risk of contamination. (Kopman EA, Sandza JG: Manipulation of the pulmonary-artery catheter after placement: maintenance of sterility. Anesthesiology 48:373-374, 1978. Reproduced with permission.)

pressure when PEEP of 10 cm H_2O or more is applied in man.[110] Roy et al, in a dog model with both open and closed thoraces, explored this further.[111] Integral to understanding this study is a reiteration of West's zones of the lung (Fig. 6-31):[112]

Zone 1: Alveolar pressure exceeds both pulmonary artery and pulmonary venous pressures, collapsing pulmonary arteries and resulting in no flow.

Zone 2: Alveolar pressure is higher than pulmonary venous pressure. Flow is then determined by the difference between pulmonary artery and alveolar pressures.

Zone 3: Pulmonary venous pressure is higher than alveolar pressures, with pulmonary capillaries being open. Flow is determined by the difference between pulmonary artery and pulmonary venous pressure.

A flow-directed catheter would not spontaneously enter zone 1, but, particularly with a turn to the left lateral decubitus position, a catheter originally in a zone 2 or 3 may lie in zone 1 (see above).

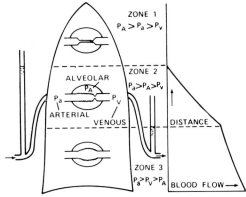

Fig. 6-31 West's zones of the lung to explain the uneven distribution of pulmonary blood flow. P_A = alveolar pressure; Pa = pulmonary arterial pressure; P_V = pulmonary venous pressure. (West JB: Respiratory Physiology: The Essentials. 2nd Ed. © 1979 The Williams & Wilkins Co., Baltimore. p 43)

Roy et al showed that when the PAC is vertically below the left atrium, wedge pressure and left atrial pressure are not significantly different except with an open thorax and PEEP > 10 cm H_2O (Fig. 6-32).[112] Alternatively, when the PAC is vertically above the left atrium, wedge pressure and left atrial pressure are significantly different

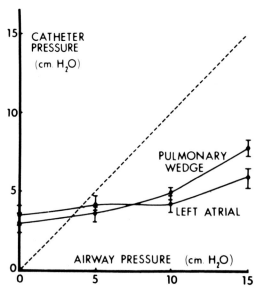

Fig. 6-32 Relationship of PCWP to left atrial pressure. PAC tip is below the left atrium; at 15 cm H$_2$O of PEEP, PCWP and LAP differed significantly. (Roy R, Powers SR, Feustel PJ, Dutton RE: Pulmonary wedge catheterization during positive end-expiratory pressure ventilation in dog. Anesthesiology 46:385-390, 1971. Reproduced with permission.)

with PEEP > 5 cm H$_2$O (Fig. 6-33). Presumably, the pressure transducer has been zeroed with respect to atmospheric pressure at the level of the left atrium. In this case, the hydrostatic head of fluid between the transducer and the catheter tip is balanced by the head of fluid between catheter tip and left atrium. These hydrostatic pressures cancel, thereby yielding a true reading of mean left atrial pressure. Artificially raising alveolar pressure (with PEEP) will not affect this pressure until alveolar pressure exceeds the absolute vascular pressure at the catheter tip. That is, a catheter tip 10 cm below the left atrium would require an alveolar pressure increase greater than 10 cm H$_2$O before any increase in pressure was seen by the transducer. It is for this reason that a catheter deep in zone 3 accurately reflects left atrial pressure even with 10 cm H$_2$O PEEP. If, however, the catheter is in zone 2, each in-

crement of PEEP will be transmitted to the transducer since the initial downstream pressure is alveolar pressure. Kane et al confirmed this, finding that with placement of a PAC in zone 1 each increment of PEEP produced an identical increase in wedge pressure.[113] Accurate determination of pulmonary capillary wedge pressure during application of PEEP therefore requires that the tip of the PAC be low in zone 3. As with other hemodynamic measurements, no single measurement is sufficient—trends and changes in other clinical measurements in response to therapy must be depended upon.[109]

Timing during the respiratory cycle of measurement of pulmonary artery pressure may also affect the pressure obtained. This has been graphically shown by Berryhill et al (Fig. 6-34).[114] It can be seen that mean wedge pressure may fluctuate widely during the ventilatory cycle. It has, therefore, been recommended that measurement of pulmonary

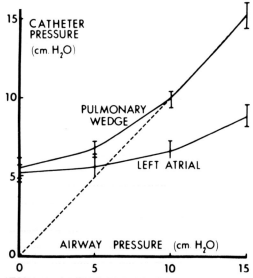

Fig. 6-33 Relationship of PCWP to LAP. PAC tip is above the left atrium; at levels of PEEP>5 cm H$_2$O, PCWP and LAP differed significantly. (Roy R, Powers SR, Feustel PJ, et al: Pulmonary wedge catheterization during positive end-expiratory pressure ventilation in dog. Anesthesiology 46:385-390, 1971. Reproduced with permission.)

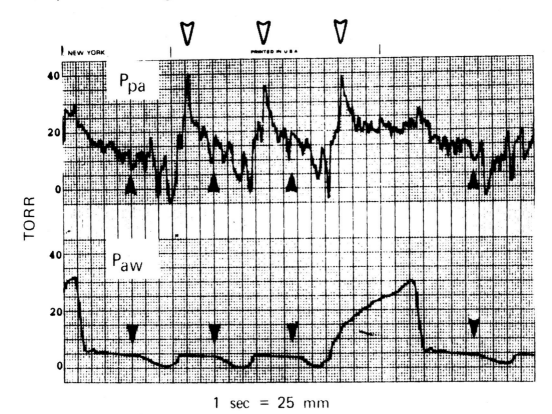

Fig. 6-34 Respiratory cycle influences on PCWP measurement. P_{pa} = pulmonary artery pressure; P_{aw} = airway pressure; closed arrows = end exhalation; open arrows = first heart beat following spontaneous inspiration. Note elevation of P_{pa} with first heart beat following spontaneous inspiration. Mean wedge pressure is seen to vary widely during the ventilatory cycle. Mean P_{pa} and PCWP should be obtained at the end of exhalation. (Berryhill RE, Benumof JL, Rauscher LA: Pulmonary vascular pressure reading at the end of exhalation. Anesthesiology 49:365-368, 1978. Reproduced with permission.)

artery and wedge pressures be obtained at the end of exhalation when there is no air flow and intrapleural pressure is at a static baseline with respect to influence on pulmonary hemodynamics.[114,115]

A PAC may serve an additional useful function in patients undergoing thoracic surgery. McCloud et al have shown that a sudden and rapid elevation of pulmonary artery pressure may be accompanied by the development of a pneumothorax even when the PAC tip is in the opposite side of the chest from the pneumothorax.[116] In the postoperative period after thoracic surgery, such changes may indicate faulty chest tube func-

tion or the development of a major airway leak.

Since the advent of invasive hemodynamic monitoring, concern has been evoked about the hemodynamic consequences of the act of catheter insertion, especially in the awake patient. Bedford has stated: "The act of introducing a Swan-Ganz catheter has been associated with excessive anxiety and potentially dangerous increases in myocardial oxygen consumption . . ."[117] Documentation for this viewpoint is difficult to find, and has, in fact, been refuted in studies by Waller and Quintin.[118,119] Waller found that after premedication with diazepam, mor-

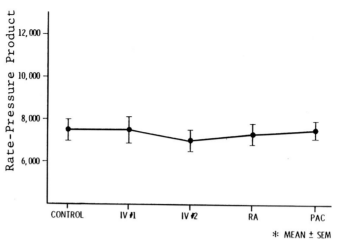

Fig. 6-35 Rate-pressure product in patients undergoing coronary artery bypass grafting at the following times: (1) control; (2) IV #1: time of insertion of first peripheral IV; (3) IV #2: time of insertion of second peripheral IV; (4) RA: radial artery catheter inserted; (5) PAC: Swan-Ganz catheter inserted. No significant change is seen from control, indicating safety of performing these procedures under local anesthesia. (Waller JL, Zaidan JR, Kaplan JA: Hemodynamic effects of vascular cannulation by residents. Anesthesiology 53:S118, 1980. Reproduced with permission.)

phine, and scopolamine and with the use of local anesthetic, insertion of a PAC in patients scheduled for elective coronary artery bypass grafting procedures caused no increase in myocardial oxygen consumption, as estimated by changes in the blood pressure and heart rate (Fig. 6-35). No patient experienced angina or ECG changes indicative of myocardial ischemia. Therefore, placing PACs in awake, premedicated patients with use of local anesthesia is recommended.

The PAC has other uses besides measurement of pulmonary artery pressures. Foremost among these is determination of cardiac output by the thermodilution method. Of the various methods for determining cardiac output (dye dilution, direct Fick principle, thermodilution, echocardiography, uptake of inert gases), thermodilution is the least cumbersome to use in the operating room. The direct Fick method is the standard for steady-state measurements of cardiac output and is said to be accurate within ± 10 percent. The Fick principle states:

$$CO = \frac{\dot{V}_{O_2}}{a-\dot{V}_{O_2}\ \text{difference}}$$

where CO = Cardiac output (ml/min)
$\dot{V}_{O_2}$ = Oxygen uptake per minute (ml/min)
$a-\dot{V}_{O_2}$ = Arteriovenous oxygen difference (ml/ml of blood)

The method requires, however, knowledge of oxygen uptake (which may be determined intraoperatively with the mass spectrometer), arterial oxygen content, and mixed venous oxygen content. The latter variable requires sampling from the pulmonary artery, as streaming of venous return and incomplete mixing make the right atrium and right ventricle unacceptable sampling sites. Thermodilution outputs require a PAC (with thermistor), a computer for cardiac output determination, and the ability to inject a bolus of fluid into the right atrium. For a clinical Fick determination the PAC would be in place anyway for mixed venous sampling, and clearly thermodilution is a less cumbersome technique. The same can be said with respect to dye dilution, which requires injection of dye into the atrium and a timed withdrawal of blood through a cuvette and densitometer, after which the area under the dye dilution curve must be calculated by exponential extrapolation, a "fore-n'-aft" triangle method, or a computer. The thermodilution technique is easier to perform in the operating room.

The dye dilution technique has been shown to correlate well with the Fick method.[120] Similarly, the thermodilution method has been shown to produce results comparable with the dye dilution method. Correlation coefficients have varied from r = .90 (after cardiac surgery) to r = .97 (in pigs) to r = .99 (in humans).[121–123] Cardiac output as determined by a thermodilution method is around 7 percent higher than that obtained by the dye method.[122,124] At lower flow ranges, areas of particular interest, thermodilution may be more accurate than dye, in part because the thermal curve becomes steeper and covers a larger area owing to lack of dilution of the cold bolus, while the dye curve becomes flatter owing to a lack of movement of the dye to the peripheral circulation.[122]

The theory and calculations of the thermodilution method assume:

1. Complete mixing of indicator (cold bolus) with blood
2. A constant flow rate
3. That the indicator passes the detector (thermistor) once and only once
4. That the injected indicator was delivered as a bolus (<4 second injection time)

If the catheter is in such a position that there is either no flow or a partial occlusion of flow past the thermistor (i.e., it is wedged or in a "constant wedge" position), unreliable outputs will be obtained. If the catheter is in the up lung during thoracotomy and the lung is

deflated (both maneuvers altering blood flow to the lung), cardiac outputs probably will not be reliable. However, no data are known to exist on this theoretical point.

The distal pressure port on the PAC may be used for withdrawal of blood for mixed venous oxygen tension–saturation determinations as well as for pressure monitoring. A decreasing $P\bar{v}O_2$ during anesthesia may indicate increased oxygen consumption (light anesthesia, lack of muscular relaxation), decreased oxygen delivery (inadvertent endobronchial intubation, decreased cardiac output, problems with O_2 inflow), or inadequate hypoxic pulmonary vasoconstriction.[123] Maneuvers which would increase $P\bar{v}O_2$ (decreasing oxygen consumption, increasing cardiac output, increasing FIO_2, etc.) may be of benefit. Increases in $P\bar{v}O_2$ above resting may represent decreased $\dot{V}O_2$ and/or the anesthetic state. Increases in $P\bar{v}O_2$ should be noted during administration of sodium nitroprusside, since one of the effects of cyanide is to poison cellular respiration with an inability of the cell to utilize oxygen.

Assessment of mixed venous oxygen tension–saturation may also be accomplished with an indwelling catheter specially designed for this purpose. Armstrong evaluated a specially-designed flow-directed catheter with a Clark-type polarographic oxygen sensor at the tip (Fig. 6-36).[125] The in vitro and in vivo measurements were within 3 mmHg of each other, and the probes had a useful life of around 48 hours. Placement of the catheter in the pulmonary artery was successful only 77 percent of the time, owing to a loss of the balloon flotation properties of the catheter with the placement of the PO_2 transducer at the tip. This latter problem has been obviated by the Opticath produced by Oximetrix (Mountain View, CA), which contains the usual PAC features plus two fiberoptic filaments to permit continuous monitoring of mixed venous oxygen saturation ($S\bar{v}O_2$) by a companion oximeter. Waller found that the in vivo $S\bar{v}O_2$ corre-

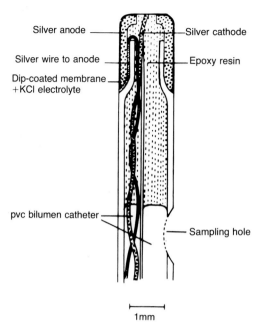

Silver anode

Silver wire to anode

Dip-coated membrane
+KCl electrolyte

Silver cathode

Epoxy resin

pvc bilumen catheter

Sampling hole

├─1mm─┤

Fig. 6-36 Catheter tip P_{O_2} transducer. (Armstrong RF, Moxham J, Cohen SL, et al: Intravascular mixed venous oxygen tension monitoring: an analysis of electrode performance in 100 patients. Br J Anaesth 53:89-96, 1981. Reproduced with permission.)

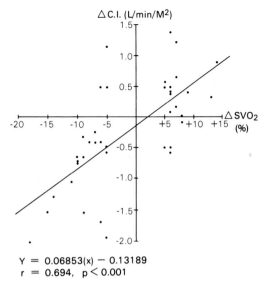

$$Y = 0.06853(x) - 0.13189$$
$$r = 0.694, \quad p < 0.001$$

Fig. 6-37 Change in cardiac index (ΔC.I.) is plotted against change in pulmonary arterial oxygen saturation (ΔSVO_2). A highly significant correlation between the two is seen, i.e., a decrease in SVO_2 indicates a decrease in C.I. (Waller JL, Kaplan JA, Bauman DI, et al: Clinical evaluation of a new fiberoptic catheter oximeter. Anesthesiology 55:A133, 1981. Reproduced with permission.)

lated well (r = .90) with in vitro measurements.[126] Additionally, a good correlation was seen between changes in $S\bar{v}O_2$ and cardiac index (Fig. 6-37). Changes in $S\bar{v}O_2$ therefore not only were accurate, but reflected changes in cardiac output. The usage of this apparatus may reduce the need for routine cardiac output determinations. Rather, as can be seen in Figure 6-37, a change in $S\bar{v}O_2$ of 5 percent or more could provide the warning as to when to determine cardiac output. This method might be less susceptible to false alterations in cardiac output determinations than thermal methods, for as long as there is any blood flow past the sensor, regardless of its intrathoracic position, the $S\bar{v}O_2$ can be determined. Alterations in pulmonary artery pressure due to being placed in zone 1 would still be evident.

Newer versions of the PACs have the capability of providing endocardial pacing.

The multipurpose Swan-Ganz catheter produced by American Edwards Laboratories is shown in Fig. 6-38. In addition to the usual PAC features, there are fine electrodes (three atrial and two ventricular) which may provide for atrial, ventricular, or atrioventricular (A-V) pacing. Zaidan has evaluated this catheter and found that A-V sequential pacing was possible 73 percent of the time, while atrial pacing was possible 80 percent and ventricular pacing was successful 93 percent of the time.[127]

Other Invasive Devices

Arterial cannulae and CVP or Swan-Ganz catheters and their derivatives are not the only invasive monitoring devices available. Attempts have been made to continuously monitor both arterial oxygen and car-

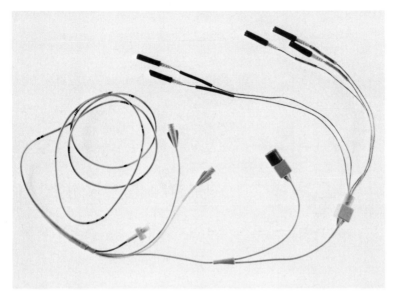

Fig. 6-38 Multipurpose Swan-Ganz catheter. Features include (left to right): balloon inflation port; right atrial port; pulmonary artery port; thermistor connection; two ventricular electrodes (proximal, distal); three atrial electrodes (proximal, central, distal). The electrodes allow atrial, ventricular, or A-V sequential pacing.

bon dioxide tensions with an indwelling device (Sentor Gas Analyzer, Ohio Medical Products). The Sentor device consists of a gas chromatograph connected to a thin heparin-coated probe which is inserted into a peripheral artery through an 18-gauge catheter. Oxygen and carbon dioxide diffuse through the probe membrane, equilibrating in 3 to 4 minutes, after which the gases are aspirated into the gas chromatograph and analyzed. Carlon et al, in comparing Sentor results with blood gases analyzed on a Corning TL 175 analyzer, found a high correlation between the results, but with a 10 to 20 percent error in the Sentor data.[128] Hall et al also found the Sentor readings to be consistently low as compared with those obtained by standard analytical techniques.[129] They also found diminished or eliminated perfusion around the probe after radial artery insertion in all but one of 17 patients in whom angiograms were performed after probe insertion. This is not unexpected after radial artery cannulation with an 18-gauge catheter. Although data from the Sentor may correlate with conventional analysis (despite erring on the low side), the incidence of arterial complications and the long time required for analysis as compared with mass spectrometry preclude widespread use of the device.

Table 6-8
Minimum Monitoring for Thoracic Anesthesia

- Electrocardiogram
  Preferably multiple lead capability
- Blood pressure monitoring
  Whether cuff, automated, or intra-arterial
- Breath sounds/heart beat
  Precordial or esophageal stethoscope
- Core temperature
  Rectal, nasopharyngeal, or esophageal
- Oxygen delivery
  O_2 monitor

Table 6-9
Current Monitoring Techniques Used for Various Types of Cases

	ECG	Non-invasive BP	Stethoscope P=precordial E=esophageal	Temperatures R=rectal NP=nasopharyngeal E=esophageal	O₂ Delivery	Urine output	Invasive BP	ABG	CVP	PAP	W*	CO
Bronchoscopy Flexible	✓	✓	P	Skin surface	✓							
Bronchoscopy Rigid	✓	✓	P	R, NP	✓		±	±				
Mediastinoscopy/ mediastinotomy	✓	✓	E	R, NP, E	✓		±	±				
Laryngoscopy	✓	✓	P	R, NP	✓		±	±				
Chamberlain thoracotomy	✓	✓	P or E	R, NP, E	✓		✓	✓	±			
Lobectomy/wedge resection	✓	✓	E	R, NP, E	✓	✓	✓	✓	✓			
Pneumonectomy	✓	✓	E	R, NP, E	✓	✓	✓	✓	✓	✓	✓	✓
Pulmonary Lavage	✓	✓	E	R, NP, E	✓		✓	✓	✓	✓	✓	✓
Tracheostomy/ tracheal reconstruction	✓	✓	E	R, NP, E	✓		✓	✓	±			
Esophageal surgery	✓	✓	P	R	✓	✓	✓	✓	✓	±	±	±
Mediastinal surgery	✓	✓	E	R, NP, E	✓	±	±	±	✓	✓	✓	
Thoracic trauma	✓	✓	P or E	R, NP, E	✓	✓	✓	✓	✓	✓	✓	✓
Pacemakers Endocardial	✓	✓	P	Skin surface	✓		±	±		±	±	±
Pacemakers Epicardial	✓	✓	E	R, NP, E	✓	✓	✓	✓	✓	±	±	±

* PCWP

Table 6-10
Recommendations for Specific Monitoring Devices

ECG: Mandatory in all cases. Problems with V_5 placement for left thoracotomy may be avoided by using needle electrodes.

Esophageal ECG: May aid in detection of complex dysrhythmias regardless of type of surgery. Esophageal surgery precludes its use.

Blood pressure cuff: Mandatory. Liability of lack of beat-to-beat information.

Automated blood pressure determination: More frequent determination, but not beat-to-beat and ABGs not available.

Precordial stethoscope: Useful except when interferes with the surgical field.

Esophageal stethoscope: Useful except during esophageal surgery.

Urinary catheter: For procedures greater than 1 to 2 hours in duration.

Temperature monitoring: Some form of core temperature monitoring is required for all cases employing general anesthesia. If sedation is employed (flexible bronchoscopy, endocardial pacemakers), core temperature assessment is difficult.

Neural blockade monitors: Useful in any case where neuromuscular blockade is employed.

EEG: Of particular use in thoracic anesthesia during cases involving cross-clamping the ascending aorta.

Transesophageal echocardiography: A potentially useful noninvasive monitor of ventricular function and cardiac output. Precluded during esophageal surgery.

Oxygen analyzers: Indicated during virtually every anesthetic.

Digital oximeters/transcutaneous O_2 monitors: Need further development prior to widespread use.

Mass Spectrometer: Initial expense is great. Particularly useful to assess breath-by-breath gas exchange after lobectomy or pneumonectomy. Provides uncomplicated information for extubation, based on gas exchange, not simply mechanical function. Overall, useful if available but not mandatory.

Arterial cannulation:
- For blood pressure: indicated where beat-to-beat changes may occur (any open chest) and where sudden volume loss (laceration of pulmonary artery during mediastinoscopy) may occur.
- For blood sampling: primarily for ABGs—justifiable in virtually any pulmonary thoracic case as gas exchange may be altered. Certainly necessary for one-lung anesthesia. Patient condition for pacemaker or bronchoscopy may indicate usage. If 3 or more ABGs are anticipated, it may be less traumatic to cannulate the artery.

Central Venous Pressure: For use in the young without heart disease in whom large fluid-volume shifts are anticipated (e.g., trauma, colon interposition, thymectomy). In others where endocardial pacemakers are being or have been placed, the CVP cannula should not become entangled in the pacemaker wires.

Pulmonary artery catheter: Indications for use are listed in Table 6-7. See text for specific problems relating to thoracic anesthesia.

Recommendations

It goes without saying that all monitoring techniques are not required for all patients. A thorough knowledge by the anesthesiologist of the operation intended, potential complications, patient characteristics, and facility of the surgeon is required to make a rational decision as to what monitoring to use. Institutional facilities may vary and influence one's decision. For instance, we have mass spectrometry available in each operating room and use it in virtually every case. Information garnered from the mass spectrometer can be obtained from other sources (arterial blood gas analysis, end-tidal gas analysis, etc.) and it would be foolish to have such an expensive device available only for rare specific events.

Basic "minimum monitoring" for thoracic anesthesia is shown in Table 6-8. The monitoring devices or techniques listed should be available and utilized on every case. Table 6-9 shows what we currently utilize as monitoring techniques for various types of cases. A summary of indications for certain devices and/or techniques is tabulated in Table 6-10. Specific indications as

well as monitoring devices will change as
technology advances and knowledge about
specific disease states increases.

REFERENCES

1. Spierdijk J, Nandort A: The difference between measurement and monitoring: What is
   worth measuring? In Feldman SA, Lugh J,
   Spierdyk J, Eds. Measurement in Anesthesia,
   Leiden University Press, 1974
2. Lee AS: Technical aspects of monitoring systems: A study in information transfer. Crul
   JF, Payne JP, Eds. Patient Monitoring. Ex-
   cerpta Medica, Amsterdam, 1970
3. Piepenbrock S, Hempelmann G: Intraoperative and postoperative monitoring of car-
   diocirculatory function in pediatric and adult
   cardiosurgical patients. Int Anesthesiol Clin
   14:3, 49-62, 1976
4. Lindop MJ: Monitoring of the cardiovascular
   system during anesthesia. Int Anesthesiol
   Clin 19:1, 1-30, 1981
5. Burchardi H, Electronische Patientenüber-
   wachung, Krankenhausartz 7:246, 1969 (cited
   in Piepenbrock and Hempelmann, Reference 3.)
6. Gersch BJ: Measurement of intravascular
   pressures, pp. 511-530. Prys-Roberts C, Ed.
   The Circulation in Anaesthesia: Applied
   Physiology and Pharmacology, Blackwell Scientific Publications, London, 1980
7. Cannard TM, Dripps RD, Helwig J et al: The
   ECG during anesthesia and surgery. Anesthesiology 21:194-202, 1960
8. Russell PM, Coakley CS: Electrocardiographic observation in the operating room.
   Anesth Analg (Cleve) 48:784-788, 1969
9. Blackburn H: The exercise electrocardiogram: technical, procedural and conceptual
   developments. In Blackburn H, Ed.: Measurements and Exercise Electrocardiography,
   Charles C Thomas, Springfield, Ill., 1967
10. Mason RE, Likar I, Biern RO et al: Multiple
    lead exercise electrocardiography. Circula-
    tion 36:517-525, 1967
11. Foëx P, Prys-Roberts C: Anaesthesia and the
    hypertensive patient. Br J Anaesth 46:575-
    588, 1974
12. Kaplan JA, King SB: The precordial elec-
    trocardiographic lead (V_5) in patients with

coronary artery disease. Anesthesiology
45:570-574, 1976
13. Dalton B: A precordial ECG lead for chest
    operations. Anesth Analg (Cleve) 55:740-741,
    1976
14. Kistner JR, Miller ED, Epstein RM: More
    than V_5 needed. Anesthesiology 47:75, 1977
15. Bazaral M, Norfleet E: Comparison of V_5 and
    CB_5 leads for intraoperative monitoring.
    Anesth Analg 60:849-853, 1981
16. Erhard LR, Sjögren A, Wahlberg I: Single
    right side precordial lead in the diagnosis of
    right ventricular involvement in inferior
    myocardial infarction. Am Heart J 91:571-
    583, 1976
17. Erhardt LR: Right ventricular involvement in
    acute myocardial infarction. Eur J Cardiol
    4:411-418, 1976
18. Kistin AD, Bruce JC: Simultaneous esopha-
    geal and standard electrocardiographic leads
    for the study of cardiac arrhythmias. Am
    Heart J 53:65-73, 1957
19. Copeland GD, Tullis IF, Brody DA: Clinical
    evaluation of a new esophageal electrode with
    particular reference to the bipolar
    esophageal electrocardiogram. Part II. Obser-
    vations in cardiac arrhythmias. Am Heart J
    57:874-885, 1959
20. Kates RA, Zaidan JR, Kaplan JA: Evalua-
    tion of the esophageal ECG lead during
    CABG surgery. Anesth Analg, in press, 1982
21. Kaplan JA: Principles of management of pa-
    tients with coronary artery disease. Int An-
    esthesiol Clin 18:4, 137-180, 1980
22. Hales S: Statical Essays: Vol 2 Containing
    Haemastatics. Winnip, London, P. 1 cited in
    Paulus DA: Noninvasive blood pressure mea-
    surement. Med Instrum 15:2, 91-94, 1981
23. Paulus DA: Noninvasive blood pressure mea-
    surement. Med Instrum 15:2, 91-94, 1981
24. Tinker JH: personal communication.
25. Bates B: A Guide to Physical Examination. J
    B Lippincott Co., Philadelphia, 1974, p. 139
26. Smith C: An endo-oesophageal stethoscope.
    Anesthesiology 15:566, 1954
27. Schwartz AJ, Downes JJ: Hazards of a simple
    monitoring device, the esophageal stetho-
    scope. Anesthesiology 47:64, 1977
28. Simpson S: Temperature range in the mon-
    key in ether anaesthesia. J Physiol (Lond),
    Proceedings R Soc Lond (Biol) 28:37-40, 1902
29. Vale RJ: Monitoring of temperature during

anesthesia. Int Anesthesiol Clin 19:1, 61-83, 1981

30. Leonard PF: Principles of electricity I: The electric meter and thermistor. Anesth Analg (Cleve) 45:246-249, 1966

31. Vaughan RW, Vaughan MS, Cork RC: Postoperative inaccuracy of liquid crystal thermometry. Anesthesiology 53, S166, 1980

32. Holdcroft A, Hall GM: Heat loss during anesthesia. Br J Anaesth 50:157-164, 1978

33. Benzinger M, Benzinger TH: Tympanic membrane temperature. JAMA 209:1207-1211, 1969

34. Cabanac M, Caputa M: Open loop increase in trunk temperature produced by face cooling in working humans. J Physiol (Lond) 289:163-174, 1979

35. Gilston A: Anaesthesia for cardiac surgery. Br J Anaesth 43:217-232, 1971

36. Scurr C, Feldman S: Scientific Foundations of Anaesthesia, Year Book Medical Publishers Inc., Chicago 1974, p 80

37. Waller JL: personal communication

38. Morris RM: Influence of ambient temperature on patient temperature during intra-abdominal surgery. Ann Surg 173:230-233, 1971

39. Morris RM, Wilkey BR: The effects of ambient temperature on patient temperature during surgery not involving body cavities. Anesthesiology 32:102-107, 1970

40. Roizen MF, Sohn YJ, L'Hommedieu CS et al: Operating room temperature prior to surgical draping: Effect on patient temperature in recovery room. Anesth Analg (Cleve) 59:852-855, 1980

41. Noback CR, Tinker JH: Hypothermia after cardiopulmonary bypass in man: amelioration by nitroprusside induced vasodilation during rewarming. Anesthesiology 53:277-280, 1980

42. Morris RM, Kumar A: The effect of warming blankets on maintenance of body temperature of the anesthetized paralyzed adult patient. Anesthesiology 36:408-411, 1972

43. Noback CR, Tinker JH: Efficacy of warming blankets in cardiovascular surgery. Anesthesiology 55:A118, 1981

44. Scott SM: Thermal blanket injury in the operating room. Arch Surg 94:181, 1967

45. Johnstone RE: Malignant heating pad. Anesthesiology 41:307, 1974

46. Ben-Zvi S: A possible cause of temperature probe failure. Anesthesiology 53:523, 1980

47. Schneider AJL, Apple HP, Braun RT: Electrosurgical burns at skin temperature probes. Anesthesiology 47:72-74, 1977

48. Haldane JS: Methods of Air Analysis. Griffin, London, 1920

49. Scholander PF: Analyser for accurate estimation of respiratory gases in one-half cubic centimetre samples. J Biol Chem 167:235-250, 1947

50. Scurr C, Feldman S: Scientific Foundations of Anaesthesia. Year Book Medical Publishers Inc., Chicago, 1974, pp. 85-97

51. Van Slyke DP, Neill JM: The determination of gases in blood and other solutions by vacuum extraction and manometric measurement. J Biol Chem 61:523-573, 1924

52. Pauling L, Wood RE, Studivant JH: An instrument for determining the partial pressure of oxygen in a gas. J Am Chem Soc 68:796-798, 1946

53. Wilson RS, Laver MB: Oxygen analysis: advances in methodology. Anesthesiology 37:112-126, 1972

54. Westenkow DR, Jordan WS, Jordan RB, et al: Evaluation of oxygen monitors for clinical use. Anesthesiology 53:S382, 1980

55. Westenkow DR, Jordan WS, Jordan RB, et al: Evaluation of oxygen monitors for use during anesthesia. Anesth Analg (Cleve) 60:53-56, 1981

56. Piernan S, Roizen MF, Severinghaus JW: Oxygen analyzer dangerous—senses nitrous oxide as battery fails. Anesthesiology 50:146-149, 1979

57. Mazza N, Wald A: Failure of battery-operated alarms. Anesthesiology 53:246-248, 1980

58. Klick JM, duMoulin GC: An oxygen analyzer as a source of *Pseudomonas*. Anesthesiology 49:293-294, 1978

59. Sarnquist FH, Todd C, Whitcher C: Accuracy of a new noninvasive oxygen saturation monitor. Anesthesiology 53:S163, 1980

60. Whitcher C, Flynn M: Use of a digital oximeter in resident training. Anesthesiology 53:S355, 1980

61. Sergejev IP: Monitoring of respiratory function during anesthesia. Int Anesthesiol Clin 19:31-60, 1981

62. Patel KP, Vonus B, Pratap KS, Konchigeri

HN: Cutaneous Po_2 monitoring during pediatric cardiac surgery. Anesthesiology 53:S343, 1980

63. Gothgen I, Jacobsen E: Transcutaneous oxygen tension measurement II. The influence of halothane and hypotension. Acta Anaesthesiol Scand, [Suppl] 67, 71-75, 1978

64. Lane GL, Samra SK, Tait AR, et al: How reliable is transcutaneous Po_2 during anesthesia? Anesthesiology 53:S329, 1980

65. Whitesell RC, Saeed Dhamee M, Munchi C: Transcutaneous Po_2 monitoring in adults. Anesthesiology 53:S372, 1980

66. Cooper JB, Newbower RS, Long CD, et al: Preventable anesthesia mishaps: A study of human factors. Anesthesiology 49:399-406, 1978

67. Emergency Care Research Institute: Anesthesia ventilators: health devices 8:151-164, 1979

68. McEwen JA, Small CF, Saunders BA, et al: Hazards associated with the use of disconnect monitors. Anesthesiology 53:S391, 1980

69. Sodal FE, Swansen GD: Mass spectrometry: current technology and implications for anesthesia, pp 167-182. In Aldrete JA, Lowe HJ, Virtue RW, Eds.: Low Flow and Closed System Anesthesia, Grune & Stratton, New York, 1979

70. Frazier WT, Paulsen AW, Odom SH: Evaluation of a multi-patient mass-spectrometer for monitoring during anesthesia. International Congress Series no. 538. Anaesthesiology, 599-601, 1980

71. Weingarten M: Synoposis of the application of the mass spectrometer to the practice of anesthesia. Low Flow and Closed System Anesthesia, Aldrete JA, Lowe HJ, Virue RW, Eds. Grune & Stratton, New York, 1979, pp 183–191

72. Operating Instructions, Puritan-Bennett/Datex CO_2 monitor and recorder.

73. Ohlson KB, Westenskow DR, Jordan WS: Feedback control of ventilation using expired CO_2. Anesthesiology 53:S387, 1980

74. Zauder HL: Medical jargon—a few lines about "lines." Anesthesiology 53:271, 1980

75. Frank O: Kritik der elastischen Manometer: Z Biol 44:445-613, 1903

76. Lambert EH, Wood EH: The use of a resistance wire strain gauge manometer to measure intra-arterial pressure. Proc Soc Exp Biol Med 64:186-190, 1947

77. Shinozaki T, Deane RS, Mazuzan JE: The dynamic responses of liquid-filled catheter systems for direct measurements of blood pressure. Anesthesiology 53:498-504, 1980

78. Gardner RM: Direct blood pressure measurement-dynamic response requirements. Anesthesiology 54:227-236, 1981

79. Prys-Roberts C, Meloche R: Management of anesthesia in patients with hypertension or ischemic heart disease. Int. Anesth Clin 19:181-217, 1980

80. Miller MG, Hedley-White J: Intra-arterial monitoring: a routine and safe procedure, pp 257-265. In Eckenhoff JE, Ed. Controversy in Anesthesiology. W. B. Saunders Co., Philadelphia, 1979

81. Bedford RF, Wollman H: Complications of percutaneous radial artery cannulation: an objective prospective study in man. Anesthesiology 38:228-236, 1973

82. Bedford RF: Long-term radial artery cannulation: effects on subsequent vessel function. Crit Care Med 6:64-67, 1978

83. Davis FM, Stewart JM: Radial artery cannulation: a prospective study in patients undergoing cardiothoracic surgery. Br J Anaesth 52:41-47, 1980

84. Downs JB, Rackstein AD, Klein EF, Jr, et al: Hazards of radial-artery catheterization. Anesthesiology 38:283, 1973

85. Bedford RF: Radial artery function following percutaneous cannulation with 18 and 20 gauge catheters. Anesthesiology 47:37-39, 1977

86. Allen EV: Thromboangitis obliterans: methods of diagnosis of chronic occlusive arterial lesions distal to the wrist with illustrative cases. Am J Med Sci 178:237-244, 1929

87. Peters KR, Chapin JW: Allen's test—positive or negative? Anesthesiology 53:85, 1980

88. Messick JM; Allen's test—neither positive nor negative. Anesthesiology 54:523, 1981

89. Ryan J, Raines J, Dalton BC et al: Arterial dynamics of radial artery cannulation. Anesth Analg (Cleve) 52:1017-1023, 1973

90. Bedford RF: Wrist circumference predicts the use of radial arterial occlusions after cannulation: Anesthesiology 48:377-378, 1978

91. Bedford RF: Removal of radial artery thrombi following percutaneous cannulation for monitoring. Anesthesiology 46:430-432, 1977

92. Schlossman D: Thrombogenic properties of vascular catheter materials in vivo. Acta Radiol [Diagn] (Stockh) 14:186-192, 1973

93. Blitt CD: Invasive monitoring techniques and indications. Presented at Bay-Cap V: Evaluation of the cardiac patient, Houston, Texas, November 14, 1980

94. Jacoby J: Intra-arterial monitoring is not a routine procedure, pp. 266-274. In Eckenhoff, JE, Ed.: Controversy in Anesthesiology. W. B. Saunders Co., Philadelphia, 1979

95. Lowenstein E, Little JW, Lo HH: Prevention of cerebral embolization from flushing radial-arterial cannulas. N Engl J Med 285:1414-1415, 1971

96. Marshall G, Edelstein G, Hirshman CA: Median nerve compression following radial arterial puncture. Anesth Analg (Cleve) 59:953-954, 1980

97. Jones RM, Hill AB, Nahrwold ML et al: A comparison of methods of radial artery cannulations. Anesthesiology 53:S207, 1980

98. Shapiro BA, Harrison RA, Walton JR: Clinical Application of Blood Gases. 2nd Ed. Year Book Medical Publishers, Chicago, 1977

99. Kaplan JA: Hemodynamic Monitoring, pp 71-115. In Kaplan JA Ed.: Cardiac Anesthesia. Grune & Stratton, New York, 1979

100. Risk C, Rudo N, Falltrick R et al: Comparison of right atrial and pulmonary capillary wedge pressures. Crit Care Med 6:172-175, 1978

101. Katz JD, Cronau LM, Barash PG et al: Pulmonary artery flow-guided catheters in the perioperative period: indications and complications. JAMA 237:2832-2834, 1977

102. Geha DG, Davis NJ, Lappas DG: Persistent atrial arrhythmias associated with placement of a Swan-Ganz catheter. Anesthesiology 39:651-653, 1973

103. Pace NL: A critique of flow-directed pulmonary artery catheterization. Anesthesiology 47:455-465, 1977

104. Humphrey CB, Oury JH, Virgilio RW et al: An analysis of direct and indirect measurement of left atrial filling pressures. J Thorac Cardiovasc Surg 41:643-647, 1976

105. Lappas D, Lell WA, Gabel JC et al: Indirect measurement of left atrial pressure in surgical patients—pulmonary capillary wedge pressure and pulmonary artery diastolic pressure compared with left atrial pressure. Anesthesiology 38:394-397, 1973

106. Benumof JL, Saidman LJ, Arkin DB, et al: Where pulmonary arterial catheters go: intrathoracic distribution. Anesthesiology 48:336-338, 1977

107. Kronberg GM, Quan SF, Schlobohm RM et al: Anatomic locations of the tips of pulmonary-artery catheters in supine patients. Anesthesiology 51:467-469, 1979

108. Kopman EA, Sandza JG: Manipulation of the pulmonary-artery catheter after placement: maintenance of sterility. Anesthesiology 48:373-374, 1978

109. Geer RT: Interpretation of pulmonary-artery wedge pressure when PEEP is used. Anesthesiology 46:383-384, 1977

110. Lozman J, Powers SR, Older T et al: Correlation of pulmonary wedge and left atrial pressures. Arch Surg 109:270-277, 1974

111. Roy R, Powers SR, Feustel PJ, et al: Pulmonary wedge catheterization during positive end-expiratory pressure ventilation in the dog. Anesthesiology 46:385-390, 1971

112. West JB: Respiratory Physiology: the essentials. 2nd Ed. Williams & Wilkins, Baltimore, 1979. p. 43

113. Kane PB, Askanazi J, Neville JF et al: Artifacts in the measurement of pulmonary artery wedge pressure. Crit Care Med 6:36-38, 1978

114. Berryhill RE, Benumof JL, Rauscher LA: Pulmonary vascular pressure reading at the end of exhalation. Anesthesiology 49:365-368, 1978

115. Civetta JM: Measurements in assessing circulatory function, pp 73-80. In Hershey SG, Ed.: Refresher Courses in Anesthesiology. Vol. 3. JB Lippincott, Philadelphia. 1975

116. McLoud TC, Barash PG, Ravin CE, et al: Elevation of pulmonary artery pressure as a sign of pulmonary barotrauma (pneumothorax). Crit Care Med 6:81-84, 1978

117. Bedford RF: "Invasive monitoring—complication" presented at Bay-Cap V: Evaluation of the cardiac patients, Houston, Texas, Nov 14, 1980

118. Waller JL, Zaidan JR, Kaplan JA, et al: Hemodynamic responses to preoperative vascular cannulation in patients with coronary artery disease. Anesthesiology 56:219-221, 1982

119. Quintin L, Walley DG, Wynands JE et al: The effect of vascular catheterization upon heart rate and blood pressure before aorto-coronary bypass surgery. Can Anaesth Soc J 28:244-248, 1981

120. Taylor SH: Measurement of the cardiac output in man. Proc R Soc Med 59: Suppl: 35, 1966

121. Kohanna FH, Cunningham JN: Monitoring of cardiac output by thermodilution after open heart surgery. J. Thorac Cardiovasc Surg 73:451-457, 1977

122. Bredgaard Sørenson M, Bille-brahe NE, Engell HC: Cardiac output measurement by thermal dilution: reproducibility and comparison with the dye-dilution technique. Ann Surg 183:67-72, 1976

123. Weisel RD, Berger RL, Hectman HB: Measurement of cardiac output by thermodilution. N Engl J Med 292:682-684, 1975

124. Rahimtoola SH, Swan HJC: Calculation of cardiac output from indicator dilution curves in the presence of mitral regurgitation. Circulation 31:711-718, 1965

125. Armstrong RF, Moxham J, Cohen SL, et al: Intravascular mixed venous oxygen tension monitoring—an analysis of electrode performance in 100 patients. Br J Anaesth 53:89-96, 1981

126. Waller JL, Kaplan JA, Bauman DI, et al: Clinical evaluation of a new fiberoptic catheter oximeter. Anesthesiology 55:A133, 1981

127. Zaidan JR: Experience with the pacing pulmonary artery catheter. Anesthesiology 53:S118, 1980

128. Carlon GC, Kahn RC, Ray C, et al: Evaluation of an "in vivo" Pao_2 and $Paco_2$ monitor in the management of respiratory failure. Crit Care Med 8:410-413, 1980

129. Hall JR, Poulton TJ, Downs JB et al: In vivo blood gas analysis: an evaluation. Crit Care Med 8:414-417, 1980

PART III.

CARDIOPULMONARY PHYSIOLOGY

Jonathan L. Benumof, M.D.

7
The Pulmonary Circulation

Knowledge of all aspects of the pulmonary circulation is important for the rational and intelligent administration of anesthesia for thoracic surgery. Appreciation of the functional anatomy of the pulmonary macro- and microcirculations is necessary in order to understand the impact of lung manipulations and surgical events on the well-being of the patient. An understanding of pulmonary vascular physiology is essential for the maintenance of hemodynamic and gas-exchange stability during the administration of any kind of anesthesia, but this is particularly true for the safe conduct of one-lung anesthesia. Because manipulations and handling of pulmonary vessels are involved, knowledge of pulmonary vascular reflexes is desirable. Awareness of the pharmacologic, metabolic, and other special functions of the pulmonary circulation is generally important for the safe management of a patient through the perioperative period, but it is especially important in patients who have biogenically active secretory lung tumors and who are receiving medications preoperatively which may have potentially harmful intraoperative anesthetic interaction implications. The final common pathway for expression of severe disease or malfunction of the pulmonary circulation consists of pulmonary hypertension and an increased pulmonary resistance. An awareness of the differential diagnosis of pulmonary hypertension, which is based on all the above considerations, is essential for swift recognition and treatment of the underlying cause(s). This chapter therefore discusses all these aspects and characteristics of the pulmonary circulation and generally does so in the order presented above.

FUNCTIONAL ANATOMY

The Pulmonary Macrocirculations

THE PULMONARY CIRCULATION[1]

The pulmonary artery and mainstem bronchus of each lung are next to one another as they enter the parenchyma of the lung. After entering the lung parenchyma, both the bronchi and arteries run within a connective tissue sheath, formed by an invagination of the pleura at the hilum and ending at the level of the bronchioles (Fig. 7-1). A potential perivascular (and peribronchial) space exists between the arteries (and the bronchi) and the connective tissue sheath

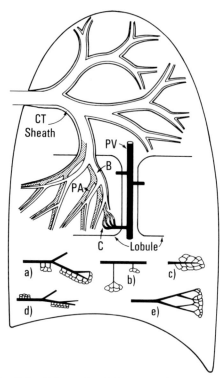

Fig. 7-1 Schematic of the general arrangement of the perivascular and peribronchial connective tissue (CT) sheath, the pulmonary arteries (PA), the pulmonary capillaries (C), the pulmonary veins (PV), and the bronchi (B). Five types of capillary network arrangements (*a* through *e*) are shown. See text for full explanation.

in much the same way as a potential pleural space lies between the two layers of the pleura. Lymphatics also run in the sheath and are therefore exposed to arterial pulsations, which, in conjunction with lymph valves, help to propel lymph proximally towards the hilum (see below). Distal to the bronchiolar level of pleural tissue penetration, both the arteries and bronchi are attached directly to the lung substance.

The negative pressure in the pulmonary tissues and the structural properties of the tissue surrounding the perivascular connective tissue sheath exert a radial traction force on the sheath. The radial traction is transmitted to the bronchi and arteries, tending to hold them open and increase their diame-

ters.[2] In the presence of pulmonary edema, fluid accumulates in the perivascular space, thereby partially isolating the artery from the bronchi. The diameter of the artery decreases, with a consequent rise in vascular resistance at that level. Because the arterial tree is elastic and filled with fluid under pressure, it physically helps to support the shape of the lung.

The main bronchus enters the lung hilum and by a series of dichotomous divisions gives rise to about 25,000 terminal bronchioles, each of which supplies an acinus. At each division the diameters of the bronchi decrease but at a rate which is less than the increase in the numbers of bronchi, so that the summed cross-sectional area at any given level increases down the bronchial tree (and therefore airway resistance decreases down the bronchial tree). Within the acinus, further dichotomous division continues down to and including the first generation of alveolar ducts, but thereafter branching is more profuse and irregular. Reduction of diameter at each division is less than before so that there is a very rapid increase in summed cross-sectional area with respect to distance down the acinus.

The pulmonary artery branches in similar fashion to and follows very closely the bronchial tree. Within the acinus, the pulmonary artery is applied closely to the respiratory bronchioles along their nonalveolated sides. This anatomical arrangement has an important functional consequence; it has been shown that blood may actually become oxygenated in small pulmonary arteries owing to the ability of oxygen to diffuse directly across the small distance between the contiguous air spaces and vessels.[3] This direct access which gas in the airways has to small arteries makes possible a very rapid and localized vascular response to changes in gas composition. Thus, a decreased PO_2 and increased PCO_2 in the airways due to regional hypoventilation can produce localized vasoconstriction and normalization of the local alveolar ventilation/perfusion (V_A/Q)

ratio. Conversely, the possibility exists that chemical or humoral substances, carried in the pulmonary arterial blood or produced in the vessel wall per se, can reach the adjoining bronchus directly and cause localized bronchoconstriction.[3]

The pulmonary artery finally gives rise to precapillary branches of variable length (Fig. 7-1), which then break up into capillary nets which course over the rounded surface of the alveoli. As in the bronchial tree, arterial branches decrease in diameter at each dichotomy down to the pericapillary branches, while the summed cross-sectional area increases. Although the two trees are similar, the arteries branch somewhat more profusely than the bronchi, especially peripherally, where they give off branches to supply alveoli on respiratory bronchioles as well as immediately adjacent alveoli of neighboring acini.

Figure 7-1 shows the various modes of origin of the capillary nets. Arrangement *a* is by far most common, where short pericapillary vessels arise at right angles from larger branches; in *b* the precapillary vessels may be long or short; in *c* arteries sometimes may terminate by breaking up abruptly into capillary loops or, as in *e*, may merge imperceptibly into the capillary network; and in *d* capillaries may arise directly from the sides of surprisingly large arteries. The functional anatomy of the pulmonary microcirculation (capillaries) will be discussed below in detail.

The pulmonary veins arise from capillaries at alveolar duct junctions, as well as on respiratory bronchioles, on the pleura, and in connective tissue septae. Those veins which start within the acinus course centrifugally to the periphery of the lobule. There they join at right angles veins running between the lobules (Fig. 7-1). The interlobular veins are therefore situated away from the conducting airways and arteries. Unlike arteries, veins do not have a perivascular space, so that veins within the lung are connected directly to the lung substance and are held open by elastic forces. The veins only come together

with the arteries and airways as these three structures approach the hilum. Casts of arteries and veins show that the venous system has a larger volume than the arterial system (ratio 2:1) and at any given level has a larger cross-sectional area. The larger cross-sectional area of the veins results in a very low resistance system, which can still function with the low driving pressure available. Under experimental conditions the extra-alveolar pulmonary veins can actually be observed changing in volume with each heartbeat, taking up temporary differences between the outputs of the right and left ventricles.

THE BRONCHIAL CIRCULATION[4]

In the adult, the bronchial arteries arise from one or two aortic trunks. There may also be supplementary or accessory bronchial arteries, which are derived from the subclavian, upper intercostal, internal mammary, and diaphragmatic arteries or the abdominal aorta. Discrete bronchial arterial branches can be identified as far as third-, fourth-, or fifth-order bronchi and then they form a peribronchial network which extends to the periphery of the lobule. Throughout their course the bronchial arteries give off the vasa vasorum of the pulmonary arteries.

The bronchial veins form two distinct systems. The superficial bronchial veins drain the main and lobar bronchi and empty into the azygos vein on the right side and the hemiazygos and mediastinal veins on the left side. The deep bronchial veins drain segmental and distal bronchi and empty into pulmonary veins.

The bronchial circulation undergoes brisk local development with new vessel formation in certain pulmonary and bronchial disease conditions. These conditions include prolonged infections, cavitation, neoplastic vessel growth, and atelectasis of the lung. The proliferation of the bronchial circulation under the above-mentioned pathological conditions is often responsible for repeated,

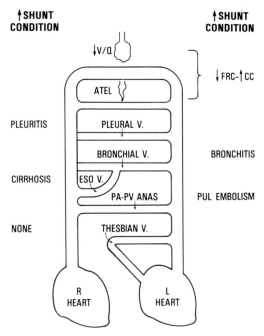

SHUNT CONDITION

↓V/Q

ATEL

PLEURITIS — PLEURAL V.

BRONCHIAL V.

CIRRHOSIS — ESO V.

PA-PV ANAS

NONE — THESBIAN V.

R HEART   L HEART

SHUNT CONDITION

↓FRC-↑CC

BRONCHITIS

PUL EMBOLISM

Fig. 7-2 Pulmonary shunt pathways. Schematic representation of all possible right (R) heart to left (L) heart shunt pathways and the pathological conditions during which these shunt pathways are increased. The bronchial and pleural arteries do not arise from the right heart outlet but rather from systemic arteries; therefore, the corresponding bronchial and pleural veins, which empty into the pulmonary veins, contain desaturated blood. V/Q = ventilation to perfusion ratio; ATEL = atelectasis; FRC = functional residual capacity; CC = closing capacity; V = vein; ESO = esophageal; PA = pulmonary artery; PV = pulmonary vein; ANAS = anastomosis; PUL = pulmonary.

sometimes serious episodes of hemoptysis. Connections between the pulmonary and bronchial arteries have been demonstrated in man and guinea pigs. Pulmonary artery to bronchial artery, capillary to capillary, and vein to vein, as well as bronchial artery to pulmonary vein connections exist. Thus, almost any part of the lung may potentially be supplied by blood from either artery and be drained by either set of veins. The bronchial artery to pulmonary vein connections are very important, particularly in such lesions as pulmonary stenosis and pul-

monary embolism. Under these two circumstances, bronchial collateral supply of tissues distal to blocked arteries helps to maintain a normal VA/Q ratio. However, even though the bronchial circulation may participate in this way in gas exchange, it is still composed of systemic vessels which vasodilate when exposed to hypoxia and are therefore incapable of local active pulmonary autoregulation (see hypoxic pulmonary vasoconstriction).[5]

OTHER RIGHT-TO-LEFT CIRCULATIONS

Figure 7-2 shows all the possible pathways for blood to travel from the right heart to the left heart and the pathologic (increased shunt) conditions during which blood flow through these pathways is significantly increased. Increased blood flow through poorly ventilated alveoli (low V/Q regions at FIO_2 < 30 percent) has a right-to-left shunt effect on oxygenation, and increased blood flow through nonventilated alveoli (atelectatic or consolidated regions at all FIO_2) is a source of true right-to-left shunt. Low V/Q and atelectatic lung units occur in conditions in which the functional residual capacity (FRC) is less than the closing capacity (CC) of the lung.*

There are several right-to-left heart vascular pathways that do not pass by or involve alveoli at all. The bronchial and pleural circulations originate from systemic arteries

---

* Complete description of the FRC-CC relationship is beyond the scope of this chapter; but, in brief, FRC equals the volume of lung that exists at the end of exhalation, and CC equals the volume of lung at which some airways start to close. When FRC is greater than CC, then no airways are closed at any time during tidal breathing, and this is a normal FRC-CC relationship (Fig. 7-3). When FRC is less than CC but CC is within tidal ventilation, then some airways are closed for part of tidal ventilation; they have less chance to participate in fresh gas exchange and they therefore function as low V/Q units. When FRC is less than CC but CC is greater than the whole of tidal ventilation, then some airways are closed all the time and they are therefore atelectatic.[6]

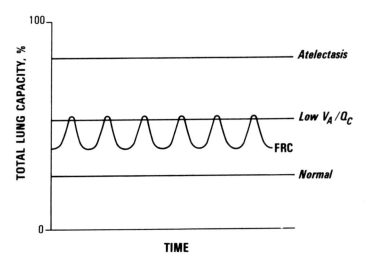

Fig. 7-3 Schematic representation of the various possible relationships between functional residual capacity (FRC) and closing capacity (CC). The sine wave depicts a patient breathing at approximately 40 percent of total lung capacity. A normal FRC-CC relationship exists when FRC > CC. Atelectasis is present when CC > FRC during the whole of tidal ventilation. A low ventilation/perfusion relationship (VA/Q) exists when CC > FRC but CC occurs within the tidal ventilation.

and empty into the left side of the heart without being oxygenated, constituting the 1 to 3 percent true right-to-left shunt normally present. With chronic bronchitis, the bronchial circulation may carry 10 percent of the cardiac output, and with pleuritis the pleural circulation may carry 5 percent of the cardiac output. Consequently, there may be as much as a 10 percent and 5 percent obligatory right-to-left shunt present, respectively, under these conditions. Intrapulmonary arteriovenous anastomoses are normally closed, but in the face of acute pulmonary hypertension such as may be caused by a pulmonary embolus, they may open and cause a direct increase in right-to-left shunt. Esophageal to mediastinal to bronchial to pulmonary vein pathways have been described and may explain in part the hypoxemia associated with portal hypertension and cirrhosis. There are no known conditions which selectively increase Thesbian channel blood flow (Thesbian vessels nourish the left heart myocardium and originate and empty into the left heart).

Pulmonary Microcirculation

SHEET FLOW

The pulmonary capillaries arise at right angles from the pulmonary arterioles. Classical anatomists have described the geometry of the pulmonary capillaries in terms of long branching tunnels (Fig. 7-4A).[7] However, and more realistically, the capillaries really spread out over the alveolar surface in a complex, interconnecting pattern, which is confined to or contained within the two dimensions of the alveolar surface plane (Fig. 7-4B).[7] In such a plane view, the capillaries may occupy up to half the surface of an alveolar wall and expose to the alveolar gas an enormous capillary surface area for gas exchange. Because of the above anatomical characteristics, the geometry of the pulmonary capillaries has been likened to the appearance of an underground parking garage as viewed from within the garage (Fig. 7-5).[7] The top and bottom of the garage are flat endothelial surfaces, which are held together

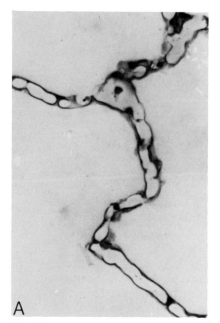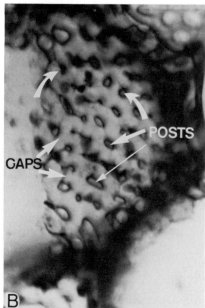

Fig. 7-4 (A) A classical histologic view of a pulmonary capillary surrounded on each side by an alveolus, the capillary appearing as a long, branching tunnel. (B) A histologic view that was cut tangential to the rounded surface of an alveolus shows that the pulmonary capillaries (CAPS) spread out in a complex, interconnecting pattern. Individual capillaries divide and meet around connective tissue posts, which join the two possible endothelial plates together. See text for full explanation. Reproduced with permission from Fung YC: The microcirculation as seen by a red cell. Microvasc. Res. 10:246-264, 1975.

and supported by columns or "posts" of connective tissue. An alveolus is on the other side of each of the endothelial surfaces. The connective tissue columns between the endothelial plates have been called posts because of their structural support function, as well as "struts" because they require one alveolus on one side of the capillary to expand if the other alveolus on the other side of the capillary collapses. The connective tissue posts occupy the circular clear spaces between the interlacing capillary network seen in Fig. 7-4B.

The endothelial surfaces form the boundaries of the two-dimensional capillary, and blood flow through this two-dimensional world has been called *sheet flow.*[8] In this model, red blood cells must wind their way through, in, and amongst the posts, much as

a car would negotiate the garage in bumper-to-bumper traffic. The sheet flow theory of the pulmonary microcirculation is consistent with experimental data and, in brief, disassociates resistance from flow as these two terms are normally related by Poiseuille's formula for fluid dynamics in a cylinder.[8] The precise flow pattern from post to post has been modeled as a function of the perfusion pressure.[9]

FLUID EXCHANGE

A cross-section through any capillary channel shown in Figure 7-4 would reveal a vascular channel lined by endothelium which usually contained one, or at most two or three, red blood cells (Fig. 7-6).[10] A summary schematic of the ultrastructural appearance of the capillary wall shown in Fig-

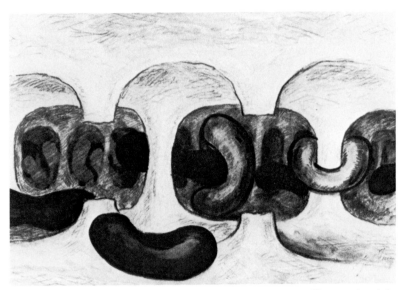

Fig. 7-5 Imaginary view of the inside of a pulmonary capillary as it might appear to a red blood cell. The view is similar to that seen when one stands inside a modern underground parking garage. Endothelial plates form the top and bottom of the garage and the plates are held together and supported by connective tissue columns or "posts." On the other side of each of the endothelial surfaces would be an alveolus, which is not shown. Reproduced with permission from Fung YC: The microcirculation as seen by a red cell. Microvasc. Res. 10:246-264, 1975.

ure 7-6 and constructed from other examples from Szidon et al is shown in Figure 7-7.[11, 12] Capillary blood is separated from alveolar gas by a series of anatomic layers: capillary endothelium, endothelial basement membrane, interstitial space, epithelial basement membrane, and alveolar epithelium. On one side of the alveolar septum [the thick, fluid- and gas-exchanging side (upper side in Fig. 7-7)], the epithelial and endothelial basement membranes are separated by an interstitial space of variable thickness containing connective tissue fibrils, elastic fibers, fibroblasts, and macrophages. The opposite side [the thin, gas-exchanging side (lower side in Fig. 7-7)] contains only fused epithelial and endothelial basement membranes. Between individual endothelial and epithelial cells are holes (slits or junctions) that provide a potential pathway for fluid to move from the intravascular space to the interstitial space

and finally from the interstitial space to the alveolar space. The endothelial junctions are 5 times the width of the epithelial junctions, and, therefore, the former are referred to as "loose" and the latter as "tight." Pulmonary capillary permeability (K) is a direct function of the size of the holes in the endothelial and epithelial linings.

It has been estimated that, in man, alveolar blood vessels (primarily capillaries) have a luminal surface area on the order of 80 m[2].[13] However, these early calculations of surface area assumed a more or less regular rounded shape of capillaries having smooth luminal surfaces. It is now evident that the capillary surfaces are not smooth but are covered with irregular complex projections (Fig. 7-8).[14] The projections are approximately 300 nm in diameter and may reach 3,000 nm in length. Some projections come to blunt ends, while others bud, branch, or

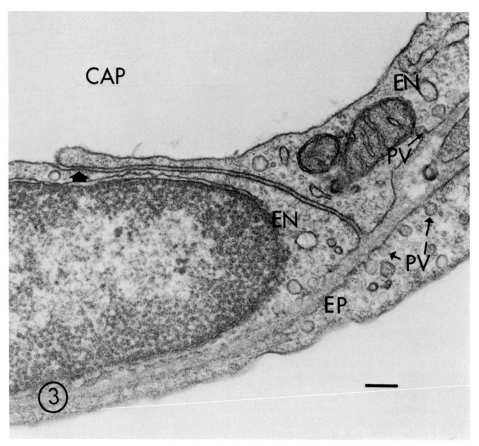

Fig. 7-6   Electron photomicrograph of an alveolar capillary membrane. EN = endothelium; EP = epithelium; CAP = capillary; dark arrow points to endothelial cell junction; PV = plasmalemmal vesicles. (Pietra GG: The basis of pulmonary edema with emphasis on ultrastructure. pp 215-234. In: The Lung: IAP Monograph No. 19. © 1978 The Williams & Wilkins Co., Baltimore.)

reflect back on the main body of the cell. The size and density of the endothelial projection meshwork is such that an eddy flow of cell-free plasma occurs along the endothelial lining cell.[15] This feature has extremely important implications for the exchange of metabolites between endothelium and blood (see Pharmacology section below).[15] The endothelial cells also contain a large population of plasmalemmal (pinocytotic) vesicles (Figs. 7-6 and 7-8), many of which communicate freely with the vascular lumen (see figures in Pietra, Reference 10 and Szidon et al, Reference 11). These endothelial vesicles and cavities function both as mass carriers of fluid

and solutes across the endothelium and as generators of transendothelial channels by fusion and fission with each other and with both endothelial domains (vascular and tissular). Therefore, owing to the presence of endothelial vesicles and the endothelial projections into the lumen of the capillary, it would appear that the true surface area of capillary endothelial cells (at least for metabolism) is much larger than previously estimated.

The pericapillary interstitial space is continuous with the interstitial tissue space that surrounds terminal bronchioles and vessels. There are no lymphatics in the intersti-

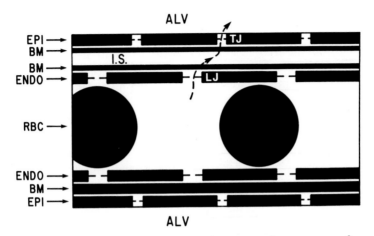

Fig. 7.7 Schematic summary of the ultrastructural appearance of a pulmonary capillary. RBC = red blood cell; ENDO = endothelium; BM = basement membrane; IS = interstitial space; EPI = epithelium; LF = loose junction; TJ = tight junction; ALV = alveolus. The upper side of the capillary has the endothelial and epithelial basement membranes separated by an interstitial space, whereas the lower side of the capillary contains only fused endothelial and epithelial basement membranes. The arrows indicate a potential pathway for fluid to move from the intravascular space to the interstitial space and from the interstitial space to the alveolar space. (Modified with permission from Fishman AP: Pulmonary edema: the water-exchanging function of the lung. Circulation 46:390-408, 1972. By permission of the American Heart Association, Inc.)

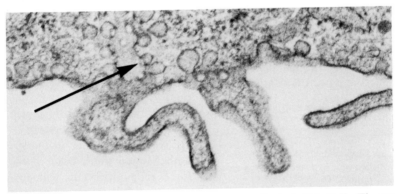

Fig. 7-8 Heath D, Smith P: The Pulmonary Endothelial Cell. Thorax 34:200–208, 1979.

tial space of the alveolar septum. Instead, lymphatic capillaries first appear in the interstitial space surrounding terminal bronchioles and small arteries. Interstitial fluid is normally removed from the alveolar interstitial space into the lymphatics by a "sump" (pressure gradient) mechanism, which is caused by the presence of a more negative pressure surrounding the larger arteries and bronchi.[16, 17] The sump mechanism is aided by the presence of valves in the lymph vessels as well as by the massaging action of the nearby arterial pulsations. When formation of interstitial fluid is excessive and the fluid cannot be cleared adequately by the lymphatics, it will accumulate in the perialveolar space and the interstitial connective tissue compartment around the large vessels and airways, forming peribronchial and periarteriolar edema fluid cuffs.* Subsequently, with increased driving force, fluid will cross the relatively impermeable epithelial wall, and the alveolar space will fill.

The hemodynamic forces that govern net transcapillary fluid movement are as follows. The net transcapillary flow of fluid (F) out of pulmonary capillaries is equal to the difference between pulmonary capillary hydrostatic pressure (P_{inside}) and the interstitial fluid hydrostatic pressure ($P_{outside}$); and to the difference between the capillary colloid osmotic pressure (π_{inside}) and the interstitial colloid osmotic pressure ($\pi_{outside}$). These four forces will produce a steady-state fluid flow (F) while a constant capillary permeability (K) obtains, according to the relationship:

$$F = K[P_{inside} - P_{outside}) - (\pi_{inside} - \pi_{outside})]$$

K is a capillary filtration coefficient expressed in ml/min per mmHg per 100 g. The filtration coefficient is the product of the effective capillary surface area in a given mass of tissue and the permeability per unit surface area of the capillary wall to filter the fluid. Under normal circumstances and at a vertical height in the lung that is at the junction of zones 2 and 3, the intravascular colloid osmotic pressure (about 26 mmHg) acts to keep water in the capillary lumen, and, working against this force, the intravascular hydrostatic pressure (about 10 mmHg) acts to force water across the loose endothelial junctions into the interstitial space. If these forces were the only ones operative, the interstitial space and, consequently, the alveolar surfaces would constantly be dry and there would be no lymph flow. In fact, the alveolar surfaces are moist, and lymphatic flow from the interstitial compartment is constant (approximately 500 ml/day). This can be explained in part by the $\pi_{outside}$ (8 mmHg) and in part by the studies that indicate that interstitial $P_{outside}$ is uniquely negative (8 mmHg) and thereby promotes, by suction, a slow loss of fluid across the endothelial holes.[21] Relative to the vertical level of the zone 2–zone 3 junction, as lung height decreases (lung dependency), absolute P_{inside} increases and fluid has a propensity to transudate, and as lung height increases (lung nondependency), absolute P_{inside} decreases and fluid has a propensity to be reabsorbed. However, fluid transudation induced by an increase in P_{inside} is limited by a concomitant dilution of proteins in the interstitial space and therefore a decrease in $\pi_{outside}$.[22] Any change in the size of the endothelial junctions, even if the above four forces remain constant, will change the magnitude and perhaps even the direction of fluid movement; increased size of endothelial junctions (increased permeability) promotes transudation, and decreased size of endothelial junctions (decreased permeability) promotes reabsorption.

---

* There is now good evidence which indicates that one of the mechanisms of hypoxemia during pulmonary edema is as follows. The perialveolar interstitial edema compresses alveoli and acutely reduces FRC. The peribronchial edema fluid cuffs compress bronchi and acutely increase closing capacity (CC).[18–20] The decreased FRC and increased CC must create areas of low V_A/Q or atelectasis (see previous footnote and Fig. 7-3). Intra-alveolar edema fluid will additionally cause alveolar collapse and atelectasis.

PULMONARY VASCULAR PHYSIOLOGY: DETERMINANTS OF VASCULAR RESISTANCE AND BLOOD FLOW DISTRIBUTION

Gravity[23-26]

The contraction of the right ventricle imparts kinetic energy to the blood in the main pulmonary artery. As some of the kinetic energy in the main pulmonary artery is dissipated in overcoming the downward pull of gravity, the absolute pressure in the pulmonary artery (Ppa) (absolute pressure = intraluminal pressure relative to atmospheric) decreases by 1 cm H_2O per centimeter of vertical distance up the lung (Fig. 7-9). At some vertical level absolute Ppa becomes zero (atmospheric), and still higher in the lung the absolute Ppa becomes negative (less than atmospheric). In this region of the lung, alveolar pressure (PA) exceeds Ppa and pulmonary venous pressure (Ppv) (which is very negative at this vertical height), causing collapse of the pulmonary vessels and cessation of blood flow (zone 1) (Fig. 7-9). Thus, zone 1 conditions are present whenever PA exceeds Ppa and Ppv (PA > Ppa > Ppv).

Descending to a lower vertical level in the lung, absolute Ppa will become positive at some point and blood flow will begin when Ppa exceeds PA (zone 2). Thus, zone 2 conditions are present whenever Ppa exceeds PA but PA exceeds Ppv (Ppa > PA > Ppv). Consequently, the amount of blood flow in zone 2 is determined by the Ppa − PA difference rather than by the more conventional Ppa − Ppv difference (see below). Since instantaneous Ppa and PA change dynamically during the cardiac and respiratory cycles, blood flow at any actual point or vertical level within zone 2 may be intermittent and will depend precisely on the phase relationships between cardiac systole and diastole and respiratory systole and diastole. Several names have been applied to the phenomenon of intermittent zone 2 blood flow, including the *waterfall*, *weir*, and *Starling resistor* phenomena and the *sluice effect*. However, since mean Ppa increases linearly down this region of the lung but mean PA remains constant, the driving pressure (Ppa − PA) increases linearly and therefore blood flow increases linearly.

Still lower down in the lung there is a vertical level where absolute Ppv becomes positive and also exceeds PA (zone 3). Thus, zone 3 conditions are present whenever both Ppa and Ppv exceed PA (Ppa > Ppv > PA). Consequently, the amount of blood flow in zone 3 is governed by the pulmonary arteriovenous pressure difference (Ppa − Ppv), and, in this zone the capillary systems are permanently open and blood flow is continuous. Descending zone 3 causes both absolute Ppa and Ppv to increase at the same rate so that the perfusion pressure (Ppa − Ppv) is unchanged. However, the pressure immediately outside the vessels, namely pleural pressure (Ppl), increases at a slower rate than the absolute vascular pressure, so that the transmural distending pressures (Ppa − Ppl and Ppv − Ppl) (transmural pressure = intraluminal pressure relative to pleural pressure) increase down zone 3, the vessel radii increase, vascular resistance decreases, and blood flow therefore further increases.[27]

Finally, whenever absolute Ppv is very high, as it would be in mitral stenosis or a region of the lung which was extremely dependent or below the vertical level of the left atrium, fluid may transudate out of the pulmonary capillaries and veins into the pulmonary interstitial compartment (see balance of forces across the capillary endothelial junctions in section above). The transudated pulmonary interstitial fluid fills the pulmonary interstitial space and may eliminate the normally present negative and radially expanding interstitial tension on the extraalveolar pulmonary vessels (Fig. 7-10). The expansion of the pulmonary interstitial space by fluid may progress to a point where pulmonary interstitial pressure (Pisf) becomes positive and exceeds Ppv (zone 4).[28] In addition, the vascular resistance of extraalveolar ves-

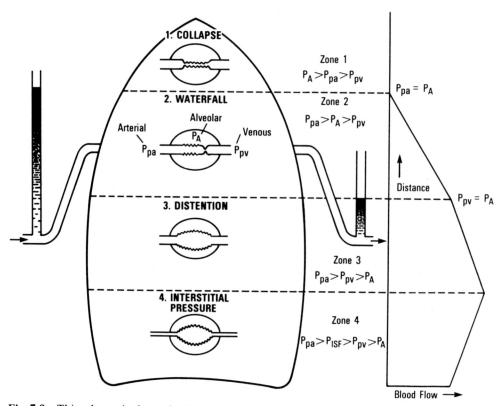

Fig. 7-9 This schematic shows the distribution of blood flow in the upright lung. In zone 1, alveolar pressure (PA) exceeds pulmonary artery pressure (Ppa) and no flow occurs because the intraalveolar vessels are collapsed by the compressing alveolar pressure. In zone 2, arterial pressure exceeds alveolar pressure but alveolar pressure exceeds venous pressure (Ppv). Flow in zone 2 is determined by the arterial-alveolar pressure difference (Ppa − PA) and has been likened to a river waterfall (blood pressure) over a dam (alveolar pressure). Since Ppa increases down zone 2 and PA remains constant, the perfusion pressure increases and flow steadily increases down the zone. In zone 3, pulmonary venous pressure exceeds alveolar pressure and flow is determined by the arterial-venous pressure difference (Ppa − Ppv), which is constant down this portion of the lung. However, the transmural pressure across the wall of the vessel increases down this zone so that the caliber of the vessels increases (resistance decreases), and so does flow. Finally, in zone 4, pulmonary interstitial pressure becomes positive and exceeds both pulmonary venous pressure and alveolar pressure. Consequently, flow in zone 4 is determined by the arterial-interstitial pressure difference (Ppa − Pisf). (Redrawn by permission from West JB: Ventilation/Blood Flow and Gas Exchange. 2nd Ed. Blackwell Scientific Publications, Oxford, 1970.

sels may be increased at a very low lung volume (i.e., the residual volume), where the tethering action of the pulmonary tissue on the vessels is lost, causing Pisf to increase positively (see lung volume discussion below).[29, 30] Thus, zone 4 conditions are present whenever Ppa exceeds Pisf, but Pisf exceeds Ppv and PA (Ppa > Pisf > Ppv > PA).[31] Consequently, the amount of zone 4 blood flow is governed by the arterio-interstitial pressure difference (Ppa − Pisf), which is less than the Ppa − Ppv difference, and therefore zone 4 blood flow is less than zone 3 blood flow. In summary then, zone 4 is a region of the lung which has transudated a large amount of fluid into the pulmonary in-

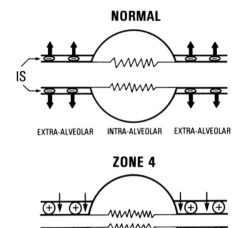

NORMAL

EXTRA-ALVEOLAR   INTRA-ALVEOLAR   EXTRA-ALVEOLAR

ZONE 4

Fig. 7-10 This figure shows the effect of lung volume on extra-alveolar vessels. In normal lungs (upper panel), lung distention creates a negative pressure around the extra-alveolar vessels, which tethers or keeps them open. When either pulmonary interstitial fluid accumulates or lung volume is extremely low, pulmonary interstitial pressure may become positive, exceed both pulmonary venous and alveolar pressure, and create a zone 4 of the lung (where flow is proportional to the pulmonary artery pressure/pulmonary interstitial pressure difference).

terstitial compartment or is possibly at a very low lung volume. Both these circumstances produce a positive interstitial pressure, causing extraalveolar vessel compression, increased extraalveolar vascular resistance, and decreased regional blood flow.

It has been demonstrated that the absolute pressure in similar-sized vessels at all vertical levels of the pulmonary circulation is not the same because of the influence of gravity. In addition, since pulmonary vascular and alveolar pressures change dynamically with the respiratory and cardiac cycles, a given small region in the lung may change zones from moment to moment. A simple numerical example will further illustrate this point (assume lung volume equals FRC and alveolar pressure is constant). In a man of ordinary height, the distance between the top and the bottom of the lung is

(apex) and the bottom (base) of the lung is about 30 cm. If the main pulmonary trunk is midway between the apex and base in the erect position, there is a column of blood 15 cm high between the pulmonary trunk and arterioles in the apex and a similar column of blood between it and arterioles in the base. A column of blood 15 cm high is equivalent to a column of mercury 11 mm high. If the absolute pressure in the main pulmonary artery is 22/9 mmHg, there is an adequate pressure to produce apical flow during systole, when apical pressure would be $22 - 11 = 11$ mmHg (zone 2 or 3) but not during diastole, when it would be $9 - 11 = -2$ mmHg (zone 1). The blood pressure at the base would be $22 + 11 / 9 + 11$, or 33/20 mmHg.

On the other hand, as *mean* Ppa and Ppv increase, two important changes take place in the pulmonary circulation: (1) recruitment or opening of previously unperfused vessels; and (2) distention or widening of previously perfused vessels.[32, 33] Thus, as mean Ppa increases, zone 1 vessels may become zone 2 vessels; in other words, new zone 2 arteries are recruited from previous zone 1 arteries. As mean Ppv increases, zone 2 vessels may become zone 3 vessels; in other words, new zone 3 veins are recruited from previous zone 2 veins. The increase in both mean Ppa and Ppv distends zone 3 vessels according to their compliance and decreases the resistance to flow through them. Zone 3 vessels may become so distended that they leak fluid and become converted to zone 4 vessels. In general, recruitment is the principal change as Ppa increases from low to moderate levels, whereas distention is the principal change as Ppa increases from moderate to high levels of vascular pressure.

Lung Volume

The functional residual capacity is the lung volume that exists at the end of normal exhalation after a normal tidal volume and when there is no air flow (no pressure differ-

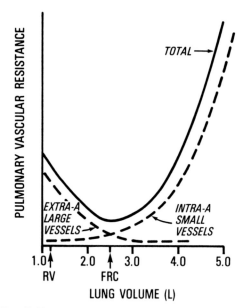

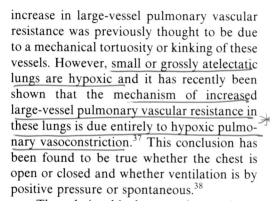

Fig. 7-11 An asymmetrical U-shaped curve relates total pulmonary vascular resistance to lung volume. The trough of the curve occurs when lung volume equals functional residual capacity. Total pulmonary vascular resistance is the sum of resistance in the intraalveolar (intra-A) small vessels, which is increased by increasing lung volume, and in the extraalveolar (extra-A) large vessels, which is increased by decreasing lung volume. RV = residual volume. The curve represents a composite of data from References 34 through 37.

ence between alveoli and atmosphere). Total pulmonary vascular resistance is increased when lung volume is either increased or decreased from FRC (Fig. 7-11).[34, 36] The increase in total pulmonary vascular resistance above FRC is due to alveolar compression of small intraalveolar vessels, resulting in an increase in pulmonary vascular resistance of small intraalveolar vessels (i.e., creation of zone 1 or zone 2). As a relatively small mitigating or counterbalancing effect, the large extraalveolar vessels may be expanded by the increased negativity of the perivascular pressure at high FRC. The increase in total pulmonary vascular resistance below FRC is due to an increase in pulmonary vascular resistance of large extraalveolar vessels. The

increase in large-vessel pulmonary vascular resistance was previously thought to be due to a mechanical tortuosity or kinking of these vessels. However, small or grossly atelectatic lungs are hypoxic and it has recently been shown that the mechanism of increased large-vessel pulmonary vascular resistance in these lungs is due entirely to hypoxic pulmonary vasoconstriction.[37] This conclusion has been found to be true whether the chest is open or closed and whether ventilation is by positive pressure or spontaneous.[38]

The relationship between lung volume and pulmonary vascular resistance also determines the regional distribution of pulmonary blood flow as a function of regional lung volume within a given single lung. At total lung capacity, all alveoli are homogeneously large, and the small intraalveolar vessels are homogeneously compressed (Fig. 7-9), while the large extraalveolar vessels are homogeneously expanded (Fig. 7-10). Since Ppa and Ppv increase down the upright lung, blood flow simply increases down the upright lung at total lung capacity. At residual volume dependent alveoli are much smaller than nondependent alveoli. Since the large extraalveolar vessels in the dependent lung are more constricted (nonexpanded) than the large extraalveolar vessels in the nondependent lung, blood flow *decreases* slightly down the upright lung at residual volume, even though Ppa and Ppv are increasing.[29, 30]

Alveolar Hypoxia

Alveolar or environmental hypoxia of in-vivo and in-vitro whole lung, unilateral lung, lobe, or lobule of lung causes pulmonary vasoconstriction. This phenomenon is called *hypoxic pulmonary vasoconstriction (HPV)* and is due to either a direct action of alveolar hypoxia on the pulmonary vasculature or an alveolar hypoxia-induced release of vasoactive substance(s).[39-43] These two mechanisms for the production of HPV are not necessarily mutually exclusive.

First, since the HPV response occurs primarily in the pulmonary arterioles of about 200 μm diameter, these vessels are advantageously situated anatomically in relation to bronchi and alveoli to permit direct detection of alveolar hypoxia. Hypoxia appears to stimulate metabolic activity of pulmonary vascular smooth muscle and accelerate production of ATP, whereas in systemic vascular beds, the action of hypoxia on metabolism is depressant. Low oxygen tension also maintains the membrane of pulmonary vascular smooth muscle cells in a state of partial depolarization and influences the role of calcium in excitation-contraction coupling.[39] Additionally or alternatively, alveolar hypoxia may cause the release of vasoconstrictor substance(s), and in the past 10 years many vasoactive substances have been proposed as the mediators of HPV (e.g., prostaglandins, catecholamines, serotonin, histamine), but none has been proved to be primarily involved in the process.[43]

There are three ways in which HPV operates in humans. First, life at high altitude or whole-lung respiration of a low inspired oxygen concentration (FIO_2) increases Ppa. This is true for newcomers, for the acclimatized, and for natives.[42] The vasoconstriction is considerable, and in normal people breathing 10 percent O_2 doubles Ppa while pulmonary wedge pressure remains constant.[44] The increased Ppa increases perfusion of the apices of the lung (recruitment of previously unused vessels) and results in gas exchange in a region of the lung not normally utilized (i.e., zone 1). Thus, with a low FIO_2, the PaO_2 is greater and the alveolar-arterial O_2 tension difference and dead-space/tidal volume ratio are less than would be expected or predicted on the basis of a normal (sea level) distribution of ventilation and blood flow. The high-altitude pulmonary hypertension is an important component in the development of mountain sickness subacutely (hours to days) and cor pulmonale chronically (weeks).[45] In fact, there is now good evidence that in patients

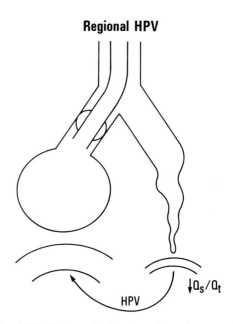

Regional HPV

$\downarrow Q_s/Q_t$

HPV

Fig. 7-12 Schematic drawing of one-lung ventilation and regional hypoxic pulmonary vasoconstriction (HPV) occurring in the other hypoxic atelectatic lung. HPV in the hypoxic lung causes a redistribution of blood flow away from the hypoxic lung to the normoxic lung, thereby diminishing the amount of shunt flow (Qs/Qt) that can occur through the hypoxic lung.

with chronic obstructive pulmonary disease, even nocturnal episodes of arterial oxygen desaturation (caused by episodic hypoventilation) are accompanied by elevations in Ppa and may account for or lead to sustained pulmonary hypertension and cor pulmonale.[46] Second, hypoxic ventilation ($FIO_2 = 0.1$) or atelectasis of one lung and one lobe generally causes a 30 to 40 or 50 to 60 percent diversion, respectively, of blood flow from hypoxic to nonhypoxic lung (Fig. 7-12).[47, 48] This is of great importance in minimizing transpulmonary shunt during diseases of one lung, one-lung anesthesia, and inadvertent intubation of a mainstem bronchus.[49, 50] In regard to one-lung anesthesia in the lateral decubitus position, it is important to note that the strength of the HPV response in man is sufficient to overcome significant vertical hydrostatic gradients.[51] Third, in patients with chronic obstructive pulmonary disease, asthma, pneumonia, and mitral stenosis who do not have bronchospasm, administration of pulmonary vasodilator drugs such as isoproterenol, sodium nitroprusside, nitroglycerin, and aminophylline cause a decrease in PaO_2 and pulmonary vascular resistance and an increase in right-to-left transpulmonary shunt.[52-66] The mechanism for these drug-induced changes is thought to be deleterious inhibition of preexisting and, in some of the lesions, geographically widespread HPV without a concomitant and beneficial bronchodilatation.[67] In accordance with the latter two lines of evidence (one-lung or regional hypoxia and vasodilator drug effects on whole-lung or generalized disease), HPV is thought to divert blood flow away from hypoxic regions of the lung, thereby serving as an autoregulatory mechanism that protects PaO_2 by favorably adjusting regional V_A/Q ratios (Fig. 7-12).[67]

Inhibition of regional HPV (Fig. 7-13) might impair arterial oxygenation by permitting increased venous admixture from hypoxic or atelectatic areas of the lung. Clinical factors that may directly vasodilate hypoxically constricted lung vessels are use of certain anesthetics, infusion of vasodilator drugs, the presence of infection in the hypoxic lung, extremely low mixed venous PO_2, and hypocapnia. Anesthetic drugs will be considered first. Most studies have found a small but consistent inhibition of HPV by N_2O.[68-70] Halothane does not inhibit HPV in dogs, but there is one report on humans which indicates that halothane does inhibit HPV.[68, 69, 71, 72] Enflurane has been studied only in animals and does not inhibit HPV.[69] Isoflurane and fluroxene exhibit dose-dependent inhibition of HPV, as do methoxyflurane, trichlorethylene, and diethyl ether.[68, 69, 73-76] Various injectable and intravenous (nonvolatile) anesthetic drugs and adjuvants, including thiopentone, ketamine, pethidine, lidocaine, chlorpromazine, fentanyl, droperidol, diazepam, pentazocine, and pentobarbitone seem to be with-

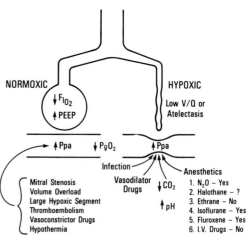

INHIBITION OF HPV

Fig. 7-13 The figure summarizes various clinical conditions and events which may inhibit regional hypoxic pulmonary vasoconstriction (HPV). Blood flow reduction to atelectatic lung is presumed to be by the same mechanism as for nitrogen-ventilated lung (as indicated in the upper right corner of the figure). Direct inhibitors of regional HPV are listed in the lower right corner of the figure. Clinical conditions which can inhibit HPV by causing increased pulmonary artery pressure (Ppa) are listed in the lower left corner of the figure. Within the normoxic lung, a low FIO_2 and high airway pressure may increase normoxic lung pulmonary vascular resistance and prevent a redistribution of blood flow away from the hypoxic lung to the normoxic lung. Finally, an extremely low mixed venous PO_2 (PvO_2) may lower normoxic lung alveolar PO_2 and cause off-setting and competing HPV in the "normoxic" lung.

out deleterious influence on HPV.[68, 78-80] However, either these latter studies have been performed on animals or, if conducted in humans, the experimental design precluded assessment of direct effects or comparison of one drug (e.g., ketamine) with any other anesthetic drug[68, 78-80] (see Ch. 8).

All systemic vasodilator drugs probably inhibit HPV.[67] Specifically tested and very potent in this regard are intravenous sodium nitroprusside, nitroglycerin, isoproterenol, aminophylline, and aerosolized beta-adrenergic agonists.[52-67] When no bronchospasm has been present in diseased lungs, these vasodilator drugs have inhibited HPV, increased shunt, and decreased arterial oxygenation. Therefore, when no bronchospasm is present, vasodilator drugs may simply convert small and autoregulating shunt units to large and nonautoregulating shunt units. When bronchospasm is present in diseased lung, these vasodilators may have no effect or may increase oxygenation because concomitant bronchodilatation may increase regional ventilation and regional alveolar PO_2, eliminating the need for and cause of the regional HPV. Therefore, when bronchospasm is present, vasobronchodilator drugs may convert small shunt units to normal gas-exchanging units.

In situations in which there is a large hypoxic compartment, extreme decreases in the mixed venous PO_2 can cause the alveolar PO_2 of the remaining, supposedly "normoxic" lung to be depressed to levels which cause competing and therefore inhibiting HPV.[81] Decreases in P_ACO_2 and $PaCO_2$ below 30 mmHg inhibit HPV.[82] Metabolic alkalemia causes pulmonary vasodilatation and also blunts HPV, while acidemia of both respiratory and metabolic origin causes pulmonary vasoconstriction.[13] The stimulus with acidemia is probably hydrogen ion and not molecular carbon dioxide. Hypoxia and acidemia act additively, and, in some studies, synergistically to cause pulmonary vasoconstriction, although the particular vascular segments upon which they act may differ.[13, 41] Finally, there is some evidence that certain types of infection, particularly granulomatous and pneumococcal infections, may inhibit HPV.[83, 84]

The pulmonary circulation is poorly endowed with smooth muscle, and even hypoxically-constricted vessels will dilate when exposed to pressures exceeding 16 to 18 mmHg.[85] Thus, the intraluminal vascular pressure against which the pulmonary vessels must constrict is a major determinant of the magnitude of HPV.[86] Clinical conditions that increase pulmonary vascular pressure, and therefore inhibit HPV (or at least clinically inhibit effective redistribution of blood flow away from hypoxic lung), are mitral stenosis, volume overload, administration of vasopressor drugs, ligation of pulmonary vessels, thromboembolism, and large hypoxic lung segments.[47, 48, 81, 86-89] Finally, a decrease in normoxic lung F_IO_2 (below 0.5) and an increase in normoxic lung airway pressure (i.e., PEEP), can cause an increase in normoxic lung vascular resistance which would prevent a redistribution of blood flow away from the hypoxic to the normoxic lung.[81, 88, 90, 91]

Cardiac Output

The passive effects of changes in cardiac output on the pulmonary circulation are as follows. As cardiac output increases, pulmonary vascular pressures increase (Fig. 7-14).[13] Since the pulmonary vasculature is distensible, an increase in pulmonary artery pressure increases the radius of the pulmonary vessels, causing pulmonary vascular resistance to decrease. The exactly opposite effect applies to the passive effect of a decrease in cardiac output on the pulmonary circulation. As cardiac output decreases, pulmonary vascular pressures decrease. The decrease in pulmonary artery pressure decreases the radius of the pulmonary vessels, causing pulmonary vascular resistance to increase.

Understanding the relationship between pulmonary vascular resistance, pulmonary artery pressure, and cardiac output during passive events is a prerequisite to recognition of active vasomotion in the pulmonary circulation (Fig. 7-15). Active vasoconstriction occurs at any time cardiac output decreases and pulmonary artery pressure either remains constant or increases. Increased pulmonary artery pressure and pulmonary vascular resistance have been found to be "a universal feature of acute respiratory failure."[92] Therefore, active pulmonary vaso-

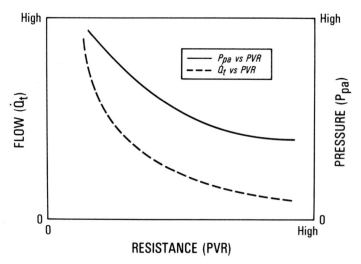

Fig. 7-14 The relationship between flow, pressure, and resistance in the pulmonary circulation. See text for full explanation. (Redrawn with permission from Fishman AP: Dynamics of the pulmonary circulation. pp 1167-1743. In Hamilton WF, Dow P, Eds: Handbook of Physiology. Vol. 2, Sect. 2, Circulation. American Physiological Society, Washington, 1963.)

constriction may play an important role in the genesis of the adult respiratory distress syndrome.[93] Active vasodilatation occurs any time cardiac output increases and pulmonary artery pressure either remains constant or decreases. When deliberate hypotension is achieved with sodium nitroprusside, cardiac output often remains constant or increases, but pulmonary artery pressure decreases, and therefore so does pulmonary vascular resistance.

PULMONARY VASCULAR REFLEXES

Cardiopulmonary receptors, whose afferent fibers course in the cardiac sympathetic nerves, have been described in both right-sided cardiac chambers (75 percent), both vena cavae (10 percent), the pulmonary veins (5 percent), the extrapulmonic portions of the pulmonary artery (5 percent), and the coronary vessels (5 percent).[94] Measurement of conduction velocity in these cardiac sympathetic afferent nerves showed that most were medullated A-fibers and some were

nonmedullated B-fibers.[95] Most medullated fibers exhibit cardiac rhythmicity, whereas nonmedullated afferents discharge irregularly and with no apparent relation to cardiac events. The discharge frequency of these cardiopulmonary sympathetic afferent fibers is augmented when the area containing the receptor is stretched by outflow occlusion, volume infusion, or inflation of an intracavity balloon and decreased during an acute hemorrhage.[96-98] However, in contrast to the effect of carotid and aortic baroreceptor function (↑ systemic blood pressure → ↑ baroreceptor discharge → ↑ inhibition of medullary cardiovascular center → systemic vasodilatation; and conversely, ↓ systemic blood pressure → ↓ baroreceptor discharge → ↓ inhibition of medullary cardiovascular center → systemic vasoconstriction), most studies have shown that stimulation of the central cardiopulmonary sympathetic afferents has a pressor effect on the cardiovascular system.[99-101] Pulmonary vascular distention causes no change or only mild changes in airway tone.[102]

It has become clear that the pulmonary

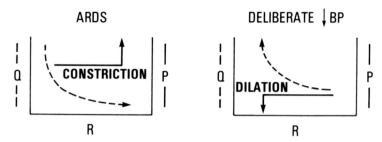

Fig. 7-15 The pulmonary circulation and vasomotion. Relationships between flow (Q), pressure (P), and resistance (R) in the pulmonary circulation in the adult respiratory distress syndrome (ARDS) (left-hand panel) and during deliberate hypotension (↓ BP). Active vasoconstriction is present in the pulmonary circulation whenever cardiac output decreases and pressure remains constant or increases; these findings are common in ARDS. Active vasodilatation is present in the pulmonary circulation whenever cardiac output increases and pressure remains constant or decreases; these findings are often present with deliberate hypotension.

efferent sympathetic nerves are part of an extensive control system, which can be stimulated centrally and reflexly to modify pulmonary vascular tone.[103-105] The effect of sympathetic stimulation is predominantly due to alpha-adrenergic receptor stimulation (alpha-receptors predominate both numerically and functionally in the pulmonary circulation) and results in diminished distensibility (stiffening) of the pulmonary arterial tree.[105] The effects of pulmonary sympathetic nerve stimulation on the pulmonary vascular resistance (as opposed to distensibility) are usually not large, but in special circumstances they can be important. For example, distention of the main pulmonary artery by balloon inflation in the conscious dog reflexly produces constriction of pulmonary arterioles and possibly venules (pressure distal to the balloon increased from 21/6 to 43/14 mm Hg) and is due to excitation of receptors located in the pulmonary artery or possibly the right side of the heart or both.[102]

Although the effects of pulmonary sympathetic nerve stimulation are not ordinarily quantitatively large, they are vital for homeostasis during stress and exercise and for maintaining a precise balance between right

and left ventricular outputs. An increase in right ventricular output causes an increase in pulmonary sympathetic nerve activity. The resultant increase in stiffness of the large pulmonary arteries increases the rate of transmission of a pulse wave of a given right ventricular beat to a level sufficiently rapid to cause an increase in the stroke volume of the subsequent left ventricular beat.[106]

Without this type of automatic adjustment, the increase in heart rate and cardiac output during exercise or excitement would alter the synchrony of the two ventricles and upset the balance in ventricular outputs. In canine studies, an abrupt onset of exercise (treadmill) without previous warning produces an increase in right ventricular stroke volume, which precedes an increase in left ventricular stroke volume by several beats.[107] Because of this asynchrony between the two ventricles, pulmonary blood volume has to increase. However, when dogs are trained to anticipate the start of exercise and sympathetic nervous activity is presumably heightened, the ventricular outputs change exactly in phase. Direct measurements in man are consistent with these observations in dogs, since it has been shown that the pulmonary blood volume remains virtually unchanged during exercise.[108] In addition, it is now clear that during experimental excitation of the hypothalmic integrative area, which is necessary in order to produce or stimulate the defense reaction, the pulmonary sympathetic nerves are stimulated to produce moderate pulmonary vasoconstriction, with presumably similar secondary effects on balancing ventricular outputs.[103-104] On the other hand, there is virtually no effect of vagal stimulation on the pulmonary circulation.

PHARMACOLOGY

General Considerations[109]

It is now well established that the pulmonary circulation has two fundamentally and physiologically important pharmacokinetic functions. First, the pulmonary circulation can inactivate or remove vasoactive substances from the venous blood [hydroxytryptamine (5-HT), bradykinin, norepinephrine (NE), prostaglandins (PGs E_1, E_2, and F_2)], whereas other substances, often very closely related to each other as well as to the above substances, are allowed free passage [epinephrine (E), angiotensin II, oxytocin, and vasopressin]. This function seems to be appropriate for the lung because in contrast to all other organs, it receives the total venous return and is therefore in an ideal position to regulate the concentration of vasoactive substances in venous blood before they reach the arterial circulation and have profound systemic effects.

The removal of some substances but not of others has led to the classification of vasoactive hormones as local or as circulating, depending upon whether they were removed by the lungs. A local hormone is released at or near the target cells, has its local effect, and is inactivated before reaching the arterial circulation. The inactivation of the hormone occurs either immediately in the tissues, within a few seconds in the venous blood, or within a few more seconds in the pulmonary circulation. It is now apparent that both enzymatic degradation (5-HT, NE) and uptake processes (PGs) play a part in the pulmonary inactivation mechanism for these substances. Defects in this metabolic function of the lung are definitely implicated in the causation of some clinical conditions. For example, potentiation of the cardiovascular effects of NE produced by some drugs (e.g., cocaine, tricyclic antidepressants, some steroids, and certain antihypertensive drugs) may be due to inhibition of pulmonary removal of NE in addition to interference with uptake and storage of NE in peripheral tissues.

On the other hand, a circulating hormone is released into the venous blood and then distributed through the arterial circulation without loss of activity on passage through the lungs. By definition, it is not possible for the lung to malfunction in its handling of a circulating hormone. At present there are no known conditions wherein the lung begins to inactivate previously unmetabolized hormones.

The presence of luminal endothelial projections and plasmalemmal cavities, with histochemical verification of the presence of enzymes at these endothelial locations, invites the functional anatomical picture of enzymes in the luminal membrane of the endothelial cell being washed and bathed with substrates which are in a continuously flowing liquid phase.[110-113] The enzyme-substrate interface is enormous at the level of the capillary bed, a condition that favors efficient metabolism by relatively small amounts of enzyme. The presence of intracellular and membrane cavities very likely explains how the metabolic products of some of the substrates (adenine nucleotides, PG) are returned to the circulation with no apparent delay or uptake by tissue.

The lungs have a number of ways in which they may influence the quantity of endothelial enzymes exposed to circulating substrates. The number of capillaries open at any given time and therefore the amount of endothelial surface exposed to blood flow are complex functions of right-to-left shunting, pulmonary venous pressure, posture, exercise (cardiac output), depth of ventilation, the composition of inhalants, and several other factors, not the least of which is the structural integrity of the lungs themselves. It might be expected that factors which significantly increase or decrease mean transit time of blood through the lungs (e.g., cardiac output, viscosity) could affect the amount of endothelial enzyme-substrate interaction. Changes in inspired oxygen tension have produced somewhat variable and not dramatic changes in the amount of lung modification of most vasoactive substances, angiotensin I conversion being an exception.[114–117]

The second important pharmacokinetic function of the pulmonary circulation is an endocrine one in that the lung is an organ which can contribute vasoactive hormones to the circulation as well as remove them. Historically, this understanding of the pulmonary circulation began with the demonstration that rapid conversion of angiotensin I to the much more active angiotensin II takes place not in the venous bloodstream per se, as previously supposed, but in the pulmonary vascular bed and that the lung is a rich source of the peptidase or converting enzyme involved. In addition, anaphylaxis has been shown to be one of the conditions in which biologically-active substances are released from the lungs. Indeed, in humans the lung seems to be the major shock organ of anaphylaxis and source of mediators. Some of the mediators released during anaphylaxis are also released by damage to lung tissue, such as is caused by overinflation, pulmonary embolism, or physical manipulation. Finally, biologically-active substances are also released from the lung when various pharmacologic agents are injected or infused into the pulmonary circulation. Table 7-1 summarizes many of the above considerations and the way in which the pulmonary

capillary bed handles biologically-active materials.

Inactivation of Endogenous Amines[109, 113, 118–121]

The biogenic amines norepinephrine, epinephrine, dopamine, 5-hydroxytryptamine, histamine (H), and acetylcholine (Ach) all have profound excitatory or inhibitory actions on a wide variety of organs and physiologic functions. The degree of removal of these amines from venous blood varies widely. Infused NE, histamine, serotonin, and dopamine all cause pulmonary vasoconstriction; E causes pulmonary vasodilatation in small doses and vasoconstriction in large doses; and Ach causes pulmonary vasodilatation.[122–123]

NOREPINEPHRINE (NE)

Approximately 20 to 35 percent of exogenously administered NE is removed on passage through the pulmonary circulation. The removal is caused by enzymatic metabolism [monamine oxidase (MAO)] on the luminal surface of the capillary endothelium. The presence of an inactivating system for NE in the pulmonary circulation, which is operative at low physiologic concentrations of NE, strongly suggests a physiologic role for this system in controlling and limiting levels of NE that reach the arterial circulation. Several clinical conditions are known or at least strongly suspected to interfere with this regulatory function.

Although the concentration of circulating NE is low under normal conditions, it can increase up to 4 μg/ml in a patient with a pheochromocytoma, a concentration that would be expected to saturate pulmonary metabolic mechanisms. Several different drugs have been found to inhibit pulmonary removal of NE. The steroids, estradiol and corticosterone inhibit metabolism of NE, and

Table 7-1

Handling of Biologically Active Materials in the Pulmonary Capillary Bed

Metabolized at endothelial surface without uptake from plasma
    Bradykinin—inactivated
    Adenine nucleotides—inactivated
    Angiotensin I—activated

Metabolized intracellularly after uptake from plasma
    Serotonin (hydroxytryptamine or 5-HT)
    Norepinephrine
    Prostaglandins E and F

Unaffected by traversing lungs
    Epinephrine
    Prostaglandin A
    Angiotensin II
    Dopamine
    Vasopressin
    (Acetylcholine)*
    Oxytocin

Synthesized within lung and released into blood
    Prostaglandins E & F

Discharged from intrapulmonary stores into blood
    Histamine
    Prostaglandins
    Slow-reacting substance of anaphylaxis
    Kallikreins
    Eosinophil leukocyte chemotactic factor of anaphylaxis

* The parentheses around acetylcholine indicates that normally very little or none reaches the lungs owing to peripheral tissue and blood cholinesterase hydrolysis. However, 90% of what little acetylcholine does reach the lungs is unaffected by passage through the pulmonary circulation.

imipramine (25 mg 3 times daily) has caused a four- to-eightfold potentiation of the pressor response to an intravenous NE infusion. Electrocardiographic abnormalities and dysrhythmias of various types after tricyclic antidepressants are well documented in man and may be due to inhibition of pulmonary uptake of NE, causing a greater than normal concentration of NE in the coronary circulation.

Anesthetic drugs and adjuvants may interfere with pulmonary metabolism of NE. In isolated lungs, NE metabolism is inhibited by cocaine, halothane, and nitrous oxide; and in anesthetized dogs halothane has abolished pulmonary inactivation of NE.[124] In man, this effect could be responsible for the higher incidence of catecholamine-induced dysrhythmias with halothane. This could also be important in surgery involving hypothermia and halothane, when pulmonary removal mechanisms would be expected to be depressed. In patients with pulmonary hypertension secondary to valvular heart disease, significantly more NE is removed from the pulmonary circulation than in patients with normal pulmonary artery pressures, perhaps reflecting an increased endothelial surface area available for metabolism and increased endothelial cell contact time (decreased transit time). Finally, total cardiopulmonary bypass in man increases pulmonary removal of NE from 23 to 50 percent. Thus, use of an amine that is not removed by the lung (e.g., epinephrine) after bypass may be preferable to administration of NE. Alternatively, left atrial, as opposed to intravenous, administration of norepinephrine might be desirable.

5-HYDROXYTRYPTAMINE (5-HT OR SEROTONIN)

The 5-HT pulmonary removal process is extremely efficient and nearly complete (98 percent). As with NE, the removal process is by enzymatic metabolism [monamine oxidase (MAO)] on the luminal surface of the capillary endothelium. Endothelial uptake and enzyme inactivation of 5-HT is completely prevented by monamine oxidase inhibitors (e.g., proniazide), and, as with NE, 5-HT uptake is inhibited by cocaine and tricyclic antidepressant drugs. However, NE and 5-HT are probably taken up at different sites, since NE in concentrations up to 6 times normal has no effect on pulmonary uptake of 5-HT.

Steroids may inhibit the removal of 5-HT, and since 5-HT causes aggregation of platelets, it is possible that increased levels of circulating 5-HT could explain the increased tendency to formation of venous thrombi during oral contraceptive and other steroid therapy. Patients suffering from carcinoid tumors have elevated blood levels of 5-HT (1 to 3 μg/ml) and frequently have cardiac valvular lesions, which are characteristically on the right side of the heart. These blood levels should be expected to saturate pulmonary removal mechanisms. However, since the cardiac lesions and fibrosis are only right-sided, pulmonary inactivation is probably functioning and causing a right-to-left concentration gradient. In addition to the link between right-sided heart lesions in patients with carcinoid tumors and pulmonary removal of 5-HT, it has been suggested that certain symptoms of bronchial carcinoid tumors are due to bypassing normal hepatic 5-HT inactivation. However, if the lung rather than the liver is the major site of 5-HT inactivation, then these symptoms equally could reflect inefficiency of pulmonary removal of 5-HT.

Recently it was shown that in patients with pulmonary hypertension secondary to valvular heart disease, significantly more 5-HT was removed from the pulmonary circulation than in patients with normal pulmonary artery pressures. Pulmonary removal of 5-HT was also markedly increased immediately after total cardiopulmonary bypass, an effect that was not correlated with changes in pulmonary blood flow or volume.

ACETYLCHOLINE

Most acetylcholine (90 percent) present in pulmonary artery blood passes through the pulmonary circulation unchanged (some acetylcholinesterases and pseudocholinesterases are present in variable amounts in endothelial and muscle cells of the pulmonary vasculature). The absence of a significant inactivating system operating on acetylcholine in the pulmonary circulation is perhaps not surprising, since the action of acetylcholine is usually terminated by hydrolysis close to its site of release from nerve endings. Furthermore, any acetylcholine escaping into the circulation is rapidly inactivated by plasma and erythrocyte cholinesterases. Consequently, it is extremely unlikely that acetylcholine would under normal circumstances be present in the blood perfusing the pulmonary circulation. However, the pharmacokinetics of more stable quarternary esters, such as succinylcholine and methacholine, could be influenced by the presence of a pulmonary inactivating system for choline esters.

HISTAMINE

Histamine is not removed from the pulmonary circulation to any appreciable extent. However, it should be noted that histamine is present in the lungs of most species, the amount being generally related to the population of mast cells. These cells can take up and store histamine, but the uptake is a slow process and is not likely to contribute to the removal of exogenous histamine during a single passage through the pulmonary circulation. However, the uptake of histamine by mast cells could contribute to its eventual distribution after exogenous administration to the whole animal.

EPINEPHRINE, ISOPROTERENOL, AND DOPAMINE

These catecholamines are not taken up or removed by the pulmonary circulation. Therefore, they should be regarded as truly circulating and wholly systemic drugs.

Inactivation of Bradykinin and Related Peptides[109, 113, 118–121, 125, 126]

The pulmonary circulation in isolated lungs inactivates about 80 percent of bradykinin passing through it. Bradykinin inactivation is due to an enzyme (dipeptidylcarboxypeptidase), which is probably located on the plasma membrane of the endothelial cells in free communication with the vascular space. This same enzyme is also responsible for the conversion of angiotensin I to angiotensin II (converting enzyme).

Even without the participation of the lung (and the peripheral tissues) in the degradation of bradykinin, the half-life of bradykinin in the circulation would be less than 2 circulation times, owing to the presence of blood kininases. Nevertheless, the pulmonary circulation attenuates the activity of circulating kinins during their transit from the venous to the arterial side, and, therefore the kinins, like NE, 5-HT, and some PGs should be regarded as local hormones. Other polypeptide hormones such as insulin, vasopressin, oxytocin, and gastrin are not metabolized by the pulmonary circulation and should therefore be regarded as circulating hormones.

The fragments of bradykinin inactivation are known to be virtually inactive on isolated intestinal or uterine smooth muscle and are not systemic vasodepressors. Nevertheless, some of these fragments may have other bradykinin-like activities, such as an increase in capillary permeability, contraction of bronchial smooth muscle, mediation of inflammation, and ability to cause pain. Snake venom, which contains a mixture of peptides, inhibits bradykinin inactivation and therefore has been called *bradykinin-potentiating factor* (BPF). Fetal and neonatal lungs have a low level of kininase, and therefore increased circulating levels of bradykinin have been implicated in the closing of the ductus arteriosus and other circulatory changes that occur at birth.[127] These changes take some hours to complete and during such time it is an advantage to have low pulmonary inactivation, thus maintaining high arterial levels of kinin.

Angiotensin-Converting Enzyme[109, 113, 118–121, 128, 129]

There are two forms of angiotensin called *angiotensin I* and *angiotensin II*. Renin, an enzyme present in the juxtaglomerular apparatus of the kidney, acts on angiotensinogen (or renin substrate, an $\alpha2$-globulin) to form the decapeptide angiotensin I. Angiotensin I is converted to an octapeptide, angiotensin II, by converting enzyme. Angiotensin II is one of the most potent systemic vasopressor substances known (and also causes pulmonary vasoconstriction). The converting enzyme is the same one responsible for the breakdown of bradykinin and is therefore localized on the pulmonary endothelial surface. The endothelial localization accounts for the rapid in vivo conversion rate of angiotensin I to angiotensin II. Although the lung is capable of producing large quantities of angiotensin II, there is no significant metabolic breakdown of angiotensin II in the lung. Pharmacologic or physiologic activity of angiotensin II is terminated by the action of the angiotensinases, a group of enzymes with wide tissue distribution which produce a large number of sites of cleavage in the peptide molecule.

Evidence that the renin-angiotensin system may be activated in patients with severe, decompensated cardiac failure has raised the possibility that angiotensin II may be responsible for the increase in systemic vascular resistance in such patients.[130] Prevention of the formation, and thus pharmacologic activity, of endogenous angiotensin II may be accomplished by inhibitors of converting enzyme and has clinically produced salutory responses in patients with severe heart failure.[131] Captopril, a new oral converting enzyme inhibitor, has been found to have especially long-term efficacy in the treatment of advanced congestive heart failure.[132, 133]

Prostaglandin Metabolism[109, 113, 118–121, 134–137]

The prostaglandins (PG) are naturally occurring substances that are distributed throughout the entire body. Chemically, the PGs may be considered derivatives of prostanoic acid (Fig. 7-16), and the nomenclature of the PGs is based on the carbon skeleton of that acid. The several groups of PGs are distinguished by the nature and geometry of the substituent groups on the end ring (for example E, F, D) and the number of double bonds in the side chains of the acid (for example E_1, E_2, F_1, F_2, etc.). The PGs possess a

PROSTANOIC ACID

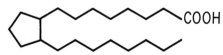
COOH

Fig. 7-16 Schematic diagram of prostanoic acid showing the carbon-carbon linkages. For the nomenclature on how carbon atom substitutions create the various prostaglandins see text.

bewildering spectrum of biologic activity, including dramatic cardiopulmonary effects in plasma concentrations, which are often as low as 10^{-7} to 10^{-8}M. PGE_1 and E_2 cause pulmonary vasodilatation, and $F_2\alpha$ causes pulmonary vasoconstriction. It is therefore not surprising to discover that the lungs possess extremely efficient enzymatic machinery for the rapid conversion of PGs to inactive metabolites and probably provide the major inactivation mechanism for PGs liberated into the venous circulation. The mechanisms for PG metabolism are extremely rapid; for example, 95 percent of infused PGE_2 is inactivated during one circulation through the lungs. The A series of PGs are not metabolized and are the only PGs likely to be circulating hormones. It is very likely that PG metabolism is caused by hydrolytic enzymes (PG dehydrogenase, PGDH), which are soluble in the cytoplasm of the endothelial cell. PG metabolism is decreased by hypoxia and increased by lipid anesthetic drugs.

If for some reason inactivation of PGs by the lung is diminished, the PGs might accumulate in the circulation in sufficient quantities to cause pharmacologic effects. Plasma levels of PGs are elevated in endotoxic shock and there is evidence that these increased levels of PGs are due to decreased PG metabolism. It is well known that the PGs can account for some of the circulatory and other changes that are a feature of this condition.

Prostaglandins are synthesized by a multienzyme complex referred to loosely as *PG synthetase*. This enzyme complex appears to be present in every mammalian tissue so far investigated (as well as in several non-mammalian tissues), and the lung contains a relative abundance of PG synthetase. Pulmonary PG synthesis may be initiated by a variety of stimuli, both physiologic and pathologic, such as vasoactive peptides, phospholipase A, anaphylactic shock, 5-hydroxytryptamine, tryptamine, and other mechanical or chemical factors. However, synthesis of PGs is unaffected by increases in inspired oxygen concentration. Release of PGs may be equated with de novo PG synthesis. They are released from the lungs in response to inflation, and, since certain PGs dilate the pulmonary vasculature, several authors have suggested that PGs might be responsible for maintaining the correct ventilation/perfusion ratio in pulmonary tissue. There is a great deal of experimental evidence that PGs are released from the lungs by a variety of traumatic stimuli, and it has been suggested that PGs may be important in the development of the clinical picture associated with immunologic reactions, pulmonary embolism, and migraine headache. The suggestion that PGs play a part in bronchial asthma has been made, since PGF_2 is a potent bronchoconstrictor.

A wide variety of compounds are known to inhibit PG synthetase, but the most clinically significant of these are members of the diverse group of aspirin-like drugs. From the literature, it is possible to suggest the following order of decreasing potency: meclofe-namic acid, niflumic acid or indomethacin, mefenamic acid, flufenamic acid, naproxen, phenylbutazone, aspirin, and ibuprofen. These aspirin-like drugs inhibit PG biosynthesis in clinical doses, and thus one might anticipate that the ability of the lungs to synthesize PGs would be impaired during therapy with these agents.

Metabolism of Chemicals and Drugs[109, 121, 138]

The chemicals and drugs that preferentially accumulate in the lung, resulting in high lung tissue-to-blood concentration ratios, have a wide variety of pharmacologic activity (Table 7-2). These chemicals include antihistamines, CNS-active drugs (such as narcotics and antidepressants), β-blockers, and herbicides (paraquat also induces lung damage). A careful examination of the chemical structures of these compounds indicates that, except for paraquat, all chemi-

Table 7-2
Accumulation of Chemicals by the Lung

Chemical	Lung/Blood Concentration Ratio[109]	Species
Antihistamines		
Cyclizine	112(4)*	Rat
Chlorcyclizine	107(3)	Rat
Diphenhydramine	100(1)	Guinea pig
Antipsychotics		
Fluphemazine	100(19)	Dog
Tricyclic antidepressants		
Imipramine	150(10), 10(24)	Rabbit
Anorectic drugs		
Chlorphentermine	53(1), 30(24)	Rat
Phentermine	40(1), 3(24)	Rat
Amphetamine	33(1)	Rat
Analgesics		
Methadone	100(3)	Rat
Beta-adrenergic blocking agents		
Propranolol	25(½)	Monkey
Propranolol	125(1)	Rabbit
Herbicide		
Paraquat	4(1), 14(32)	Rat

* Numbers in parentheses are hours after ingestion

cals listed in Table 7-2 are amines with pk_as greater than 8.

In one study, propranolol uptake in conscious ambulant dogs after a single passage through the pulmonary circulation was 53 percent; this increased to 81 percent during anesthesia with thiopental, nitrous oxide, and halothane and to 64 percent during anesthesia with thiopental, nitrous oxide, and fentanyl.[139] Interaction between lipid-soluble anesthetic agents and pulmonary endothelial cell membranes may be an important factor in increasing lung uptake of lipophilic propranolol (as it is with the PGs), although alteration in pulmonary perfusion associated with a reduction in cardiac output during general anesthesia (increased contact time) may play a part. Therefore, the pharmacologic effects of propranolol administered during general anesthesia may be somewhat unpredictable. Methadone and amphetamine accumulate in, and are extensively degraded by, the lung; while imipramine and cholorcyclizine, which also accumulate in the lung, are not degraded. Since imipramine is an inhibitor of lung MAO, it may prevent the metabolic degradation of 5-HT and NE by the lung. Cardiovascular toxicities have been reported for various tricyclic antidepressants, and frequent cardiovascular complications have been seen in poisoning by antidepressants. Pulmonary hypertension observed with the use of anorexic drugs can be related to inhibition of the detoxication of vasoactive substances by the lung.[140] Toxicity produced by paraquat is characterized by lung fibrosis and death.[141, 142] This toxicity appears to be related to both accumulation of paraquat in the lung and generation of free radicals by the lipid peroxidation of paraquat.

Anaphylaxis and Release of Chemical Mediators[109, 113, 119, 120, 121, 143, 144]

The signs of anaphylaxis in man include acute respiratory distress, asphyxia, angioneurotic edema, severe hypotension, and vascular collapse. The respiratory distress may result from upper airway obstruction caused by laryngeal edema and/or severe bronchospasm. Postmortem examination of the lungs of humans dying in anaphylactic shock reveals hyperinflation with alternating areas of emphysema and collapse. Similar changes are seen in patients dying of status asthmaticus.

During human anaphylaxis, the lung releases histamine (which is stored in lung mast cells in a complex with protein and heparin), slow-reacting substance of anaphylaxis (SRS-A, stored in a preformed state), PGs E_1, E_2, and F_2 (release of PGs during anaphylaxis must be from de novo synthesis), and possibly bradykinin. However, since histamine and SRS-A are known to cause release of lung PGs and the amount of PG released during anaphylaxis is not related to the antigen dose, PG release may be secondary to that of the primary mediators, namely histamine and SRS-A. Since these two primary mediators also cause release of catecholamines from the adrenal medulla, the catecholamines must be regarded as secondary mediators of anaphylaxis.

Histamine directly causes bronchoconstriction due to H_1 receptor stimulation. However, this effect is somewhat attenuated in vivo owing to concomitant histamine-induced adrenal medullary release of bronchodilating catecholamines. Histamine is a potent pulmonary artery vasoconstrictor and may contribute to the pulmonary edema that occurs in anaphylaxis or following pulmonary embolism since it increases pulmonary (and systemic) vascular permeability. These changes may be attributed to partial disconnection of the endothelial cell junctions. Histamine released during anaphylactic shock and subsequent pulmonary damage may in turn contribute to the release of PGs. SRS-A is a potent human bronchoconstrictor and is perhaps more important in humans than any other species studied. The exact role of PGs released from lung tissue by anaphylaxis seems hard to define, since both E- and F-type PGs are released and they have directly opposing actions on some smooth muscles. For example, E_2 is a bronchodilator and vasodilator, and F_2 is a bronchoconstrictor with variable and species-dependent hemodynamic effects. Perhaps one of the actions of PGs released in the lung is to sensitize bronchial and vascular smooth muscle to the actions of the other mediators. Bradykinin causes bronchoconstriction, systemic hypotension, and increased capillary permeability, and perhaps PG release.

The release of the mediators of anaphylaxis can be pharmacologically inhibited, and many of these release inhibitors are also physiologic antagonists. In humans, histamine and SRS-A release are inhibited by β-adrenergic drugs, methylxanthines, and disodium cromoglycate. Release of PGs is inhibited by the aspirin-like drugs and disodium cromoglycate.

Lung Lesions and Physical and Chemical Stimuli[119, 145]

It is possible that any substance the lung is capable of synthesizing and/or storing may, under certain conditions, be released into the pulmonary circulation.[107, 143, 144] Table 7-3 shows that neoplastic lung disease may produce almost any biologically-active polypeptide and the associated characteristic clinical syndrome caused by the polypeptide. Mechanical stimulation of the lung, such as stroking of the lung surface or retraction during surgery, may cause release of various vasoconstrictor and vasodilator substances, respectively. Hyper- or hypoinflation of the lung may cause release of PGs.[47, 148-151] Chemical stimulation of the lung, such as by alveolar hypoxia, also causes release of PGs, which may then serve to normalize V/Q rela-

Table 7-3

Polypeptide Hormone Secretion in Pulmonary Disease: Resultant Syndromes and Commonly Associated Lesions

Hormones	Syndrome	Lung Lesion
ACTH	Hypokalemic alkalosis, edema, Cushing's syndrome	Oat-cell carcinoma, adenoma
ADH (arginine vasopressin)	Hyponatremia (SIADH)	Oat-cell carcinoma, adenoma, tuberculosis, pneumonia, aspergillosis
PTH or related peptide	Hypercalcemia	Squamous-cell carcinoma, adenocarcinoma, and large-cell undifferentiated carcinoma
Gonadotropins	Gynecomastia (adults), precocious puberty (children)	Large-cell anaplastic carcinoma
VIP or related peptide	Watery diarrhea or no symptoms	Squamous-, large-, or oat-cell carcinoma
? Growth hormone, serotonin, kinins (and PGs, other)	Hypertrophic osteoarthropathy, "carcinoid"	Squamous-cell carcinoma, bronchial adenoma, oat-cell carcinoma
Insulin-like peptide	Hypoglycemia	Mesenchymal cell tumors
Glucagon or related peptide	Hyperglycemia	Fibrosarcoma
Prolactin	Galactorrhea (or no symptoms)	Anaplastic-cell carcinoma
Combinations of above	Multiple syndromes	Anaplastic-cell carcinoma

Abbreviations: ACTH = adrenocorticotropic hormone; SIADH = syndrome of inappropriate secretion of antidiuretic hormone; PTH = parathyroid hormone; PGs = prostaglandins; VIP = vasoactive intestinal polypeptide

tionships.[152, 153] Many of the biogenic amines and peptides are capable of provoking release of one another during passage through the pulmonary circulation.

OTHER SPECIAL FUNCTIONS OF THE PULMONARY CIRCULATION[154-156]

Reservoir for Left Ventricle

The pulmonary vessels contain about 900 ml of blood, of which more than half is in readily distensible veins. Since these veins are an extension of the left atrium, they constitute a blood reservoir which supplies blood to fill the left ventricle and maintain its output, even when the right ventricular pump falls behind for a few beats. Thus, the left ventricular stroke volume (output per beat) has been shown to remain unchanged for several beats, even when the pulmonary artery is completely blocked by a balloon. The larger the left atrium and the more distended the pulmonary veins, the more capacious will be the reservoir.

Protective Function

The pulmonary vessels act as a filter to trap and prevent emboli from reaching and blocking systemic arteries, arterioles, or capillaries. Because the lungs can adequately perform their gas exchange function in the presence of a reduced number of conducting and exchanging vessels, blockage of some pulmonary vessels is far better tolerated than blockage of most systemic vessels (e.g., the coronary or cerebral vessels). Pulmonary embolism due to venous thrombosis is not uncommon (500,000 patients per year) and has led to the recommendation that all patients who risk development of perioperative thrombosis (patients with vascular diseases, malignancy, heart failure, varicose veins, immobility, obesity,

advanced age, increased blood viscosity) should be treated with low-dose heparin.[156] Pulmonary fibrin and fat embolism are encountered as a complication of skeletal fractures and burns. Fat emboli may activate the hemostatic mechanism, resulting in a progressively increasing obstruction of the pulmonary microcirculation. Pulmonary platelet emboli are encountered as a complication of a consumption coagulopathy (as in sepsis, abruptio placentae, dead fetus syndrome, amniotic fluid embolism, malignancy, severe hypotension, and in patients with massive blunt trauma). These emboli only dissolve in those disease states in which intravascular clotting was associated with generalized intravascular fibrinolysis, and therefore they usually remain in the microcirculation and can usually be demonstrated at autopsy. The respiratory distress syndrome in premature infants seems to be a combination of hypoxia- and acidosis-induced intravascular clotting, with a failure of the pulmonary fibrinolytic system (which is present in the pulmonary artery endothelial cells) to be activated.

Nutrition

The lungs have an additional arterial blood supply through the bronchial vessels of the systemic circulation. Thus, a lung does not die when its pulmonary artery is ligated. However, recent studies of animals after unilateral pulmonary artery occlusion demonstrated that many alveoli become hemorrhagic and collapse within 1 to 3 days, although they recover later and appear almost normal after some months. Blood flow through the alveolar capillaries is therefore essential for the nutrition of the alveoli and alveolar ducts. In its absence, the bronchial arteries can provide an adequate blood supply to these capillaries through new or expanded channels, but this requires several weeks to fully develop.

MECHANISMS OF PULMONARY ARTERIAL HYPERTENSION IN CLINICAL SITUATIONS

The preceding sections discussed the functional anatomy, physiology, neural reflexes, pharmacology, and special functions of the pulmonary circulation. Pathology or excessive changes in any or all of these characteristics or functions of the pulmonary circulation can result in pulmonary hypertension. The major consequences of pulmonary hypertension are cor pulmonale, formation of pulmonary edema and congestion, and inhibition of pulmonary autoregulation.[11, 12, 45, 86]

Increased Pulmonary Blood Flow (See Cardiac Output Section)

When the cardiac output *acutely* increases (i.e., pharmacologic manipulation, volume loading), pulmonary perfusion pressure should increase. In most studies, flow increases more than the difference between pulmonary artery and pulmonary arterial wedge pressures (the perfusion pressure), so a decrease in vascular resistance is observed. The decrease in vascular resistance may be due both to distention of previously perfused vessels and to recruitment of new vessels. During graded exercise, the pulmonary artery pressure increases maximally during the first level of work load; with subsequent increased levels of exercise, the pressure does not increase substantially. In prolonged exercise with a constant cardiac output, the pulmonary artery pressure slowly decreases from an initially high level, due to decreases either in pulmonary resistance or in left atrial pressure. Another condition associated with a sudden increase in flow in a main pulmonary artery is the acute occlusion or ligation of the other main pulmonary artery. Flow and pressure increase in the only open artery; however, in this circumstance the vascular resistance is probably not decreased.[157]

In *chronic* conditions of increased pulmonary blood flow, the pulmonary artery pressure may remain completely normal. For example, this is the case after pneumonectomy, even in older patients, or after many years in the same patient.[158] Another example of this situation occurs in some congenital heart diseases, especially in pre-tricuspid shunts such as an atrial septal defect, in which a flow of 2 to 3 times normal is associated with a normal pulmonary artery pressure. In these chronic conditions of increased pulmonary blood flow, pulmonary artery pressure is normal and there is a large decrease in pulmonary vascular resistance.

Increased Left Atrial Pressure

An increase in left ventricular pressure, such as occurs with myocardial infarction and other ventricular diseases, causes back-distention and pressure and a passive increase in wedge and pulmonary arterial pressures. The evolution of pulmonary hypertension with mitral stenosis is different and complex. At the beginning of mitral stenosis, there is only a passive transmission of the elevated left atrial pressure to the pulmonary tree. However, even at this stage of the disease, there may be vasoconstriction of the muscular part of the pulmonary vessels. In the second stage, anatomical changes appear in the pulmonary vessels in response to the sustained passive hypertension. These anatomical changes include medial hypertrophy of the muscular arteries and intimal thickening and fibrosis, causing a large gradient from pulmonary arterial diastolic to wedge pressure. It is also possible that an increase in interstitial pressure contributes to the elevation of pulmonary artery pressures. Finally, pulmonary venous occlusive disease should be included as a postcapillary cause of pulmonary hypertension.[157, 159]

Anatomical Changes

Changes in the structure of the arterial wall of the pulmonary vessels may be secondary to a chronic increase in pressure, as in mitral stenosis. However, there are other conditions which are associated with anatomical changes in the pulmonary vessels. In some cases of congenital cardiac defects, especially of the post-tricuspid types (ventricular septal defect, persistent ductus arteriosus), pulmonary hypertension is present from birth. In these cases, the normal decrease in the thickness of the media with decreasing vessel size is interrupted, and medial hypertrophy and increase in smooth muscle in the vascular wall occur.

In many of the hundreds of cases of primary pulmonary hypertension of unknown etiology that have been described, the same pathological changes have been observed without any associated heart defect. However, in addition to intimal fibrosis, an arteritis and a plexiform angiomatoid lesion may be present. The etiology of primary pulmonary hypertension is not known, but suggestions have included persistence of the fetal circulation, collagen vascular disease, familial transmission, and drug-induced or dietary (ingestion of the Crotalaria plant) causes.[138] Recently, abnormalities in the pulmonary circulation in smokers dying suddenly without apparent significant cardiopulmonary disease have been demonstrated for the first time.[160, 161] The changes consisted of thickening of the media of pulmonary arteries less than 500 μm in diameter, increased intimal fibrosis, particularly in arteries less than 200 μm in diameter, and an increase in the number of muscular pulmonary arteries less than 200 μm in diameter. The last observation was attributed to muscularization of partially muscular or wholly nonmuscular pulmonary arteries. Changes in the pulmonary arteries were closely related to both severity of small airway disease and centrilobular emphysema. The arterial changes probably represent a response to regional alveolar hypoxia due to small airway disease and/or emphysema.

Obstruction of Vessels

In diseases associated with the obstruction of pulmonary vessels [thromboembolism, fat embolism, tumor embolism, parasites (schistosomiasis)] an increase in pressure and resistance may be observed.[162] The mechanism of pulmonary hypertension in thromboembolism is due, at least in part, to simple mechanical occlusion of a sufficient number of vessels [in addition to compression of vessels by pulmonary interstitial edema, release of vasoconstrictive substances (e.g., platelet release of serotonin), HPV, or neural reflex vasoconstriction].[162]

Hypoxic Pulmonary Vasoconstriction

This topic was considered in detail in a prior section. The most common and important causes of HPV-induced pulmonary hypertension are acute and chronic severe lung disease and prolonged residence at high altitudes.

Mechanical Compression of Pulmonary Vessels

Pulmonary vessels may be compressed by interstitial fluid or blood and by high positive alveolar pressure. If cardiac output is kept relatively constant, then pulmonary artery hypertension will occur. High positive alveolar pressure may directly compress pulmonary vessels, and there is now evidence to also indicate that excessive distention of a region of the lung (e.g., a lobe) will excessively stretch the extraalveolar vessels in this region, causing a fluid leak into the pulmo-

nary interstitial space.[163] The interstitial fluid
may compress the pulmonary vasculature
and increase pulmonary vascular resistance
(zone 4 conditions).

Transmission of Pressure from the Bronchial Circulation

It is considered likely that in some diseases (bronchiectasis, neoplastic diseases) the
development of anastomosis between the
high-pressure bronchial arteries and the low-
pressure pulmonary circulation could be a
mechanism explaining an increase in pulmonary artery, venous, and wedge pressures.

REFERENCES

1. Horsfield K: Functional morphology of the
   pulmonary circulation, pp 1-18. In Cumming
   G, Bonsignore G, Eds.: Pulmonary Circulation in Health and Disease. Plenum Press,
   New York, 1980
2. Hughes JMB, Glazier JB, Maloney JE, et al:
   Effect of lung volume on the distribution of
   pulmonary blood flow in man. Respir Physiol
   4:58-72, 1968
3. Reid L: Structural and functional reappraisal
   of the pulmonary arterial system. In: The Scientific Basis of Medicine Annual Reviews.
   Athlone Press, London, 1968
4. Blasi A: Bronchial circulation: anatomical
   viewpoint, pp 19-26. In Cumming G, Bonsignore G., Eds: Pulmonary Circulation in
   Health and Disease. Plenum Press, New
   York, 1980
5. Lilker ES, Nagy EJ: Gas exchange in the pulmonary collateral circulation of dogs: effects
   of alveolar hypoxia and systemic hypoxemia.
   Am Rev Respir Dis 112:615-620, 1975
6. Benumof JL: Anesthesia and respiratory
   physiology. In: Miller R, Ed.: Anesthesia.
   Churchill Livingston, New York, 1981
7. Fung YC: The microcirculation as seen by a
   red cell. Microvasc Res 10:246-264, 1975
8. Fung YC, Sobin SS: Theory of sheet flow in
   lung alveoli. J Appl Physiol 26(4):472-488,
   1969
9. West JB, Schneider AM, Mitchell M: Recruitment in networks of pulmonary capillaries. J Appl Physiol 39:976-984, 1975
10. Pietra GG: The basis of pulmonary edema
    with emphasis on ultrastructure, pp. 215-234.
    In: The Lung: IAP Monograph No. 19. Wil-
    liams & Wilkins, Baltimore, 1978
11. Szidon JP, Pietra GG, Fishman AP: The al-
    veolar-capillary membrane and pulmonary
    edema. N Engl J Med 286:1200-1204, 1972
12. Fishman AP: Pulmonary edema: the water
    exchanging function of the lung. Circulation
    46:390-408, 1972
13. Fishman AP: Dynamics of the pulmonary
    circulation, pp. 1167-1743. In Hamilton WF,
    Dow P, Eds: Handbook of Physiology. Vol. 2,
    Sect. 2, Circulation. American Physiological
    Society, Washington, 1963
14. Heath D, Smith P: The pulmonary endothe-
    lial cell. Thorax 34:200-208, 1979
15. Smith U, Ryan JW: Electron microscopy of
    endothelial components of the lungs: correla-
    tions of structure and function. Fed Proc
    32:1957-1966, 1973
16. Permutt S: Effect of interstitial pressure of the
    lung on pulmonary circulation. Med Thorac
    22:118-131, 1965
17. Staub NC: "State of the Art" review. Patho-
    genesis of pulmonary edema. Am Rev Respir
    Dis 109:358-372, 1974
18. Hales CA, Kazemi H: Small airways function
    in myocardial infarction. N Engl J Med
    290:761-768, 1974
19. Harken AH, O'Conner NE: The influence of
    clinically undetectable edema on small air-
    way closure in the dog. Ann Surg 184:183-
    188, 1976
20. Biddle TL, Yu PN, Hodges M, et al: Hypoxe-
    mia and lung water in acute myocardial in-
    farction. Am Heart J 92:692-699, 1976
21. Guyton AC: A concept of negative interstitial
    pressure based on pressures in implanted per-
    forated capsules. Circ Res 12:399-410, 1963
22. Staub NC: Pulmonary edema: physiologic
    approaches to management. Chest 74:559-
    564, 1978
23. West JB, Dollery CT: Distribution of blood
    flow and ventilation-perfusion ratio in the
    lung measured with radioactive CO_2. J Appl
    Physiol 15:405-410, 1960
24. Permutt S, Bronberger-Barnea B, Bane HN:
    Alveolar pressure, pulmonary venous pres-
    sure, and the vascular waterfall. Med Thorac
    19:239-266, 1962

25. West JB, Dollery CT, Naimark A: Distribution of blood flow in isolated lung, relation to vascular and alveolar pressures. J Appl Physiol 19:713-724, 1964

26. West JB: Ventilation/Blood Flow and Gas Exchange. 2nd Ed. Blackwell Scientific Publications, Oxford, 1970

27. Hoppin FG Jr, Green ID, Mead J: Distribution of pleural pressure surface pressure. J Appl Physiol 27:863-873, 1969

28. West JB, Dollery CT, Heard BE: Increased pulmonary vascular resistance in the dependent zone of the isolated dog lung caused by perivascular edema. Circ Res 17:191-206, 1965

29. Hughes JMB, Glazier JB, Maloney JE, et al: Effect of lung volume on the distribution of pulmonary blood flow in man. Respir Physiol 4:58-72, 1968

30. Hughes JM, Glazier JB, Maloney JE, et al: Effect of extra-alveolar vessels on the distribution of blood flow in the dog lung. J Appl Physiol 25:701-709, 1968

31. West JB, Ed.: Regional Differences in the Lung. Academic Press, New York, San Francisco, London, 1977

32. Permutt S, Caldini P, Maseri A et al.: Recruitment versus distensibility in the pulmonary vascular bed, pp. 375-387. In Fishman AP, Hecht H, Eds: The Pulmonary Circulation and Interstitial Space. University of Chicago Press, Chicago, 1969.

33. Maseri A, Caldini P, Harward P et al.: Determinants of pulmonary vascular volume. Recruitment versus distensibility. Circ Res 31:218-228, 1972

34. Simmons DH, Linde CM, Miller JH et al.: Relation of lung volume and pulmonary vascular resistance. Circ Res 9:465-471, 1961

35. Burton AC, Patel DJ: Effect on pulmonary vascular resistance of inflation of the rabbit lungs. J Appl Physiol 12:239-247, 1958

36. Wittenberger JL, McGregor M, Berglund E et al: Influence of state of inflation of the lung on pulmonary vascular resistance. J Appl Physiol 15:878, 1960.

37. Benumof JL: Mechanism of decreased blood flow to the atelectatic lung. J Appl Physiol 46:1047-1048, 1978

38. Pirlo AF, Benumof JL, Trousdale FR: Atelectatic lobe blood flow: open vs. closed chest, positive pressure vs. spontaneous ventilation. J Appl Physiol 50:1022-1026, 1981

39. Bohr D: The pulmonary hypoxic response. Chest 71(2 Feb. Suppl), 244-246, 1977

40. Bergofsky EH: Ions and membrane permeability in the regulation of the pulmonary circulation, pp 269-285. In Fishman AP, Hecht H, Eds: The Pulmonary Circulation and Interstitial Space. 1969

41. Bergofsky EH: Mechanisms underlying vasomotor regulation of regional pulmonary blood flow in normal and disease states. Am J Med 57:378-391, 1974

42. Fishman AP: Hypoxia on the pulmonary circulation—how and where it works. Circ Res 38:221-231, 1976

43. Benumof JL, Mathers JM, Wahrenbrock EA: The pulmonary interstitial compartment and the mediator of hypoxic pulmonary vasoconstriction. Microvas Res 15(1):69-75, 1978

44. Doyle JT, Wilson JS, Warren JV: The pulmonary vascular responses to short-term hypoxia in human subjects. Circulation 5:263-270, 1952

45. Fishman AP: State of the Art. Chronic cor pulmonale. Am Rev Respir Dis 114:775-794, 1976

46. Boysen PG, Block AJ, Wynne JW et al.: Nocturnal pulmonary hypertension in patients with chronic obstructive pulmonary disease. Chest 76:536-542, 1979

47. Zasslow MA, Benumof JL, Trousdale FR: Hypoxic pulmonary vasoconstriction and the size of the hypoxic compartment. Anesthesiology 55:A379, 1981

48. Marshall BE, Marshall C: Continuity of response to hypoxic pulmonary vasoconstriction. J Appl Physiol 49(2):189-196, 1980

49. Grant JL, Naylor RW, Crandell WB: Bronchial adenoma resection with relief of hypoxic pulmonary vasoconstriction. Chest 77:446-449, 1980

50. Benumof JL: Physiology of the open chest and one-lung ventilation. In Kaplan JA: Thoracic Anesthesia, Churchill Livingstone, New York, 1982

51. Arborelius J Jr, Lilja B, Zauner CW: The relative effect of hypoxia and gravity on pulmonary blood flow. Respiration 31:369-380, 1974

52. Gazioglu K, Katreider N, Hyde R: Effect of isoproterenol on gas exchange during oxygen breathing in patients with chronic pulmonary diseases. Am Rev Respir Dis 104:188-194, 1971

53. Kochukoshy KN, Chick TW, Jenne JW: The

effect of nitroglycerin in gas exchange on chronic obstructive pulmonary disease. Am Rev Respir Dis 111:117-183, 1975

54. Pain MCF, Charlton GC, Read J: Effect of intravenous aminophylline on distribution of pulmonary blood flow in obstructive lung disease. Am Rev Respir Dis 95:1005-1018, 1967

55. Chick TW, Nicholson DP, Johnson AL Jr: Effects of isoproterenol on distribution of ventilation and perfusion in asthma. Am Rev Respir Dis 107:869-874, 1973

56. Knudson RJ, Constantine HP: An effect of isoproterenol on ventilation—perfusion in asthmatic versus normal subjects. J Appl Physiol 22:402-406, 1967

57. Tai E, Read J: Response of blood gas tensions to aminophylline and isoprenaline in patients with asthma. Thorax 22:543-549, 1967

58. Saunders CA, Hawthorne JW, Heitman H et al: Effect of vasopressor administration on blood gas exchange in mitral disease. Clin Res 13:351-358, 1965

59. Mookherjee S, Fulethan O, Warner RF et al: Effects of sublingual nitroglycerin on resting pulmonary gas exchange and hemodynamics in man. Am J Cardiol 57:106-110, 1978

60. Hales C, Slate J, Westphal D: Blockade of alveolar hypoxic pulmonary vasoconstriction by sodium nitroprusside and nitroglycerin (Abstr). Am Rev Respir Dis 115:335, 1977

61. Mookherjee S, Warner R, Keighley J et al: Worsening of ventilation-perfusion relationship in the face of hemodynamic improvement during nitroprusside infusion (Abstr) Am J Cardiol 39:282, 1977

62. Chatterjee K, Parmley WW, Ganz W et al: Hemodynamic and metabolic responses to vasodilator therapy in acute myocardial infarction. Circulation 48:1183-1193, 1973

63. Berkowitz C, McKeever L, Croke RP et al: Comparative responses to dobutamine and nitroprusside in patients with low output cardiac failure. Circulation 56:918-924, 1977

64. Wildsmith JAW, Drummond GB, Macrae WR: Blood gas changes during induced hypotension with sodium nitroprusside. Br J Anaesth 47:1205-1211, 1975

65. Veltzer JL, Doto JO, Jacoby J: Depressed arterial oxygenation during sodium nitroprusside administration for intraoperative hypertension. Anesth Analg (Cleve) 55:880-881, 1976

66. Brodie TS, Gray R, Swan HJC et al: Effect of nitroprusside on arterial oxygenation, intrapulmonic shunts and oxygen delivery (Abstr). Am J Cardiol 37:123, 1976

67. Benumof JL; Hypoxic pulmonary vasoconstriction and sodium nitroprusside infusion. (Editorial) Anesthesiology 50:481-483, 1979

68. Benumof JL, Wahrenbrock EA: Local effects of anesthetics on regional hypoxic pulmonary vasoconstriction. Anesthesiology 43:525-532, 1975

69. Mathers JM, Benumof JL, Wahrenbrock EA: General anesthetics and regional hypoxic pulmonary vasoconstriction. Anesthesiology 46:111-114, 1977

70. Sykes MK, Hurtig JB, Tait AR, et al: Reduction of hypoxic pulmonary vasoconstriction in the dog during administration of nitrous oxide. Br J Anaesth 49:301-307, 1977

71. Sykes MK, Gibbs JM, Loh L et al.: Preservation of the pulmonary vasoconstrictor response to alveolar hypoxia during the administration of halothane to dogs. Br J Anaesth 50:1185-1196, 1978

72. Bjertnas LJ, Hauge A, Nakken KF, et al: Hypoxic pulmonary vasoconstriction: inhibition due to anesthesia. Acta Physiol Scand 96:283-285, 1976

73. Bredesen J, Bjertnaes L, Hauge A: Effects of anesthetics on the pulmonary vasoconstrictor response to acute alveolar hypoxia. Microvasc Res 10:236-241, 1975

74. Sykes MK, Davies DM; Loh L et al.: The effect of methoxyflurane on pulmonary vascular resistance and hypoxic pulmonary vasoconstriction in the isolated perfused cat lung. Br J Anaesth 48:191-194, 1976

75. Sykes MK, Davies DM, Chakrabarti MK, et al: The effects of halothane, trichlorethylene and ether on the hypoxic pressor response and pulmonary vascular resistance in the isolated, perfused cat lung. Br J Anaesth 45:655-663, 1973

76. Sykes MK, Arnot RN, Jastrzebski J et al: Reduction of hypoxic pulmonary vasoconstriction during trichlorethylene anesthesia. J Appl Physiol 39(1):103-106, 1975

77. Sykes MK, Hurtig JB, Tait AR, et al: Reduction of hypoxic pulmonary vasoconstriction during diethyl ether anesthesia in the dog. Br J Anaesth 49:293-299, 1977

78. Bjertnas LJ: Hypoxia-induced vasoconstriction in isolated perfused lungs exposed to in-

jectable or inhalation anesthetics. Acta Anaesthesiol Scand 21:133-147, 1977

79. Bjertnas LJ, Hauge A, Kriz M: Hypoxia—induced pulmonary vasoconstriction: effects of
fentanyl following different routes of administration. Acta Anaesthesiol Scand 24:53-57,
1980

80. Weinreich AI, Silvay G, Lumb PD: Continuous ketamine infusion for one lung anesthesia. Can Anaesth Soc J 27:485-490, 1980

81. Benumof JL, Pirlo AF, Trousdale FR: Inhibition of hypoxic pulmonary vasoconstriction
by decreased P_vO_2: a new indirect mechanism. J Appl Physiol 51:871-874, 1981

82. Benumof JL, Mathers JM, Wahrenbrock EA:
Cyclic hypoxic pulmonary vasoconstriction
induced by concomitant carbon dioxide
changes. J Appl Physiol 41:466-469, 1976

83. Irwin RS, Martinex-Gonzalez-Rio H, Thomas
HM II et al: The effect of granulomatous pulmonary disease in dogs on the response of the
pulmonary circulation hypoxia. J Clin Invest
60:1258-1265, 1977

84. Light RB, Mink SN, Wood LDH: Pathophysiology of gas exchange and pulmonary perfusion in pneumococcal lobar pneumonia in
dogs. J Appl Physiol 50(3):524-530, 1981

85. Borst HG, McGregor M, Whittenberger JL et
al: Influence of pulmonary arterial and left
atrial pressures on pulmonary vascular resistance. Circ Res 4:393-399, 1956

86. Benumof JL, Wahrenbrock EA: Blunted hypoxic pulmonary vasoconstriction by increased lung vascular pressure. J Appl Physiol 38:840-850, 1975

87. Ward CF, Benumof JL, Wahrenbrock EA:
Inhibition of hypoxic pulmonary vasoconstriction by vasoactive drugs. Abstracts of Scientific Papers, 1976 Annual Meeting, Am Soc
Anesthesiol 333-334, 1976

88. Scanlon TS, Benumof JL, Wahrenbrock EA
et al: Hypoxic pulmonary vasoconstriction
and the ratio of hypoxic lung to perfused normoxic lung. Anesthesiology 49:177-181, 1978

89. Marshall BE, Marshall C, Benumof JL, et al:
Hypoxic pulmonary vasoconstriction in dogs:
effects of lung segment size and alveolar oxygen tensions. J Appl Physiol 51:1543-1551,
1981

90. Johansen I, Benumof JL: Flow distribution in
abnormal lung as a function of F_IO_2. Anesthesiology 51(3S):369, 1979

91. Benumof JL, Rogers LSN, Moyce PR et al:
Hypoxic pulmonary vasoconstriction and
regional and whole lung PEEP in the dog.
Anesthesiology 51(6):503-507, 1979

92. Zapol WM, Snider MT: Pulmonary hypertension in severe acute respiratory failure. N
Engl J Med 296:476-480, 1977

93. Benumof JL: The pulmonary circulation: relation to ARDS. 1977 Annual Refresher
Course Lecture. American Society of Anesthesiologists 132:1-14, 1977

94. Donald DE, Shepherd JT: Reflexes from the
heart and lungs: physiological curiosities or
important regulatory mechanisms. Cardiovasc Res 12:449-469, 1978

95. Uchida Y: Afferent sympathetic nerve fibres
with mechanoreceptors in the right heart.
Am J Physiol 228:223-230, 1975

96. Malliani A, Parks M, Tuckett RP, et al: Reflex increases in heart rate elicited by stimulation of afferent cardiac sympathetic nerve
fibers in the cat. Circ Res 32:9-14, 1973

97. Hess GL, Zuperku EJ, Coon RL, et al: Sympathetic afferent nerve activity of left ventricular origin. Am J Physiol 227:543-546,
1974

98. Lombardi F, Malliani A, Pagani M: Nervous activity of afferent sympathetic fibres
innervating the pulmonary veins. Brain Res
113:197-200, 1976

99. Folkow B, Neil E, Eds, pp. 320-339. In: Circulation, Oxford University Press, Oxford,
1971

100. Malliani A, Peterson DF, Bishop VS, et al:
Spinal sympathetic cardiovascular reflexes.
Circ Res 30:158-166, 1972

101. Malliani A, Recordati G, Schwartz PJ: Nervous activity of afferent cardiac sympathetic
fibres with atrial and ventricular endings. J
Physiol 229:457-469, 1973

102. Lloyd TC, Jr: Reflex effects of left heart and
pulmonary vascular distention of airways of
dogs. J Appl Physiol 49(4):620-626, 1980

103. Anderson FL, Brown AM: Pulmonary vasoconstriction elicited by stimulation of the
hypothalamic integrative area for the defense reaction. Circ Res 21:747-756, 1967

104. Laks MM, Juratsch CE, Garner D et al:
Acute pulmonary artery hypertension produced by distention of the main pulmonary
artery in the conscious dog. Chest 68:807-
813, 1975

105. Szidon JP, Fishman AP: Autonomic control
of the pulmonary circulation, pp. 239-265.

In Fishman AP, Hecht HH, Eds: Pulmonary Circulation and Interstitial Space. University of Chicago Press, Chicago, 1969

106. Maloney JE, Bergel DH, Glazier JB et al: Transmission of pulsatile blood pressure and flow through the isolated lung. Circ Res 23:11-24, 1968

107. Franklin DL, Van Citters RL, Rushmer RF: Balance between right and left ventricular output. Circ Res 10:17-26, 1962

108. Varnauskas E: The effect of physical exercise on pulmonary blood volume, pp. 105-111. In Muller C Ed: Conference on Pulmonary Circulation. Scandinavian University Books, Oslo, 1965

109. Bakhle YUS, Vane JR, Eds: Metabolic functions of the lung. Vol 4 In: Lung Biology in Health and Disease. Marcel Dekker, Inc. New York, 1977

110. Marchesi VT, Barrnett RJ: The demonstration of enzymatic activity in pinocytotic vesicles of blood capillaries with the electron microscope. J Cell Biol 17:547-556, 1963

111. Smith U, Ryan JW: Pulmonary endothelial cells and metabolism of adenine nucleotides, kinins and angiotensin I. In Back N, Sicuteri F, Eds: Advances in Experimental Medicine and Biology. Vol 21. Vasopeptides, pp. 267-276. Plenum Press, New York, 1972

112. Tierney DF: Lung metabolism and biochemistry. Ann Rev Physiol 36:209-231, 1974

113. Fishman AP, Pietra GG: Handling of bioactive materials by the lung. N Engl J Med 291:Pt 1, 884-890, 1974

114. Tucker A, Weir KE, Grover RF, et al: Oxygen-tension-dependent pulmonary vascular responses to vasoactive agents. Can J Physiol Pharmacol 55:251-257, 1977

115. Vader CR, Mathias MM, Schatte CL: Pulmonary prostaglandin metabolism during normobaric hyperoxia. Prostaglandins Med 6:101-110, 1981

116. Harabin AL, Peake MD, Sylvester JT: Effect of severe hypoxia on the pulmonary vascular response to vasoconstrictor agents. J Appl Physiol 50(3)561-565, 1981

117. Leuenberger PJ, Stalcup SA, Mellins RB et al: Decrease in angiotension I conversion by acute hypoxia in dogs. Proc Soc Exp Biol Med 158:586-592, 1978

118. Junod AF: Metabolism of vasoactive agents in lung. Am Rev Respir Dis 115:51-57, 1977

119. Junod AF: Metabolism, production and release of hormones and mediators in the lung. Am Rev Respir Dis 112(1):92-108, 1975

120. Fishman AP, Pietra GG: Handling of bioactive materials by the lung (Part 2). N Engl J Med 291:953-959, 1974

121. Gillis CN: Metabolism of vasoactive hormones by the lung. Anesthesiology 39(6):626-632, 1973

122. Dollery CT, Glazier JB: Pharmacological effects of drugs on the pulmonary circulation in man. Clin Pharmacol Ther 7:807-818, 1966

123. Barer GR, McCurrie JR: Pulmonary vasomotor responses in the cat: the effects and interrelationship of drugs, hypoxia and hypercapnia. Q J Exp Physiol 54:156-167, 1969

124. Bakhle YS, Bloch AJ: Effects of halothane on pulmonary inactivation of noradrenaline and prostaglandin E_2 in anaesthetized dogs. Clin Sci Mol Med 50:87-90, 1976

125. Ferreira SH, Vane JR: Half-lives of peptides and amines in the circulation. Nature 215:1237-1240, 1967

126. Alabaster VA, Bakhle YS: The inactivation of bradykinin in the pulmonary circulation of isolated lungs. Br J Pharmacol 45:299-309, 1972

127. Melmon KL, Cline MJ, Hughes T, et al: Kinins: Possible mediators of neonatal circulatory changes in man. J Clin Invest 47:1279-1302, 1968

128. Dorer FE, Kahn JR, Lentz KE et al: Hydrolysis of bradykinin by angiotensin-converting enzyme. Circ Res 34:824-827, 1974

129. Ng KKF, Vane JR: Fate of angiotensin I in the circulation. Nature 218:144-150, 1968

130. Curtiss C, Cohn JN, Vrobel T, et al: Role of the renin-angiotensin system in the systemic vasoconstriction of chronic congestive heart failure. Circulation 58:763-770, 1978

131. Garvas H, Faxon DP, Berkoben J et al: Angiotensin converting enzyme inhibition in patients with congestive heart failure. Circulation 50:770-776, 1978

132. Davis R, Ribner HS, Keung E et al: Treatment of chronic congestive heart failure with captopril, an oral inhibitor of angiotensin-converting enzyme. N Engl J Med 301:117-121, 1979

133. Dzau VJ, Colucci WS, Williams GH et al.: Sustained effectiveness of converting-en-

zyme inhibition in patients with severe congestive heart failure. N Engl J Med 302:1373-1378, 1980

134. Hyman AL, Spannhake EW, Kadowitz PJ: Prostaglandins and the lung. Am Rev Respir Dis 117:111-136, 1977

135. Kadowitz PJ, Joiner PD, Hyman AL: Physiological and pharmacological roles of prostaglandins. Ann Rev Pharmacol 15:285-299, 1975

136. Kadowitz PJ, Spannhake EW, Knight DS, et al: Vasoactive hormones in the pulmonary vascular bed. Chest suppl, 71:257-263, 1977

137. Vane JR: Inhibitors of prostaglandin, prostacyclin and thromboxane synthesis, pp 27-44. In: Advances in Prostaglandin and Thomboxane Research, Vol IV, 1978, Raven Press, New York

138. Bakhle YS, Vane JR: Pharmocokinetic function of the pulmonary circulation. Physiol Rev 54:1007-1045, 1974

139. Pang JA, Williams TR, Blackburn JP et al.: First pass lung uptake of propranolol enhanced in anesthetized dogs. Br J Anesth 53:601-604, 1981

140. Fishman AP: Dietary pulmonary hypertension. Circ Res 35:657-660, 1974

141. Clark DG, McElligott TF, Hurst EW: The toxicity of paraquat. Br J Ind Med 23:126-132, 1966

142. Robertson B, Enhorning G, Ivemark B et al: Experimental respiratory distress induced by paraquat. J Pathol 103:239-244, 1971

143. Austen KF, Systemic anaphylaxis in the human being. N Engl J Med 291:661-664, 1974

144. Pavek K: Anaphylactic shock in the monkey: its hemodynamics and mediators. Acta Anaesthesiol Scand 21:293-307, 1977

145. Said SI: Endocrine role of the lung in disease. Am J Med 57:453-465, 1974

146. Lipsett MB: Hormonal syndromes associated with neoplasia. Adv Metab Disord 3:111-152, 1968

147. Piper PJ, Vane JR: The release of prostaglandins from the lung and other tissues. Ann NY Acad Sci 180:363-385, 1971

148. Andersen HW, Benumof JL: Intrapulmonary shunting during one-lung ventilation and surgical manipulation. Anesthesiology 55:A377, 1981

149. Said SI, Kitamura S, Vreim C: Prostaglandins: release from the lung during mechanical ventilation at large tidal volumes. J Clin Invest 51:83A, 1972

150. Kitamura S, Preskitt J, Yoshida T, et al: Prostaglandin release, respiratory alkalosis and systemic hypertension during mechanical ventilation. Fed Proc 32:341-345, 1973

151. Said SI, Yoshida T: Release of prostaglandins and other humoral mediators during hypoxic breathing and pulmonary edema. Chest 66:12S, 1974

152. Said SI, Hara N, Yoshida T: Hypoxic pulmonary vasoconstriction in cats: modification by aspirin and indomethacin. Fed Proc 34:438-444, 1975

153. Said SI, Yoshida T, Kitamura S, et al: Pulmonary alveolar hypoxia: release of prostaglandins and other humoral mediators. Science, 185:1181-1185, 1974

154. Fishman AP: Nonrespiratory functions of the lungs. Chest 72(1):84-89, 1977

155. Heinemann HO, Fishman AP: Nonrespiratory functions of the mammalian lung. Physiol Rev 49:1-47, 1969

156. Mammen EF: Blood coagulation and pulmonary function, pp 91-106. In Dal Santo G, Ed.: Nonrespiratory Functions of the Lung and Anesthesia, Vol 15, No 4, Little Brown & Company, 1977

157 Harris P, Heath D: The Human Pulmonary Circulation. Churchill Livingstone, Edinburgh, 1977

158. Denolin H: Contribution à l'étude de la circulation pulmonaire en clinique. Acta Cardiol (Brux) Suppl X, 1961

159. Wagenvoort CA, Wagenvoort N: Pathology of pulmonary hypertension. John Wiley & Sons, New York, 1977

160. Hale KA, Niewolhner DE, Cosio MG: Morphologic changes in the muscular pulmonary arteries: relationship to cigarette smoking, airways disease, and emphysema. Am Rev Respir Dis 122:273-278, 1980

161. Thurlbeck WM: Smoking, airflow limitation, and the pulmonary circulation. Am Rev Respir Dis 122:183-186, 1980

162. Enson Y: Pulmonary heart disease: relation of pulmonary hypertension to abnormal lung structure and function. Bull NY Acad Med 53:551-566, 1977

163. Albert R, Lakshminarayan KS, Kirk W, et al: Lung inflation can cause pulmonary edema in zone I of in-situ dog lungs. J Appl Physiol 49(5):815-819, 1980

Jonathan L. Benumof, M.D.

8
Physiology of the Open Chest and One-lung Ventilation

Patients undergoing thoracic surgery usually are in the lateral decubitus position under general anesthesia, have an open chest wall, and are pharmacologically paralyzed. Compared with the awake state in the upright position, all these anesthesia and surgical requirements (lateral decubitus position, general anesthesia, open pleural space, and paralysis) can cause major alterations in the distribution of perfusion (Q), ventilation (V), and ventilation-perfusion relationships (V/Q). The first part of this chapter will discuss each one of these anesthetic and surgical effects on the distribution of Q, V, and V/Q, as well as consider the physiological consequences of spontaneous ventilation with an open chest.

In addition, a good deal of thoracic surgery must be performed with the operated lung being either nonventilated (nonmoving) and/or functionally or physically separated from the ventilated, dependent lung. This is most easily accomplished by the insertion of a double-lumen tube. Via blockade of one airway lumen, the nondependent or surgical lung is deliberately not ventilated, and via the other airway lumen, the dependent or nonsurgical lung is ventilated (one-lung ventilation). One-lung ventilation imposes a new host of determinants on the distribution of blood flow (and of course ventilation), and the second part of this chapter will consider the physiology of one-lung ventilation. Based on this physiology, the initial management, as well as special and promising new one-lung ventilation management techniques, will be described.

PHYSIOLOGY OF THE OPEN CHEST

Distribution of Perfusion, Ventilation, Ventilation-Perfusion Ratio—Awake, Closed Chest

UPRIGHT POSITION

Distribution of Perfusion

The contraction of the right ventricle imparts kinetic energy to the blood in the main pulmonary artery. As some of the kinetic energy in the main pulmonary artery is dissipated in climbing a vertical hydrostatic

287

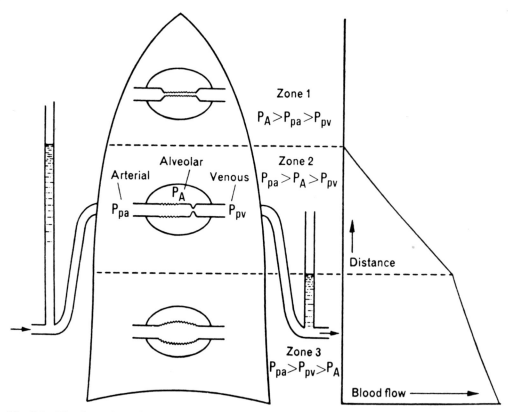

Fig. 8-1 The figure is a schematic which accounts for the distribution of blood flow in the isolated lung. In zone 1, alveolar pressure (PA) exceeds pulmonary artery pressure (Ppa) and no flow occurs because the vessels are collapsed. In zone 2, arterial pressure exceeds alveolar pressure, but alveolar pressure exceeds pulmonary venous pressure (Ppv). Flow in zone 2 is determined by the arterial-alveolar pressure difference (Ppa−PA), which steadily increases down the zone. In zone 3, pulmonary venous pressure now exceeds alveolar pressure and flow is determined by the arterial-venous pressure difference (Ppa−Ppv), which is constant down this zone of the lung. However, the pressure across the walls of the vessels increases down the zone, so that their caliber increases and so does flow. (Redrawn by permission from West JB, Dollery CT, Naimark A: Distribution of blood flow in isolated lung: Relation to vascular and alveolar pressures. J. Appl Physiol 19:713-724, 1964.)

gradient, the absolute pressure in the pulmonary artery (Ppa) decreases by 1 cm H_2O per cm of vertical distance up the lung (Fig. 8-1). At some height, Ppa becomes zero (atmospheric), and still higher in the lung it becomes negative.[1] In this region of the lung, alveolar pressure (PA) exceeds Ppa and pulmonary venous pressure (Ppv) which is very negative at this vertical height. The pulmonary vessels in this region of the lung are compressed and collapsed by the PA, and there is no blood flow (zone 1) (Fig. 8-1).

Further down the lung absolute Ppa becomes positive and blood flow begins when Ppa exceeds PA (zone 2). At this vertical level in the lung, PA still exceeds Ppv and the amount of blood flow is determined by the Ppa − PA difference rather than the more conventional Ppa − Ppv difference (see below).[2] Since Ppa increases linearly down this region of the lung but PA is constant, the driving pressure (Ppa − PA), and therefore the blood flow, increases linearly.

Finally, near the bottom of the lung

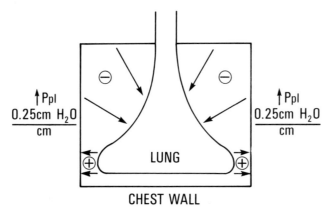

Fig. 8-2 This schematic of the lung within the chest wall shows the tendency of the lung to assume a globular shape. The tendency of the top of the lung to collapse inward creates a relative vacuum (negative pressure) at the apex of the lung, and the tendency of the bottom of the lung to spread outward creates a relatively positive pressure at the base of the lung. Thus, pleural pressure increases by 0.25 cm of water per centimeter of lung dependency.

there is a vertical level where Ppv becomes positive and also exceeds Pa. In this region of the lung blood flow is governed by the pulmonary arteriovenous pressure difference (Ppa − Ppv) (zone 3). In this zone both these vascular pressures exceed Pa, and capillary systems are thus permanently open and blood flow is continuous. Descending zone 3 causes both absolute Ppa and Ppv to increase at the same rate, so that the perfusion pressure (Ppa − Ppv) is unchanged. However, the pressure outside the vessels, namely the pleural pressure (Ppl), increases at a lower rate than Ppa and Ppv so that the transmural distending pressures [(Ppa − Ppl) and (Ppv − Ppl)] increase down zone 3. The vessel radii also increase, vascular resistance decreases, and blood flow therefore increases further.

Distribution of Ventilation

The lung is a viscoelastic organ which, if suspended at the hilum *without* the presence of a surrounding and *supporting* chest wall, would assume a globular shape, where the apex of the lung would be very narrow and the base of the lung would be very broad. The tendency to assume a globular shape in the presence of an intact chest wall is expressed by the creation of a negative pleural pressure at the top of the lung (where the lung pulls away from the chest wall) and a relatively positive pleural pressure at the bottom of the lung (where the lung is compressed against the chest wall) (Fig. 8-2).

Gravity therefore causes pleural pressure (Ppl) to increase (become more positive) as lung dependency increases.[3] Since Pa is the same throughout the lung, the Ppl gradient causes regional differences in transpulmonary distending pressures (Pa − Ppl). Since Ppl is most positive (least negative) in the dependent basilar lung regions, alveoli in these regions are more compressed and therefore are considerably smaller than the superior, relatively noncompressed apical alveoli (approximately fourfold volume difference). If the regional differences in alveolar volume are translated to a pressure-volume curve for a normal lung (Fig. 8-3), the dependent small alveoli are on the midportion and the nondependent large alveoli are on the upper portion of the S-shaped or sigmoid

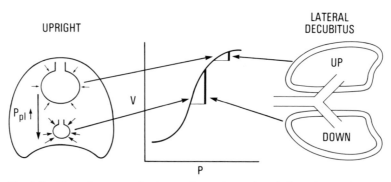

Fig. 8-3 Pleural pressure in the awake patient (closed chest) is most positive in the dependent portion of the lung, and alveoli in this region are
therefore most compressed and have the least volume. Pleural pressure is
least positive (most negative) at the apex of the lung, and alveoli in this region are therefore least compressed and have the largest volume. When
these regional differences in alveolar volume are translated over to a regional transpulmonary pressure–alveolar volume curve, the small dependent alveoli are on a steep (large-slope) portion of the curve and the large
nondependent alveoli are on a flat (small-slope) portion of the curve. In
this diagram regional slope equals regional compliance. Thus, for a given
and equal change in transpulmonary pressure, the dependent part of the
lung receives a much larger share of the tidal volume than the nondependent part of the lung. In the lateral decubitus position (right-hand side of
diagram) gravity also causes pleural pressure gradients and therefore similarly affects the distribution of ventilation. The dependent lung lies on a
relatively steep portion and the upper lung lies on a relatively flat portion
of the pressure-volume curve. Thus, in the lateral decubitus position the
dependent lung receives the majority of the tidal ventilation.

pressure-volume curve. Since the different
regional slopes of the composite curve are
equal to the different regional lung compliances, dependent alveoli are very compliant
(steep slope) and nondependent alveoli are
noncompliant (flat slope). Thus, the majority
of the tidal volume is preferentially distributed to dependent alveoli since they expand
more per unit pressure change than nondependent alveoli.[4]

Distribution of Ventilation-to-Perfusion
(V_A/Q) Ratio

The preceding two sections established
that both perfusion and ventilation increase
with lung dependency. Figure 8-4 shows that
the increase in both blood flow and ventilation (left-hand vertical axis) is linear with
distance down the normal upright lung

(horizontal axis, from the top to the bottom
of the lung).[5] Since blood flow increases
more rapidly than ventilation with distance
down the lung, the ventilation-perfusion
ratio (V_A/Q) (right-hand vertical axis),
where V_A is alveolar ventilation, decreases
rapidly at first and then more slowly. The
degree of overperfusion or underventilation
of alveoli is most conveniently expressed in
terms of the V_A/Q ratio. Thus, alveoli at the
base of the lung are somewhat overperfused
in relation to their ventilation ($V_A/Q < 1$),
whereas the alveoli at the apex are greatly
underperfused in relation to their ventilation
($V_A/Q > 1$). The relative overperfusion and
underventilation of the dependent lung
causes this region to be relatively hypoxic
and hypercapnic, whereas the relative over-
ventilation and underperfusion of the nondependent lung causes this region to be

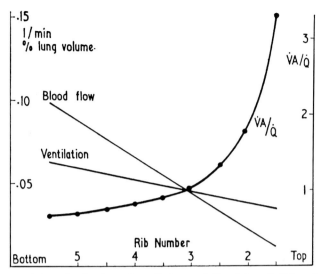

Fig. 8-4 Distribution of ventilation and blood flow (left-hand vertical axis) and the ventilation-perfusion ratio (right-hand vertical axis) in normal upright lung as a function of lung dependency (abscissa). Both blood flow and ventilation are expressed in liters/min percent alveolar volume and have been drawn as smoothed-out linear functions of vertical height. Both blood flow and ventilation increase with lung dependency but blood flow increases more than ventilation so the ventilation-perfusion ratio decreases. The closed circles mark the ventilation-perfusion ratios of horizontal lung slices (three of which are shown in Fig. 8-5). A cardiac output of 6 liters/min and a total minute ventilation of 5.1 liters/min was assumed. (Reproduced with permission from West, JB: Ventilation/Blood Flow and Gas Exchange, 2nd Ed. Blackwell Scientific Publications, Oxford and Edinburgh, 1970.)

relatively hyperoxic and hypocapnic (Fig. 8-5).[6]

LATERAL DECUBITUS POSITION

Gravity causes a vertical gradient in the distribution of pulmonary blood flow in the lateral decubitus position for the same reason that it does in the upright position. Consequently, blood flow to the dependent lung is much greater than blood flow to the nondependent lung (Fig. 8-6).

Since gravity also still causes a vertical gradient in Ppl in the lateral decubitus position, ventilation is relatively increased in the dependent lung compared with the nonde-

pendent lung. In addition, in the lateral decubitus position the dome of the lower lung diaphragm is pushed higher into the chest than the dome of the upper lung diaphragm. Consequently, the lower diaphragm is more cephalad and therefore more sharply curved than the upper diaphragm. As a result, the lower diaphragm is able to contract more efficiently during spontaneous respiration. Thus, in the lateral decubitus position in the awake patient, the lower lung is normally better ventilated than the upper lung, regardless of the side on which the patient is lying, although there remains a tendency towards greater ventilation of the larger right lung.[7] Since blood flow to the lungs is also

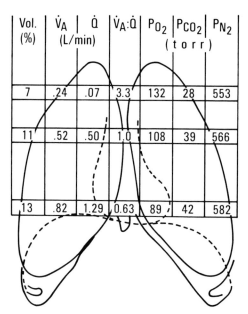

Vol. (%)	$\dot{V}_A$ (L/min)	$\dot{Q}$	$\dot{V}_A{:}\dot{Q}$	P_{O_2}	P_{CO_2}	P_{N_2} (torr)
7	.24	.07	3.3	132	28	553
11	.52	.50	1.0	108	39	566
13	.82	1.29	0.63	89	42	582

Fig. 8-5 The ventilation-perfusion ratio and the regional composition of alveolar gas. Values for the regional flow, ventilation, P_{O_2} and P_{CO_2} are derived from Figure 8-4. P_{N_2} has been obtained by the difference from the total gas pressure (which, including water vapor, equals 760 torr). The volumes of the three lung slices are also shown. Compared with the top of the lung, the bottom of the lung has a low ventilation-perfusion ratio and is relatively hypoxic and hypercapnic. (Reproduced with permission from West JB: Regional differences in gas exchange in the lung of erect man. J Appl Physiol 17:893-898, 1962.)

influenced by gravity in this position, there is also greater perfusion to the lower lung. The preferential ventilation to the lower lung, then, is matched by its increased perfusion, so that the distribution of the ventilation-perfusion ratios of the two lungs is not greatly altered when the awake subject assumes the lateral position.

Distribution of Perfusion and Ventilation—Lateral Decubitus Position, Anesthetized, Closed Chest

Compared to a patient in the lateral decubitus position in the awake state, the induction of general anesthesia alone does not cause any alteration in the distribution of pulmonary blood flow between the dependent and nondependent lungs. Thus, in the anesthetized patient, the dependent lung continues to receive relatively more perfusion than the nondependent lung. The induction of general anesthesia, however, does cause significant changes in the distribution of ventilation between the two lungs.

In the lateral decubitus position, the majority of tidal ventilation is switched from the lower lung in the awake subject to the upper lung in the spontaneously-ventilating anesthetized subject.[8,9] There are four interrelated reasons for this change in the relative distribution of ventilation between the upper and lower lung. First, the induction of general anesthesia classically causes a decrease in functional residual capacity (FRC), and both lungs share in the loss of lung volume. Since each lung occupies a different initial position on the pulmonary pressure-volume curve while the subject is awake, a general anesthesia-induced reduction in each lung's FRC causes each lung to move to a lower but still different portion of the pressure-volume curve (Fig. 8-7). The dependent lung moves from an initially steep part of the curve (with the subject awake) to a lower and flatter part of the curve (after anesthesia is induced); while the nondependent lung moves from an initially flat portion of the pressure-volume curve (with the subject awake) to a lower and steeper part of the curve (after anesthesia is induced). Thus, with the induction of general anesthesia, the lower lung moves to a less favorable (flat, noncompliant) portion and the upper lung to a more favorable (steep, compliant) portion of the pressure-volume curve. Second, if the anesthetized patient in the lateral decubitus position is also paralyzed and artificially ventilated, the high curved diaphragm of the lower lung no longer confers any advantage in ventilation (as it does in the awake state), since it is no longer actively contracting.[10] Third, the mediastinum rests upon the lower lung and physically impedes lower lung expansion, as well as selectively decreasing lower lung FRC. Fourth, the

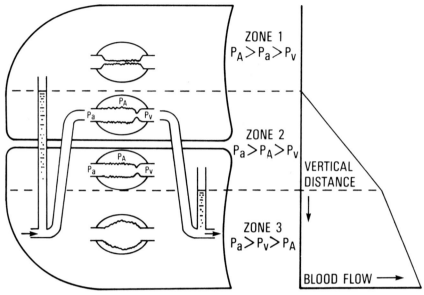

ZONE 1
$P_A > P_a > P_v$

P_A
P_a P_v

ZONE 2
$P_a > P_A > P_v$

P_A
P_a P_v

VERTICAL
DISTANCE
↓

ZONE 3
$P_a > P_v > P_A$

BLOOD FLOW ⟶

Fig. 8-6 Schematic representation of the effects of gravity on the distribution of pulmonary blood flow in the lateral decubitus position. Vertical gradients in the lateral decubitus position are similar to those in the upright position (shown in Fig. 8-1) and cause the creation of zones 1, 2, and 3. Consequently, pulmonary blood flow increases with lung dependency and is largest in the dependent lung and least in the nondependent lung.

weight of the abdominal contents pushing cephalad against the diaphragm is largest in the dependent lung, which physically impedes down-lung expansion the most and disproportionately decreases lower lung FRC. Finally, suboptimal positioning effects and procedures, such as failure to provide room for lower lung expansion and the presence of excessively inwardly projecting supporting rolls and operating table angulations, may considerably compress the dependent lung. Opening the nondependent hemithorax further disproportionately increases ventilation to the nondependent lung (see below).

In summary, the anesthetized patient, with or without paralysis, in the lateral decubitus position and with a closed chest has a nondependent lung which is well ventilated but poorly perfused and a dependent lung which is well perfused but poorly ventilated, resulting in a increased degree of inhomogeneity and mismatching of ventilation and perfusion. The application of positive end-expiratory pressure (PEEP) to both lungs restores the majority of ventilation to the lower lung.[11] Presumably, the lower lung moves back up to a steeper, more favorable part of the pressure-volume curve, and the upper lung returns to its original position on a flat, unfavorable portion of the curve.

Distribution of Perfusion and Ventilation—Lateral Decubitus Position, Anesthetized and Open Chest

Compared with the condition of the anesthetized, closed-chested patient in the lateral decubitus position, opening the chest wall and pleural space alone does not cause any significant alteration in the partitioning of pulmonary blood flow between the dependent and nondependent lung (ventilation, of course, must now be accomplished by positive pressure). Thus, in the anesthetized patient in the lateral decubitus position, the dependent lung continues to receive relatively more perfusion than the nondependent lung.

AWAKE   ANESTHETIZED

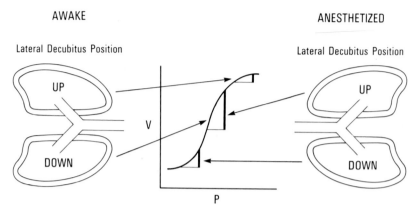

Fig. 8-7 The left-hand side of the schematic shows the distribution of ventilation in the awake patient (closed chest) in the lateral decubitus position and the right-hand side shows the distribution of ventilation in the anesthetized patient (closed chest) in the lateral decubitus position. The induction of anesthesia has caused a loss in lung volume in both lungs, with the nondependent (up) lung moving from a flat noncompliant portion to a steep compliant portion of the pressure-volume curve and the dependent (down) lung moving from a steep compliant part to a flat, noncompliant part of the pressure-volume curve. Thus, the anesthetized patient in a lateral decubitus position has the majority of the tidal ventilation in the nondependent lung (where there is the least perfusion) and the minority of the tidal ventilation in the dependent lung (where there is the most perfusion).

Opening the chest wall and pleural space, however, does have a significant impact on the distribution of positive pressure ventilation (ventilation can no longer be spontaneous) between the two lungs.

Opening the chest may cause even a further mismatching of ventilation with perfusion (Fig. 8-8).[12] If the upper lung is no longer restricted by a chest wall and the total effective compliance of that lung is equal to that of the lung parenchyma alone, it will be relatively free to expand and consequently be overventilated (and remain underperfused). Conversely, the dependent lung may continue to be relatively noncompliant and poorly ventilated and overperfused.[13] From a practical point of view, it is necessary to mention that surgical retraction and compression of the exposed upper lung can provide a partial, although nonphysiologic, solution to this problem in that if expansion of the exposed lung is mechanically or externally restricted, ventilation will be diverted to the dependent, better-perfused lung.

Theoretically, a more physiologic solution to the adverse effects of anesthesia and surgery in the lateral decubitus position on the distribution of ventilation and perfusion would be the application of selective PEEP to the dependent lung. Selective PEEP to the lower lung should increase the ventilation to this lung by moving it up to a steeper, more favorable portion of the lung pressure-volume curve. Indeed, this has been done with reasonably good success.[14] A series of 22 mechanically ventilated patients undergoing thoracotomy in the lateral decubitus position was divided into two groups. Group I patients had 10 cm H_2O of PEEP applied to the dependent lung while zero end-expiratory pressure (ZEEP) was applied to the nondependent lung. This was accomplished by using a Carlen's double-lumen endobronchial tube and a specially constructed PEEP valve circuit (Fig. 8-9). Group II (control) patients were intubated with a standard endotracheal tube and both lungs were ventilated with ZEEP. Selective PEEP to the de-

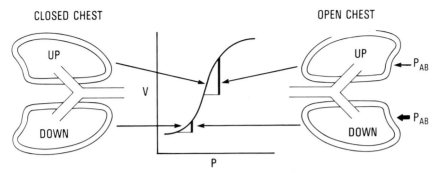

Fig. 8-8 This schematic of a patient in the lateral decubitus position compares the closed-chested anesthetized condition with the open-chested anesthetized and paralyzed condition. Opening the chest increases nondependent lung compliance and reinforces or maintains the larger part of the tidal ventilation going to the nondependent lung. Paralysis also reinforces or maintains the larger part of tidal ventilation going to the nondependent lung because the pressure of the abdominal contents (P_{AB}) pressing against the upper diaphragm is minimal and it is therefore easier for positive pressure ventilation to displace this lesser resisting dome of the diaphragm.

pendent lung in group I patients resulted in an adequate Pao_2 with a lower inspired O_2 concentration during surgery and a smaller alveolar-arterial oxygen difference at the end of surgery than when both lungs were ventilated with ZEEP. The use of this technique, however, requires great caution and frequent arterial blood gas monitoring, since selective PEEP to the lower lung may selectively increase vascular resistance in this lung and result in blood flow being shunted to the non-ventilated upper lung.[15]

Distribution of Perfusion and Ventilation—Lateral Decubitus Position, Anesthetized, Open Chest and Paralyzed

In the open-chested anesthetized patient in the lateral decubitus position, the induction of paralysis alone does not cause any significant alteration in the partitioning of pulmonary blood flow between the dependent and nondependent lung. Thus, in the paralyzed anesthetized patient in the lateral decubitus position with an open chest, the dependent lung continues to receive relatively more perfusion than the nondependent lung. There are, however, strong theoretical

and experimental considerations that indicate that paralysis might cause significant changes in the distribution of ventilation between the two lungs under these conditions.

In the supine and lateral decubitus positions, the weight of the abdominal contents pressing against the diaphragm is greatest on the dependent part of the diaphragm (posterior lung and down lung, respectively) and least on the nondependent part of the diaphragm (anterior lung and up lung, respectively) (Fig. 8-8). In the awake, spontaneously breathing patient, the normally present active tension in the diaphragm overcomes the weight of the abdominal contents, and the diaphragm moves the most (largest excursion) in the dependent portion and least in the nondependent portion. This is a healthy circumstance because this is another factor which causes or maintains the greatest amount of ventilation where there is the most perfusion (dependent lung) and the least amount of ventilation where there is the least perfusion (nondependent lung). During paralysis and positive-pressure breathing, the passive and flaccid diaphragm is displaced preferentially in the nondependent portion, where the resistance to diaphragmatic movement by the abdominal contents is least and the diaphragm is displaced minimally in the

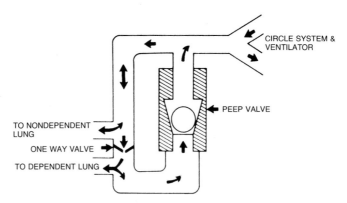

Fig. 8-9 Schematic representation of the circuit used to apply selective positive end-expiratory pressure (PEEP) to the dependent lung while ventilating the nondependent lung with zero end-expiratory pressure. The one-way valve in the circuit separates the nondependent lung limb from the dependent lung limb. The PEEP valve is a spring-loaded device. The volume of the circuit is 50 ml. (From Brown DR, Kafer ER, Roberson VD et al: Improved oxygenation during thoracotomy with selective PEEP to the dependent lung. Anesth Analg 56:26-31, 1977.)

dependent portion where the resistance to diaphragmatic movement by the abdominal contents is greatest.[16] This is an unhealthy circumstance because the greatest amount of ventilation may occur where there is the least perfusion (nondependent lung) and the least amount of ventilation may occur where there is the most perfusion (dependent lung).[16]

The Open Chest-Mediastinal Flap, and Paradoxical Respiration

An examination of the physiology of the open chest during spontaneous ventilation reveals why controlled positive-pressure ventilation is the only practical way to provide adequate ventilation during thoracotomy. In the spontaneously breathing, closed-chested patient in the lateral decubitus position, there is equal negative pressure in each hemithorax on each side of the mediastinum. However, the weight of the mediastinum still causes some compression of the lower lung. With the nondependent hemithorax open, atmospheric pressure in that cavity exceeds the negative pressure in the dependent

hemithorax; this imbalance of pressure on the two sides of the mediastinum causes a further downward displacement of the mediastinum into the dependent thorax. During inspiration the caudad movement of the dependent-lung diaphragm increases the negative pressure in the dependent lung and causes a still further displacement of the mediastinum into the dependent hemithorax. During expiration, as the dependent-lung diaphragm moves cephalad, the pressure in the dependent hemithorax becomes relatively positive, and the mediastinum is pushed upward out of the dependent hemithorax (Fig. 8-10).[17] Thus the tidal volume in the dependent lung is decreased by an amount equal to the inspiratory displacement caused by mediastinal movement. This phenomenon is called *mediastinal shift* and is one mechanism which results in impaired ventilation in the open-chested spontaneously-breathing patient in the lateral decubitus position. The mediastinal shift can also cause circulatory changes and reflexes which result in a clinical picture similar to shock; the patient is hypotensive, pale, and cold, with dilated pupils. Local anesthetic infiltration of the pulmo-

EXPIRATION

Pneumothorax

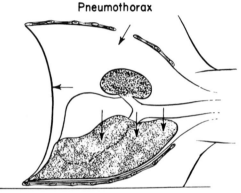

INSPIRATION

Pneumothorax

Fig. 8-10 Schematic representation of mediastinal shift in the spontaneously breathing open-chested patient in the lateral decubitus position. During inspiration, negative pressure in the intact hemithorax causes the mediastinum to move downward. During expiration, relative positive pressure in the intact hemithorax causes the mediastinum to move upward (From Tarhan S, Moffitt EA: Principles of thoracic anesthesia. Surg Clin North Am 53:813-826, 1973.)

nary plexus at the hilum and the vagus nerve in the neck can diminish these reflexes. Controlled positive pressure ventilation abolishes these ventilatory and circulatory changes associated with mediastinal shift.

When a pleural cavity is exposed to atmospheric pressure, the lung is no longer held open by negative intrapleural pressure and it tends to collapse because of unopposed elastic recoil. Thus, the lung in an open chest is at least partially collapsed. It has long been observed that during spontaneous ventilation with an open hemithorax, lung collapse is accentuated during inspiration, and, conversely, the lung expands during expiration. This reversal of lung movement with an open chest has been termed *paradoxical respiration*. The mechanism of paradoxical respiration is similar to that of mediastinal shift. During inspiration, the descent of the diaphragm on the side of the open hemithorax causes air from the environment to enter the pleural cavity on that side through the thoracotomy opening and fill the space around the exposed lung. The descent of the hemidiaphragm on the closed-chest side causes gas to enter the closed-chest lung in the normal manner. However, gas also enters the closed-chest lung, which has an increased negative pressure, from the open-chest lung, which remains at atmospheric pressure, resulting in further reduction in the size of the open-chest lung during inspiration. During expiration the reverse occurs, with the collapsed, open-chest lung filling from the intact lung and air moving back out of the exposed hemithorax through the thoracotomy. The phenomenon of paradoxical respiration is illustrated in Figure 8-11.[17] Paradoxical breathing is increased by a large thoracotomy and by increased airway resistance in the intact lung. Paradoxical respiration may be prevented either by manual collapse of the open-chest lung or, more commonly, by controlled positive-pressure ventilation.

PHYSIOLOGY AND TECHNIQUE OF ONE-LUNG VENTILATION

Two-Lung Versus One-Lung Ventilation

As summarized in Figure 8-12, the preceding section has developed the concept that the anesthetized patient in the lateral decubitus position, with an open chest and paralyzed, may have a considerable ventila-

EXPIRATION

Pneumothorax

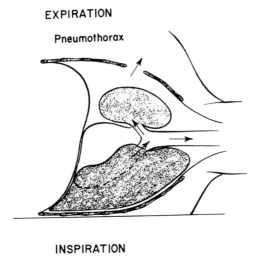

INSPIRATION

Pneumothorax

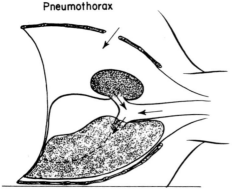

Fig. 8-11 Schematic representation of paradoxical respiration in the spontaneously breathing open-chested patient in the lateral decubitus position. During inspiration movement of gas from the exposed lung into the intact lung and movement of air from the environment into the open hemithorax causes collapse of the exposed lung. During expiration the reverse occurs, and the exposed lung expands. (From Tarhan S, Moffitt EA: Principles of thoracic anesthesia. Surg Clin North Am 53:813-826, 1973.)

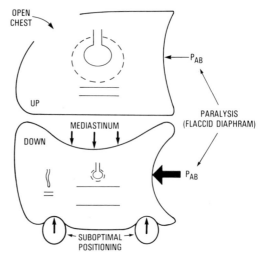

Fig. 8-12 Schematic summary of ventilation-perfusion relationships in the anesthetized patient in the lateral decubitus position, with an open chest, paralyzed, and suboptimally positioned. The nondependent lung is well ventilated (as indicated by the large dashed lines), but poorly perfused (small perfusion vessel) and the dependent lung is poorly ventilated (small dashed lines) but well perfused (large perfusion vessel). In addition, the dependent lung may also develop an atelectatic shunt compartment (indicated on the left side of the lower lung) because of the circumferential compression of this lung.

tion-perfusion mismatch, consisting of good ventilation but poor perfusion to the nondependent lung and poor ventilation but good perfusion to the dependent lung. The blood flow distribution was seen to be mainly and simply determined by gravitational effects. The relatively good ventilation of the up lung was seen to be caused, in part, by the open-chest and paralyzed conditions. The relatively poor ventilation of the dependent lung was seen to be caused, in part, by the loss of dependent-lung volume with general anesthesia and by compression of the dependent lung by the mediastinum, abdominal contents, and suboptimal positioning effects. In addition, poor mucociliary clearance and absorption atelectasis with an increased F_IO_2 may cause further dependent-lung volume loss. Consequently, two-lung ventilation under these circumstances may result in an increased $P(A-a)o_2$ and less than perfect oxygenation.

However, if the nondependent lung is nonventilated, as during one-lung ventilation, then any blood flow to the nonventilated lung becomes shunt flow, in addition to whatever shunt flow might exist in the down

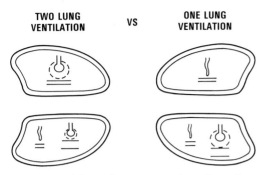

TWO LUNG VENTILATION VS **ONE LUNG VENTILATION**

Fig. 8-13 Schematic representation of two-lung ventilation versus one-lung ventilation. The essential difference is that during one-lung ventilation the nonventilated lung has some blood flow and therefore has an obligatory shunt which is not present during two-lung ventilation.

lung (Fig. 8-13). Thus, one-lung ventilation creates an obligatory right-to-left transpulmonary shunt through the nondependent lung which is not present during two-lung ventilation. Consequently, it is not surprising to find that when oxygenation is compared during the two-lung versus one-lung ventilation, given the same FIO_2 (and the same hemodynamic and metabolic status, etc.), one-lung ventilation with the obligatory up-lung shunt flow results in a somewhat lower PaO_2 than two-lung ventilation. This contention is best supported by one study which compared two-lung with one-lung ventilation and oxygenation with each patient serving as his or her own control.[18]

Although one-lung ventilation imposes an oxygenation handicap, carbon dioxide removal is usually not a problem. Blood passing through underventilated alveoli tends to retain its CO_2 and does not take up enough O_2; blood traversing overventilated alveoli gives off an excessive amount of CO_2 but cannot take up a proportionately increased amount of O_2 owing to the flatness of the oxyhemoglobin dissociation curve in this region. Hence, a single overventilated lung can eliminate enough CO_2 but cannot take up enough O_2 to compensate for the nonventilated lung. In addition, there is a great disparity between the venous-to-arterial O_2 and

CO_2 tension differences (60 and 6 mmHg, respectively), and a shunt will cause a much larger change in PaO_2 than in $PaCO_2$. Thus, with one-lung ventilation, $PACO_2$ to $PaCO_2$ gradients are small, and PAO_2 to PaO_2 gradients are usually large.

Indications for One-Lung Ventilation[19]

There are several absolute, as well as strong relative, indications for provision of one-lung anesthesia (Table 8-1). Isolation of one lung from the other is absolutely necessary to prevent spillage or contamination from an infected (abscessed) or bleeding lung to the noninvolved lung. The presence of a large bronchopleural fistula that is treated with a chest tube, a bronchopleural cutaneous fistula, or a giant unilateral lung cyst requires the use of a double-lumen endotracheal tube in order to safely provide adequate selective ventilation to the noninvolved side. Finally, one-lung anesthesia is absolutely necessary in order to perform unilateral bronchopulmonary lavage in patients with pulmonary alveolar proteinosis (and, rarely, asthma or cystic fibrosis).

One-lung anesthesia is relatively indi-

Table 8-1
Indications for One-Lung Anesthesia

A. Absolute
  1. Prevention of spillage or contamination from diseased to nondiseased lung
    a. Infection
    b. Massive hemorrhage
  2. Control the distribution of ventilation
    a. Bronchopleural fistula
    b. Bronchopleural cutaneous fistula
    c. Giant unilateral lung cyst
  3. Unilateral bronchopulmonary lavage
    a. Pulmonary alveolar proteinosis
B. Relative
  1. Surgical exposure—high priority
    a. Thoracic aortic aneurysm
    b. Pneumonectomy
  2. Surgical exposure—low priority
    a. Esophageal resection
    b. Lobectomy

cated when collapse of one lung confers a critical benefit to the performance of surgery by facilitating surgical exposure. Thus, pneumonectomy, upper lobectomy (which is technically the most difficult lobectomy), and repair of a thoracic aortic aneurysm may be made much easier by eliminating ventilation to the lung on the side of the procedure and are therefore high-priority relative indications. Indications for the use of one-lung anesthesia for some other procedures, such as lower lobectomy or esophageal resection, are less firm and therefore lower priority relative indications (see Ch. 11).

Determinants of the Distribution of Perfusion during One-lung Ventilation

Although the benefits of one-lung anesthesia in terms of isolating one diseased lung from the other or optimizing operating conditions are obvious and often mandatory, a very large and variable alveolar-to-arterial oxygen tension difference $[P(A-a)O_2]$ is a necessary consequence of this intervention.[18-24] The enlarged $P(A-a)O_2$ often results in systemic hypoxemia. The most important reason for the increased $P(A-a)O_2$ and hypoxemia during one-lung anesthesia is that there is continued perfusion to the nondependent, nonventilated (atelectatic) lung, creating an increase in transpulmonary shunt.[18,20,22,23] The reason for the variability in the degree of the $P(A-a)O_2$ and hypoxemia during one-lung ventilation is that there are multiple factors involved in determining the amount of perfusion to the upper, nonventilated lung. The factors which determine, independent of gravity, the amount of perfusion to the atelectatic lung are: (1) the degree of active vasoconstriction in the hypoxic, atelectatic lung (hypoxic pulmonary vasoconstriction, or HPV); (2) the degree of surgical compression, retraction, and manipulation of the atelectatic lung; (3) the preop-

erative and intraoperative condition of the dependent lung; and (4) the method used to ventilate the dependent lung. The latter three influences on the distribution of pulmonary blood flow operate, at least in part, by effects on HPV. Figure 8-14 is a one-lung ventilation pathophysiologic flow diagram which outlines some of the important components of these four major influences on HPV, as well as the relationship of one influence to another.

HYPOXIC PULMONARY VASOCONSTRICTION

Hypoxic pulmonary vasoconstriction diverts blood flow away from hypoxic regions of the lung and thereby minimizes the amount of transpulmonary shunt flow. Recently, it has been shown that the mechanism of decreased blood flow to an atelectatic lobe, whether the chest is open or closed and whether ventilation in the rest of the lung is spontaneous or controlled, is entirely due to HPV.[25,26] Although the following discussion is primarily concerned with nondependent-lung HPV, it is important to realize that the dependent lung may have a shunt compartment and therefore HPV. Thus, any factor which inhibits nondependent-lung as well as dependent-lung HPV will have a deleterious effect on the distribution of blood flow during one-lung ventilation and will impair gas exchange (see Figs. 8-12 and 8-13).

Clinical conditions that may directly vasodilate hypoxically constricted lung vessels are use of certain anesthetics, infusion of vasodilator drugs, presence of infection in the nondependent lung, and hypocapnia.[27-34] In all species tested, isoflurane, fluroxene, and nitrous oxide dose-dependently inhibit HPV.[27,28,34] Halothane does not inhibit HPV in dogs, but there is one report on humans which indicates that halothane does inhibit HPV.[27,28,36,37] Enflurane has been studied only in animals and does not inhibit HPV.[27] Injectable and intravenous anesthetics probably do not inhibit HPV.[28,38-40] All

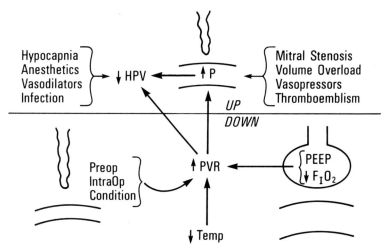

Fig. 8-14 Pathophysiologic diagram of the determinants of blood flow distribution during one-lung ventilation. All pathways shown have some influence on hypoxic pulmonary vasoconstriction (HPV). Surgical manipulation, retraction, and compression comprise a complex variable and are not shown. See text for full explanation of each pathway.

systemic vasodilator drugs probably inhibit HPV.[29–31] Specifically tested and very potent in this regard are sodium nitroprusside, nitroglycerin, isoproterenol, and aminophylline.[31] Decreases in P_ACO_2 and $PaCO_2$ below 30-mm Hg inhibit HPV.[34] Finally, there is some evidence that certain types of infections, particularly granulomatous and pneumococcal infections, may inhibit HPV[32, 33] (see Ch. 7).

The pulmonary circulation is poorly endowed with smooth muscle, and even hypoxically constricted vessels will dilate when exposed to pressures exceeding 16 to 18 mmHg.[41] Thus, the intraluminal vascular pressure against which the pulmonary vessels must constrict is a major determinant of the magnitude of HPV.[42] Clinical conditions that increase pulmonary vascular pressure and therefore inhibit HPV (or at least inhibit effective or clinically significant amounts of blood flow redistribution away from the hypoxic lung) are mitral stenosis, volume overload, administration of vasopressor drugs, ligation of pulmonary vessels, thromboembolism, and large hypoxic lung segments.[29, 42–45]

SURGICAL MANIPULATION

Although HPV is responsible for the majority of blood flow redistribution away from the nonventilated atelectatic lung, it is certainly possible that severe nondependent-lung compression (directly compressing lung vessels) and severe nondependent-lung retraction (causing kinking and tortuosity of lung vessels) may further reduce nondependent-lung blood flow. This lung manipulation component of blood flow reduction will be variable with respect to both time and magnitude.

On the other hand, recent evidence indicates that physical trauma to pulmonary tissue may cause local release of vasodilator prostaglandins.[46] Indeed, one study has shown that moderate degrees of surgical manipulation of the nonventilated lung significantly increase the shunt fraction compared with two-lung ventilation with the chest open and one-lung ventilation with the chest closed.[47] Thus, depending on the exact nature of the physical stimulus, it appears that the delicate HPV mechanism may be enhanced or inhibited.

The pulmonary vascular resistance in the ventilated compartment of the lung also determines the ability of the ventilated, and supposedly normoxic, lung to accept redistributed blood flow from the hypoxic lung.[43, 48–50] Clinical conditions that are independent of specific dependent-lung disease, but which may still increase dependent (nonhypoxic) lung pulmonary vascular resistance and therefore may inhibit nondependent (hypoxic) lung HPV, are a low (but above room air) inspired oxygen tension in the dependent lung and hypothermia.[48–51]

However, the existence of a significant hypoxic compartment within the ventilated dependent lung is an important cause of increased dependent-lung pulmonary vascular resistance.[43] For the purpose of this discussion, the hypoxic compartment in the dependent lung may have been present preoperatively, or may have developed intraoperatively as a consequence of the surgical and anesthetic experience.

The extent of disease in the dependent lung preoperatively determines, at least initially, the vascular resistance and the amount of shunting in the dependent lung. In addition, there are numerous causes and mechanisms for the development of disease in the dependent lung intraoperatively which would be accompanied by increased dependent-lung vascular resistance and increased shunting.[52–54] Absorption atelectasis can occur in regions of the dependent lung which have low V/Q ratios when they are exposed to high inspired oxygen concentrations.[55, 56] Loss of dependent-lung volume due to the induction of anesthesia and paralysis, compression from the weight of the mediastinum, suboptimal positioning effects, and difficulty in secretion removal may cause the development of poorly ventilated and atelectatic areas. Finally, maintaining the lateral decubitus position for prolonged periods of time may cause fluid to transudate in the dependent lung and cause further decreased dependent-lung volume (FRC) and increased airway closure in the dependent lung.[57] A decrease in FRC and an increase in closing volume in the dependent lung will create areas which have a low ventilation/perfusion ratio or atelectasis.

In view of the factors listed above which can affect the amount of nondependent-lung blood flow, the method used to ventilate the dependent lung is important in this regard. First, if the dependent lung is hyperventilated, then the resultant hypocapnia may inhibit HPV. Second, if the dependent-lung method of ventilation involves an excessive amount of airway pressure, due either to use of high PEEP levels or to very large tidal volumes, the deleterious effects of increased dependent-lung airway pressure, namely increasing dependent-lung vascular resistance (which would increase nondependent-lung blood flow), may outweigh the beneficial effects of the opening of atelectatic and low V/Q areas in the dependent lung. Third, a high inspired oxygen concentration to the dependent lung may cause vasodilatation in it, enhancing nondependent-lung HPV; however, absorption atelectasis is promoted by a high inspired oxygen concentration to low V/Q areas in the dependent lung.[43, 50, 55, 56]

Still other factors may contribute to hypoxemia during one-lung ventilation. Hypoxemia due to mechanical failure of the O_2 supply system or the anesthesia machine is a recognized hazard of any kind of anesthesia.[58–63] Gross hypoventilation of the dependent lung can be a major cause of hypoxemia. Malfunction of the dependent-lung airway lumen (blockage by secretions) and malposition of the double-lumen endotracheal tube and right upper lobe slot are other common causes of an increased $P(A-a)O_2$ and hypoxemia. The anesthesiologist must pay special attention to the position of the double-lumen endotracheal tube after each change in the patient's position, since a tube previously correctly positioned in the trachea may enter a bronchus after the patient or his head has been turned or moved into a new position.[64]

For example, it is well known that flexion of the head causes caudad movement and extension of the head causes cephalad movement of an endotracheal tube.[64, 65] Consequently, it is not surprising that as high as a 50 percent incidence of main-stem bronchus intubation may occur with a single-lumen tube following institution of a 30-degree Trendelenberg position.[66] In this latter study, cephalad shift of the carina during the Trendelenberg position caused the previously "fixed" endotracheal tube to be located in a main-stem bronchus. Resorption of residual oxygen from the clamped nonventilated lung is time-dependent and may account for a gradual increase in shunt and decrease in PaO_2 after one-lung ventilation is initiated.[52]

With all other anesthetic and surgical factors constant, anything that decreases the mixed venous partial pressure of oxygen (PvO_2) [decreased cardiac output, increased oxygen consumption (excessive sympathetic nervous system stimulation, hyperthermia, shivering)] will cause an increased $P(A-a)O_2$.[67, 68]

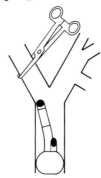

Fig. 8-15 The upper left-hand corner shows a left lung double-lumen endotracheal tube in place while surgery of the right lung (as represented by the clamp) is being performed. The upper right-hand corner shows a right lung double-lumen endotracheal tube in place while left lung surgery is being performed. Note the slot in the right lung double-lumen tube which allows ventilation of the right upper lobe. The bottom panel shows a left lung double-lumen endotracheal tube pulled back into a main tracheal position where both lumens ventilate the right lung during left lung surgery.

Technique of Double-Lumen Tube Insertion (see Ch. 11)

A left-lung double-lumen endotracheal tube is used for operations on the right lung which require nonventilation of the right lung and ventilation of the left lung (Fig. 8-15).[69] For operations on the left lung, which require nonventilation of the left lung and ventilation of the right lung, either a left- or right-sided tube may be used, although the use of a right-sided tube for the purpose of selective right-lung ventilation (and left-lung isolation) introduces the very real risk of obstruction and inadequate ventilation of the right upper lobe.[69] In order to avoid this complication, some anesthesiologists utilize a left-sided tube for all cases requiring one-

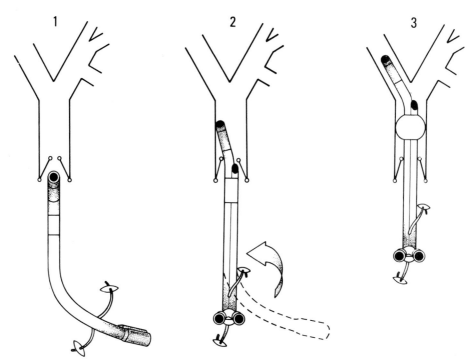

Fig. 8-16 Schematic diagram of the passage of the left lung Robertshaw tube. The distal curvature should be concave anteriorly initially (as tube tip advances through glottis), and the proximal curve should be off to the right and parallel to the floor (in the supine patient). After the tube tip passes the vocal cords, the entire tube should be rotated 90 degrees so that the proximal curvature is now concave anteriorly and the distal curvature is off to the left and parallel to the floor. The tube should be pushed in until a moderate resistance to further passage is encountered and most of the tube is inside the mouth (close to the parting of the individual lumens from the common molding).

lung anesthesia. If clamping of the left main-stem bronchus is necessary, the tube can be withdrawn at that time into the trachea and the right lung ventilated through both the right and left lumens of the tube (Fig. 8-15). However, if the left main-stem bronchus is involved in the disease process (i.e., left main-stem endobronchial tumor, extrinsic compression) then the left lung should not be instrumented and a right-sided double-lumen tube should be used (see Ch. 11).

Prior to intubation with a double-lumen endotracheal tube, both cuffs and all connections should be checked. The tube is coated with a lubricating jelly (preferably containing a local anesthetic), and a lubricated stylette is passed into the left lumen until the tip

of the stylette is just proximal to the end of the most distal lumen and shaped so that the natural curvature of the distal part of the tube is preserved as concave anteriorly. The patient is then anesthetized and paralyzed as described in other chapters in this book. A curved, open-flanged blade (MacIntosh) should be used for laryngoscopy since it provides the largest possible area through which to pass the double-lumen tube.

A double-lumen tube, such as the Robertshaw tube (no carinal hook), is passed with the distal curvature initially concave anteriorly (Fig. 8-16). After the tube tip passes the larynx, the tube is rotated 90 degrees (so that the proximal curve is now concave anteriorly and the distal curve is pointing either to the left or right side) to allow endobronchial intubation on the appropriate side. Double-lumen endotracheal tubes that contain a carinal hook (e.g., Carlens tube) are first inserted through the vocal cords with the hook facing posteriorly. When the tip of the tube has passed the vocal cords, the entire tube is rotated 180 degrees so that the hook passes anteriorly through the glottis. After the tube tip and hook pass the larynx, the tube is rotated 90 degrees so that the tube tip enters the appropriate bronchus. Advancement of a double-lumen endotracheal tube is halted when moderate resistance to further passage is encountered, indicating that the tube tip has been firmly seated in the main-stem bronchus or that the carinal hook, when present, has engaged the carina. Double-lumen endotracheal tubes may also be passed successfully via a tracheostomy, although it should be remembered that the tracheal cuff may lie outside the trachea in this situation.[70, 71]

Once the tube tip is thought to be endobronchial, a checklist is carried out to ensure proper functioning of the tube. One technique to accomplish this is shown in Figure 8-17 (see Ch. 11 for another method). The tracheal cuff is inflated and several short, rapid, positive-pressure ventilations delivered in order to best determine, both by auscultation and by observation of the chest, that both lungs are being ventilated (Fig. 8-17, 1). If only unilateral breath sounds or chest movements are present, it is likely that both the endotracheal tube lumina have entered a mainstem bronchus. In this situation, the tube is withdrawn 2 to 3 cm at a time and ventilation reassessed after each withdrawal.

The subsequent steps that are performed when using a left double-lumen endotracheal tube are designed to assure functional separation of the two lungs by the double-lumen tube (Figs. 8-17,2,3). The right (tracheal) connecting tube is clamped proximal to the right lumen suction cap and the right lumen suction cap is opened. The left lung is inflated via the left lumen, and while

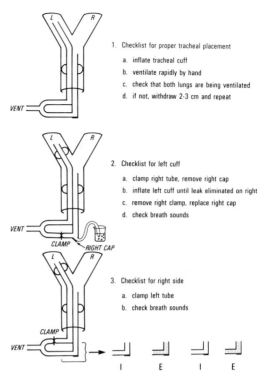

1. Checklist for proper tracheal placement
   a. inflate tracheal cuff
   b. ventilate rapidly by hand
   c. check that both lungs are being ventilated
   d. if not, withdraw 2-3 cm and repeat

2. Checklist for left cuff
   a. clamp right tube, remove right cap
   b. inflate left cuff until leak eliminated on right
   c. remove right clamp, replace right cap
   d. check breath sounds

3. Checklist for right side
   a. clamp left tube
   b. check breath sounds

Fig. 8-17 Schematic representation of one technique to ensure proper functioning of a left double-lumen endotracheal tube: (1) checklist for proper tracheal placement; (2) checklist for left cuff; (3) checklist for right side. See text for full explanation.

listening, feeling (hand, cheek), or looking (bubble through water method, see Ch. 12) for a leak from the open right lumen cap, the bronchial (left) cuff is inflated until the leak is eliminated. The right cap is replaced and the right connecting tube clamp removed while listening for bilateral breath sounds. If bilateral breath sounds are not heard, the entire procedure must be repeated, beginning with the inflation of the tracheal cuff. If bilateral breath sounds are present, the right connecting tube is clamped once again while listening to and observing the right chest. Right-sided breath sounds should disappear while left-sided breath sounds should remain unchanged. Next, the right connecting tube is unclamped and the left connecting tube clamped while listening to and observing the left chest. Left-sided breath sounds should disappear while right-sided breath sounds should remain unchanged. The left connecting tube should then be unclamped, bilateral breath sounds reascertained, and the tube secured in place. The same sequence of steps is used for a right-sided tube, except that the laterality of clamping, opening, and closing caps, etc. must be reversed. Use of a clear (nonopaque) double-lumen tube allows observation of the tidal movement of respiratory moisture (Fig. 8-17, 3), which may serve as a quick check or confirmation of ventilation in a particular lung

Confidence in proper placement may be increased by several procedures. Auscultation of the lungs in the axillary regions minimizes transmitted breath sounds. Fiberoptic confirmation of double-lumen tube position is very precise, rapid and, most importantly, repeatable after the patient is turned into the operating position (see Ch. 12). Finally, functional separation of the two lungs can be assured by the air bubble leak detection method.

Management of One-Lung Ventilation

The previous discussion of the respiratory physiology of one-lung ventilation indicated that this technique incurs a high risk of causing systemic hypoxemia. Thus, it is extremely important that the ventilation of the one (dependent) lung be managed optimally. This section considers the management of one-lung ventilation in terms of the most appropriate tidal volume, respiratory rate, inspired oxygen concentraton, and dependent-lung PEEP level that should be used.

The effect of systematic change in dependent-lung tidal volume on arterial oxygenation during one-lung anesthesia has been studied (Fig. 8-18).[23] Measurement of blood gases and transpulmonary shunt were performed at the following times: sample 1, lateral decubitus position with the chest

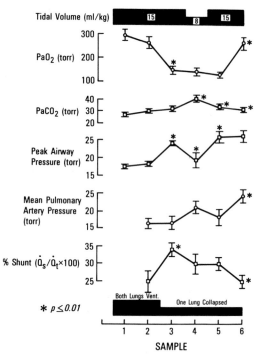

Fig. 8-18 The effects of changing tidal volume on arterial blood gas values, peak airway pressure, pulmonary artery pressure, and shunt during one-lung anesthesia. Arterial PO_2 and percent shunt are not significantly affected by changing tidal volume from 15 ml/kg to 8 ml/kg or vice versa. (Redrawn and reprinted by permission from Flacke JW, Thompson DS, Reed RC: Influence of Tidal Volume and Pulmonary Artery Occlusion on Arterial Oxygenation During Endobronchial Anesthesia. South. Med. J. 69:619-626, 1976.)

closed and two-lung tidal volume of 15 mg/kg; sample 2, chest open with the same two-lung (upper lung included) ventilation; sample 3, 10 minutes after collapse of the upper lung and with dependent-lung tidal volume of 15 ml/kg; sample 4, 10 minutes after tidal volume to the dependent lung was reduced from 15 to 8 ml/kg; sample 5, 10 minutes after dependent-lung tidal volume was increased from 8 to 15 ml/kg; sample 6, 10 minutes after occlusion of the pulmonary artery to the upper lung. This study reported a consistent decrease in PaO_2 and increase in shunt during one-lung anesthesia (sample 3 compared with sample 2) and noted that these PaO_2 decreases and shunt increases were significantly related to the patient's preoperative PaO_2 and vital capacity. Changes in PaO_2 with alterations in the tidal volume (sample 4 compared with samples 3 and 5) in individual patients were variable and unpredictable in both degree and direction (although the mean value for the group did not change). After the pulmonary artery to the upper lung was clamped (sample 6), shunt decreased while PaO_2, peak airway pressure, and mean pulmonary artery pressure increased. Thus, it appears that changing the tidal volume from 15 ml/kg to 8 ml/kg during one-lung ventilation has an unpredictable but usually not great impact on arterial oxygenaton.

It is a general finding that elimination of CO_2 is not usually a problem during one-lung anesthesia.[52, 72–74] Figure 8-18 shows that lowering the minute ventilation by approximately one-half (tidal volume reduced from 15 ml/kg to 8 ml/kg while the respiratory rate was constant) has little effect on arterial $PaCO_2$. Thus, on the commencement of one-lung anesthesia, a tidal volume of 8 to 12 ml/kg is used and it is only necessary to change the respiratory rate slightly (approximately 20 pecent) in order to maintain the $PaCO_2 \cong 40$ mmHg. This intermediate range of dependent-lung tidal volume is used in the hope of avoiding dependent-lung atelectasis while at the same time not excessively increasing dependent-lung vascular resistance. Since the compliance of the lower lung is decreased and the dependent-lung tidal volume of 8 to 12 ml/kg represents an increase in tidal volume to that lung, peak dependent-lung inspiratory pressure is usually moderately increased.[52]

Although the theoretical danger of dependent-lung absorption atelectasis exists, a high inspired concentration of oxygen is used in order to minimize the risk of hypoxemia during one-lung anesthesia.[19–24, 52] However, it should be realized that although increasing the inspired oxygen concentration has a very beneficial effect when the shunt is small, the effect is not nearly as dramatic when a large shunt is present, as in one-lung anesthesia. Thus, excellent oxygenation can rarely be achieved during one-lung anesthesia, and the adequacy of oxygenation must be monitored by frequent blood gas determinations.[18, 19, 22, 23, 53] Intermittent ventilation to the upper lung for short periods of time may be required if severe hypoxemia occurs.[18, 19, 52]

Several investigators have studied the effects of selective dependent-lung PEEP during one-lung anesthesia.[23, 75, 76] In these studies the effects of PEEP during one-lung anesthesia have depended on the amount of PEEP, the tidal volume used, and where the lung was initially on its pressure-volume curve. In one study, 10 cm H_2O PEEP caused a decrease in PaO_2 in most patients. This was attributed to an increased shunt through the nondependent, atelectatic lung and to a decreased cardiac output.[24] However, the tidal volume used was not stated and it is therefore difficult to interpret the results. In another study, 5 cm H_2O PEEP had no significant effect on cardiorespiratory function.[75] The patients in this study had one lung ventilated with volumes normally recommended for two-lung ventilation. Since these patients already had a relatively high mean airway pressure due to the initial tidal ventilation, it is not surprising that additional beneficial effects were not observed with the application of only a low level of PEEP. Other studies have shown that high tidal volumes, variations in the inspiratory-to-expiratory ratio, and intermittent manual hyperventilation of the lower lung are not beneficial.[21, 76]

An approach to obtaining adequate oxygenation during one-lung anesthesia is outlined in Table 8-2. Two-lung ventilation should be maintained for as long as possible. When one-lung ventilation is commenced, a tidal volume of 8 to 12 ml/kg is used and the respiratory rate is adjusted so that $PaCO_2 \cong 40$ mmHg. A high inspired oxygen concentration is used and arterial gases are moni-

Table 8-2

Ventilatory Management of One-Lung Anesthesia

1. Maintain two-lung ventilation as long as possible
2. Begin one-lung ventilation with a tidal volume of 8 to 12 ml/kg
3. Adjust the respiratory rate so that $PaCO_2 \cong 40$ mmHg
4. Use high FIO_2
5. Utilize frequent or continuous arterial PO_2 and PCO_2 monitoring
6. If hypoxemia occurs,
   a. Cautiously introduce nondependent and/or dependent lung PEEP; check frequently for benefit by blood gases, or
   b. Utilize occasional two-lung ventilation
7. Clamp the pulmonary artery to the nonventilated lung as early as possible (for pneumonectomy)

tored frequently. If severe hypoxemia is present and there is a reasonable suspicion that the dependent lung is diseased, a low level of dependent-lung PEEP is cautiously instituted. Alternatively, the nondependent lung may be intermittently ventilated (two-lung ventilation) as long as operating conditions permit. Finally, most of the ventilation-perfusion imbalance can be eliminated by clamping of the nonventilated lung's pulmonary artery as early as possible during pneumonectomy.

It should be noted that the need for a quiet surgical field for short periods of time may arise during a thoracotomy in which a standard endotracheal tube and two-lung ventilation are employed. This can be accomplished relatively safely by using the principle of apneic mass movement oxygenation. If ventilation is stopped during the administration of 100 percent oxygen and the airway is left connected to a fresh oxygen supply, oxygen will be drawn into the lung by mass movement to replace that which crossed the alveolar capillary membrane. If 100 percent oxygen has been previously used, there is usually no difficulty in maintaining an adequate arterial PO_2 during at

least 20 minutes of apneic mass movement oxygenation. This technique, however, causes retention of all the CO_2 produced. The arterial PCO_2 rises by approximately 6 mmHg in the first minute, and then 3 to 4 mmHg each minute thereafter. Based on these considerations, if a patient had a normal CO_2 production and was hyperventilated to produce a $PaCO_2$ of 30 mmHg and then made apneic, the $PaCO_2$ after 10 minutes would be 63 to 72 mmHg. Indeed, one report described a series of eight patients in whom apneic mass movement oxygenation was employed after normal ventilation for a period of 18 to 55 minutes.[77] Although the lowest arterial saturation that resulted was 98 percent, the $PaCO_2$ in five patients in whom it was measured ranged from 103 to 250 mmHg and the pH ranged from 6.72 to 6.97. Severe degrees of hypercapnia and respiratory acidosis may be well-tolerated in some healthy patients, but it appears that the safe period of apneic oxygenation during thoracotomy would lie under 10 minutes.

Special New Techniques to Improve Oxygenation during One-Lung Ventilation

FIBEROPTIC CONFIRMATION OF DOUBLE-LUMEN TUBE LOCATION

Conventional methods, such as auscultation and inspection, can provide a reasonable degree of confidence in the correctness of double-lumen tube position. However, if the clinical signs of location are confusing, as they often are in clinical practice, passing a fiberoptic scope down both the lumens of the endotracheal tube will provide direct inspection of tube location. The methods for this procedure are presented in Chapter 12. If there is any reason to suspect incomplete functional separation of the two lungs, the air bubble leak method described in Chapter 12 can confirm or rule out this possibility.

Recently, two reports, one on humans and one on dogs, have shown that application of PEEP with 100 percent oxygen (O_2 PEEP) without tidal ventilation to only the nonventilated lung significantly increased arterial oxygenation.[78, 79] The study in dogs was performed with electromagnetic flow probes on both main pulmonary arteries and showed that low levels of O_2 PEEP (5 and 10 cm H_2O) without tidal ventilation to the nondependent lung greatly increased PaO_2 and decreased shunt while blood flow to the nonventilated lung remained unchanged. Therefore, low levels of O_2 PEEP simply maintained the patency of nondependent-lung airways, allowing some distention of the nondependent-lung alveolar space and thereby permitting oxygen exchange to take place in the nonventilated lung (Fig. 8-19). On the other hand, 15 cm H_2O of O_2 PEEP caused similar PaO_2 and shunt changes while blood flow to the nondependent, nonventilated lung significantly decreased. Therefore, high levels of O_2 PEEP act by permitting oxygen exchange in the nonventilated lung, as well as by causing blood flow diversion to the ventilated lung, where both oxygen and carbon dioxide exchange can take place (Fig. 8-19). Since low levels of O_2 PEEP are as efficacious as high levels of O_2 PEEP and have less hemodynamic impact, use of only a low level of O_2 PEEP to the nondependent lung is recommended when severe hypoxemia is resistant to standard and usual methods of resolution. Oxygen insufflation at ZEEP did not improve arterial PaO_2 and is not recommended. The lack of efficacy of O_2 insufflation is probably due to the inability of a zero transbronchial airway pressure to maintain airway patency so that the insufflated oxygen cannot reach the gas-exchanging alveolar region of the lung.

Relatively simple systems can provide O_2 PEEP without tidal respiration to the

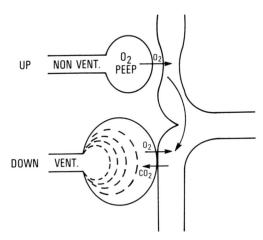

Fig. 8-19 This schematic diagram shows that selective up-lung PEEP (without tidal ventilation) can cause uptake of oxygen by the nonventilated lung with blood flow by allowing oxygen to reach the gas-exchanging alveolar regions of the lung and/or by increasing nonventilated lung pulmonary vascular resistance, which can divert blood flow away from the nonventilated lung to the ventilated lung, where oxygen and carbon dioxide exchange can take place.

nondependent lung. An example of a system is shown in Figure 8-20. The pressure relief valve limits the escape of the inflowing oxygen and thereby creates a constant distending pressure to the nonventilated, nondependent lung.[78] However, constant observation of the nonventilated lung is necessary to ensure that untoward occlusion of the pressure relief valve does not result in excessive and dangerous inflation of the operated lung. Alternatively, a simple, lightweight-plastic portable PEEP device has been recently described and can be simply and directly attached to the nondependent-lung airway to provide 5 to 10 cm H_2O of O_2 PEEP.[80] Above these levels of PEEP, the device generates high noise levels due to the turbulence of oxygen flow and is not recommended. Very recently, a double-lumen tube adapter has been developed which greatly facilitates the application of nondependent-lung and differential-lung PEEP.[81]

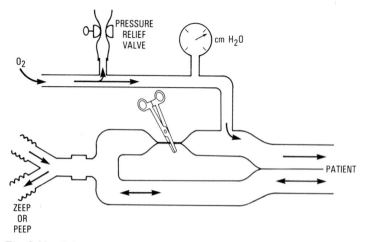

Fig. 8-20 Schematic of a simple, selective up-lung PEEP system. The fresh inflow of oxygen is restricted or limited by a pressure release valve and therefore a constant distending airway pressure to the nonventilated lung occurs.

HIGH-FREQUENCY VENTILATION

High-frequency ventilation has been used in intensive care units, during anesthesia for operations on the upper airway, and, most importantly, in patients undergoing thoracotomy and open-chest surgery.[82-88] Pleural pressure remains either negative or only slightly positive throughout the ventilatory cycle during high-frequency ventilation, and therefore this form of mechanical support has little hemodynamic impact. In addition—and this factor is most relevant to the performance of thoracic surgery—high-frequency ventilation creates excellent operating conditions for the surgeon in that the lung is only slightly distended and nonmoving.

Although not yet reported at the time of this writing, the combination of high-frequency ventilation to only the up (nondependent) lung with conventional ventilation of the down (dependent) lung would appear to create excellent thoracic operation conditions. First, the operative field would be nonmoving. Second, the nonmoving lung would exchange oxygen and carbon dioxide instead of just oxygen, as is the case with selective up-lung PEEP. Third, the hemodynamic consequences of up-lung high frequency ventilation should be minimal. Fourth, dependent-lung atelectasis could be minimized.

DIFFERENTIAL LUNG PEEP

Differential lung PEEP, that is the application of a different (and ideally optimal) amount of PEEP to each lung, has been used in intensive care units.[89-93] The application of differential lung PEEP during one-lung ventilation and thoracic surgery would then simply be a variation of selective up-lung PEEP, wherein the down (dependent) lung is ventilated with a PEEP that results in improved dependent-lung ventilation-perfusion relationships while a static (no ventilation) level of PEEP (5 to 10 cm H_2O) is applied to the up, nonventilated lung. If the nondependent lung can be ventilated during surgery, then PEEP with conventional tidal ventilation can be applied to the up lung while the down lung receives perhaps a different, but more importantly an optimal, level of PEEP and tidal ventilation. Ideally, the application of differential lung PEEP should cause equal functional residual capacities in the two lungs. Theoretically, in order to achieve equal functional residual capacities in the two lungs, the amount of PEEP applied to each lung should be inversely proportional to the compliance of each lung. The use of differential lung PEEP avoids applying high levels of PEEP to (and therefore excessively distending) a compliant lung as would otherwise be necessary to adequately expand the remaining and least compliant lung. Consequently, the application of differential lung PEEP has also been found to have less hemodynamic impact than the use of conventional two-lung PEEP. In addition, there is now good evidence to indicate that excessive distention of a normal region of the lung (ie, a lobe) causes not only an increased shunt but also interstitial edema in that region.[15, 94, 95]

PULMONARY ARTERY BALLOON
INFLATION IN THE DISEASED
(NONVENTILATED) LUNG

Blood flow to a hypoxic region of the lung can be diminished by hypoxic pulmonary vasoconstriction. The magnitude of the reduction of blood flow is approximately 50 percent for a single whole lung and perhaps 60 percent for a single lobe, but factors that are inhibitory to HPV are often present (see above discussion) and the reduction in blood flow is sometimes much less than 50 percent.[43, 44] Recently, it has been shown that blood flow to a hypoxic lung can be diminished on a mechanical basis by the nonocclusive inflation of a pulmonary artery catheter balloon which is located in the ipsilateral (on the same side as the diseased or nonventilated lung) main pulmonary artery.[79, 96–98] With nonocclusive inflation of the pulmonary artery catheter balloon, the balloon is inflated until the pulse pressure of the phasic pulmonary artery pressure trace just begins to dampen or until 0.8 to 1.0 ml of air has been used. Under these circumstances, the inflated balloon causes a mechanical resis-

tance to nonventilated or diseased lung blood flow, and right-to-left transpulmonary shunt can be reduced by approximately 15 percent. Since the vast majority of pulmonary artery catheters locate in the right lung when floated to a wedge position blindly (without the use of fluoroscopy), the pulmonary artery balloon inflation method of favorably manipulating the distribution of pulmonary blood flow is only technically feasible (without fluoroscopy) when the right lung is the nonventilated or diseased lung.[99] The method has been used moderately successfully during periods of lung drainage in the course of unilateral lung lavage procedures (see Ch. 12), in critically ill infants with unilateral lung disease, and in dogs to favorably redistribute pulmonary blood flow during one-lung ventilation.[79, 96–98] Thus, the desired flow diversions (and perhaps augmentation of HPV) caused by pulmonary artery balloon inflation may be uniquely useful in situations in which oxygen PEEP to the nonventilated lung is impractical (e.g., surgical interference, pulmonary hemorrhage) or impossible (e.g., pulmonary lavage). However, since inflation of a pulmonary artery catheter balloon *in addition* to any level of O_2 PEEP *does not* significantly change PaO_2 or Qs/Qt (but still significantly decreases blood flow to the nonventilated or nondiseased lung) and may potentially cause damage to pulmonary vessels, O_2 PEEP should be applied as the *primary response* to severe hypoxemia during one-lung ventilation, and pulmonary artery balloon inflation should be reserved as a secondary response to severe hypoxemia in the above-mentioned situations.

In summary, this chapter has described the physiology of the open chest and the consequences of being in the lateral decubitus position, anesthetized, and paralyzed. It appears that this set of conditions does not result in perfect oxygenation but is still more efficient or provides better oxygenation than one-lung ventilation. However, one-lung ventilation has mandatory, as well as strong relative indications, and, therefore, knowledge of the physiology of one-lung ventilation is important in order to properly manage this condition. The determinants of the blood flow distribution during one-lung ventilation have been described in terms of hypoxic pulmonary vasoconstriction, surgical manipulation on the operated lung, and the condition of the down (dependent) lung, as well as the method used to ventilate the dependent lung. The recommended technique and management of one-lung ventilation is based on these determinants of blood flow distribution. Finally, special new techniques to correct severe hypoxemia during one-lung ventilation have been described; they include new forms of ventilation such as selective up-lung PEEP, high-frequency ventilation, and differential lung PEEP, as well as attempts to favorably manipulate the distribution of pulmonary blood flow by pulmonary artery catheter balloon inflation. Thus, at the present time it is technically and theoretically possible to achieve oxygenation that is equal to two-lung ventilation even though one lung is being operated on, is nonmoving, and may be diseased. These latest developments in anesthesia for thoracic surgery have resulted in the application of techniques in the operating room that were created outside the operating room in the ICUs, such as high-frequency ventilation, differential lung PEEP, and fiberoptic bronchoscopy; they have also resulted in the application of techniques outside the operating room that were created in the operating room such as the use of modern double-lumen tubes and adapters and pulmonary artery balloon inflation manipulation of pulmonary blood flow.

REFERENCES

1. West JB, Dollery CT, Naimark A: Distribution of blood flow in isolated lung: relation to vascular and alveolar pressures. J Appl Physiol 19:713-724, 1964
2. Permutt S, Bromberger-Barnea B, Bane HN: Alveolar pressure, pulmonary venous pressure and the vascular waterfall. Med Thorac 19:239-260, 1962
3. Hoppin FG Jr, Green ID, Mead J: Distribution of pleural surface pressure. J Appl Physiol 27:863-873, 1969
4. Milic-Emili J, Henderson JAM, Dolovich MB et al: Regional distribution of inspired gas in the lung. J Appl Physiol 21:749-759, 1966
5. West JB: Ventilation/Blood Flow and Gas Exchange. 2nd Ed. Blackwell Scientific Publications, Oxford and Edinburgh, 1970
6. West JB: Regional differences in gas exchange in the lung of erect man. J Appl Physiol 17:893-898, 1962
7. Svanberg L: Influence of posture on lung volumes, ventilation and circulation in normals. Scand J Clin Lab Invest 9: suppl 25, 1-95, 1957
8. Rheder K, Sessler AD: Function of each lung in spontaneously breathing man anesthetized with thiopental-meperidine. Anesthesiology 38:320-327, 1973
9. Potgieter SV: Atelectasis: its evolution during upper urinary tract surgery. Br J Anaesth 31:472-483, 1959
10. Rheder K, Hatch DJ, Sessler AD et al: The function of each lung of anesthetized and paralyzed man during mechanical ventilation. Anesthesiology 37:16-26, 1972
11. Rheder K, Wenthe FM, Sessler AD: Function of each lung during mechanical ventilation with ZEEP and with PEEP in man anesthetized with thiopental-meperidine. Anesthesiology 39:597-606, 1973
12. Nunn JF: The distribution of inspired gas during thoracic surgery. Ann R Coll Surg Engl 28:223-237, 1961
13. Wulff KE, Aulin I: The regional lung function in the lateral decubitus position during anesthesia and operation. Acta Anaesthesiol Scand 16:195-205, 1972
14. Brown DR, Kafer ER, Roberson VO et al: Improved oxygenation during thoracotomy with selective PEEP to the dependent lung. Anesth Analg (Cleve) 56:26-31, 1977
15. Benumof JL, Rogers SN, Moyce PR et al: Hypoxic pulmonary vasoconstriction and regional and whole-lung PEEP in the dog. Anesthesiology 51:503-507, 1979
16. Froese AB, Bryan CA: Effects of anesthesia

and paralysis on diaphragmatic mechanics in man. Anesthesiology 41:242-255, 1974

17. Tarhan S, Moffitt EA: Principles of thoracic anesthesia. Surg Clin North Am:813-826, 1973

18. Tarhan S, Lundborg RO: Carlens endobronchial catheter versus regular endotracheal tube during thoracic surgery: a comparison of blood gas tensions and pulmonary shunting. Can Anaesth Soc J 18:594-599, 1971

19. Alfery DD, Benumof JL: Anesthesia for thoracic surgery. In Miller R, Ed, Anesthesia, Churchill Livingstone, New York, 1981.

20. Torda TA, McCulloch CH, O'Brien HD et al: Pulmonary venous admixture during one-lung anesthesia: the effect of inhaled oxygen tension and respiration rate. Anaesthesia 29:272-279, 1974

21. Khanom T, Branthwaite MA: Arterial oxygenation during one-lung anesthesia (1): A study in man. Anaesthesia 28:132-138, 1973

22. Kerr JH, Smith AC, Prys-Roberts C et al: Observations during endobronchial anesthesia. II. Oxygenation. Br J Anaesth 46:84-92, 1974

23. Flacke JW, Thompson DS, Read RC: Influence of tidal volume and pulmonary artery occlusion on arterial oxygenation during endobronchial anesthesia. South Med J 69:619-626, 1976

24. Tarhan S, Lundborg RO: Effects of increased expiratory pressure on blood gas tensions and pulmonary shunting during thoracotomy with use of the Carlens catheter. Can Anaesth Soc J 17:4-11, 1970

25. Benumof JL: Mechanism of decreased blood flow to atelectatic lung. J Appl Physiol 46:1047-1048, 1979

26. Pirlo AF, Benumof JL, Trousdale FR: Atelectatic lobe blood flow: open vs. closed chest, positive pressure vs. spontaneous ventilation. J Appl Physiol 50:1022-1026, 1981

27. Mathers JM, Benumof JL, Wahrenbrock EA: General anesthetics and regional hypoxic pulmonary vasoconstriction. Anesthesiology 46:111-114, 1977

28. Benumof JL, Wahrenbrock EA: The local effects of general anesthetics on regional hypoxic pulmonary vasoconstriction. Anesthesiology 43:525-532, 1975

29. Ward CF, Benumof JL, Wahrenbrock EA: Inhibition of hypoxic pulmonary vasoconstriction by vasoactive drugs. Abstracts of Scientific Papers, 1976 Annual Meeting, Am Soc Anesthesiol 333-334, 1976

30. Johansen I, Benumof JL: Reduction of hypoxia induced pulmonary artery hypertension by vasodilator drugs. Am Rev Respir Dis 199:375, 1979

31. Benumof JL: Hypoxic pulmonary vasoconstriction and sodium nitroprusside infusion (Editorial) Anesthesiology 50:481-483, 1979

32. Irwin RS, Martinez-Gonzalez-Rio H, Thomas HM III et al: The effect of granulomatous pulmonary disease in dogs on the response of the pulmonary circulation to hypoxia. J Clin Invest 60:1258-1265, 1977

33. Light RB, Mink SN, Wood LDH: Pathophysiology of gas exchange and pulmonary perfusion in pneumococcal lobar pneumonia in dogs. J Appl Physiol 50(3):524-530, 1981

34. Benumof JL, Mathers JM, Wahrenbrock EA: Cyclic hypoxic pulmonary vasoconstriction induced by concomitant carbon dioxide changes. J Appl Physiol 41:466-469, 1976

35. Hurtig JB, Tait AR, Loh L, Sykes MK: Reduction of hypoxic pulmonary vasoconstriction by nitrous oxide administration in the isolated perfused cat lung. Can. Anaesth Soc J 24:540-549, 1977

36. Sykes MK, Gibbs JM, Loh L et al: Preservation of the pulmonary vasoconstrictor response to alveolar hypoxia during the administration of halothane to dogs. Br J Anaesth 50:1185-1196, 1978

37. Bjertnas LJ, Hauge A, Nakken KF, Bredesen JE: Hypoxic pulmonary vasoconstriction: inhibition due to anesthesia. Acta Physiol Scand 96:283-285, 1976

38. Bjertnas LJ: Hypoxia-induced vasoconstriction in isolated perfused lungs exposed to injectable or inhalation anesthetics. Acta Anesthesiol Scand 21:133-147, 1977

39. Bjertnas LJ, Hauge A, Kriz M: Hypoxia-Induced pulmonary vasoconstriction: effects of fentanyl following different routes of administration. Acta Anaesthesiol Scand 24:53-57, 1980

40. Weinreich AI, Silvay G, Lumb PD: Continuous ketamine infusion for one-lung anesthesia. Can Anaesth Soc J 27:485-490, 1980

41. Borst HG, McGregor M, Whittenberger JL et

al: Influence of pulmonary arterial and left atrial pressures on pulmonary vascular resistance. Circ Res 4:393-399, 1956

42. Benumof JL, Wahrenbrock EA: Blunted hypoxic pulmonary vasoconstriction by increased lung vascular pressures. J Appl Physiol 38:840-850, 1975

43. Scanlon TS, Benumof JL, Wahrenbrock EA et al: Hypoxic pulmonary vasoconstriction and the ratio of hypoxic lung to perfused normoxic lung. Anesthesiology 49:177-181, 1978

44. Marshall BE, Marshall C: Continuity of response to hypoxic pulmonary vasoconstriction. J Appl Physiol 49(2):189-196, 1980

45. Marshall BE, Marshall C, Benumof JL, Saidman LJ: Hypoxic pulmonary vasoconstriction in dogs: effects of lung segment size and alveolar oxygen tensions. J Appl Physiol 51:1543-1551, 1981

46. Piper P, Vane J: The release of prostaglandins from lung and other tissues. Ann NY Acad Sci 180:363-385, 1971

47. Andersen HW, Benumof JL: Intrapulmonary shunting during one-lung ventilation and surgical manipulation. Anesthesiology 55:A377, 1981

48. Benumof JL, Pirlo AF, Trousdale FR: Inhibition of hypoxic pulmonary vasoconstriction by decreased P_vO_2: a new indirect mechanism. J Appl Physiol 51:871-874, 1981

49. Pease RD, Benumof JL: P_AO_2 and P_vO_2 interaction on hypoxic pulmonary vasoconstriction. J Appl Physiol (in press)

50. Johansen I, Benumof JL: Flow distribution in abnormal lung as a function of F_IO_2. Anesthesiology 51(3S):369, 1979

51. Benumof JL, Wahrenbrock EA: Dependency of hypoxic pulmonary vasoconstriction on temperature. J Appl Physiol 42:56-58, 1977

52. Kerr JH: Physiological aspects of one-lung (endobronchial) anesthesia. Int Anesthesiol Clin 10:61-78, 1972

53. Craig JOC, Bromley LL, Williams R: Thoracotomy and the contralateral lung: A study of the changes occurring in the dependent and contralateral lung during and after thoracotomy in lateral decubitus. Thorax 17:9-15, 1962

54. Benumof JL: Respiratory physiology and respiratory function during anesthesia. Ch 22. In Miller, R. Ed.: Anesthesia. Churchill-Livingstone, New York 1981

55. Dantzker DR, Wagner PD, West JB. Instability of lung units with low V/Q ratios during O_2 breathing. J Appl Physiol 38:886-895, 1975

56. Lumb PB, Silvay G, Weinreich AI et al: A comparison of the effects of continuous ketamine infusion and halothane on oxygenation during one-lung anesthesia in dogs. Can Anaesth Soc J 26:394-401, 1979

57. Ray JF III, Yost L, Moallem S et al: Immobility, hypoxemia and pulmonary arteriovenous shunting. Arch Surg 109:537-541, 1974

58. Ward CS: The prevention of accidents associated with anesthetic apparatus. Br J Anaesth 40:692-701, 1968

59. Mazze RI: Therapeutic misadventures with oxygen delivery systems: the need for continuous in-line oxygen monitors. Anesth Analg (Cleve) 51:787-792, 1972

60. Epstein RM, Rackow H, Lee ASJ et al: Prevention of accidental breathing of anoxic gas mixture during anesthesia. Anesthesiology 23:1-4, 1962

61. Sprague DH, Archer GW: Intraoperative hypoxia from an erroneously filled liquid oxygen reservoir. Anesthesiology 42:360-362, 1975

62. Eger EI, Epstein RM: Hazards of anesthetic equipment. Anesthesiology 25:490-504, 1964

63. Benumof JL: Monitoring respiratory function during anesthesia, pp. 31-51. In Saidman, LF and Smith, NT, Eds.: Monitoring in Anesthesia. John Wiley Sons, Inc., New York 1978

64. Martin JT: Positioning in Anesthesia and Surgery. W.B. Saunders Co., Philadelphia, London, Toronto, 1978

65. Conrady PA, Goodman LR, Cainge R et al. Alteration of endotracheal tube position. Flexion and extension of the neck. Crit Care Med 4:8-12, 1976

66. Heinonen J, Takki S, Tammisto T: Effect of the Trendelenburg tilt and other procedures on the position of endotracheal tubes. Lancet 1:850-853, 1969

67. Kelman GF, Nunn JF, Prys-Roberts C, Greenbaum R: The Influence of the Cardiac Output on Arterial Oxygenation: A Theoretical Study. Br J Anaesth 39:450-458, 1967

68. Prys-Roberts C: The metabolic regulation of circulatory transport, pp. 87-96. In Scurr C. and Feldman S., Eds. Scientific Foundations

of Anesthesia. Sec II, Part A, Ch 2. FA Davis Co, Philadelphia, 1970

69. Pappin JC: The current practice of endobronchial intubation Anaesthesia 34:57-64, 1979

70. Simpson PM: Tracheal intubation with a Robertshaw tube via a tracheostomy. Br J Anaesth 48:373-375, 1976

71. Seed RF, Wedley JR: Tracheal intubation with a Robertshaw tube via a tracheostomy (letter). Br J Anaesth 49:639, 1977

72. Bachand R, Audet J, Meloche R et al: Physiological changes associated with unilateral pulmonary ventilation during operations on one lung. Can Anaesth Soc J 22:659-664, 1975

73. Kerr J, Smith AC, Prys-Roberts C et al: Observations during endobronchial anaesthesia. I. Ventilation and carbon dioxide clearance. Br J Anaesth 45:159-167, 1973

74. Hatch D: Ventilation and arterial oxygenation during thoracic surgery. Thorax 21:310-314, 1966

75. Aalto-Setala M, Heinonen J, Salorinne Y: Cardiorespiratory function during thoracic anesthesia: a comparison of two-lung ventilation and one-lung ventilation with and without PEEP. Acta Anaesthesiol Scand 19:287-295, 1975

76. Khanam T, Branthwaite MA: Arterial oxygenation during one-lung anesthesia (2). Anaesthesia 28:280-290, 1973

77. Frumin MJ, Epstein RM, Cohen G: Apneic oxygenation in man. Anesthesiology 20:789-798, 1959

78. Capan LM, Turndorf H, Patel C et al: Optimization of arterial oxygenation during one-lung anesthesia. Anesth Analg (Cleve) 59:847-851, 1980

79. Alfery DD, Benumof JL, Trousdale FR: Improving oxygenation during one-lung ventilation: the effects of PEEP and blood flow restriction to the nonventilated lung. Anesthesiology 55:381-385, 1981

80. Zamost BG, Alfery DD, Johanson I: Description and clinical evaluation of a new continuous positive airway pressure device. Crit Care 9:109-113, 1981

81. Andersen, HW, Benumof JL, Ozaki GT: New improved double-lumen tube adaptor. Anesthesiology 56:54-56, 1982

82. Bjerager K, Sjostrand U, Wattwill M: Long-term treatment of two patients with respiratory insufficiency with IPPV/PEEP and HFPPV/PEEP. Acta Anaesthesiol Scand, suppl 64:55-68, 1977

83. Carlon G, Ray C, Klain M, McCormack P: High frequency positive pressure ventilation in management of a patient with bronchopleural fistula. Anesthesiology 52:160-162, 1980

84. Butler WJ, Bohn DJ, Bryan AC, Froese AB: Ventilation by high frequency oscillation in humans. Anesth Analg (Cleve) 59:577-584, 1980

85. Sjostrand U: High frequency positive pressure ventilation (HFPPV): a review. Crit Care Med 8:345-364, 1980

86. Borg U, Eriksson I, Sjostrand U: High frequency positive pressure ventilation (HFPPV): a review based upon its use during bronchoscopy and for laryngoscopy and microlaryngeal surgery under general anesthesia. Anesth Analg (Cleve) 59:594-603, 1980

87. Eriksson I, Nilsson L-G, Nordstrom S, Sjostrand U: High frequency positive pressure ventilation (HFPPV) during transthoracic resection of tracheal stenosis and during perioperative bronchoscopic examination. Acta Anaesthesiol Scand 19:113-119, 1975

88. Malina JR, Nordstrom SG, Sjostrand UH, Wattwill LM: Clinical evaluation of high frequency positive pressure ventilation (HFPPV) in patients scheduled for open chest surgery. Anesth Analg (Cleve) 60:324-330, 1981

89. Venus B, Pratap KS, Op'Tholt T: Treatment of unilateral pulmonary insufficiency by selective administration of continuous positive airway pressure through a double-lumen tube. Anesthesiology 52:74-77, 1980

90. Sachdeva SP: Treatment of post-operative pulmonary atelectasis by active inflation of the atelectatic lobe(s) through an endobronchial tube. Acta Anaesthesiol Scand 18:65-67, 1974

91. Glass DD, Tonnesen AS, Gabel JC et al: Therapy of unilateral pulmonary insufficiency with a double lumen endotracheal tube. Crit Care Med 4:323-326, 1976

92. Powner DJ, Eross B, Grenvik A: Differential lung ventilation with PEEP in the treatment of unilateral pneumonia. Crit Care Med 5:170-172, 1977

93. Trew F, Warren BR, Potter WA et al: Differ-

ential lung ventilation in man. Crit Care Med 4:112, 1976

94. Carlon GC, Kahn R, Howaland WS et al: Acute life threatening ventilation-perfusion inequality: an indication for independent lung ventilation. Crit Care Med 6:380-383, 1978

95. Albert RK, Lakshminarayan S, Kirk W, Buttler J: Lung inflation can cause pulmonary edema in zone 1 of in-situ dog lungs. J Appl Physiol 49:815-819, 1980

96. Alfery DD, Zamost BG, Benumof JL: Unilateral lung lavage: blood flow manipulation by ipsilateral pulmonary artery balloon inflation. Anesthesiology 55:376-381, 1981

97. Benumof JL, Spragg RG, Alfery DD: Pulmonary artery balloon manipulation of pulmonary blood flow during unilateral lung lavage. Anesthesiology 55:A376, 1981

98. Petersen BM: Balloon directed pulmonary blood flow. Crit Care Med 9:540-543, 1981

99. Benumof JL, Saidman LJ, Arkin DB, Diamant M: Where pulmonary artery catheters go: intrathoracic distribution. Anesthesiology 46:336-338, 1977

PART IV.

SPECIFIC ANESTHETIC CONSIDERATIONS

Patrick E. Curling, M.D.

9
Anesthesia for Thoracic Diagnostic Procedures

The choice of anesthesia for laryngoscopy, fiberoptic bronchoscopy, rigid bronchoscopy, mediastinoscopy, mediastinotomy, esophagoscopy, and thoracoscopy involves surgical, anesthetic, and patient factors that enter into the selection of a suitable technique. The patient's pathological lesion and its pathophysiological impact on the airway during anesthesia are the ultimate elements to be considered.

The preoperative evaluation and preparation of the patient undergoing thoracic surgery have been discussed in Chapters 4 and 5; they are equally applicable to the patient scheduled for a diagnostic procedure.

General anesthesia for thoracic diagnostic procedures can be very challenging. Not only does the airway have to be shared with the surgeon, but often the same instrument, e.g., a ventilating bronchoscope. Prior communication with the surgeon concerning the patient's status and the proposed surgical plan cannot be overemphasized. Close cooperation and communication, which are vital intraoperatively, are initiated by this preoperative contact.

The selection of regional blocks and

topical anesthesia is an equal challenge. Proper patient selection, skill at performing the block, and choice of correct doses and drugs are the demands placed on the anesthesiologist.

The objectives of general anesthesia include analgesia, unconsciousness, skeletal muscle relaxation, and control of excessive sympathetic or parasympathetic activity to noxious stimuli. However, only analgesia, sedation, and control of excessive reflex activity are required during local or regional block procedures.

LARYNGOSCOPY

Preoperative Evaluation

The usual concerns of preoperative evaluation of the patient with upper airway or pulmonary disease have been emphasized in Chapter 4. In addition, there are special considerations in airway evaluation for laryngoscopy. The presence of stridor in a resting state suggests significant airway obstruction. Dysphonia may also be a symptom

319

of obstruction but is related to the site of infiltration of a tumor. Findings on *indirect* laryngoscopy should be part of the preoperative evaluation. Sellers divides patients into three groups on this basis, as outlined in Table 9-1.[1]

The patient with the compromised airway should have a posterior-anterior and lateral neck x-ray as a minimum, and these should be personally reviewed by the anesthesiologist. Xeroradiographs that utilize a highly charged selenium plate give more definite resolution.[2] Good definition of size and location can be achieved by tomograms, while computerized axial tomography, or CAT scan, offers the highest degree of resolution. The technique giving the highest resolution that is available in a particular institution should be done preoperatively. An example of an anterior mediastinal mass impinging on the airway is illustrated in the x-ray in Figure 9-1.

Regardless of whether general anesthesia or topical and regional block is selected, the patient deserves the same preoperative workup. Proctor suggests that diagnostic procedures should not be considered "minor" surgical procedures and the patients should not receive "minor" general anesthetics.[3] This author would emphasize there are no "minor" regional or local anesthetics either, having been involved in the resuscitation of patients undergoing surgery with local anesthesia.

The Stimulus of Laryngoscopy During General Anesthesia

The marked tachycardia, hypertension, laryngospasm, and patient movement induced by laryngoscopy and endotracheal intubation under a light level of anesthesia are a vivid learning experience for any anesthesiologist.[4] Studies in the artificially ventilated cat demonstrate that mechanical stimulation of the laryngeal and tracheobronchial regions causes reflex tracheobronchial con-

Table 9-1

Classification of Preoperative Airway Obstruction

Group I	Unobstructed airway at rest and a small lesion
Group II	Mild degree of respiratory obstruction at rest or a large lesion
Group III	Gross airway obstruction at rest

Sellers SL, Augoustides TA: Anesthesia for laryngeal surgery. Otolaryngo 5:203–206, 1976. With permission of the author and publisher.

striction, while similar stimulation of the epipharynx and nasal mucosa causes reflex bronchodilatation. Stimulation of the nose, epipharynx, laryngopharynx, and tracheobronchial tree also causes a reflex increase in systemic blood pressure.[5]

MAC EI_{50} has been defined as the anesthetic concentration needed by 50 percent of the population to permit laryngoscopy, easy visualization of the glottis, relaxation of the vocal cords, absence of extremity movement, and absence of bucking after tracheal intubation.[6] In children at sea level, this is calculated for halothane at 1.3 percent. Thus there is an objective clinical level of anesthesia to aim for, albeit wrong in 50 percent of cases. MAC EI_{50} for enflurane at sea level is 2.9 percent.[7] MAC BAR_{50} as defined by Roizen et al is the age-adjusted dose of anesthesia that blocks the adrenergic response in 50 percent of individuals to a skin incision; MAC BAR_{95} blocks the response in 95 percent of individuals.[8] Thus it is possible to compare the MAC_{50}, MAC_{95}, MAC EI_{50}, MAC EI_{95}, MAC BAR_{50}, and MAC BAR_{95} (Table 9-2). These data are from healthy unpremedicated children and adults.

Complications such as pulmonary edema and ventricular tachycardia have been reported secondary to endotracheal intubation during light anesthesia in sick patients.[9] Mechanical manipulation of the airways can lead to excessive sympathetic stimulation and cardiac dysrhythmias or even sudden death.[10-13] Parasympathetically-mediated mechanical stimuli can also produce dysrhythmias, e.g., vagal arrest.[5, 12, 14]

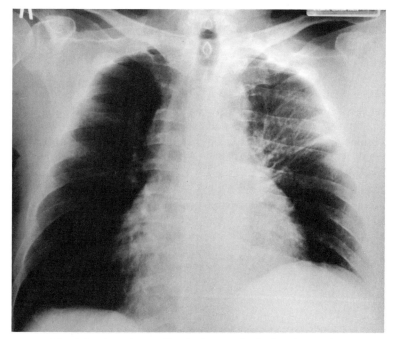

Fig. 9-1 Anterior mediastinal mass displacing the trachea.

To provide a "stress-free" general anesthetic for laryngoscopy, MAC EI_{95} or perhaps MAC BAR_{95} must be achieved to prevent harmful reflex sympathetic or parasympathetic cardiac complications. However, Roizen points out that anesthetic depth to MAC BAR_{50} and MAC BAR_{95} to diminish or abolish the intraoperative stress response has to be balanced against the greater depression of myocardial and respiratory function at the deeper levels of anesthesia.[8]

Regional Block and Topical Anesthesia for Laryngoscopy or Bronchoscopy

TOPICAL INSTILLATION

Lidocaine, tetracaine, and cocaine are the usual drugs selected for topical anesthesia.[3, 15–17] Cocaine is often used since it produces vasoconstriction by inhibiting reuptake of norepinephrine.[18] All these drugs should be applied topically over 10 to 15

Table 9-2
Comparison of MAC, MAC_{EI}, and MAC_{BAR}

	Halothane	Enflurane
MAC_{50}	1.0 MAC (0.74 ± 0.03%)	1.0 MAC (1.68 ± 0.04%)
MAC EI_{50}	1.3 MAC	1.4 MAC
MAC BAR_{50}	1.5 MAC	1.6 MAC
MAC_{95}	1.2 MAC	1.1 MAC
MAC EI_{95}	1.7 MAC	1.9 MAC
MAC BAR_{95}	2.1 MAC	2.6 MAC

These values have been age-adjusted.

Adapted from: Roizen MF, Horrigan RW, Frazer BM: Anesthetic doses blocking adrenergic (stress) and cardiovascular responses to incision—MAC BAR. Anesthesiology 54:390–398, 1981. With permission of the author and publisher.

minutes to avoid very high blood levels (see below).

Using the traditional dropper technique, the oropharynx is first sprayed and then, by using a curved cannula, progressive instillation of drug is made to the base of the tongue, both valleculae, the epiglottis, and the adducted vocal cords. Indirect mirror laryngoscopy can be used to aid placement. The tongue is retracted with a gauze held by the patient or an assistant.[19, 20]

The internal laryngeal nerve can be anesthetized by applying a small cotton swab soaked in anesthetic into each pyriform fossa or by placing drops in the valleculae.[19, 20] Another alternative is to use pledgets soaked in anesthetic, which are progressively placed into the pharynx by using Magill forceps. Then, by using gentle traction with a Macintosh laryngoscope blade to depress the tongue, swabs can be applied to the uvula and soft palate. Finally, the vocal cords are sprayed under direct vision.[21]

NEBULIZATION

Ultrasonic nebulization of lidocaine with the patient spontaneously breathing is popular for fiberoptic bronchoscopy, and can be used for laryngoscopy as well.[22-24] With a DeVilbiss Model 900 ultrasonic nebulizer used with 4 percent lidocaine for analysis of particle size, a mean size of 6.3 microns has been determined, 80 percent of the particles being below 10 microns. Theoretically, this would deliver 55 percent of the mass of the aerosolized anesthetic to the larynx and tracheobronchial tree, as illustrated in Figure 9-2.[22] This method delivers topical anesthesia to all the bronchial tree that the fiberoptic bronchoscope reaches and overcomes the problems seen with earlier methods of topical anesthesia.[25] Ultrasonic nebulization can be combined with gargling or swallowing viscous lidocaine or swallowing liquid lidocaine to produce topical anesthesia of the esophagus for fiberoptic esophagoscopy as well as bronchoscopy.[26]

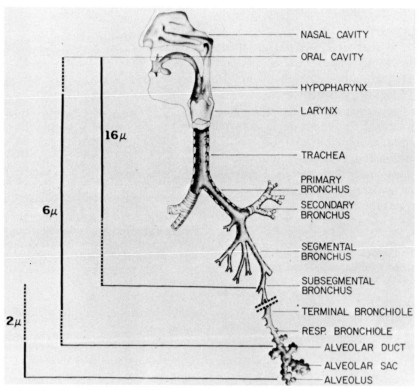

Fig. 9-2 Theoretical deposition of various sized particles in the respiratory tract. (Christoforidis AJ, Tomashefsk JF, Mitchell MS: Use of an ultrasonic nebulizer for the application of oropharyngeal, laryngeal and tracheobronchial anesthesia. Chest 59:629-633, 1971.)

TRANSCRICOID PUNCTURE

Percutaneous transcricoid puncture provides topical anesthesia to the upper and lower respiratory tract. The technique is contraindicated in a patient with an enlarged thyroid, carcinoma or tuberculosis of the tracheobronchial tree, a bleeding diathesis, or obscured landmarks.[21] The skin should be infiltrated with local anesthesia via a 25-gauge needle and the membrane punctured with a 22-gauge catheter and needle; aspiration of air confirms the correct position. The needle is withdrawn, a syringe is firmly attached to the catheter, air is again aspirated, and xylocaine is injected as the patient *forcefully inspires*. The use of a 22-guage, 1-inch long over-the-needle Teflon catheter unit ensures prevention of needle breakage or vessel laceration when the patient coughs.[27] Transcricoid puncture with larger needles has been associated with serious hemorrhage or death.[28, 29] The complication rate for transcricoid puncture has been reported at 0.3 to 0.6 percent, with broken needles, local hematomas, local infection and abscess, and subcutaneous emphysema being the most common complications.[28]

SPECIFIC NERVE BLOCKS FOR LARYNGOSCOPY

Superior Laryngeal Nerve Block

The superior laryngeal nerve arises from the vagus nerve at the nodose ganglion, descends inferiorly and anteriorly toward the larynx, and then divides into an external motor branch to the cricothyroid muscle and an internal sensory branch, the target of the block. The internal branch is located anteriorly, accompanied by the superior laryngeal artery. Together they penetrate the thyroid membrane midway between the hyoid and thyroid cartilages and 1 cm anterior to the cornu of the thyroid (Fig. 9-3).[27, 30, 31] Once the internal branch of the superior laryngeal nerve penetrates the thyrohyoid membrane, it breaks into sensory branches to

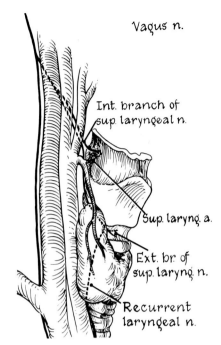

Fig. 9-3 Nerve supply of the larynx. (Gaskill JR, Gillies DR: Local anesthesia for peroral endoscopy. Arch Otolaryngol 84:654-657, 1966. Copyright 1966, American Medical Association)

the mucosa of the larynx, the laryngeal surface of the epiglottis, and part of the posterior larynx.

With the patient supine, the anesthesiologist's finger is placed under the superior cornu of the thyroid cartilage and retracts the carotid sheath posteriorly (Fig. 9-4). A long 26-gauge needle is advanced until the thyrohyoid membrane is felt or "popped"; 2 ml of 1% lidocaine is then injected after aspiration for blood or air. Sharp ear pain may occur from stimulation by the needle of the auricular branch of the nerve (Arnold's nerve). The block is then repeated on the opposite side.[30]

Glossopharyngeal Plexus Block

The glossopharyngeal plexus is composed of the glossopharyngeal nerve and minor contributions from branches of the vagus nerve, the sympathetic chain, and possibly the superior laryngeal nerve.[27] Thus,

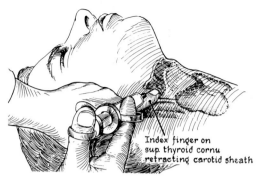

Fig. 9-4 Block of the internal branch of the superior laryngeal nerve. (Gaskill JR, Gillies DR: Local anesthesia for peroral endoscopy. Arch Otolaryngol 84:654-657, 1966. Copyright 1966, American Medical Association.)

the glossopharyngeal nerve block should more correctly be termed the glossopharyngeal *plexus* block.[32] The technique described below blocks the tactile and pressure receptors of the afferent limbs of the gag reflex. Bilateral glossopharyngeal plexus blocks are necessary for total abolition of the gag reflex since there is overlap of innervation on both sides. Classically, the glossopharyngeal nerve supplies sensory innervation of the uvula, soft palate, posterior pharyngeal wall, lateral pharyngeal wall, and posterior third of the tongue.

The glossopharyngeal plexus is usually blocked with an angled tonsillar needle (Fig. 9-5). The tongue is depressed and the needle inserted at the midpoint of the posterior tonsillar pillar and advanced laterally to a maximum depth of 1 cm. After aspiration, 3 ml of 1% lidocaine is injected.[31]

BLOOD LEVELS AND TOXICITY (TABLE 9-3)

Lidocaine

Central nervous system toxicity is seen with serum concentrations greater than 9 to 10 μg/ml.[33-35] By using 4% topical lidocaine or an endotracheal spray, Bromage showed peak blood concentrations at 5 to 25 minutes. He recommended a maximum topical dose

below 6 mg/kg, since that dose produced toxic blood levels in 5 percent of patients.[34] After 5 minutes, an 18.2 μg/ml blood level was noted in one patient who received 360 mg of lidocaine (body weight of patient not given).[34] This emphasizes that an occasional patient may become toxic with these "safe" levels. In another study, a dose of 3 mg/kg administered via a commercial aerosol dispenser with freon (no longer available) gave peak arterial levels of 2.5 μg/ml and venous levels of 3.2 μg/ml.[35] Since the volume of distribution of lidocaine varies among subjects, differences in blood levels reflect a varying rate of absorption.[36-38] During fiberoptic bronchoscopy, nebulized lidocaine, 280 mg via IPPB plus additional 2% lidocaine jelly to the nostril, and 1 to 2% lidocaine instilled via the bronchoscope (total doses ranging from 600 to 1,190 mg) resulted in the highest peak plasma concentration of 8.7 μg/ml and a mean peak concentration time between 5 and 30 minutes. These doses are higher than recommended but surprisingly were not associated with toxic levels. These doses also helped to avoid major dysrhythmias during fiberoptic bronchoscopy.[39] Studies by deJong and others have shown that diazepam can be used to raise the seizure threshold and abort local anesthetic-induced convulsions when large doses of local anesthetic are used.[40-45]

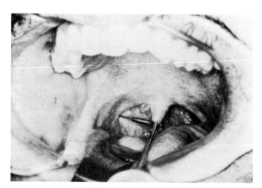

Fig. 9-5 Glossopharyngeal plexus block with angled tonsillar needle. (Cooper M, Watson RL: An improved regional technique for peroral endoscopy. Anesthesiology 43:372-374, 1974.)

Tetracaine

Tetracaine, in a dose of 30 to 40 mg, was used for topical and transtracheal anesthesia in a series of 1,000 bronchoscopies.[46] There were 12 minor reactions, including hypotension and bradycardia, which were treated with Trendelenberg position and oxygen, and impending convulsions, which were treated with thiopental. There were seven severe reactions, six convulsions, and one pronounced bronchospasm. These patients were premedicated with 120 mg of phenobarbital. Blood levels of tetracaine were not available. This incidence of side reactions is probably unacceptable today.

Cocaine

Cocaine is absorbed from all sites of application, and enhanced absorption occurs in the presence of inflammation. It is a potent local anesthetic and central nervous system stimulant and also blocks reuptake of catecholamines at adrenergic nerve endings.[18] The usually-stated maximum dose is 200 mg, although toxicity may be seen with as little as 20 mg, and ventricular fibrillation has been reported with a dose as low as 30 mg.[47] It is topically applied in 5 to 10% solution, and epinephrine should not be used with it. A fatal oral dose is considered to be 1.2 g in a 70-kg person, the LD_{50} being 500 mg. The half-life in plasma is approximately 1 hour.[4, 17, 47, 48]

BRONCHOSCOPY

Landa has reviewed the indications for bronchoscopy and the instruments of choice (Table 9-4 and 9-5).[49]

Fiberoptic Bronchoscopy

The introduction of the fiberoptic bronchoscope (FOB) has complemented techniques developed for the rigid bronchoscope.[50, 51] Snider believes that the fiberoptic bronchoscope has revolutionized bronchoscopy by removing discomfort, the risk of broken teeth, and vasovagal reactions with extreme extension of the neck.[52] Its smaller size permits examination of the fifth order of branching of the bronchi, and the transbronchial brush and forceps have increased diagnostic acumen. The FOB may also be used for selective bronchography.[53]

PHYSIOLOGICAL CHANGES DURING FIBEROPTIC BRONCHOSCOPY

Hypoxemia develops during FOB (in healthy volunteers and sick patients), with an average decline of the PaO_2 by 20 mmHg, and lasts for 1 to 4 hours following the procedure.[54–58] This is treated by raising the FIO_2 by oxygen supplementation with either a nasal cannula held in the mouth, a modified venturi mask, an oxygen mask providing 28 percent O_2 for CO_2-retaining patients, or an endotracheal tube with a T-piece adapter.[59, 60]

Patients, but not healthy controls, develop increased airway obstruction after FOB.[56] These changes in pulmonary function tests are probably secondary to direct mechanical activation of cough and irritative reflexes in the airway and possibly mucosal edema.[61] Abnormalities in pulmonary function tests are usually transient and are back to baseline within 24 hours.[56, 61]

Patients given atropine by injection or aerosol demonstrate significant bronchodilator effects that help to overcome some of the deleterious effects of FOB on pulmonary function.[61] The bronchodilatation produced by atropine has been known for some time, but the common misconception of anesthesiologists is that atropine will dry bronchial secretions, especially in asthmatics.[62] The literature does not document a deleterious effect of atropine on secretions in patients with obstructive lung disease but rather a beneficial bronchodilator effect.[63, 64] Therefore, atropine is recommended in the premedication regime for FOB. Neuhaus has demonstrated that atropine-pretreated patients undergoing FOB do not develop deterioration in pulmonary function immediately after bronchoscopy when compared with baseline. These effects are illustrated in Figures 9-6 through

Table 9-3
Suggested Maximum Doses of Local Anesthetics

| Drug | Topical | | Regional Block | |
	Concentrations, %	Dose	Concentrations, %	Dose
Cocaine	5–10	200 mg	—	—
Tetracaine	1–2	80 mg	0.1 –0.25	100 mg
			(rarely used)	
Lidocaine	2–4	200 mg	0.5 –2	500 mg
Bupivicaine	—	—	0.25–0.75	200 mg

Data from Ritchie JM, Cohen PJ, Dripps RD: Cocaine, procaine, and other local anesthetics. In Goodman LS, Gilman A, Eds: The Pharmacological Basis of Therapeutics, 4th ed. Copyright © 1970 by Macmillan Publishing Co., Inc., New York.

9-9.[61] The efficacy of atropine would be most beneficial in patients with reactive airways or in compromised patients who can ill afford further deterioration in pulmonary function.[61] Topical lidocaine aerosol has been shown to decrease forced vital capacity prior to FOB, but atropine reversed this effect as well.[61]

Isoproterenol hydrochloride by aerosol, in general, reversed the effects of FOB. However, isoproterenol was associated with an increased frequency of palpitations, whereas atropine only produced occasional difficulty in voiding in patients receiving these drugs preoperatively for 3 weeks.[65] To summarize these data, isoproterenol is not recommended and atropine appears to be the premedicant of choice for fiberoptic bronchoscopy.[66-68]

A preliminary report of ventilation and perfusion scans in six healthy volunteers undergoing a saline lobar lavage through a cuffed FOB demonstrated the development of defects on the perfusion scan and delayed washout on the ventilation scan.[57] Three of the six volunteers also had delayed washout in other lobes. Thus, saline lobar lavage may induce ventilation abnormalities in areas of the lung *other* than the area lavaged. These ventilation and perfusion defects returned to

Table 9-4
Indications for Bronchoscopy

Diagnostic Indications	Therapeutic Indications
Cough	Foreign bodies
Hemoptysis	Accumulated secretions
Wheeze	Atelectasis
Atelectasis	Aspiration
Unresolved pneumonia	Lung abscess
Diffuse lung disease	Reposition endotracheal tubes
Preoperative evaluation	Placement of endobronchial tubes
Rule out metastasis	
Assess local disease recurrence	
Abnormal chest x-ray findings	
Recurrent laryngeal nerve paralysis	
Diaphragm paralysis	
Acute inhalation injury	
Exclude tracheo-esophageal fistula	
During mechanical ventilation	
Selective bronchography	

Adapted from: Landa JF: Indications for bronchoscopy. Chest 73 (suppl.): 686–690, 1978. With permission of author and publisher.

Table 9-5
Instruments of Choice for Bronchoscopy

OPEN TUBE
Foreign bodies
Massive hemoptysis
Vascular tumors
Small children
Endobronchial resections

FLEXIBLE INSTRUMENT
Mechanical problems of the neck
Upper lobe and peripheral lesions
Limited hemoptysis
During mechanical ventilation
Pneumonia, for selective cultures

COMBINATION
Positive cytology with negative chest x-ray

Landa JF: Indications for bronchoscopy. Chest 73 (Suppl): 686–690, 1978. With permission of author and publisher.

normal more slowly than those in the area of lavage. In addition, the ventilation and perfusion defects returned to normal more slowly than the hypoxemia.[57]

Major cardiac dysrhythmias, defined as a sinus bradycardia $\leq$ 40 beats per minute (BPM), atrial fibrillation with a rapid ventricular response $\geq$ 120 BPM, supraventricular tachycardia $\geq$ 140 BPM, or premature ventricular contractions (PVCs) $\geq$ 50/hour,

developed in 11 percent of 70 patients during FOB and correlated with a PaO_2 less than 60 mm Hg.[69] None was treated and all were self-limited. Elguindi et al using 777 $\pm$ 40 mg of nebulized lidocaine, only reported an increase in minor dysrhythmias and a decrease in major dysrhythmias (serum lidocaine levels were in the therapeutic range 5.0 $\pm$ 0.6μg/ml.)[39] In patients with coronary artery disease who received an average lidocaine dose of 274 mg and 0.5 mg of atropine, no increase in PVCs was seen.[70]

Suctioning via the 2-mm suction port of the FOB at 760 mm Hg removes 14.2 liters/minute of air and will thus lower FIO_2 and FAO_2. Suctioning during FOB should be brief and at 100 mmHg maximum pressure to prevent unacceptable hypoxemia and cardiac dysrhythmias.[71, 72]

When the FOB is advanced into the trachea through an endotracheal tube, the effective ventilating area of the endotracheal tube lumen is reduced. With a standard 5.7 mm ED FOB, a number 8.0 mm ID endotracheal tube or larger must be used.[73] This is illustrated with data from Lindholm (Fig. 9-10 and Table 9-6).[74]

Carden and Raj have designed an adult tube made of silicone in a Cole-type design

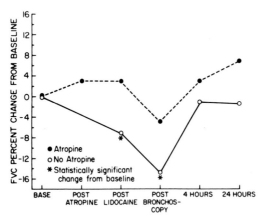

Fig. 9-6 Changes in forced vital capacity (FVC) during FOB. (Neuhaus A, Markowitz D, Rotman HH et al: The effects of fiberoptic bronchoscopy with and without atropine on pulmonary function in humans. Ann Thorac Surg 25:393-398, 1978.)

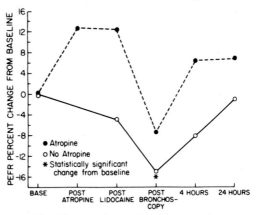

Fig. 9-7 Changes in peak expiratory flow rate (PEFR) during FOB. (Neuhaus A, Markowitz D, Rotman HH et al: The effects of fiberoptic bronchoscopy with and without atropine on pulmonary function in humans. Ann Thorac Surg 25:393-398, 1978.)

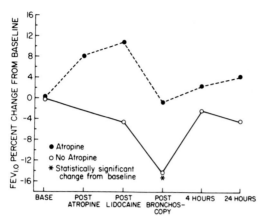

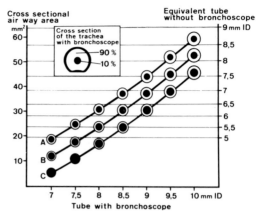

Fig. 9-8 Changes in forced expiratory volume in 1 second (FEV_1) during FOB. (Neuhaus A, Markowitz D, Rotman HH et al: The effects of fiberoptic bronchoscopy with and without atropine on pulmonary function in humans. Ann Thorac Surg 25:393-398, 1978.)

Fig. 9-10 Diagram of cross-sectional areas of endotracheal tubes holding fiberoptic bronchoscopes. Different caliber tubes (outer circle) containing three different size bronchoscopes (filled center) as shown: (A) 5 mm ED; (B) 5.7 mm ED; (C) 6.0 mm ED. White area within the tubes shows available cross-sectional airway area. Insert: Relation between available cross-sectional airway area of the trachea and the bronchofiberscope in nonintubated normal patients. (Lindholm CE, Ollman B, Snyder JV et al: Cardiorespiratory effects of flexible fiberoptic bronchoscopy in critically ill patients. Chest 74:362-368, 1978.)

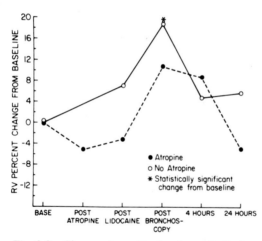

Fig. 9-9 Changes in residual volume (RV) during FOB. (Neuhaus A, Markowitz D, Rotman HH et al: The effects of fiberoptic bronchoscopy with and without atropine on pulmonary function in humans. Ann Thorac Surg 25:393-398, 1978.

with a smaller diameter of tube that passes through the cords (Fig. 9-11).[75] The high resistance to flow only occurs in the narrow section that is now only a quarter of the total length of the tube, which allows the use of an FOB in a patient who can only accept a 7.5 mm endotracheal tube.[76] They have also de-

signed a swivel adapter which seals the FOB without leakage when used through an endotracheal tube (Figs. 9-12 and 9-13).

FIBEROPTIC BRONCHOSCOPY IN THE CRITICALLY ILL PATIENT

Studies have shown that FOB is diagnostically and therapeutically useful for assessing airway patency, airway damage, management of atelectasis and retained secretions, or occasionally for removing foreign bodies.[62] Mechanical ventilation can continue during FOB, but the cardiovascular and respiratory changes that occur must be understood in order to prevent acute cardiopulmonary deterioration. The introduction of the FOB will result in a decreased PaO_2, and the PEEP effect from the reduced cross-

Table 9-6
Relationship of endotracheal tube size to PEEP produced by insertion of 5.7 mm FOB

ET Tube Size, mm ID	Cross-Sectional Area, % Occupied by the 5.7 mm FOB	Maximum Measured PEEP in Patients, cm H_2O
7	66	35
8	51	20
9	40	—

Lindholm CE, Ollman B, Snyder JV et al.: Cardiorespiratory effects of flexible fiberoptic bronchoscopy in critically ill patients, Chest 74:362–368, 1978. With permission of author and publisher.

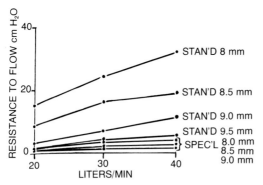

Fig. 9-11 Resistance to flow through standard and Carden (SPEC'L) endotracheal tubes with fiberoptic bronchoscope in place. (Carden E, Raj P: Special new low-resistance-to-flow tube and endotracheal tube adapter for use during fiberoptic bronchoscopy. Ann Otol Rhinol Laryngol 84:631-634, 1975.)

sectional area may cause barotrauma (Fig. 9-14). Excessive suctioning may further decrease tidal volume, functional residual capacity, and FIO_2, producing severe hypoxemia. Cardiac output is usually increased if the patient has adequate cardiac reserve (Fig. 9-15).

In the critically ill patient on mechanical ventilation, PEEP should be discontinued during FOB and the FIO_2 increased to 1.0. Adequate ventilation should be monitored by visual chest excursion and arterial blood gases.[74] Suction at 100 mmHg should be used only for minimal time periods. A chest x-ray should be obtained after the procedure to rule out mediastinal emphysema and pneumothorax.[51, 74, 77]

Complications

From retrospective reviews of 24,251 and 48,000 fiberoptic bronchoscopies a number of conclusions can be drawn.[79–80] Tetracaine was specifically implicated as having a narrow range of safety and was associated with a high mortality rate. Lidocaine had a much wider margin of safety and toxicity was likely only from a massive overdose. Laryngospasm and bronchospasm due to inadequate anesthesia caused life-threatening emergencies. Other complications were as expected from this type of procedure: broken brushes, hemorrhage, pneumothorax, and hypoxemia.

A prospective Russian series compared 1,146 fiberoptic bronchoscopies performed under topical tetracaine and procaine anesthesia with 3,449 rigid bronchoscopies done with general anesthesia using hexobarbital.[80] More of the anesthetic complications were attributable to the toxic effects of tetracaine than to the general anesthetic. However, rigid bronchoscopy produced more major life-threatening complications. These authors noted that the largest number of complications developed in patients with bronchial asthma. Table 9-7 summarizes data on complication rates from a number of series during FOB.[78–81]

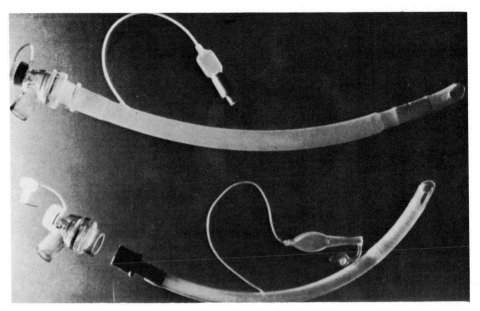

Fig. 9-12 Standard and special low-resistance endotracheal tube (Carden) with adapter. (Carden E. Recent improvements in techniques for general anesthesia for bronchoscopy. Chest 73:697-700, 1978.)

Rigid Bronchoscopy, Alone or With Fiberoptic Bronchoscopy

Techniques of ventilation for rigid bronchoscopy include use of the ventilating bronchoscope along with:

1. Apnea with intermittent ventilation[82-84]
2. The Sanders attachment with venturi injection[82-87]
3. The Carden side-arm injection system[86-89]
4. The Bronchoflator injection system[90-91]
5. The Venti-bronchoscopes I and II[92]
6. The addition of nitrous oxide or halothane to the Carden technique[93-94]
7. A mechanical ventilator, eg: Bird Mark II[95]
8. Ventilation with gases delivered via the side arm[96-97]
9. High frequency positive pressure ventilation[98-100]

Systems other than the ventilating bronchoscope which may be used in rigid bronchoscopy include:

1. Insufflation via a catheter in an apneic patient[94, 101]
2. Cuirass ventilation or external chest compression[102,103]
3. A small endotracheal tube alongside the bronchoscope[104]
4. A ventilating catheter placed alongside the bronchoscope[105]

Ventilation during the first rigid bronchoscopies was done by the apneic technique or with intermittent ventilation between the visualization periods of the surgeon. In general, the Sanders techniques and their later modifications have improved ventilation during anesthesia, especially for prolonged bronchoscopies. Anesthetic techniques had usually consisted of intravenous barbiturates and succinylcholine for relaxation. The Sanders techniques and its modifications reduced the degree of hypercarbia and hypoxia and made it possible to add nitrous oxide or halogenated agents to the anesthetic technique.

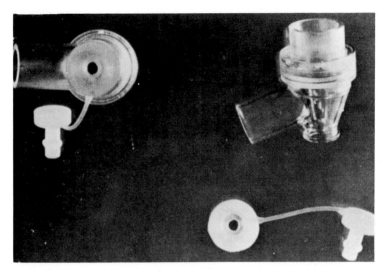

Fig. 9-13 Endotracheal tube adapters for FOB. (Carden E: Recent improvements in techniques for general anesthesia for bronchoscopy. Chest 73:697-700, 1979.)

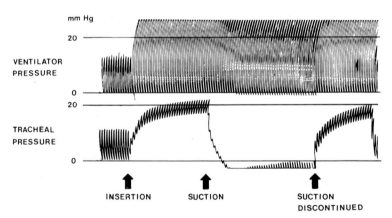

Fig. 9-14 Ventilation of a dog via a 7.0 mm ID endotracheal tube; insertion of 5.7 mm ED bronchoscope; simultaneous recording of ventilator and intratracheal pressure. Insertion of the bronchoscope resulted in an immediate elevation of the peak respiratory pressure due to airway obstruction; tracheal pressure showed a gradual elevation of peak respiratory pressure and a PEEP effect of 16 mm Hg at 1 minute. A negative pressure of 62 mmHg was applied to the suction port of the FOB; in six breaths the intratracheal pressure was continuously negative, indicating removal of air from the lung in spite of unchanged ventilator function. (Lindholm CE, Ollman B, Snyder JV et al: Cardiorespiratory effects of flexible fiberoptic bronchoscopy in critically ill patients. Chest 74:362-368, 1978.)

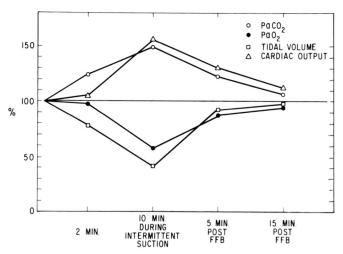

Fig. 9-15 Cardiorespiratory variables during FOB in patients being mechanically ventilated. Changes in four variables during FOB in six critically ill patients during ongoing controlled mechanical ventilation. Prebronchoscopy values are 100 percent. Measurements were repeated at 2 minutes after insertion of the bronchoscope, at 10 minutes during ongoing intermittent suctioning, and at 5 and 15 minutes following FOB. (Lindholm CE, Ollman B, Snyder JV, et al: Cardiorespiratory effects of flexible fiberoptic bronchoscopy in critically ill patients. Chest 74:362-368, 1978.)

APNEIC OXYGENATION

Denitrogenation and subsequent apneic oxygenation in eight healthy patients with an FiO_2 of 1.0 for 30 minutes resulted in maintenance of arterial oxygen saturation (lowest level, 98 percent), hypercapnia (highest recorded $PaCO_2$ = 250 mmHg), and acidosis (lowest pH = 6.88) in a classic study.[106] These patients were not truly apneic, as the onset of ventilation was used as a sign for more muscle relaxant. The rate of rise of $PaCO_2$ was 3 to 5 mmHg per minute.

Fraioli et al emphasized the importance of the functional residual capacity (FRC) to body weight ratio and demonstrated that patients with low FRC/weight ratios could not tolerate apnea for more than 5 minutes.[107] In their study, two groups of patients were denitrogenated for 10 minutes and then subjected to apneic oxygenation with 6 liters/minute of oxygen through either a na-

sopharyngeal cannula or an endotracheal tube. Group II had an FRC/weight ratio of 36.7 ±9ml/kg, whereas Group I had an FRC/weight ratio of 53.3 ±7 ml/kg. Because of the smaller FRC and larger body mass in Group II, accumulation of alveolar nitrogen resulted in a higher PAN_2 and lower PAO_2. This resulted in a significant difference between the two groups starting at 4 minutes of apnea (Figs. 9-16 and 9-17). The authors recommended that only patients with predicted FRC/weight ratios greater than *50 ml/kg* have apneic oxygenation for longer than *5 minutes.*

VENTILATION THROUGH A RIGID
VENTILATING BRONCHOSCOPE

If the principles of apnea outlined above are followed, then intermittent ventilation through a side-arm bronchoscope with inhalational agents added can be safely done for

Table 9-7
Complication Rates for Fiberoptic Bronchoscopy[78-81]

Author	Year	Type of Study	Number of Procedures	Complications		
				Deaths	Major	Minor
Lukomsky	1981	Prospective	1,146	0	0.3%	5.4%
Credle	1974	Retrospective	24,251	1	0.8%	0.01%
Pereira	1978	Prospective	908	1	1.7%	6.5%
Suratt	1976	Retrospective	48,000	12		

These series are comparable but definitions for minor and major complications vary.

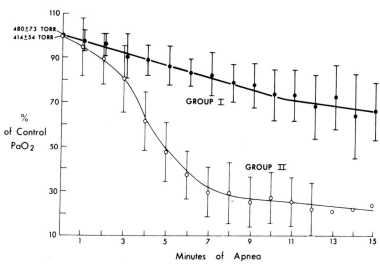

Fig. 9-16 Effects of apneic oxygenation in relation to FRC/weight ratio. Mean percentages of PaO_2 for group I (FRC/weight ratio of 53.3 ±7 ml/kg) and group II (FRC/weight ratio of 36.7 ±9 ml/kg) are shown. PaO_2's for group II had declined to 50 percent of control after 5 minutes of apneic oxygenation, whereas group I patients still had PaO_2's that were 90 percent of control. A significant difference between the two groups occurred by 4 minutes. Mean zero-time PaO_2's are shown. (Fraioli RL, Sheffe LA, Steffanson JL: Pulmonary and cardiovascular effects of apneic oxygenation in man. Anesthesiology 39:588-596, 1973.)

a short bronchoscopy. However, longer bronchoscopies and poor blood gases in some patients have led to the development of other techniques.

Sanders first presented his technique to the Academy of Anesthesiology in 1966 and published it in 1967.[82] This revolutionized the method of ventilation during rigid bronchoscopy. His idea of utilizing the Venturi effect to entrain air and halothane was later developed by others.

The jet of gas under high pressure at the proximal end of the tube generates a negative pressure and entrains air at the inlet (Fig. 9-18).[84, 108] The volume delivered at the outlet is the sum of the jet volume and the entrained volume. For each combination of driving pressure and jet orifice and tube diameters, a maximal inflating pressure is obtained that is largest with the distal end obstructed.[87] The flow characteristics of the particular blowgun used must be considered.[101] In Figures 9-19 and 9-20 from Sanders' original paper, the 8 × 40 Negus bron-

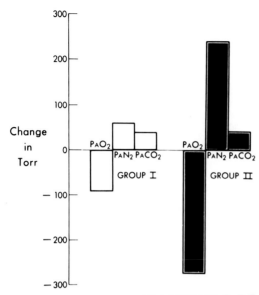

Fig. 9-17 Changes in alveolar gas after 15 minutes of apneic oxygenation in man. Group I has an FRC/weight ratio of 53.3 ±7 ml/kg and group II has an FRC/weight ratio of 36.7 ±9 ml/kg. The decrease in P_{AO_2} was nearly totally accounted for by the increases in P_{AN_2} and P_{ACO_2}. The P_{ACO_2}'s were essentially the same in the two groups. P_{AN_2} in group II patients was significantly greater, thereby accounting for the different declines of P_{AO_2}. (Fraioli RL, Sheffe LA, Steffenson JL: Pulmonary and cardiovascular effects of apneic oxygenation in man. Anesthesiology 39:588-596, 1973.)

choscope (the usual scope) delivered a 20 mmHg pressure at 50 psi with a flow of 160 L/min through a jet orifice of 0.043 inches.[82] Giesecke et al compared the intermittent ventilating bronchoscope technique with the Sanders injection technique and demonstrated that better ventilation was achieved with the Sanders bronchoscope.[84] They confirmed the earlier finding by Morales that the anesthesiologist's estimate of minute ventilation using the intermittent ventilation technique often leads to respiratory acidosis.[84, 109] These data are illustrated in Table 9-8.

The Sanders technique resulted in improved ventilation, but in patients with poor compliance, problems with hypercarbia and hypoxia were reported.[108, 110] Smith et al re-

ported a PaO_2 of 18 mmHg and $PaCO_2$ of 60 mmHg in a patient with carcinoma infiltrating both lungs.[110] Thus it was obvious that the Sanders technique needed to be improved by increasing the FiO_2 from 0.25 or 0.35 and by providing a means to ventilate the patient with decreased compliance.

Komesaroff in Australia developed the Bronchoflator, which allowed an FiO_2 of 0.60 to 0.80, and Carden in Canada at about the same time, developed his side-arm injector that gave an FiO_2 of 0.90 to 1.0.[77, 88–90, 93, 97, 111] In the poorly compliant patient, the Carden system can develop 55 cm H_2O pressure in the bronchoscope. This technique has been used in over 1,000 bronchoscopies without a pneumothorax.[88] Moreover, N_2O can be added through a Bird oxygen blender with maintenance of good blood gases (Table 9-9).[93]

Sullivan increased the Sanders jet size to 0.087 inches from 0.045 inches, which allows delivery of 40 cm H_2O at 50 psi to aid in ventilation of patients with decreased compliance.[112] Keep used a 38-cm tube that ran almost to the end of the bronchoscope and used Entonex (50% N_2O/50% O_2) as his driving gas.[91] Blood levels of N_2O reach a plateau in 9 to 15 minutes.[94] The incidence of

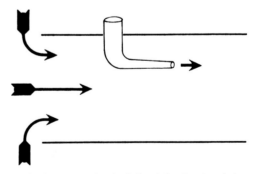

Fig. 9-18 Venturi principle of the Sanders injector. A jet of gas placed near the end and parallel to the long axis of an open tube produces a negative pressure, and air is entrained from behind the jet. The outflow from the tube is equal to the volume of gas flow through the jet plus the air entrained. (Diaz PM: Anesthesia for bronchoscopy. Anesthesiology Review, 10-14, June 1975.)

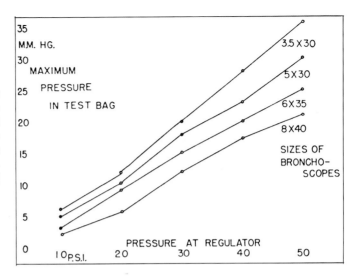

Fig. 9-19 Maximum pressures developed in a test bag by Sanders injectors with different psi pressure sources and different-sized bronchoscopes. (Sanders RD: Two ventilating attachments for bronchoscopes, Del Med J 39:170-175, 192, 1967.)

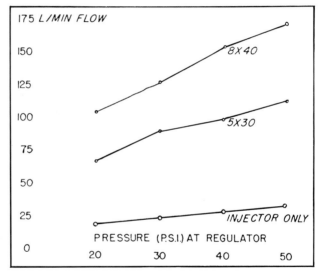

Fig. 9-20 Total flow through 8 × 40 and 5 × 30 Pilling bronchoscopes compare with flow through the injector only. (Sanders RD: Two ventilating attachments for bronchoscopes. Del Med J 39:170-175, 192, 1967.)

awareness had been reported as 4 percent during apneic oxygenation for bronchoscopy, and this stimulated the trend for inhalation supplementation of intravenous techniques.[113] The Bird Mark II ventilator was also used instead of a blowgun as a driving pressure source.[87, 95, 111]

In prolonged procedures a combination of rigid and fiberoptic bronchoscopy under general anesthesia is often undertaken.[114] In the United Kingdom prolonged bronchoscopies with the side-arm Venturi technique have proven satisfactory.[96] Halothane can

also be entrained from the side arm when using the unmodified Sanders technique. However, prolonged bronchoscopies using the Sanders technique have been reported to reverse a left-to-right intracardiac shunt to a right-to-left shunt owing to high airway pressures.[115] A small endotracheal tube (4 mm) can be used alongside a rigid bronchoscope with a 50-psi driving source, which is a modification of older methods of manual ventilation.[116] Ventilation by the rigid bronchoscope and the small endotracheal tube simultaneously via a Y in the inhalation arm

Table 9-8

Comparison of Blood Gases with Ventilating Bronchoscopes and Injection Bronchoscopes

	Control			During Bronchoscopy		
	n	pH	$PaCO_2$	PaO_2	pH	$PaCO_2$	PaO_2
Ventilating							
Morales	11	7.39	40	78	7.25	80	300
Giesecke (reference study)	21	7.40	38	81	7.31	48	176
Weighted mean	32	7.40	39	82	7.29	60	220
Injection							
Mette	20	—	38	80	—	32	200
Morales	14	7.39	40	98	7.35	42	200
Pender	11	7.41	40	77	7.47	32	228
Giesecke (reference study)	21	7.38	38	81	7.36	38	116
Weighted mean	66	7.39	39	81	7.38	36	187

n = patient number

Adapted from: Giesecke AH, Gerbershagen HU, Dortman C et al.: Comparison of the ventilating and injection bronchoscopes. Anesthesiology 38:298–303, 1973. With permission of author and publisher.

enables bilateral ventilation even when the bronchoscope is in one of the main bronchi.[104] An inflation catheter made from a nasogastric tube or Foley catheter inside or outside the rigid bronchoscope can be used in place of an endotracheal tube.[105] General anesthesia during the fiberoptic bronchoscopy is simple as long as the principles of correct endotracheal tube size for the size of the bronchoscope are followed.[117] The modified Carden tube can also be used during this part of the combined procedure.[75]

HIGH-FREQUENCY POSITIVE PRESSURE VENTILATION

High-frequency positive pressure ventilation (HFPPV) using a ventilator of negligible internal compliance, an insufflation frequency of 60 per minute, and a relative insufflation time of 22 percent can be used during either rigid or fiberoptic bronchoscopy. No air entrainment occurs through the proximal end of the bronchoscope and there is continuous exhalation during the procedure.[99] The suction biopsy channel of the FOB has been used for HFPPV; however, a pneumothorax has been reported during FOB when the side arm is used to deliver the gases.[99, 118] Simple nomograms are available for the equipment, which is now starting to appear in the United States.[100]

GENERAL ANESTHESIA FOR BRONCHOSCOPY

Once the choice of general anesthesia for bronchoscopy has been made, then the technique of ventilation and selection of drugs should be based on the status of the patient and the skill and speed of the surgeon. For example, a patient with hypertension and documented coronary artery disease with an estimated FRC/weight ratio of 55 ml/kg could be ventilated intermittently via the side-arm technique if the surgeon only took 5 minutes for a rigid bronchoscopy. However, if the surgery was prolonged by a combined procedure, e.g., rigid and fiberoptic bronchoscopy, by teaching or photography, or by a slower surgeon, then a Sanders injector technique assures better blood gases

Table 9-9
Arterial Blood Gas Values before and during Bronchoscopy with 60 to 70 percent N_2O

	Patient 1	Patient 2	Patient 3	Patient 4	Patient 5	Patient 6	Average ± SEM
Age (years), sex	72, M	63, M	35, M	69, F	62, M	55, M	
Bronchoscope size (mm)	8 × 40	7 × 40	8 × 40	8 × 40	8 × 40	8 × 40	
Before bronchoscopy							
$\quad PaO_2$ (torr)	70	72	81	76	72	92	77 ± 3
$\quad PaCO_2$ (torr)	34	39	44	33	39	36	38 ± 2
$\quad pH$	7.47	7.44	7.42	7.43	7.44	7.45	
N_2O (per cent)	75	70	70	70	60	70	
After 10 minutes of bronchoscopy							
$\quad PaO_2$ (torr)	74	126	120	91	185	117	114 ± 8 (70 percent)
$\quad PaCO_2$ (torr)	45	33	28	30	25	18	29 ± 4
$\quad pH$	7.35	7.47	7.60	7.49	7.58	7.65	

Carden E, Schwesinger WB: The use of nitrous oxide during ventilation with the open broncho-scope. Anesthesiology 39: 551–555, 1973. With permission of author and publisher.

than the intermittent ventilation technique.

This same patient would probably not tolerate the cardiovascular depression with halothane or enflurane at MAC BAR_{95} necessary to obtund the sympathetic response to bronchoscopy.[9, 119] In fact, 3 of 40 healthy patients in Roizen's study did not tolerate MAC BAR_{95} levels with enflurane.[8] Also, in the study by Calverley et al healthy volunteers did not tolerate greater than 1.5 MAC of enflurane with controlled ventilation.[120]

The choice of a muscle relaxant would depend upon the anticipated length of the procedure, the cardiovascular effects of the drug, and whether or not further surgery, e.g., lobectomy, was planned following the bronchoscopy.

The first bronchoscopies were performed with thiopental or methohexital infusions along with succinylcholine. The technique is still useful today when supplemented with some of the drugs shown in Table 9-10.[121–132] This "balanced technique" allows a sufficient depth of anesthesia to be achieved without the associated cardiovascular depression of a pure inhalational technique.

MEDIASTINOSCOPY

Mediastinoscopy allows for determining the extent of disease in the mediastinum with a relatively low morbidity and mortality compared with an exploratory thoracotomy.[133] The lymphatics of the lung drain first to the subcarinal and paratracheal areas and then to the sides of the trachea, the supraclavicular areas, and finally the thoracic duct.[134] Mediastinoscopy is used mainly for carcinoma of the lung but it is also useful for diagnosis of other clinical conditions (Table 9-11).[135] Contraindications to mediastinoscopy are shown in Table 9-12. The morbidity for various series has ranged from 1.5 to 3 percent and the mortality has been reported as 0.09 percent (see Table 9-13).[136–146]

In addition to the routine anesthetic preoperative workup, checks should be made for the following prior to a mediastinoscopy.

1. The presence of an impaired cerebral circulation when a history of transient ischemic attacks, stroke, or a carotid bruit is present
2. The adequacy of the airway

Table 9-10
Useful Drugs for Control of the Sympathetic Response and Cough Reflex

Induction	Maintenance	Supplemental Drugs
Diazepam	Morphine	Intravenous lidocaine[121-124]
Fentanyl	Fentanyl	Topical and regional anesthesia
Midazolam	Meperidine	Endotracheal lidocaine[125]
Thiopental	Alphaprodine	Prior treatment with beta-blockers[126]
Althesin	Halogenated agents	Propranolol[123, 126-128]
Ketamine		Practolol[129]
		Oral viscous lidocaine[130]
		Intravenous sodium nitroprusside[131]
		Intravenous nitroglycerin
		Droperidol[132]

3. The presence of the myasthenic syndrome secondary to carcinoma[137]
4. The presence of an ascending aortic aneurysm—laboratory tests should be ordered to exclude syphilis[138]
5. Adequate blood cross-matched and available[139]

In addition to the usual monitors, the *right* radial artery pulse should be monitored by palpitation, plethysmography, or a direct

Table 9-11
Mediastinal Lesions

Benign	Malignant
Thymus	
Cysts	
Lipoma	Primary
Hyperplasia	Lymphoma
Cysts	Others
Tracheal	Bone
Bronchial	Vascular
Enterogenous	Connective tissue
Tumors	
Nervous System	
Neuroma	
Thyroid	
Retrosternal goiter	Secondary
Aneurysms	Lung
Ascending aorta	Pericardium
Lymph nodes	
Sarcoidosis	

Vaughan RS: Anesthesia for mediastinoscopy. Anesthesia 33:195–198, 1978. With permission of author and publisher.

arterial pressure recording (if the patient's status warrants it) to detect compression of the innominate artery. Petty detected decreases in the right radial artery pulse in four of seven patients, with alterations in pressure lasting 15 to 300 seconds.[140] The right carotid artery can be monitored by a doppler, or theoretically, the electroencephalogram could be monitored. The threat of an air embolism with a venous tear, especially in the superior vena cava, makes precordial doppler monitoring reasonable.

Knowledge of the anatomy, cardiorespiratory physiology, and the patient's disease allows for planning the anesthetic management and predicting the potential complications of the mediastinoscopy. For example, the presence of a superior mediastinal venous obstruction would make an intravenous in the lower extremity advisable, since a laceration of the superior vena cava would require blood administration via the inferior vena cava.

Mediastinoscopy can be performed in a patient who is suitably premedicated by using lidocaine to infiltrate the suprasternal area, the strap muscles, and the periosteum of the posterior surface of the clavicles and sternum.[147] Transtracheal lidocaine can be used to abolish the cough reflex since displacement of the trachea causes the only significant discomfort.[148] Blunt dissection of the mediastinum is relatively pain-free as there are few pain fibers to the trachea.[147, 148] In

Table 9-12

Anesthetic and Surgical Contraindications to Mediastinoscopy

Relative	Absolute
Superior vena caval obstruction	Inoperability
Thoracic inlet obstruction	Recurrent laryngeal nerve involvement
	Cardiac status precluding anesthesia
	Aneurysm of the ascending aorta
	Previous mediastinoscopy

Adapted from: Vaughan RS: Anesthesia for mediastinoscopy. Anesthesia 33:195–198, 1978. With permission of author and publisher.

fact, some authors have reported abandoning general anesthesia because of the success of this technique.

General anesthesia involves standard intravenous and inhalational techniques with attention to the potential complications. An armored endotracheal tube is sometimes used to avoid tracheal compression from the mediastinoscope. The potential for bradycardia, hypotension, or dysrhythmias due to mechanical stimulation of the aorta, ventricle, or trachea must be kept in mind.[139] Variations from the standard mediastinoscopy approach, such as parasternal mediastinotomy or anterior mediastinoscopy in the second intercostal space, have also been reported.[149, 150]

THORACOSCOPY

Thoracoscopy was developed by Jacobeus for diagnosis and treatment of tuberculous effusions in 1910 and is now being used as a purely diagnostic tool.[151, 152] Of all the diagnostic techniques, thoracoscopy allows the most complete examination of the thorax.[153] It is currently used for diagnosis of pleural disease, pleural effusions, parenchymal disease, infectious diseases, particularly in immunosuppressed patients; for staging procedures of suspected neoplasmas; for chemical pleurodesis; and in children.[154–160]

Anesthesia of the lateral thoracic wall for thoracoscopy can be achieved by local anesthetic infiltration or intercostal nerve blocks two spaces above and below the usual sixth intercostal space. The intercostal blocks also anesthetize the parietal pleura. Retraction of the visceral pleura often stimulates the cough reflex during visualization of the posterior pulmonary hilum and can be prevented by a stellate ganglion block.[151] By avoiding general anesthesia and positive pressure ventilation, a sufficient pneumothorax for adequate thoracoscopy is maintained.

Table 9-13

Complications of Mediastinoscopy

Hemorrhage:
    Venous
    Arterial
    Tumor
    Myocardial
    Aneurysm
Tracheal rupture
Tracheal collapse after extubation
Pneumothorax
Pneumomediastinum
Pneumopericardium
Damage to the thoracic duct (chylothorax)
Nerve damage:
    Left recurrent laryngeal nerve
    Phrenic nerve
Cardiac arrest
Simulated cardiac arrest (compression of the innominate artery)
Air embolism
Cardiac biopsy
Dysrhythmias
Hypertension
Bradycardia
Hypotension
Transient hemiparesis
Infection (late)
Tumor invasion of skin incision (late)

However, general anesthesia with an endobronchial tube and one-lung ventilation can be used and was first reported by Friedel in 1970.[161] General anesthesia with an endobronchial tube allows for complete reexpansion of the lung if pleurodesis is done and avoids the pain of instillation of talc for recurrent pneumothorax.[162] A high FiO_2 is necessary with either local or general anesthesia to overcome the pathophysiological effects of the pneumothorax.

ESOPHAGOSCOPY

Esophagoscopy is an essential part of the investigation of patients with symptoms suggestive of an esophageal lesion or of a hiatus hernia. Iatrogenic perforation of the upper esophagus is the major risk and carries a mortality rate ranging from 34 to 84 percent.[163] Factors contributing to instrument perforation are: the relatively thin wall of the esophagus (absence of serosa); the gap in longitudinal muscle fibers of the inferior constrictor of the pharynx and upper esophagus; the pressure of the lower cervical vertebrae against the esophagus (cervical spondylosis increases the danger); the length of the procedure; and, of course, the age and general condition of the patient and presence of concomitant disease.[164, 165]

Practical points during esophagoscopy include: (1) attempting to protect against regurgitation in the symptomatic patient by the use of oral antacids, cimetidine, and a rapid sequence induction technique with cricoid pressure; (2) use of an anesthetic technique that ensures paralysis and absence of bucking; and (3) selection of a small-sized endotracheal tube to prevent anterior compression of the esophagus during instrumentation.

REFERENCES

1. Sellers SL, Augoustides, TA: Anesthesia for endolaryngeal surgery. J Otolaryngol 5:203-206, 1976

2. Moorthy SS, LoSasso AM, King H et al.: Evaluation of larynx and trachea by xeroradiography. Anesth Analg (Cleve) 55:598-600, 1976

3. Proctor DF: Anesthesia for peroral endoscopy and bronchography. Anesthesiology 29:1025-1036, 1968

4. Denlinger JK, Messner JT, D'Orazio DJ et al.: Effect of intravenous lidocaine on the circulatory response to tracheal intubation. Anesthesiol Rev 3, No. 2, 13-16, 1976

5. Tomori Z, Widdicombe JG: Muscular, bronchomotor and cardiovascular reflexes elicited by mechanical stimulation of the respiratory tract. J Physiol 200:25-49, 1969

6. Yakaitis RW, Blitt CD, Angiulo JP: End-tidal halothane concentration for endotracheal intubation. Anesthesiology 47:386-388, 1977

7. Yakaitis RW, Blitt CD, Angiulo JP: End-tidal enflurane concentration for endotracheal intubation. Anesthesiology 50:59-61, 1979

8. Roizen MR, Horrigan RW, Frazer BM: Anesthetic doses blocking adrenergic (stress) and cardiovascular responses to incision—MAC BAR. Anesthesiology 54:390-398, 1981

9. Fox E, Sklar GS, Hill CH et al.: Complications related to the pressor response of endotracheal intubation. Anesthesiology 47:524-525, 1977

10. Converse JG, Landmesser CM, Harmel MH: Electrocardiographic changes during extubation. Anesthesiology 13:163-168, 1952

11. King BD, Elder JD, Proctor DF et al.: Reflex circulatory responses to tracheal intubation performed under topical anesthesia. Anesthesiology 15:231-238, 1954

12. Strong MS, Vaughn CW, Mahler DL et al.: Cardiac complications of microsurgery of the larynx: etiology, incidence and prevention. Laryngoscope 84:908-920, 1974

13. Katz PL, Bigger JT: Cardiac arrhythmias during anesthesia and operation. Anesthesiology 33:193-213, 1970

14. Paintal AS: Vagal sensory receptors and their reflex effects. Physiol Rev 53:159-227, 1973

15. Perry LB: Topical anesthesia for bronchoscopy. Chest 73: suppl, 691-693, 1978

16. Cooper M, Watson RL: An improved regional anesthetic technique for peroral endoscopy. Anesthesiology 43:372-374, 1975

17. Ritchie JM, Greene NM: Local anesthetics. In Gilman AG, Goodman LS, Gilman A, Eds.: The Pharmacological Basis of Therapeutics. 6th Ed. Macmillan, New York, 1980.

18. Smith RB: Cocaine and catecholamine inter-action: a review. Arch Otolaryngol 98:139-141, 1973

19. Fry WA: Techniques of topical anesthesia for bronchoscopy. Chest 73: Suppl, 694-696, 1978

20. Wilton TNP: Anesthesia for peroral endos-copy, pp. 400-437. In Mushin WW, Ed.: F.A. Davis Company, Philadelphia, 1963

21. Duncan JAT: Intubation of the trachea in the conscious patient. Br J Anaesthesia 49:619-623, 1977

22. Christoforidis AJ, Tomashefski JF, Mitchell MS: Use of an ultrasonic nebulizer for the application of oropharyngeal, laryngeal and tracheobronchial anesthesia. Chest 59:629-633, 1971

23. Plummer M, George B: Personal communica-tion

24. Kandt D, Schlegel M: Bronchologic examina-tions under topical ultrasonic aerosol inhala-tion anesthesia. Scand J Respir Dis 54:65-70, 1973

25. Grant WB: Correspondence. Br Med J 4:464, 1974

26. Jafek BW, Bauknight S, Calcaterra TC: Per-cutaneous anesthesia for endoscopy. Arch Surg 104:658-661, 1972

27. Stiffel P, Hameroff SR: A modified technique for transtracheal anesthesia. Anesthesiology 51:274-275, 1979

28. Lung JA, Muir RW, Hopeman AR: Percu-taneous polyethylene tube tracheostomy complicated by serious intratracheal hemor-rhage. Am Surg 34:694-696, 1968

29. Unger KM, Moser KM: Fatal complication of transtracheal aspiration. Arch Intern Med 132:437-439, 1973

30. Gaskill JR, Gillies DR: Local anesthesia for peroral endoscopy. Arch Otolaryngol 84:654-657, 1966

31. Cooper M, Watson RL: An improved re-gional anesthetic technique for peroral endos-copy. Anesthesiology 43:372-374, 1974

32. Barton S, Williams JD: Glossopharyngeal nerve block. Arch Otolaryngol 93:186-188, 1971

33. Patterson JR, Blaschke TF, Hunt KK: Lido-caine blood concentrations using fiberoptic bronchoscopy. Am Rev Respir Dis 112:53-57, 1975

34. Bromage PR, Robson JG: Concentrations of lidocaine in the blood after intravenous, in-tramuscular, epidural and endotracheal ad-ministration. Anaesthesia 16:461-478, 1961

35. Pelton DA, Daly M, Cooper PD et al.: Plasma lidocaine concentrations following topical aerosol application to the trachea and bron-chi. Can Anaesth Soc J 17:250-255, 1970

36. Hug CC, Jr.: Personal communication

37. Viegas O, Stoelting RK: Lidocaine in arterial blood after laryngotracheal administration. Anesthesiology 43:491-493, 1975

38. Chu SS, Rah KH, Brannan MD: Plasma con-centration of lidocaine after endotracheal spray. Anesth Analg (Cleve) 54:438-441, 1975

39. Elguindi AS, Harrison GN, Abdulla AM et al.: Cardiac rhythm disturbances during fi-beroptic bronchoscopy: a prospective study. J Thorac Cardiovasc Surg. 77:557-561, 1979

40. deJong RH, Heavner JE: Diazepam prevents local anesthetic seizures. Anesthesiology 34:523-531, 1971

41. deJong RH, Heavner JE: Diazepam prevents and aborts lidocaine convulsions in monkeys. Anesthesiology 41:226-230, 1974

42. Maekawa T, Sakabe T, Takeshita H: Diaze-pam blocks cerebral metabolic and circula-tory responses to local anesthetic-induced sei-zures. Anesthesiology 41:389-391, 1974

43. deJong RH, Heavner JE: Local anesthetic seizure prevention: Diazepam vs. pentobarbi-tal. Anesthesiology 36:449-457, 1972.

44. deJong RH, DeRosa RA: Benzodiazepine treatment of seizures from supra-convulsant doses of local anesthetics: Reg Anes 6:51-54, 1981

45. deJong RH: Toxic effects of local anesthetics. JAMA 239:1166-1168, 1978

46. Weisel W, Tella RA: Reaction to tetracaine used as topical anesthetic in bronchoscopy. JAMA 147:218-222, 1951

47. Ritchie JM, Cohen PJ, Dripps RD: Cocaine, procaine and other synthetic local anesthetics. In Goodman LS, Gilman A, Eds: The Phar-macological Basis of Therapeutics. 4th Ed. MacMillan, New York, 1970

48. Gay GR, Inaba DS, Rappolt RT et al.: "An' ho, ho, baby, take a whiff on me." la dama blanca cocaine in current prospective. Anesth Analg (Cleve) 55:582-587, 1976

49. Landa JF: Indications for bronchoscopy. Chest 73: suppl., 686-690, 1978

50. Barrett CR: Flexible fiberoptic bronchoscopy in the critically ill patient. Chest 73: suppl., 746-749, 1978

51. Raj PP, Forestner J, Watson TD et al: Tech-niques for fiberoptic laryngoscopy in anesthe-sia. Anesth Analg (Cleve) 53:708-714, 1974

52. Snider GL: When not to use the broncho-scope for hemoptysis. Chest 76:1-2, 1979

53. Simelaro JP, Marks B, Meals R et al.: Selective bronchography following fiberoptic bronchoscopy. Chest 70:240-241, 1976

54. Zavala DC: Complications following fiberoptic bronchoscopy, the "good news" and the "bad news." Chest 73:783-785, 1978

55. Albertini RE, Harrell JH, Kurihara N et al.: Arterial hypoxemia induced by fiberoptic bronchoscopy. JAMA 230:1666-1667, 1974

56. Salisbury BG, Metzger CF, Altose MD et al: Effect of fiberoptic bronchoscopy on respiratory performance in patients with chronic airway obstruction. Thorax 30:441-446, 1975

57. Burns DM, Francoz RA, Kalafer ME et al.: Ventilation and perfusion changes following saline lobar lavage in normal adults. Am Rev Respir Dis 117: suppl.: 97, 1978

58. Dubrawsky C, Awe RJ, Jenkins DE: The effect of bronchofiberoptic examination on oxygen status. Chest 67:137-140, 1975

59. Harless KW, Scheinhorn DJ, Tannen RL et al.: Administration of oxygen with mouth-held nasal prongs during fiberoptic bronchoscopy. Chest 74:237-238, 1978

60. Sanderson DR, McDougall JC: Transoral bronchofiberoscopy. Chest 73: suppl., 701-703, 1978

61. Neuhaus A, Markowitz D, Rotman HH et al.: The effects of fiberoptic bronchoscopy with and without atropine premedication on pulmonary function in humans. Ann Thorac Surg 25:393-398, 1978

62. Wilkinson PL, Haur J, Miller RD eds: Clinical Anesthesia. CV Mosby Company, St. Louis, 1980, pp. 8-12.

63. Chamberlain DA, Muir DCF, Kennedy KP, Atropine methonitrate and isoprenaline in bronchial asthma. Lancet 2:1019-1021, 1962

64. D'Autrebande L: Aerosols medicamenteux. III. Possibilités de traitement des états asthmatiformes par aerosols de substances dites bronchodilatrices. Arch Int Pharmacodyn Ther 46:379, 1941

65. Klock LE, Miller TD, Morris AH et al.: A comparative study of atropine sulfate and isoproterenol hydrochloride in chronic bronchitis. Am Rev Respir Dis 112:371-376, 1975

66. Crompton GK: A comparison of responses to bronchodilator drugs in chronic bronchitis and chronic asthma. Thorax 23:46-55, 1968

67. Astin TW: Reversibility of airway obstruction in chronic bronchitis. Clin Sci Mol Med 42:725-733, 1972

68. Belen J, Neuhaus A, Markowitz D et al.: Modification of the effect of fiberoptic bronchoscopy on pulmonary mechanics. Chest 79:516-519, 1981

69. Shrader DL, Lakshminarayan S: The effect of fiberoptic bronchoscopy on cardiac rhythm. Chest 73:821-824, 1978

70. Luck JC, Messeder OH, Rubenstein MJ: Arrhythmias from fiberoptic bronchoscopy. Chest 74:139-143, 1978

71. Lampton LM: Bronchoscopy: Caution! JAMA 73:138, 1978

72. Miller EJ: Hypoxemia during fiberoptic bronchoscopy. Chest 75:103, 1979

73. Grossman E, Jacobi AM: Minimal optimal endotracheal tube size for fiberoptic bronchoscopy. Anesth Analg (Cleve) 53:475-476, 1974

74. Lindholm CE, Ollman B, Snyder JV et al.: Cardiorespiratory effects of flexible fiberoptic bronchoscopy in critically ill patients. Chest 74:362-368, 1978

75. Carden E, Raj P: Special new low resistance to flow tube and endotracheal tube adapter for use during fiberoptic bronchoscopy. Ann Otol Rhinol Laryngol 84:631-634, 1975

76. Carden E: Recent improvements in techniques for general anesthesia for bronchoscopy. Chest 73: suppl., 697-700, 1978

77. Lindholm CE: Flexible fiberoptic bronchoscopy in the critically ill patient. Ann Otol Rhinol Laryngol 83:786-794, 1974

78. Credle WF, Smiddy JF, Elliott RC: Complications of fiberoptic bronchoscopy. Am Rev Respir Dis 109:67-72, 1974

79. Suratt PM, Smiddy JF, Gruber B: Deaths and complications associated with fiberoptic bronchoscopy. Chest 69:747-751, 1976

80. Lukomsky GI, Ovchinnikov AA, Bilal A: Complications of bronchoscopy: Comparison of rigid bronchoscopy under general anesthesia and flexible fiberoptic bronchoscopy under topical anesthesia. Chest 79:316-321, 1981

81. Pereira W, Kovnat DM, Snider GL: A prospective cooperative study of complications following flexible fiberoptic bronchoscopy. Chest 73:813-816, 1978

82. Sanders RD: Two ventilating attachments for bronchoscopes. Del Med J 39:170-175, 192, 1967

83. Morales ES, Krumperman LW, Cohen JG: Bronchoscopy under diazepam anesthesia. Anesth Analg (Cleve) 52:414-421, 1973

84. Giesecke AH, Gerbershagen HU, Dortman C et al.: Comparison of the ventilating and injection bronchoscopes. Anesthesiology 38:298-303, 1978

85. Duvall AJ, Johnsen AF, Buckley J: Bronchoscopy under general anesthesia using the Sanders ventilating attachment. Ann Otol Rhinol Laryngol 78:490-498, 1969

86. Carden E: Recent improvements in anesthetic techniques for use during bronchoscopy. Ann Otol Rhinol Laryngol 83:777-785, 1974

87. Spoerel WE: Ventilation through an open bronchoscope. Can Anaesth Soc J 16:61-65, 1969

88. Carden E: Positive pressure ventilation during anaesthesia for bronchoscopy: a laboratory evaluation of two recent advances. Anesth Analg (Cleve) 52:402-406, 1973

89. Carden E, Trapp WG, Oulton J: A new and simple method for ventilating patients undergoing bronchoscopy. Anesthesiology 33:454-458, 1970

90. Komesaroff D, McKie B: The "bronchoflator": a new technique for bronchoscopy under general anaesthesia. Br J Anaesth 44:1057-1068, 1972

91. Keep PJ: A method of ventilation with Entonox during bronchoscopy. Br J Anaesth 46:970-972, 1974

92. Lee ST: A ventilating bronchoscope for inhalation anesthesia and augmented ventilation. Anesth Analg (Cleve) 52:89-93, 1973

93. Carden E, Schwesinger WB: The use of nitrous oxide during ventilation with the open bronchoscope. Anesthesiology 39:551-555, 1973

94. Hinds CJ, Ellis RH, Saloojee Y: Blood levels of nitrous oxide during bronchoscopy. Anaesthesia 33:784-787, 1978

95. Bennetts FE: Automatic ventilation during bronchoscopy: Experience with a Bird Mark 2 ventilator. Br J Anaesth 49:1061-1064, 1977

96. Fuller WR, Davies DM, Stradling P: Anaesthesia for bronchoscopy prolonged by teaching and photography. Anaesthesia 27:292-300, 1972

97. Carden E, Burns WW, McDevitt NB et al.: A comparison of venturi and side-arm ventilation in anesthesia for bronchoscopy. Can Anaesth Soc J 20:569-574, 1973

98. Smith RB, Lindholm CE, Klain M: Jet ventilation for fiberoptic bronchoscopy under general anesthesia. Acta Anaesthesiol Scand 20:111-116, 1976

99. Satyanarayana T, Capan L, Ramanathan S et al.: Bronchofiberscopic jet ventilation. Anesth Analg (Cleve) 59:350-354, 1980

100. Borg U, Eriksson I, Sjöstrand U: High frequency positive-pressure ventilation (HFPPV): A review based upon its use during bronchoscopy and for laryngoscopy and microlaryngeal surgery. Anesth Analg (Cleve) 59:594-603, 1980

101. Poling HE, Wolfson B, Siker ES: A technique of ventilation during laryngoscopy and bronchoscopy. Br J Anaesth 47:382-384, 1975

102. Sleath GE, Graves HB: The use of the cuirass respirator during laryngoscopy and bronchoscopy under general anesthesia. Can Anaesth Soc J 5:330-336, 1958

103. Shane SS, Ashman H, Welfeld A et al: General anesthesia in bronchoscopy employing the Emerson "raincoat" respirator. Laryngoscope 68:25-31, 1958

104. Hoffman S, Bruderman I: Blood pressure and blood-gas changes during anesthesia for bronchoscopy using a modified method of ventilation. Anesthesiology 37:95-98, 1972

105. Gillick JS: The inflation-catheter technique for ventilation during bronchoscopy. Anesthesiology 40:503-506, 1974

106. Frumin J, Epstein R, Cohen G: Apneic oxygenation in man. Anesthesiology 20:789-798, 1959

107. Fraioli RL, Sheffer LA, Steffenson JL: Pulmonary and cardiovascular effect of apneic oxygenation in man. Anesthesiology 39:588-596, 1973

108. Diaz PM: Anesthesia for bronchoscopy. Anesth Rev. 10-14, June 1975

109. Morales GA, Epstein BS, Cinco B et al.: Ventilation during general anesthesia for bronchoscopy. J Thorac Cardiovasc Surg 57:873-878, 1969

110. Smith C, Shroff PF, Steele JD: General anesthesia for bronchoscopy. Ann Thorac Surg 8:348-354, 1969

111. Carden E, Galido J: Foot-pedal control of jet ventilation during bronchoscopy and mi-

crolaryngeal surgery. Anesth Analg (Cleve) 54:405-406, 1975

112. Sullivan MT, Neff WB: A modified Sanders ventilating system for rigid-wall bronchoscopy. Anesthesiology 50:473-474, 1979

113. Barr AM, Wong RM: Awareness during general anesthesia for bronchoscopy and laryngoscopy using the apneic oxygen technique. Br J Anaesth 45:894-900, 1973

114. Perry LB, Sanderson DR: Anesthesia for prolonged bronchoscopy. Ann Thorac Surg 19:248-253, 1975

115. Rao TLK, Mathru M, Azad C et al.: Bronchoscopy and reversal of intracardiac shunt. Anesthesiology 51:558-560, 1979

116. El-Naggar M: The use of a small endotracheal tube in bronchoscopy. Br J Anaesth 47:390-392, 1975

117. Tahir AH: General anesthesia for bronchofiberoscopy. Anesthesiology 37:564-566, 1977

118. Britton RM, Nelson KG: Improper oxygenation during bronchofiberoscopy. Anesthesiology 40:87-89, 1974

119. Prys-Roberts C, Greene LT, Meloche R et al.: Studies of anaesthesia in relation to hypertension. II: Hemodynamic consequences of induction and endotracheal intubation. Br J Anaesth 43:531-546, 1971

120. Calverley RK, Smith NT, Prys-Roberts C et al.: Cardiovascular effects of enflurane anesthesia during controlled ventilation in man. Anesth Analg (Cleve) 57:619-628, 1978

121. Steinhaus JE, Gaskin L: A study of intravenous lidocaine as a suppressant of cough reflex. Anesthesiology 24:285-290, 1963

122. Steinhaus JE, Howland DE: Intravenously administered lidocaine as a supplement to nitrous oxide-thiobarbiturate anesthesia. Anesth Analg (Cleve) 37:40-46, 1958

123. Prys-Roberts C, Meloche R: Management of anesthesia in patients with hypertension or ischemic heart disease, p. 181. In Prys-Roberts C, Ed.: Hypertension, Ischemic Heart Disease and Anesthesia. Int Anesthesiol Clin. Little, Brown & Company, Boston, 1980

124. Denlinger JK, Messner JT, D'Orazio DJ et al.: Effect of intravenous lidocaine on the circulatory response to tracheal intubation. Anesthesiol Rev 3:13-15, 1976

125. Denlinger JK, Ellison N, Ominsky AJ: Effects of intratracheal lidocaine on circula-

tory responses to tracheal intubation. Anesthesiology 41:409-412, 1974

126. Prys-Roberts C, Foex P, Biro GP et al.: Studies of anaesthesia in relation to hypertension. V. Adrenergic beta-receptor blockade. Br J Anaesth 45:671-681, 1973

127. Johnstone M: Propranolol (inderal) during halothane anaesthesia. Br J Anaesth 38:516-529, 1966

128. Prys-Roberts C: Adrenergic mechanisms, agonist and antagonist drugs. pp. 375-428. In Prys-Roberts C, Ed.: The Circulation In Anaesthesia. Blackwell Scientific Publications, Oxford, 1980

129. Jenkins AV: Adrenergic beta-blockade with ICI 50, 172 (practolol) during bronchoscopy. Br J Anaesth 42:59-63, 1970

130. Stoelting RK: Circulatory response to laryngoscopy and tracheal intubation with or without prior oropharyngeal viscous lidocaine. Anesth Analg (Cleve) 56:618-621, 1977

131. Stoelting RK: Attenuation of blood pressure response to laryngoscopy and tracheal intubation with sodium nitroprusside. Anesth Analg (Cleve) 58:116-119, 1979

132. Keller R, Waldovogel H, Herzog H: Neurolept analgesia for bronchoscopic examinations. Chest 67:315-319, 1975

133. Philips PA, Van de Water J: Mediastinoscopy vs. exploratory thoracotomy. Arch Surg 105:48-51, 1972

134. Flynn TJ, Rossi NP, Lawton RL: Significance of mediastinoscopy in carcinoma of the lung. Arch Surg 94:243-246, 1967

135. Vaughan RS: Anaesthesia for mediastinoscopy. Anaesthesia 33:195-198, 1978

136. Ashbaugh DF: Mediastinoscopy. Arch Surg 100:568-572, 1970

137. Fassoulaki A: Anesthesia for mediastinoscopy. Anaesthesia 34:75-76, 1978

138. Weissberg D, Herczed E: Perforation of thoracic aortic aneurysm—a complication of mediastinoscopy. Chest 78:119-120, 1980

139. Roberts JT, Gissen AJ: Management of complications encountered during anesthesia for mediastinoscopy. Anesthesiol Rev 6:31-35, 1979

140. Petty C: Right radial artery pressure during mediastinoscopy. Anesth Analg (Cleve) 58:428-430, 1979

141. Lee CM, Grossman LB: Laceration of the left pulmonary artery during mediastinos-

copy. Anesth Analg (Cleve) 56:226-227, 1977

142. Foster ED, Munro DD, Dobell ARC: Mediastinoscopy. Ann Thorac Surg 13:273-286, 1972

143. Baggs KJ, Braun RA: An evaluation of mediastinoscopy as a guide to diagnoses and therapy. Arch Surg 111:703-706, 1976

144. Trinkle JK, Bryant LR, Hiller AJ: Mediastinoscopy—experience with 300 consecutive cases. J Thorac Cardiovasc Surg 60:297-300, 1970

145. Barash PG, Tsai B, Kitahata LM: Acute tracheal collapse following mediastinoscopy. Anesthesiology 44:67-68, 1976

146. Lee JH, Salvatore A: Innominate artery compression simulating cardiac arrest during mediastinoscopy: a case report. Anesth Analg (Cleve) 55:748-749, 1976

147. Morton JR, Guinn GA: Mediastinoscopy using local anesthesia. Am J Surg 122:696-698, 1971

148. Ward PH, Stephenson SE, Harris PF, Exploration of the mediastinum under local anesthesia. Ann Otol Rhinol Laryngol 75:368-379, 1966

149. Jolly PL, Hill LD, Lawless PA et al.: Parasternal mediastinotomy and mediastinoscopy. J Thorac Cardiovasc Surg 66:549-556, 1973

150. Jolly PL, Li W, Anderson RP: Anterior and cervical mediastinoscopy for determining operability and predicting resectability in lung cancer. J Thorac Cardiovasc Surg 79:366-371, 1980

151. Jacobeus HC: Possibility of the use of the cystoscope for investigation of serous cavities. Muench Med Wochenschr 57:2090, 1910

152. Idem: Endopleural operations by means of a thorascope. Beitr Klin Tuberk 35:1, 1915

153. Rodgers BM, Ryckman FC, Moazam F et al.: Thoracoscopy for intrathoracic tumors. Ann Thorac Surg 31:414-420, 1981

154. Canto A, Blasco E, Casillas M et al.: Thoracoscopy in the diagnosis of pleural effusion. Thorax 32:550-554, 1977

155. Bloomberg AE: Thoracoscopy in perspective. Surg Gynecol Obstet 147:433-443, 1978

156. Rodgers BM, Moazam F, Talbert JL: Thoracoscopy in children. Ann Surg 189:176-180, 1979

157. Lewis RJ, Kunderman PJ, Lewis RJ et al.: Direct diagnostic thoracoscopy. Ann Thorac Surg 21:536-540, 1976

158. Miller JI, Hatcher CR: Thoracoscopy: a useful tool in the diagnosis of thoracic disease. Ann Thorac Surg 26:68-72, 1978

159. Rodgers BM, Talbert JL: Thoracoscopy for diagnosis of intrathoracic lesions in children. J Pediatr Surg 11:703-708, 1976

160. Radigan LR, Glover JL: Thoracoscopy. Surgery 82:425-428, 1977

161. Friedel H: Importance of bronchological examination in cases of pleural diseases. Bronchos 20:77, 1970

162. Weissberg D, Kaufman M: Diagnostic and therapeutic pleuroscopy. Chest 78:732-735, 1980

163. Steyn JH, Brunner PL: Perforation of cervical oesophagus at oesophagoscopy. Scott Med J 7:494-497, 1962

164. Wooloch Y, Zer M, Dintsman M et al.: Iatrogenic perforations of the esophagus. Arch Surg 108:357-360, 1974

165. Aniansson G, Hallen O: Perforation of the esophagus. Acta Otolaryngol (Stock) 59:554-558, 1965

George Silvay, Ph.D., M.D.
Avron I. Weinreich, M.D.
James B. Eisenkraft, M.D.

10
Anesthesia for Pulmonary Surgery

The challenges confronting the thoracic anesthesiologist include the pneumothorax produced by the thoracotomy, ventilation in the lateral position, and control of secretions from one lung to the other. The introduction of positive pressure ventilation via a double-lumen tube represents the major advance in addressing these problems. The routine use of endobronchial intubation for pulmonary surgery was advocated twenty years ago by Bjork, Carlens, and Newman.[1,2] Despite the apparent advantages of this technique, its use still remains controversial. In response to a questionnaire (unpublished) concerning the current practice of anesthesia for pulmonary surgery in the major medical centers of North America in 1981, it was evident that the majority (70%) of anesthesiologists employ an endotracheal tube, rather than an endobronchial tube, a volatile inhaled anesthetic agent (74%), controlled respiration and intermittent suction.

The reluctance to accept the routine use of one-lung ventilation (OLV) is based upon

concern regarding hypoxemia, increased resistance to gas flow, and technical difficulties in passing the double-lumen tube. However, most authorities believe that patients undergoing a thoracotomy for pulmonary surgery should be managed using an endobronchial technique, since this method permits ventilation of one or both lungs at any time during the procedure and provides medical, surgical, and physiologic advantages. If an endotracheal tube is used for pulmonary surgery with the patient in the lateral position, there may be some situations where the patient is deprived of optimal care during the operation.

There are special circumstances in which protection of the "down" lung can be achieved only with OLV. This category includes bronchiectasis, bronchopleural fistula (with or without empyema), lung abscess, and hemoptysis (traumatic; A-V malformations of lung, traumatic bronchoscopy). In these situations, sudden flooding of the healthy lung could result in dire consequences not unlike those following massive aspiration of gastric contents.

Further advantages of OLV over endotracheal anesthesia are found in the anesthetic management of bullous emphysema, giant pulmonary air cyst, and chronic (recurrent) spontaneous pneumothorax, where air tamponade could develop with effects similar to those of a tension pneumothorax. The use of OLV is mandatory for bronchial sleeve resection and resection of carinal tumors (see Chs. 8, 11).

In addition to protecting the healthy lung from necrotic tumor, purulent or bloody secretions, and air tamponade, the endobronchial tube offers certain technical advantages to the surgeon. Total collapse of the "up" lung allows better exposure to the hilar structures, provides superior operating conditions (a "quiet lung"), and thus reduces the duration of surgery. Use of the stapler for wedge resections is facilitated, and open inspection of the bronchus can be made easily without interrupting ventilation. Postoperative pulmonary complications are reduced by using OLV since trauma to the lung, due to surgical retraction and excessive handling, is minimized.

The acceptability of OLV depends upon the extent to which hypoxemia may occur and whether the latter outweighs the above-stated advantages. The earlier objection to increased airway resistance due to the relatively small lumina of the double-lumen tube today may be considered in a more positive light. The work of inflating the lung is performed by a volume-controlled ventilator; and the passive expiratory resistance due to the tube provides a modest degree of positive end-expiratory pressure which helps to increase functional residual capacity (FRC) in the "down" lung. There are many techniques available to correct hypoxemia during OLV (see Ch. 8). The recent development of high-frequency positive-pressure ventilation (HFPPV) will ultimately lead to its use in the operating room during thoracic surgery with

OLV. Malina et al from Sweden recently reported on the use of HFPPV in 10 patients undergoing thoracotomy.[3] They demonstrated that it could be used safely in man with maintenance of good blood gases, and a lower mean intrathoracic pressure than during regular controlled ventilation. The application of HFPPV to the "up" lung to improve oxygenation during OLV will surely follow.

This chapter emphasizes the pharmacology of anesthetic drugs used during thoracic surgery and the anesthetic management of some of the more difficult situations seen during chest surgery. (Preoperative evaluation and preparation are discussed in Chapters 4 and 5, and the physiology of OLV in Chapter 8.)

PHARMACOLOGY OF ANESTHETIC DRUGS

The objectives of general anesthesia are to produce controlled levels of narcosis, analgesia, and relaxation so that the particular operative procedure will be tolerated by the patient with a minimum of adverse effects. When considering these goals in relation to pulmonary surgery, certain aspects of the pharmacology of anesthesia drugs assume a greater importance. The patients commonly have some impairment of lung function and may also show evidence of cardiovascular dysfunction so that knowledge of how these systems may be affected by anesthetic agents is essential. When the organ of gas exchange is also the target of surgery, the anesthesiologist and the surgeon may have a conflict of interests. A compromise must be reached so that surgery is possible while adequate oxygenation is assured.

Oxygen flows from the environment, or in this case the anesthesia circuit, down a gradient of partial pressures to reach the tissues. This gradient has been called the "oxygen cascade." There are a number of general ways in which anesthetic drugs may affect the oxygen cascade which should be considered in discussing pharmacology.

Anesthetics may alter the normal awake responses to hypoxemia and hypercapnia. Thus, alveolar ventilation may be disturbed as a result of changes in respiratory rate, tidal volume, or both. Anesthetics may change the work of breathing by affecting compliance, responses to changes in compliance, and also by influencing bronchial mucus, bronchomotor tone, and hence airway resistance. The normal response to an increase in the work of breathing may be obtunded, leading to hypoventilation.

Within the lung there are various mechanisms which attempt to match ventilation and ‧ perfusion so that neither is wasted. These mechanisms may be altered by anesthetics. The hypocapnic bronchoconstrictor reflex functions to reduce ventilation to areas of the lung which are poorly perfused and to preferentially ventilate areas which are well perfused.[4] This tends to make the excretion of carbon dioxide more efficient. Depression of this mechanism allows ventilation of poorly perfused areas of the lung, leading to an increase in physiological dead space and "wasted ventilation."

Pulmonary perfusion is a function of cardiac output and pulmonary vascular resistance, both of which may be affected by anesthetic drugs. Within the lung there is a mechanism which acts to direct blood flow to areas which are well-oxygenated. This is the hypoxic pulmonary vasoconstrictor (HPV) reflex which diverts blood away from areas which are poorly oxygenated.[5] By directing perfusion to well-oxygenated areas, the tendency for "shunting" and venous admixture is reduced. It is well known that during general anesthesia venous admixture increases and contributes to the production of a reduced PaO_2. Depression of hypoxic vasoconstriction may be a contributing factor here.

Hypoxic vasoconstriction becomes particularly important during one-lung anesthesia since the collapsed or "up lung" represents a very large potential right-to-left shunt.[6] Many investigators have studied the effects of anesthetics on HPV with a view to minimizing venous admixture during OLV. Volatile inhalational anesthetic agents appear to depress HPV; intravenous agents do not appear to have as much effect (see Ch. 8).[7,8]

Oxygen delivery from the lungs to the tissues is effected via the blood stream and cardiovascular system. Oxygen delivery or oxygen flux is the concept of the rate of oxygen availability to the tissues per minute.[9] This is a function of hemoglobin concentration, saturation, and cardiac output (CO) in particular.

O_2 Flux:
Hemoglobin $\times$ Saturation $\times$ 1.34 $\times$ Cardiac Output $\times$ $1/100$.*
ml O_2/min = gm/100 ml $\times$ % ml O_2 (combining with 1 gm of Hb when fully saturated)

If Hb is 15gm/100 ml, saturation is 97%, and cardiac ouput is 5 L/min

O_2 Flux = 15 $\times$ 0.97 $\times$ 1.34 $\times$ 5000 $\times$ 0.01 = Approx. 1000 ml O_2/minute

Since O_2 flux represents the "bottom line" when it comes to oxygen delivery, the effects of anesthetic drugs on the cardiovascular system, especially cardiac output, must be considered. The latter may be affected by changes in rate, rhythm, and stroke volume—all well-known targets of anesthetic agents.

The anesthetic drugs will be discussed in relation to how they may affect oxygenation and oxygen flux during anesthesia and the perioperative period. The reader should consult other textbooks of pharmacology and anesthesiology for further information and discussion of the actions of these agents on the other systems of the body.

---

* Since Hb concentration is in gm/100 ml.

Inhalational Anesthetics

The inhalational anesthetics to be discussed are the gas, nitrous oxide, and the volatile anesthetic agents. Table 10-1 shows some important physical properties of these drugs.

NITROUS OXIDE

Nitrous oxide is a sweet-smelling, nonirritating, colorless gas. It is a weak anesthetic agent with a MAC of 110 percent.[10] This means that the partial pressure of nitrous oxide which is required to produce anesthesia in 50 percent of subjects is in excess of 760 mmHg (one atmosphere). Thus it cannot be used as the sole anesthetic agent under normal ambient pressure conditions. However, since anesthetic effects are additive, nitrous oxide at concentrations of less than one MAC may be used to supplement other anesthetic agents at concentrations of less than their MAC to produce one MAC equivalent of anesthesia.

Nitrous oxide may affect oxygenation in a number of ways. Since it is only a weak anesthetic, higher concentrations are required and the concentrations of N_2O needed to produce anesthesia may, by necessity and Dalton's Law, produce hypoxia (low FiO_2). During pulmonary surgery, high inspired oxygen concentrations are often needed which means that N_2O can only be used in relatively low concentrations, if at all, and thus it may only supplement the anesthetic state. Low concentrations of N_2O can produce analgesia (20% N_2O).[11] Higher concentrations (50%) will produce some amnesia, but not reliably, so that awareness can be a problem. In any event, supplementation with other anesthetic agents is necessary.

During the introduction of nitrous oxide into the anesthetic circuit, it is rapidly taken up from the alveoli. Oxygen given along with nitrous oxide will be concentrated—the so-called "concentration effect," as nitrous oxide enters the blood, leaving relatively

more oxygen in the alveoli and raising the PaO_2.[12] This concentrating effect of N_2O on oxygen or any other concomitantly administered inhaled agent lasts for up to ten minutes and may help improve oxygenation during this time.

When nitrous oxide is discontinued, the opposite effect is seen. Nitrous oxide rapidly leaves the blood to enter the alveoli and dilutes the gases present in the alveoli. As a result, the oxygen present is "diluted" by the emerging nitrous oxide. If the patient is not given increased concentrations of oxygen to breathe during this time, diffusion hypoxia (Fink effect) may be produced.[13,14] Diffusion hypoxia usually occurs if the patient is allowed to breathe room air after a nitrous oxide anesthetic. The hypoxia and desaturation last for about 15 minutes and may be significant in high-risk patients.[14]

Nitrous oxide may decrease chest wall compliance if given in association with a narcotic analgesic. Truncal rigidity can be produced, which may require neuromuscular blocking agents and ventilation for its treatment.[15-17] Nitrous oxide seems to have little effect on bronchial tone, but it does have a depressant effect on mucociliary flow in the trachea which may theoretically increase airway resistance due to accumulation of secretions.

The response to hypercapnia is not depressed by nitrous oxide, and indeed respiration may actually be increased.[18] The load-compensating response, the mechanism whereby respiratory effort increases if airways resistance is increased or chest compliance decreased, is usually depressed by general anesthesia. Added inspiratory resistance depresses the ventilatory response to CO_2, but this response is not depressed further by N_2O.

Nitrous oxide does have a depressant effect on the respiratory response to hypoxia, and a further depression of the response is observed if an inspiratory resistance is added.[19] A blunted hypoxic response may play a part in the diffusion hypoxia syn-

Table 10-1
Physical Properties of the Commonly Used Inhalational Anesthetics

Agent	Formula	Odor	MWT.	Boiling Point (°C) at 760 mmHg	Vapor Pressure (mmHg) at 20°C	Partition Coefficients at 37°C Blood/gas	Oil/gas	MAC %
Enflurane	$\begin{array}{c} \text{Cl F} \quad\text{F} \\ \mid\;\mid\quad\mid \\ \text{H-C-C-O-C-H} \\ \mid\;\mid\quad\mid \\ \text{F F}\quad\text{F} \end{array}$	Pungent ethereal	184.5	56.5	171	1.91	98.5	1.7
Halothane	$\begin{array}{c} \text{Br F} \\ \mid\;\mid \\ \text{H-C-C-F} \\ \mid\;\mid \\ \text{Cl F} \end{array}$	Pungent sweet	197.4	50.2	244	2.3	224	0.76
Isoflurane	$\begin{array}{c} \text{F Cl}\quad\text{F} \\ \mid\;\mid\quad\mid \\ \text{F-C-C-O-C-H} \\ \mid\;\mid\quad\mid \\ \text{F H}\quad\text{F} \end{array}$	Ethereal	184.5	48.5	239	1.43	91	1.2
Nitrous Oxide	N_2O	Sweet	44	—	(750 psi)	0.47	1.4	110

drome mentioned above, when N_2O is discontinued in the absence of an oxygen-enriched mixture. In this situation, the only defense available to the patient is hyperventilation in response to hypoxemia, and depression of this response by N_2O may compound the hypoxic state. This effect of N_2O is observed with concentrations of 35 to 50 percent.[19]

Perhaps the most significant effect of N_2O during pulmonary surgery is its ability to enter closed air spaces.[20] Pneumothoraces, lung cysts, and the empty hemithorax following pneumonectomy may suffer expansion or increases in pressure due to nitrous oxide's solubility and diffusion properties.* Air spaces contain nitrogen, a poorly soluble gas. If the patient breathes the more soluble nitrous oxide, the blood cannot carry away significant quantities of the poorly soluble nitrogen. The blood can, however, bring considerable quantities of the soluble nitrous oxide from the lungs to the air space. The maximum theoretical increase in volume is determined by the concentration of nitrous oxide in the lungs, since, at equilibrium, an identical concentration must exist in the closed air space. If the alveoli contain 50 percent N_2O, the air space at equilibrium must also contain 50 percent N_2O. Thus a volume of N_2O equal to the initial gas volume must enter the space and the size doubles. If 80 percent N_2O is in the lungs, then 80 percent must be achieved in the air space which must expand to five times its size! The volume increases disproportionately with increasing N_2O concentrations, approaching infinite size if 100 percent N_2O were to be used. In practice, the increases in gas volume are less than predicted since equilibrium is incomplete and because nitrogen is lost from the air space to the blood.

---

* The rate of diffusion of gas through a "wet membrane" is directly proportional to the solubility of the gas (Henry's Law) and inversely proportional to the square root of the molecular weight of the gas (Graham's Law).

Nitrous oxide is contraindicated in the presence of a pneumothorax, noncommunicating air cyst, or pulmonary bleb, when a rapid increase in volume could result. The volume of an air cyst may double in 10 minutes and quadruple in 2 hours.[21] If the air space is unable to expand, the pressure within it will rise and, if transmitted to the great veins, cardiorespiratory difficulties can arise.[22] Volume increases cause mediastinal shift or other symptoms of tension pneumothorax.

Following the closure of a thoracotomy for pneumonectomy the hemithorax contains free air. Provided the space is drained by a chest tube, no dangerous rise in pressure will result if N_2O is being administered. In cases where the chest is not drained, oxygen alone should be used and the pressure in the hemithorax should be decreased to -4 to -8 cmH_2O using a needle and syringe. This negative pressure matches the intrapleural pressure on the contralateral side and prevents mediastinal shift.

It is well known that absorption atelectasis of sequestered alveoli is rapid if they contain a gas which is soluble in, or taken up by, the blood. Thus 100 percent oxygen favors atelectasis. In the same way, absorption collapse is more rapid if the alveoli contain an oxygen/N_2O mixture than if they contain an oxygen/nitrogen mixture.[23] The insoluble nitrogen "splints" the alveoli and reduces the tendency to atelectasis. Nitrous oxide, being more soluble than nitrogen, enhances collapse. Except after periods of prolonged inhalation of N_2O, the mixed venous nitrous oxide tension is usually much less than the alveolar tension which provides an alveolar-pulmonary capillary gradient favorable for the diffusion and absorption of N_2O from the sequestered alveoli. This property is significant in one-lung anesthesia when the down lung is being ventilated. This lung already has a decreased FRC and increased closing volume, favoring atelectasis and an increase in venous admixture during anesthesia and the postoperative period. The effect on hypocapnic bronchoconstriction has not been studied. In isolated perfused rat lungs, nitrous oxide was found not to reduce hypoxia-induced vasoconstriction.[8]

There is little information on the effect of N_2O alone on the cardiovascular system. Forty percent N_2O was found to cause a steady and direct depression of myocardial function during 30 minutes of N_2O/O_2 breathing in volunteers.[24] Blood pressure was maintained, however, due to an increase in peripheral vasoconstriction. In clinical practice the depressant effects may be marked, necessitating a reduction in or withdrawal of N_2O. If cardiac output is depressed, oxygen flux may be compromised, leading to tissue hypoxemia.

More recently, the subacute effects of nitrous oxide have become apparent. These include neurological symptoms, hemopoietic effects, possible teratogenic and mutagenic effects, and an inhibition of methionine synthetase, an enzyme which is involved in the pathway for DNA synthesis.[25-28] While much of the evidence is epidemiological, it has caused a lot of controversy about a gas which was, until recently, thought to be totally inert and harmless.[29] Air-oxygen mixtures may be used in the future if nitrous oxide proves to be a significant hazard. Indeed, the authors have used air/oxygen mixtures plus intravenous agents for pulmonary surgical anesthesia and found them satisfactory (unpublished data).

Valuable aspects of nitrous oxide include its rapid onset of action and its lack of dysrhythmogenicity. Provided the various caveats to its use are borne in mind, nitrous oxide may still be usefully employed in some forms of pulmonary surgery.

VOLATILE ANESTHETIC AGENTS

The only volatile anesthetics in common use today are the halogenated hydrocarbons halothane, enflurane, and isoflurane. Methoxyflurane will not be discussed, since it is no longer in common use following reports of dose-related nephrotoxicity. These agents are liquids at room temperature, but vaporize enough to have an anesthetically useful vapor phase.

The volatile agents are complete anesthetics, since all the objectives of general anesthesia are attained if an appropriate concentration is used. The concentration necessary, however, may produce undesirable depressant side effects so that these agents are commonly used in lower doses in conjunction with muscle relaxants and nitrous oxide. In this way the unwanted effects may, to some extent, be avoided. When a high inspired oxygen concentration is required to ensure adequate arterial oxygenation, the volatile agents may be used only with a relaxant to provide the amnesic, analgesic, and relaxation components of the anesthetic triad.

The volatile agents have basically similar effects on the cardiorespiratory systems, but they differ in degree. All depress respiration, the responses to carbon dioxide, hypoxemia, respiratory "loading," etc. These aspects will now be considered in relation to each agent.

Halothane

Halothane, an alkane, was developed in the mid-1950s as a result of the predictions about the molecular structure that would provide nonflammability and low solubility (halogenation), molecular stability (CF_3 moiety), and anesthetic potency. It is a result of the fluoride technology that also facilitated the separation of uranium isotopes for the atomic bomb.

Halothane is a colorless liquid with a sweet, nonirritant odor. It is nonflammable, nonexplosive and the prototype for all the currently used volatile agents. It is a respiratory depressant and, in volunteers, it causes $PaCO_2$ to rise from an awake value of 35 mmHg to progressively higher levels as the concentration of halothane is increased.[30] Tidal volume is reduced and respiratory rate is increased, possibly by stimulation of stretch receptors in the lung.[31] The overall effect is a decrease in alveolar ventilation. At concentrations of 1.0 to 1.5 percent halothane, the apneic threshold rises by a $PaCO_2$ of 9 mmHg.[32] As anesthetic depth increases, $PaCO_2$ rises and may cause release of endogenous catecholamines. Subanesthetic concentrations of halothane have no effect on the ventilatory response to hypercarbia, depression beginning only when consciousness is lost.[32]

Halothane depresses the ventilatory response to hypoxemia.[33] This depression is observed at concentrations as low as 0.1 MAC which may occur postoperatively in patients recovering from halothane anesthesia.[34] These depressant effects are very important in patients dependent on hypoxia to drive respiration (e.g., COPD patients); and these patients must be monitored carefully in the postoperative period. In spontaneously breathing patients, these effects are antagonized to some extent by surgical stimulation, but such stimulation cannot always be relied upon to normalize ventilation.

If a normal awake subject encounters an impedance to respiration such as airway obstruction or a decrease in compliance due to pressure on the chest, ventilation is decreased initially. Respiratory effort is then increased such that over the next ten breaths ventilation returns to normal. In anesthetized patients, this response to loading is obtunded and a clear airway must always be ensured. Surgical maneuvers must not be allowed to interfere with chest movement if the patient is breathing spontaneously.[35]

Halothane has been shown to have a very valuable bronchodilator effect. It reduces air flow resistance and increases airway conductance.[36] The incidence of wheezing is relatively low during halothane anesthesia, and asthmatic episodes have been effectively terminated by this drug.[37] The bronchodilator effect of halothane has actually been observed during bronchoscopy, and halothane is widely advocated for the

patient with obstructive airways disease.[38,39] Although halothane has been shown to depress mucociliary clearance in dogs, there is a very low incidence of coughing and secretions during halothane anesthesia in man.[40,41]

Since halothane is the halogenated agent in longest use, it has been widely employed in pulmonary anesthesia. Indeed, the survey of anesthesia for pulmonary surgery in 1981 showed that a volatile technique using halothane was the one most commonly employed (74%). In 1946, Von Euler and Liljestrand suggested that local pulmonary vasoconstriction in response to hypoxia normally acts to redistribute pulmonary blood flow away from poorly ventilated to more adequately ventilated regions of the lung.[5] In 1964, Buckley et al suggested that halothane anesthesia may abolish this response in the dog.[42] Since then, numerous animal studies have shown depression of hypoxic vasoconstriction by volatile anesthetic agents.[43-45] Unfortunately, there are relatively few studies in man, but Bjertnaes has demonstrated depression of this response in man using a radioisotope method.[46] He found that the damping effect of halothane (and diethyl ether) on the response to hypoxia was demonstrated at blood concentrations of halothane comparable to those used in clinical anesthesia and concluded that it was likely that inhibition of hypoxia-induced pulmonary vasoconstriction contributes to the development of arterial hypoxemia during halothane anesthesia.

Depression of HPV and the resultant increase in venous admixture by halothane is important, especially during one-lung ventilation.[7] If HPV is depressed in the "up" lung, there is a great potential for shunting of blood through this organ. Intravenous anesthetic agents have not been found to have such a depressant effect on HPV, and their use has, therefore, been advocated in place of halothane and other volatile agents in patients who are at particular risk for poor oxygenation.[7]

Bjertnaes has demonstrated in isolated

lung studies that the route of administration of drugs is important in regard to the effect on HPV.[8] Thus, when halothane is administered via the airways, the HPV response is abolished at low concentrations (as measured in pulmonary venous blood) which are from ⅓ to ½ of those reducing the response by 50 to 70 percent during administration via the pulmonary artery, under conditions of low alveolar halothane concentration.[8,47] While halothane abolishes HPV more effectively when given via the alveoli than via the blood stream, the intravenous agent fentanyl has no effect on HPV whether given in nebulized form via the lungs or by the more conventional intravenous route.

Despite its effect on hypoxic vasoconstriction, halothane has been very successfully used for one-lung anesthesia. Generally, it is used with an FiO_2 of 1.0 in order to maintain good arterial oxygenation. Adequacy of oxygenation is usually considered present if the PaO_2 is greater than 70 mmHg.[48] Khanam et al reported a mean PaO_2 of 73.5 mmHg during one-lung ventilation with halothane (1%), nitrous oxide (60%) and oxygen (40%).[49,50] Tarhan used 1 percent halothane and 99 percent oxygen for one-lung anesthesia in 14 patients and reported a mean PaO_2 of 170 mmHg.[51] Four out of the 14, however, had a PaO_2 of less than 70 mmHg. Tarhan considered that if this PaO_2 (70 mmHg) is accepted as the lowest safe level during anesthesia in patients with normal or only slightly impaired cardiovascular function, the arterial oxygenation in these four patients was inadequate.[51] Alveolar ventilation by $PaCO_2$ criteria was normal or below normal in all patients, so that the low PaO_2 was not due to underventilation.

Torda et al investigated shunting during one-lung halothane anesthesia.[52] The range of shunt before lung deflation was 3 to 29 percent, and after lung deflation was 21 to 65 percent at 20 minutes and 22 to 63 percent at 30 minutes. Halothane one-lung anesthesia is thus associated with significant degrees of shunting. Following pneumonectomy or clamping of the pulmonary artery on the collapsed side, there is a considerable improvement in the PaO_2 and a diminution in calculated shunt, demonstrating the persistence of blood flow through the unventilated lung (Table 10-2).[6]

Halothane may increase venous admixture by depression of HPV, and it may also upset the V/Q ratio by depressing the hypocapnic bronchoconstrictor mechanism.[4] This is a feature of its bronchodilator effect which allows ventilation of underperfused parts of the lung, leading to increased dead space. The effect is mediated by a nonspecific adrenergic mechanism which is not inhibited by beta-blocking agents.[4]

Halothane produces a dose-related depression of the cardiovascular system.[53] Myocardial contractility, cardiac output, and stroke volume decrease as halothane concentration increases. Heart rate tends to remain unchanged, but the blood pressure shows a dose-related fall as peripheral resistance and cardiac output decrease. The negative inotropic effect is a disadvantage in patients with poor myocardial function, since low cardiac output combined with poor arterial oxygenation results in decreased oxygen availability. In this situation, the decrease in mixed venous oxygen content together with an increased right-to-left shunt will result in further arterial desaturation.

Halothane sensitizes the myocardium to the dysrhythmic effects of catecholamines, both endogenous and exogenous. This is a feature of alkane anesthetics and is less evident with ethers. Johnston et al determined

Table 10-2

Influence of Pneumonectomy on PaO_2 and Qs/Qt (mean ± SD)

	FiO_2 0.5		
	TLV	OLV	PPN
PaO_2 (mmHg)	128 ± 37	89 ± 12	112 ± 22
Qs/Qt(%)	18 ± 5	36 ± 4	26 ± 3

TLV = two lung ventilation; OLV = one lung ventilation; PPN = post-pneumonectomy

the dose of submucosally injected epinephrine required to produce three or more premature ventricular extrasystoles in 50 percent of normocapnic patients anesthetized with 1.25 MAC concentrations of various volatile agents.[54] Halothane produced the greatest sensitization with extrasystoles being induced with 2 μg/kg body weight of epinephrine as compared to 7 μg/kg with isoflurane anesthesia.

All types of dysrhythmias have been reported with halothane; the most common include bigeminy, junctional rhythms, and junctional and ventricular extrasystoles. The management of the cardiovascular complications of halothane is described well by Hug.[55]

The controversy concerning the existence of halothane hepatitis remains unresolved, and conclusive evidence for its existence remains incomplete.[56] It has become clear, however, that a significant amount of the halothane administered to a patient is metabolized and that metabolism of anesthetics is associated with toxicity.[57]

Despite all the negative aspects described above, halothane has proven itself to be a valuable agent for pulmonary surgery in patients in whom oxygenation is not severely at risk. It is certainly the most acceptable agent for patients undergoing inhalation induction due to its sweet smell and lack of pungency. Low concentrations in association with nitrous oxide and relaxants have been widely employed for pulmonary resections with relatively few problems.[49-52,58]

Enflurane

Enflurane is an ether and was developed in 1963 during the search for an agent which would be less dysrhythmogenic than halothane. The ethers seemed a promising group, since they did not increase the incidence of ventricular dysrhythmias. It is qualitatively similar to halothane in respect to its anesthetic properties, with only a few notable exceptions.[59] High concentrations of enflurane in conjunction with hypocapnia tend to produce a seizure pattern by EEG and sometimes cause gross body movements.[60]

Enflurane is biodegraded to a lesser extent (2.6% of dose administered) than is halothane (20% of dose administered).[61,62] It is less potent than halothane, the MAC being 1.7 percent compared to 0.76 percent for halothane; and it potentiates the relaxant effects of the competitive neuromuscular blockers to a greater extent than halothane at equal depths of anesthesia (MAC equivalents).[63] From the partition coefficient and solubility data, the uptake of enflurane would be expected to be more rapid than that of halothane. In clinical practice, however, the pungency of enflurane makes it less pleasant to breathe during an inhalational induction, and the induction may take longer with enflurane than with halothane.

Enflurane is a more potent respiratory depressant than halothane.[64] As the concentration of enflurane is increased in spontaneously breathing subjects, respiration is depressed and $PaCO_2$ rises rapidly. Unstimulated patients have a $PaCO_2$ of 61 mmHg at 1.86 percent enflurane (approx. 1 MAC), 76 mmHg at 1.5 MAC, and apnea supervenes at 2 MAC.[65] As with halothane, alveolar ventilation decreases despite an increase in respiratory rate, since tidal volume is greatly reduced.[34]

The ventilatory response to hypoxia is also greatly depressed by enflurane, more so than with halothane.[66,67] Subanesthetic concentrations (0.1 MAC) of enflurane, which have no detectable effect on the response to CO_2, reduce the ventilatory responses to hypoxia and acidemia to less than half of their awake values, and light anesthesia of 1.1 MAC abolishes these responses altogether.

A study of enflurane in patients with COPD showed a higher incidence of coughing and secretions than occurred with halothane, although the differences were not statistically significant.[41] Enflurane has been reported as being clinically useful in patients with COPD, and has been favorably compared with halothane for this group.[41,68]

The effects of enflurane on bronchial tone are not well established. While enflurane has been shown to protect against bronchospasm in the asthma dog model, there are three case reports in man which suggest that it may actually cause bronchospasm.[33,69] Enflurane abolishes the hypocapnic bronchoconstrictor reflex, producing bronchodilation in dog lungs, raising the possibility of a species difference.[4] A study of the effects of enflurane on airway conductance in human volunteers revealed no change during early anesthesia (up to 8 minutes at 2.5% enflurane), but a 56 percent increase in conductance after 15 minutes at 2.5 percent.[36] Overall it would appear that enflurane usually produces bronchodilatation in normal subjects, but the irritation produced by this drug may precipitate coughing and bronchoconstriction in susceptible subjects.

The effects of enflurane on hypoxic pulmonary vasoconstriction are also not firmly established. Mathers et al, working with a dog lung model, found no depression of HPV by enflurane; while Bjertnaes did find depression of HPV in the isolated rat lung model.[44,47] Definitive data in humans has yet to be established, but it seems likely that enflurane, like other volatile agents (halothane, ether), will obtund this response.[43] There is also no clinical data on the degree of shunting associated with enflurane anesthesia during one-lung ventilation to compare with the extensive halothane data.

Like halothane, enflurane depresses the cardiovascular system in a dose-related fashion, but does not sensitize the myocardium to the dysrhythmogenic effects of catecholamines to the same extent as halothane.[54,70] Greater stability of rhythm is a worthwhile feature, although a variety of dysrhythmias have been reported with enflurane, including tachycardia, bradycardia, transient junctional rhythm, premature atrial and ventricular contractions and A–V dissociation.

At equianesthetic doses, enflurane depresses contractility, cardiac output, and blood pressure more than halothane. The effect on heart rate is variable. Interestingly, a comparison of the circulatory effects of enflurane alone with enflurane plus nitrous oxide at a given MAC level suggests that the combination produces less depression of cardiac output, stroke volume, and aortic dp/dt than does enflurane alone.[71]

Isoflurane

Isoflurane is the most recently introduced volatile agent and is an isomer of enflurane. Its physical properties most closely approach those of an ideal agent. Thus it is nonflammable at all anesthetizing concentrations, stable on storage, and its blood solubility is lower than those of the other halogenated hydrocarbons. The low blood and tissue solubility levels enable the level of anesthesia to be regulated quickly and precisely.

Isoflurane also has the distinction of being the least biodegradable of the volatile agents, only about 0.25 percent of the administered dose being metabolized.[72] From its physical properties, it might be expected that the induction of anesthesia with isoflurane is the most rapid. Its slight pungency, however, is a negative feature in this regard, and induction with halothane is more rapid since it is more acceptable to patients. The lesser solubility of isoflurane does mean, however, that it is excreted more rapidly than the other volatile agents and recovery is quicker.

Isoflurane is a profound respiratory depressant. The dose-related depression of the response to carbon dioxide is greater than that due to halothane, but less than enflurane.[30,64,73] At 1.1 MAC isoflurane, the $PaCO_2$ in spontaneously breathing volunteers was about 49 mmHg and the slope of the CO_2 response curve was 85 percent of the awake value. As with the other agents, this is due mainly to a decrease in tidal volume. Addition of nitrous oxide (which by itself has little effect on ventilation) to isoflurane decreases the ventilatory depression seen with isoflurane alone at the same depth of anesthesia (MAC equivalent).[18] This is fortunate since the addition of nitrous oxide decreases the PaO_2 and would increase the potential for hypoxia in the absence of increased ventilation.

During isoflurane anesthesia, the normal awake response to respiratory loading due to increased airway resistance or decreased chest compliance is reduced, and any increases in airway resistance will cause a parallel increase in $PaCO_2$. Surgical stimulation helps to some extent to counteract the depressant effects of isoflurane on ventilation.[74] Like the other agents, isoflurane depresses the ventilatory response to hypoxia. Depression is detectable at 0.1 MAC and the response is completely obtunded at 1.1 MAC isoflurane.

Airway resistance was found to be increased with both 1 and 2 percent isoflurane.[75] Despite this, isoflurane has been proposed as being a suitable agent for use in patients with COPD although as yet there is no published experience of its use in this group.[75] The effects on hypocapnic bronchoconstriction have also yet to be determined.

Regional hypoxic pulmonary vasoconstriction is depressed by isoflurane in the dog lung model.[44] Indeed, isoflurane significantly decreased HPV where halothane and enflurane caused only slight changes. There is no human data as yet to confirm or refute these observations; but if the results in dogs can be extrapolated to man, patients with atelectasis or those undergoing one-lung anesthesia may be at greater risk of hypoxemia if anesthetized with isoflurane.

The undesirable effects on HPV may be compensated for to some extent by a lesser depressant effect on the cardiovascular system.[76] In normal subjects, clinically useful concentrations of isoflurane (1-2 MAC) cause little or no depression of myocardial function or cardiac output, in contrast to halothane and enflurane. There is no increase in right atrial pressure at 0.9 to 1.4 MAC isoflurane, and only a slight increase at 1.9 MAC, compared to much greater increases with equivalent doses of other volatile agents. It also causes only a small change in heart rate, tending to, if anything, increase it slightly. Arterial blood pressure and peripheral resistance decrease in a dose-related manner.

Cardiac rhythm remains most stable with isoflurane. There appears to be minimal sensitization of the myocardium to exogenous doses of epinephrine compared with halothane or enflurane.[54] The cardiovascular stability due to isoflurane is not depressed by beta-adrenergic blockade.[77]

Overall clinical experience with isoflurane is still rather limited, but this agent certainly has advantageous properties in several areas. Only future trials will determine its true usefulness in pulmonary surgery. In particular, the effects on hypoxic vasoconstriction, hypocapnic bronchoconstriction, and oxygenation during one-lung anesthesia must be elucidated.

Premedication

The most important indication for preoperative medication today is to make the operating room experience as pleasant as possible for the patient under the particular circumstances. With any drug used preoperatively it is essential to ensure that the unwanted effects do not outweigh the therapeutic ones.

The ideal premedicant agent would allay anxiety, provide basal sedation, amnesia, and patient cooperation while producing minimal cardiorespiratory or other side effects. In addition, anticholinergic agents can be used preoperatively to reduce respiratory tract secretions and prevent bradycardias. Some anesthesiologists believe that it is better to treat excessive secretions if they occur, rather than to expose every patient to a drug that may not be needed. However, smokers, obese patients, and black patients are more prone than others to develop problems with secretions, and an anticholinergic appears indicated in such cases. If ketamine is to be used, then a drying agent should be given preoperatively, since ketamine produces an increase in secretions.

Although opiate premedication has been used in patients undergoing pulmonary surgery, because of the respiratory depression associated with this group of drugs, some believe there is no longer any place for them in thoracic anesthesia and that the benzodiazepines are the premedicant drugs of choice.[78]

ANTICHOLINERGICS

The use of anticholinergic premedication originated with the need to reduce the often excessive oral and respiratory tract secretions incurred during open-drop ether anesthesia. The need for anticholinergic premedication has become controversial, since modern anesthetic techniques are generally less of an irritant to the respiratory tract.[79] In a double-blind study, it was found that 97.6 percent of the unsatisfactory anesthetic ratings in the patients who did not receive an anticholinergic drug were due to excessive secretions and associated problems such as coughing and laryngospasm.[80]

On the other hand, it has been suggested that drying agents might increase the incidence of complications by decreasing the transportability of bronchial mucus due to increased viscosity. Annis et al studied the effects of atropine 0.4 mg IM given 45 minutes preoperatively on the velocity of tracheal mucus in anesthetized patients.[81] Significant decreases in mucus velocity were found at 30 minutes following induction of anesthesia. In every patient, whether given atropine or not, the trachea showed increased secretions, erythema, and edema after 75 minutes of anesthesia. They concluded that premedicant doses of atropine contribute to the impairment of this "vital host defense mechanism during general anesthesia." The decrease in mucus velocity might not be clinically important in normal individuals, but may be in those with chronic retention of secretions.

Jones and Drummond looked at the effects of atropine premedication on postoperative respiratory complications in 50 patients undergoing abdominal surgery.[82] The patients were examined on the first and third postoperative days for the presence of productive cough, axillary pyrexia ($>37\,^\circ$ C), and abnormal physical signs in the chest. No statistically significant difference was found between those patients given atropine and those not, in the frequency of any of the above complications.

Perhaps the explanation for the differing opinions regarding the value of atropine in preventing respiratory complications lies in the large variation in secretions among individuals.[83] The normal range of secretion volume is 10 to 100 ml daily, of which 95 percent is water; the volume is increased with chronic irritation. The larger the size of the glands (denoting hypertrophy), the greater the amount secreted and the less the effectiveness of atropine therapy in the prevention of sputum in chronic bronchitis.[84] Atropine mainly blocks the secretions of the mucus cells, while the serous cells are relatively less affected. This has been thought to increase viscosity and thus contribute to sputum retention.

Atropine dilates air passages, especially the larger ones. This has been shown by an increase of up to 30 percent in the anatomical dead space following 0.5 mg IM of atropine, while larger doses do not cause a greater effect.[85,86] This bronchodilation lasts up to 3 hours following atropine administration.[87] Unsedated patients can respond to the increase in anatomical dead space by an increase in minute volume, and $PaCO_2$ is unchanged.[88] Atropine does not alter the response to hypercapnia, and, although atropine has been thought to increase the alveolar-arterial oxygen gradient, this effect is still controversial.[89-92]

Although smaller airways are dilated less than larger ones, atropine reduces airway resistance and improves airway conductance in COPD, exercise, and allergic states, since there is an element of intrinsic bronchoconstriction in these situations which is mediated by the parasympathetic nervous system.[93] These useful clinical effects can be achieved equally as well using an aerosol which avoids the other side effects of atropine.[94]

With respect to the cardiovascular system, the most important effect of atropine is on the heart rate. While tachycardia is the expected response, it can be preceded by a bradycardia if small doses are used.[95] Large doses produce an increase in rate; and above a dose of 2 mg total vagal block can be assumed, since there is no further increase in rate. A completely vagally-blocked patient can be expected to have a rate of around 130 beats per minute.[96] The mechanism for the biphasic response to atropine is not clear.

Injection of atropine in healthy subjects causes an increase in cardiac output in proportion to the tachycardia. Stroke volume is unchanged and peripheral resistance falls with a decrease in mean arterial pressure.[97] The pulmonary pressure falls and there is a decrease in pulmonary blood volume, which indicates that blood is redistributed away from the lungs.[98]

Atropine may cause dysrhythmias which usually take the form of A-V dissociation with retrograde conduction, nodal rhythm, or atrial and ventricular extrasystoles.[99] The incidence varies according to the anesthetic technique, type of surgery, and whether the $PaCO_2$ is raised.

Scopolamine is also sometimes used as an anticholinergic premedicant. It has a greater effect on drying secretions and reducing postoperative nausea. It produces more sedation than atropine, produces amnesia, has a prolonged antanalgesic action, and may produce restlessness and confusion.

Glycopyrrolate, a quaternary ammonium compound, has recently come into use as a potent, long-acting anticholinergic agent which has certain advantages over atropine. Studies have shown that it is twice as potent as atropine on a weight basis. It is associated with a lower incidence of cardiac dysrhythmias and, being a quaternary ammonium compound, crosses the blood brain barrier to a smaller extent than the tertiary amine atropine.[100] This implies that there would be less in the way of CNS effects with glycopyrrolate than with atropine, which occasionally causes excitatory phenomena. Glycopyrrolate also appears to be a more effective drying agent than atropine, and is longer acting.[101] Whether this is an advantage in patients with lung disease is debatable. The main area of superiority of glycopyrrolate over atropine is in its lesser effect on increasing heart rate and lower incidence of dysrhythmias.

Parenteral Drugs Used for Premedication and/or Anesthesia

BENZODIAZEPINES

The benzodiazepine derivatives used in anesthesia include diazepam, lorazepam, and the newly introduced midazolam. All are qualitatively similar and produce CNS depression. Small doses reduce anxiety and produce sedation; larger doses induce sleep, generally with a large margin of safety.

The derivative most commonly used is diazepam, since both oral and parenteral preparations are available. It may be used for premedication, for induction of anesthesia, and as an amnesic. Premedication is satisfactory with oral administration of diazepam and this route avoids painful intramuscular injection. The usual oral dose for premedication is 0.1 to 0.2 mg/kg with a few sips of water.

Intravenous administration of diazepam is uncomfortable and associated with a high incidence of phlebitis and thrombosis. These side effects are due to the solvent in which diazepam is formulated. They can be avoided to some extent by injection into a rapidly flowing intravenous line; by drawing blood back into the syringe to dilute it; or by preceding the injection with intravenous lidocaine.

Diazepam produces mild depression of the respiratory system. Given intramuscularly as premedication it has no significant effects on respiratory rate, tidal volume, minute ventilation, dead space, VD/VT ratio, alveolar ventilation, or blood gases.[102] Respiratory depression has been reported after oral administration of 5 mg diazepam, and more significant depression has been reported after intravenous diazepam.[103] Hypoventilation is due primarily to a decrease in tidal volume; and although the rate increases, the minute volume is reduced by 20 to 30 percent.[104] Arterial PO_2 falls and $PaCO_2$ rises.[105] Rarely, the injection of diazepam may be associated with apnea, cyanosis, and unconsciousness.[106] However, Steen et al found that at doses of up to 0.66 mg/kg, diazepam given intravenously produced no statistically significant depression in the response to CO_2.[107] The basis for the variability in respiratory response is not known, but it should always be borne in mind, especially in patients at risk and in the aged.

Diazepam (5 mg IV) does not significantly affect the airway resistance in asthmatic patients; and, in patients with COPD, a dose of 0.11 mg/kg IV does not cause changes in FEV_1 or the FEV_1/FVC ratio.[108, 109] It can thus be safely used in patients with lung disease.

Diazepam has been widely used to allay preoperative anxiety, and in this role has been received very favorably. Numerous studies have shown that when compared with opiates and barbiturates it relieves anxiety with relatively few side effects.[110, 111] When compared with other premedicants, any minor differences have generally been in favor of diazepam. It produces amnesia which may be anterograde but is never retrograde. Diazepam is therefore valuable in sedating a patient whose cooperation is needed

for an awake intubation and who desires to remember little about the procedure. The amnesic effect is thought to be due to a depression of memory input rather than retrieval and is probably not due to a reduction in level of consciousness at the time of the unpleasant procedure.[112] The amnesic effect has been considered of particular value in patients undergoing bronchoscopy when a dose of 0.15 mg/kg IV reduced anxiety, induced cooperation, and increased relaxation. It did not interfere with the secretory function and the motility of the tracheobronchial tree, nor did it interfere with the cough reflex or increase the risk of laryngospasm or bronchospasm.[113]

The cardiovascular effects are generally minimal, so diazepam is very useful in critically ill patients. Diazepam produces small reductions in arterial blood pressure, and a decrease in cardiac output due to a reduction in stroke volume which is probably the result of a lowering of ventricular filling pressure rather than myocardial contractility.[104] Likewise, changes in pulmonary arterial mean pressure and total pulmonary resistance are not significant.[105] Diazepam reduces myocardial oxygen demand and myocardial oxygen consumption, a valuable feature in patients with coronary insufficiency.[114] The mechanism underlying this effect is as yet undetermined, although it may be due to a reduction in sympathetic activity associated with the anxiolytic effects.

For induction of general anesthesia, most authors agree that, in doses of 0.16 mg/kg to 0.32 mg/kg IV, blood pressure changes are minimal and respiratory effects small and transitory. Induction with diazepam is slower than with thiopental, taking as long as three minutes; and some patients may require very large doses to produce sleep. The variability in response to benzodiazepines, in general, is much greater than that to barbiturates, which may be a minor negative aspect. Dysrhythmias on induction are rare, and intravenous diazepam is considered to be an excellent alternative to thiopental, especially in poor risk patients in whom the cardiovascular effects of the barbiturates may be considered undesirable.

Diazepam is also valuable in patients when a ketamine technique is to be used. It attenuates the catecholamine response to ketamine and reduces the hypertensive reaction which might otherwise occur.[7,115] In addition, the incidence of emergence phenomena associated with ketamine anesthesia may be reduced by diazepam. Doses of 10 mg given intravenously near the end of the operation do not unduly prolong recovery, yet make the anesthesia far more acceptable to the patient.[116]

Lorazepam is one of the more recently introduced benzodiazepine derivatives, and it differs from diazepam quantitatively rather than qualitatively in its actions. Neither drug can be recommended for intravenous administration because of local irritation, and both cause a phlebitic reaction on intravenous administration.

Given orally, 4 mg of lorazepam has been compared favorably with 10 mg of diazepam as premedication. The onset of action is slower than diazepam, and no major side effects have been observed (i.e., no hypotension, tachycardia, or gross respiratory depression).[117]

Lorazepam has been found by some authors to stimulate respiration and by others to depress it.[118,119] The occurrence of periodic breathing has been reported following lorazepam (2 mg IV) in two out of 20 patients with COPD, and in one normal subject after an injection of 4 mg of lorazepam IM.[118,119] No such abnormal breathing pattern has been reported following diazepam. The pattern of periodic breathing following lorazepam is similar to that seen during the onset of sleep, and represents an alteration in respiratory control which may be a potential hazard. Adeoshun et al studied this phenomenon in 10 patients given 2 mg of lorazepam IV and observed periodic breathing in 9 out of the 10.[120] They suggested that the mechanism was either a direct effect on brain stem

respiratory control or a change in blood flow to the respiratory center.

Lorazepam provides more sedation than diazepam and it is more potent on a weight basis. Diazepam (10 mg) and lorazepam (2.5 mg) produce comparable levels of sedation.[121] The onset of action of lorazepam is slower and the duration of action three to four times longer than that of an equivalent dose of diazepam. In equivalent doses given intravenously, both drugs produce an anterograde amnesia, but the frequency of this effect is greater with lorazepam. It has been suggested that this agent impairs retrieval of information from memory, rather than input and consolidation.[121]

In respect to preventing emergence sequelae from ketamine anesthesia, lorazepam is more reliable than diazepam when given as premedication. For this purpose, lorazepam 4 mg given IV, IM, or orally is effective, while diazepam is unreliable. Since the onset of action of lorazepam is relatively slow, it must be given a sufficiently long time before ketamine, and the prolonged effect may be a disadvantage for short procedures where rapid recovery is required.[122] In contrast, the intravenous injection of diazepam towards the end of a ketamine anesthetic will reduce the emergence sequelae without producing the prolonged depressant effect seen with lorazepam.[117]

Midazolam maleate is a benzodiazepine derivative which resembles diazepam in its pharmacological properties, but it is water soluble and therefore less of an irritant. It is currently undergoing extensive clinical trials for use both as a premedicant and as an intravenous induction agent. In a dose of 0.07 mg/kg IM, it produces satisfactory anxiolysis and sedation; and in a dose of 0.2 mg/kg IV, it provides a satisfactory intravenous induction of anesthesia with no adverse side effects and with less variability in response than is seen with intravenous diazepam.[123] Because of the low incidence of pain on injection, fewer postoperative venous complications, and speedier onset and shorter duration of action than diazepam, midazolam seems to be a new induction agent with great potential.[124]

NEUROLEPTANESTHESIA

Neuroleptanalgesia is the state of apparent indifference to pain induced by the combination of a potent analgesic with a major tranquilizing drug. The patient remains conscious but is in a trance-like state, remaining immobile and pain free. With the addition of muscle relaxants and nitrous oxide, a state of neuroleptanesthesia is achieved.

Droperidol (dehydrobenzperidol), a butyrophenone, is a major tranquilizer and fulfills the neurolept criteria, which are: (1) inhibition of motor activity; (2) production of catalepsy; (3) antagonism of apomorphine-induced vomiting; and (4) antagonism of amphetamine-induced arousal. It produces a patient who has an outwardly peaceful appearance, who may be sleeping but is easily aroused, and who can obey simple commands. Appearances can be deceptive, however, for although the patient may appear placid, his subjective experience may be one of agitation and restlessness sometimes called "inner anxiety."[125]

Droperidol has no analgesic properties of its own, although it may prolong the effects of fentanyl. It has a powerful antiemetic effect which antagonizes the emetic effects of opiates, and it may occasionally produce CNS excitation as evidenced by varying degrees of dyskinesia.

Droperidol has minimal effects on the respiratory system. Soroker et al found a modest reduction in tidal volume and minute ventilation with no significant changes in respiratory rate, blood gas tensions, or other respiratory parameters following 5 mg of droperidol IM.[102] The reduction in tidal volume was secondary to a reduction in lung expansion during inspiration, but it was so slight as to not affect blood gases. The mechanisms suggested for these effects were relief of anxiety, extrapyramidal dyskinesia of respiratory muscles, and central depression.

Cardiovascular effects are also minimal, although hypotension may be induced by a central action or a peripheral alpha-adrenergic blocking effect.[126] Effects on cardiac output are variable with a decrease often being produced.[127] In addition, droperidol appears to have an antidysrhythmic effect, the mechanism of which is uncertain.[128]

Droperidol can be used in pulmonary surgical patients in combination with diazepam, both as an intravenous premedicant or a supplement to anesthesia. Herr et al studied the effects of intravenous diazepam and droperidol alone and in combination for premedication.[129] They found that the combination of droperidol (2.5 mg) with diazepam (5 mg) produced better anxiolysis, sedation, amnesia, and patient and physician acceptance, than 10 mg of either drug given alone. Increasing the proportion of droperidol produced more anxiety; larger doses of diazepam produced oversedation.

The adverse effects of ketamine are influenced variably by droperidol. Bessy et al found that the cardiovascular and psychotomimetic sequelae were obtunded, while others found little or no reduction in sequelae.[130-132]

Intravenous Anesthetic Drugs

FENTANYL

Fentanyl is a synthetic opiate-analgesic which, on a weight basis, is about 100 times more potent than morphine. After a single dose it has a shorter duration of action than other opiates, although following multiple doses a cumulative effect is observed and may be prolonged.

Fentanyl is a potent respiratory depressant. Following a dose of 0.2 mg IV, changes in respiratory pattern occur within 15 to 30 seconds; and by 120 seconds there are variable decreases in respiratory rate and tidal volume. Following larger single intravenous doses (0.5–0.8 mg), depression of tidal volume and rate occur within 90 seconds and Cheyne-Stokes breathing may be produced.[15] Respiratory depression in the awake patient can be offset by instructing him to breathe, and, therefore, small doses can be useful to sedate patients for an awake intubation. Peak depression of ventilatory rate occurs within 5 to 10 minutes and little change occurs in the next 10 minutes. The return to control levels varies according to the previous administration of narcotic analgesics.[133]

The character of respiratory depression following fentanyl differs from that due to inhalational anesthetic agents; there is a progressive decrease in respiratory rate, and, in conscious subjects, tidal volume may show a compensatory increase. The reduction in respiratory rate is due to a prolongation of the expiratory pause, the duration of inspiration being unaltered. This pattern is typical of opiate-induced respiratory depression.

Delayed respiratory depression may also be a problem after the use of fentanyl anesthesia. Adams and Pybus described three cases in which severe respiratory depression occurred several hours after apparent recovery from an anesthetic in which fentanyl was a component.[134] Becker et al showed that fentanyl has a biphasic effect on the ventilatory response to CO_2.[135] In 26 patients, respiratory depression (as evidenced by a decrease in slope of the CO_2 response curve) was maximal shortly after intravenous administration of the drug, and then decreased steadily. Continued monitoring showed a second phase of respiratory depression, occurring when the patient was in the recovery room, which was maximal at about 160 minutes after the last dose of fentanyl. It was postulated that either varying levels of stimulation during the recovery period alter the CO_2 response, or that fentanyl, being a weak base, is secreted into the stomach to be reabsorbed later on transit to the jejunum. These authors emphasized the possible risk imposed by an otherwise minor degree of airway obstruction in a patient who has little ventilatory response to a small CO_2 challenge.[135]

Fentanyl may produce truncal rigidity and decreased thoracic compliance, especially if administered rapidly and in the presence of N_2O. These effects may be severe and require treatment with muscle relaxants and controlled ventilation.[13,16] These ventilatory changes may also affect cardiovascular function by diminishing venous return.

In isolated rat lung studies, intravenous fentanyl was found not to depress HPV; further studies showed that even if fentanyl was given into the lungs in nebulized form, it still did not depress HPV.[8] Adequate amounts of fentanyl were reaching the alveoli when given in nebulized form, as documented by blood levels which were found to be high with this mode of administration. The lack of effect of these high concentrations suggested to Bjertnaes that it was unlikely that HPV in man would be affected by the concentrations of fentanyl used in anesthetic practice.[136] The lack of effect of nebulized fentanyl on HPV suggests that it is its pharmacological properties rather than the route of administration which are of importance.

Numerous studies of the cardiovascular effects of fentanyl have revealed clinically insignificant changes in hemodynamic parameters.[133] Unlike morphine, fentanyl causes no release of histamine and therefore no vasodilatation. Cardiac rate may decrease due to a vagotomimetic effect of fentanyl which can be readily antagonized by anticholinergic agents. Fentanyl in small doses may be useful in treating the minor degrees of tachycardia sometimes seen with isoflurane anesthesia. Even very large doses have been shown not to decrease myocardial contractility, but cardiac output may decrease if rate decreases.

KETAMINE

Ketamine is a phencyclidine derivative which produces a state of dissociative anesthesia. This state is characterized by catalepsy, light sedation, amnesia, and profound analgesia.

Ketamine has a rapid onset of action when given intravenously as an induction agent in a dose of 2 mg/kg. A dose of 5 to 10 mg/kg IM also produces a very rapid induction of anesthesia. Tremor and spontaneous involuntary movements are common during a ketamine induction, and hypertonus may also occur. Occasionally, failure to obtain an anesthetic effect occurs and may be associated with the absence of appropriate cerebral development in the patient.[137] Ketamine produces profound analgesia which outlasts the period of sleep and, in contrast to the barbiturates, antanalgesia does not follow its administration. Following a single intravenous dose of 2 mg/kg, consciousness usually returns in about 15 minutes. Diplopia and other visual disturbances are frequently noted on return of consciousness, and these may be very distressing to the patient. Such emergence phenomena have been one of the major problems with ketamine.

The respiratory effects of ketamine appear to be minimal and transient. Mild depression has been reported by some workers, but others have found respiratory stimulation.[138,139] When it occurs, the peak depressant effect is seen 2 minutes after intravenous induction, and it usually lasts only 5 minutes. In most patients, there is a slight increase in respiratory rate, but a decrease in tidal volume accounts for the fall in alveolar ventilation, increased $PaCO_2$ and decreased PaO_2.[140] When preceded by diazepam during anesthesia induction, intravenous ketamine may produce apnea.

Ketamine produces bronchodilation in animals and effectively antagonizes the bronchoconstrictive effects of histamine, acetylcholine, and 5-hydroxytryptamine on the trachea and bronchi.[141] Corssen and others have reported that ketamine is safe for administration to asthmatic patients and that it produces relief from bronchospasm.[142-144] Huber measured airway resistance and reported a decrease in nine out of ten asthmatic patients, and no significant change in seven non-asthmatic patients.[144] It has been suggested that the bronchodilation is due to beta-adrenergic stimulation resulting from the elevation in catecholamine levels associated with ketamine.[145] However, when airway resistance is increased using an ultrasonic aerosol, ketamine causes no change in resistance while isoproterenol, given to those patients who do not respond to ketamine, produces a rapid decrease in resistance.[146] Another mechanism suggested is based upon the observation that atropine blocks the tachycardia caused by ketamine.[147] Thus cholinergic receptors in the sympathetic neuroeffector junction may be the mechanism responsible for the observed bronchodilation, although more conclusive proof is lacking.[148]

Coughing and laryngospasm occur rarely with ketamine, and laryngeal reflexes are not markedly depressed with normal adult doses. The laryngeal protection should not be relied upon, however, since greater depression occurs as anesthesia continues.

The cardiovascular effects of ketamine are, in general, stimulatory. It increases blood pressure, heart rate, and cardiac output, although effects on stroke volume and systemic vascular resistance are variable.[149] The cardiovascular stimulation has the same time course as the anesthetic effects of ketamine, and it has been suggested that the stimulatory effects are centrally mediated via the sympathetic nervous system.[150] Stimulation is reduced by general anesthesia, but potentiated by other cardiovascular stimulatory drugs such as pancuronium. The hypertension and tachycardia associated with ketamine induction can often be modified by adequate doses of droperidol and diazepam given intravenously prior to ketamine. However, such attempts have not always proven reliable.[151]

Tweed found that the cardio-stimulatory effects were associated with a marked increase in cardiac work and thus with increased myocardial oxygen consumption.[149] While the use of ketamine in patients with atherosclerotic heart disease is relatively contraindicated for this reason, others have found that diazepam adequately modifies the response to ketamine, and the combination has been satisfactorily used in patients undergoing coronary artery bypass surgery.[115]

On the basis of its cardiovascular stimulatory effects, ketamine has been widely advocated as the drug of choice for induction in severely ill patients.[149,152] However, Waxman et al studied cardiac output and oxygen transport in response to ketamine in 12 critically ill patients and were unable to confirm the uniformly beneficial effects of ketamine induction.[153] Following a single dose of ketamine, they found decreases in cardiac and pulmonary performance and in peripheral oxygen transport in this group of patients.[153]

Ketamine increases pulmonary artery pressure and pulmonary vascular resistance which causes an increase in right heart work.[154] Indeed, the physiologic alterations to ketamine were found to be more pronounced on the pulmonary than on the systemic vascular bed, and to the right rather than the left side of the heart. The use of ketamine may therefore be contraindicated in patients with pulmonary or systemic hypertension. Gassner et al studied the effect of ketamine on the pulmonary artery pressure in animals and man and concluded that changes in the pulmonary hemodynamics are secondary to effects on cardiac output, rather than primary effects on pulmonary vasoconstriction or dilatation.[155] They also noted that the pulmonary vascular effects can be largely counteracted during cardiac catheterization by premedication with droperidol.

Little has been written about the use of ketamine in thoracic surgery. Vaughan and Stephen first described the use of ketamine in 40 patients undergoing thoracic procedures (including 12 lung resections) and found it to be a safe and adequate technique, although they did not look specifically at cardiorespiratory parameters.[156] Weinreich et al later reported the results of a continuous ketamine infusion technique during one-lung anesthesia in 110 patients undergoing elective pulmonary resection.[7] This technique provided lower values for calculated shunt and venous admixture, and fewer patients with a PaO_2 of less than 70 mmHg (4%) when compared with a halothane technique (39%). They suggested that ketamine reduces venous admixture and maintains PaO_2 both by its effects on the cardiovascular system and possibly also by not obtunding HPV (Table 10-3). However, Gooding et al found that following a dose of 2.2 mg/kg of ketamine given intravenously over one minute to 16 adult patients (not undergoing thoracic surgery), there was a transient increase in total pulmonary shunt; arterial PO_2 was not altered, and the increase in shunt was not prolonged.[154]

Emergence sequelae have been a major problem with ketamine anesthesia. The incidence varies greatly, and reliable figures are difficult to obtain. The emergence reactions include almost any kind of unpleasant emotional experience, dreams and hallucinations, and long-term psychotomimetic effects. The incidence appears to be related to dosage and is greater in women than men. Opiates, droperidol, and benzodiazapines re-

Table 10-3
Oxygenation During Ketamine Anesthesia
(mean ± SD)

Parameter	Two Lung Ventilation		One Lung Ventilation	
	F_{IO_2} 0.5	F_{IO_2} 1.0	F_{IO_2} 0.5	F_{IO_2} 1.0
PaO_2 (mmHg)	160 ± 69	340 ± 90	83 ± 26	128 ± 30
A-aDO_2 (mmHg)	164 ± 39	360 ± 40	245 ± 41	570 ± 90
Qs/Qt (%)	14 ± 4	14 ± 9	26 ± 6	36 ± 9

duce the incidence as described previously, and few patients have any memory of emergence delirium, particularly if given diazepam. In many instances, the emergence problems are more distressing to the attendants than to the patient.

When used with 66 percent nitrous oxide, the dosage requirement for ketamine is reduced by 39 percent, recovery time by 63 percent, and the incidence of unpleasant emergence reactions is also correspondingly reduced.[157] Weinreich et al reported no emergence phenomena in their 110 patients, using ketamine, nitrous oxide, droperidol, and diazepam as their technique; and they emphasized the importance of constant preoperative and postoperative reassurance for the patient.[7]

The use of a ketamine infusion or intermittent doses for maintenance of thoracic anesthesia has several potential advantages. There is less operating room pollution, long action, good analgesia, and no absolute requirement for nitrous oxide. Vaughan and Stephen used intermittent ketamine in a dose of 1.0 to 1.2 mg/kg/hour with a N_2O/Innovar/ketamine technique.[156] Lilburn, Dundee, and Moore used ketamine infusions in 200 patients for short operations and found the ketamine dosage per kg per minute varied both with time and whether the patient was being ventilated or was breathing spontaneously.[158] Weinreich et al maintained anesthesia with an infusion rate of 2 mg/kg/hour; Idvall, using 2.4 mg/kg/hour, obtained favorable hemodynamic conditions, no postoperative respiratory depression, and no recall of the procedure.[7,159]

In paralyzed patients, lower doses are required to provide anesthesia. The ketamine-pancuronium combination, however, is best avoided since there is an unacceptable degree of tachycardia.[158] A ketamine-curare combination appears to be the most useful when relaxation is required. The effects of ketamine and succinylcholine infusions have not been reported. Thus, ketamine appears to be a promising intravenous anesthetic agent for use in pulmonary surgery. Further studies in this area are needed for a more complete evaluation.

THIOPENTAL

Thiopental is described as an ultra-short-acting barbiturate, but the short duration of its effects is due to redistribution from blood and brain to other tissues, rather than to rapid elimination.

Respiration is profoundly depressed by thiopental, the degree depending upon dose, rate of administration, and whether other central depressants (such as opiates) have been given. Following a moderate dose, there is generally an increase in depth of respiration for 30 to 40 seconds, followed by momentary apnea when the cerebral concentration peaks, after which breathing resumes but with a decrease in rate and depth. In contrast to opiates, respiratory volume rather than frequency is primarily affected by barbiturates.

The response to carbon dioxide is depressed in proportion to anesthetic depth, and, in deep anesthesia, hypoxia acting via the carotid sinus is an important stimulus to the maintenance of respiration.[160,161] On this basis, preoxygenation should increase the respiratory depression following a barbiturate induction.

Thiopental anesthesia is associated with mild bronchial constriction, but secretions are not increased. Laryngospasm is common during light thiopental anesthesia due possibly to a sensitization of laryngeal reflexes. Bronchospasm, like laryngospasm, is not due directly to thiopental, but to early stimulation of the respiratory tract during too light a level of anesthesia when the reflexes are more sensitive. Once established, however, the bronchospasm may be difficult to relieve. Lorenz showed that following clinically used doses of thiopental, the plasma histamine level rose significantly by 350 percent and then fell to normal levels in 10 minutes.[162] This observation is of little clinical significance in normal subjects; marked rises in histamine even in cases of thiopental anaphylaxis have not been reported.

The parasympathomimetic effects of thiopental have been said to be contraindications to its use in patients with obstructive airways disease. The same mechanism which may precipitate laryngospasm (i.e., stimulation of the larynx when anesthesia is too light), may also precipitate bronchospasm in those already predisposed to this condition. It is recommended that if such patients are to be given thiopental, its judicious use should be preceded by an antihistamine premedicant, and that known bronchoconstrictors such as morphine be avoided.

Thiopental depresses the heart, and cardiac output decreases as the plasma level rises. Cardiac irritability is not affected, but dysrhythmias sometimes occur due to associated hypoxia or hypercarbia. In response to a single dose, there is generally a mild initial hypotension which returns to normal within a few minutes. When the drug is injected rapidly and in large doses, profound hypotension may result due to peripheral vasodilatation, vasomotor center depression, and direct depression of myocardial contractility. Such falls in blood pressure are especially marked in patients with pre-existing cardiovascular disease, hypertension, or shock.

Muscle Relaxants

Muscle relaxants are used in pulmonary surgery to facilitate intubation of the larynx, to prevent movement of the patient during light levels of anesthesia for positioning, to permit control of ventilation, and to produce diaphragmatic paralysis so that reflex responses to hilar traction are obtunded. Once the chest has been opened, it is not usually necessary to give further doses of muscle relaxants if a large dose has been given initially, especially when a volatile anesthetic agent is used. The side effects of these drugs are of particular interest.

SUCCINYLCHOLINE

This is a short-acting depolarizing muscle relaxant. Apart from paralyzing the respiratory muscles, it may produce an increase in bronchial secretions (muscarinic effect), and bronchospasm has been reported. In some cases this was associated with release of histamine, while in others it was part of an anaphylactic response.[163,164] Hemodynamic effects are minimal, although vagal stimulation may cause a bradycardia and fall in blood pressure, especially after large or repetitive doses. Dysrhythmias and asystolic cardiac arrest may also occur, but these effects can be prevented by prior administration of atropine. Because of its short duration of action, succinylcholine is useful for endotracheal or endobronchial intubation, and for producing paralysis in short procedures such as endoscopies.

D-TUBOCURARINE

This is a competitive, nondepolarizing relaxant which is often used in patients undergoing pulmonary resection. Bronchospasm may occur in asthmatics due to histamine released by this drug, although this is a very rare occurrence. Intravenous administration produces a dose-related hypotension with decreased peripheral resistance. A bradycardia is often associated with the hypotension, but a slight increase in heart rate may occur initially if a large dose is given. This is a result of histamine release which has a direct effect on the heart, releases catecholamines, and initiates a baroreceptor reflex as a result of sudden vasodilatation. The hypotensive effect of curare is also associated with blockade of sympathetic ganglia. Administration of any vasoconstrictor will help overcome these cardiovascular effects. Curare can be used in association with ketamine since it will tend to counter the tachycardia and hypertension due to the latter agent. Ketamine also appears to enhance the neuromuscular block of d-tubocurarine. This is an effect which may be related to protein binding, since it is not observed with succinylcholine or pancuronium, agents which do not bind significantly to plasma protein.[165]

DIMETHYL-TUBOCURARINE

This competitive neuromuscular blocker is more potent than d-tubocurarine as a relaxant, but is a less potent inhibitor of both vagal and sympathetic ganglionic transmission. In low doses, it produces less histamine release so that hemodynamic effects are minimal, with little or no change in heart rate or blood pressure.

PANCURONIUM

This is a synthetic, competitive, non-depolarizing relaxant. It is free of histamine-releasing properties and has been used safely in patients with high bronchial reactivity.[166] The cardiovascular effects are stimulatory with a tendency to increase heart rate, cardiac output, and systemic blood pressure.[167] There is no significant alteration of peripheral vascular resistance. While the mild tachycardia has been found useful in patients receiving propranolol therapy, it is undesirable when ketamine is being administered. Pancuronium is useful in patients who are a poor cardiovascular risk, or if a volatile agent is being used as the anesthetic technique.

ANTIDYSRHYTHMIC THERAPY

The most common cardiac complications following thoracotomy are dysrhythmias, the average incidence being about 20 percent. Dysrhythmias are particularly common in patients over 50 years of age who have undergone lung resection; the incidence is higher following right pneumonectomy than left. Most occur within the first week following surgery, and almost 90 percent occur between the second and sixth postoperative days. Beck-Nielsen reported on dysrhythmias in a series of 300 thoracotomies for lung resection, and found that atrial fibrillation occurred in 20 percent of patients with malignant disease, but in only 3 percent with benign disease.[168] In general, it is the older patient with a greater liability to develop cardiovascular depression and hypoxemia in whom the risk of dysrhythmias is greatest. The underlying mechanisms are thought to be the synergistic effects of increased vagal tone and hypoxemia.

Postoperative clinical trials have shown that quinidine is useful in patients over 45 years of age, although others have preferred to use digoxin preoperatively because of the potential toxicity of quinidine.[169,170] The basis of digitalization is that it may prevent dysrhythmias; but if not, it at least should result in a slower rate of atrial fibrillation. There are some reports that routine digitalization prior to lung resection can halve the incidence of cardiac problems in patients at greatest risk.[170,171]

Unfortunately, there is no randomized study to adequately demonstrate the value or risks of digitalis and quinidine given pre- or postoperatively. Since quinidine depresses the heart, it should probably only be used postoperatively for treatment, rather than for prophylaxis. Preoperative digitalis, however, does seem to be indicated for patients over 55 years of age who have cardiac enlargement, a history of cardiac failure, hypertension, or atherosclerotic heart disease. Many such patients will probably already be taking digitalis; but if not, prophylaxis should begin a week prior to surgery. However, the patient should be underdigitalized during surgery, since the most common dysrhythmias seen following surgery may be difficult to differentiate from digitalis toxicity. Because of this, no digoxin should be given during the 24 hours prior to surgery.

The use of digitalis in a patient with a normal heart is debatable. Against its use are the potential toxic effects of the drug and the difficulty in assessing adequacy of digitalization in the absence of heart failure. In favor of its use is the efficacy of prophylactic digoxin in reducing the incidence of potentially fatal complications in older patients. The latter view is supported by the findings of Shields and Ujiki that the incidence of post-operative dysrhythmias was significantly reduced from 14 percent in the patients who were not digitalized preoperatively, to 2.7 percent in those who were.[170] Also, in their series of 125 patients, no clinical or ECG findings of toxicity from digitalis were observed. These authors recommended routine prophylactic digitalization in older patients undergoing lung surgery. However, their recommendation is highly controversial, and not followed by most physicians.

When a patient develops a rapid ventricular rate, despite apparent adequate digitalization, and there is concern about producing toxicity if more digoxin is given, small doses of propranolol may be useful. Propranolol, 0.5 to 2.0 mg IV, is effective in reducing the ventricular rate, and the improvement in cardiac output associated with the lower rate often offsets the myocardial depressant effect of propranolol. In patients with COPD, propranolol may also increase airways resistance, and should, therefore, be used with great caution. The introduction of more specific (cardioselective) beta-blockers and slow channel calcium blockers (e.g., verapamil) represents an improvement in the treatment of dysrhythmias in patients with obstructive airways disease.

FLUIDS

Careful attention to fluid management is essential during anesthesia for thoracotomy and lung resection. As for any major operation, adequate volumes of crystalloid should be given. Some groups use 10 ml/kg during the first hour, and 5 ml/kg thereafter, with adjustments made according to the urine output, cardiovascular responses, monitoring, and the estimated blood loss.

Blood replacement during routine lung resection is usually not necessary, but extensive bleeding can occur and blood should be cross-matched and available. During thoracoplasty, pleuro-pneumonectomy, pleurec-

tomy, and decortication for mesothelioma, excessive bleeding is common and blood should be replaced from the outset of the operation. In all cases, blood should be replaced according to the assessed loss and serial hematocrit measurements. A central venous pressure catheter may be helpful in assessing the volume status. It is essential to use fluids and blood judiciously in order to maintain a constant O_2 flux. This involves keeping the cardiac output stable to minimize the venous admixture, and ensuring adequate oxygen-carrying capacity of the blood.

Intravenous fluids and blood should be warmed prior to administration, since this helps to retard the decrease in patient temperature often seen during thoracic surgery. Blood products should be filtered using a transfusion microfilter, since this may help to reduce the amount of debris reaching the lung which normally acts as a filter. This is especially important in situations where large volumes of blood are being transfused.[172]

The dangers of overhydration of patients during pneumonectomy have been discussed by Hutchin et al.[173] They found that circulatory dynamics and urine output may be improved by infusion of large fluid loads, but this occurred at the risk of developing pulmonary edema and impairment of lung mechanics. It has been shown in dog studies that giving large volumes of fluid causes a decrease in lung compliance in proportion to the fluid volume administered, and that airway resistance increases due to tracheobronchial edema.[174] The overall effect is an increase in the work of breathing. If a patient is given such fluid loads and cannot cope with the extra work of breathing, then hypoxemia, hypercapnia, and acidosis may develop. Very large infusions may eventually produce pulmonary congestion and edema if the transport capacity of the pulmonary lymphatics is exceeded.

The threshold for the production of pulmonary congestion is lowered if a lobectomy or pneumonectomy has been undertaken.

This is in part because the pulmonary vascular reserve, normally able to accommodate moderate additions to the pulmonary blood volume, has been removed along with the resected lung tissue. It should be borne in mind that the normal stress response to surgery causes an antidiuresis with further retention of fluid, so that fluids should be given with caution to patients who have undergone pneumonectomy and lobectomy.[173] In the event that congestion develops, immediate treatment with diuretics and positive pressure ventilation is indicated until normovolemia and cardiovascular homeostasis are achieved.

Fluid balance assessment by CVP or pulmonary artery catheters may not be totally reliable during thoracotomy, and patients can develop pulmonary congestion with relatively normal pressure readings.[173] There is also a syndrome of congestive atelectasis which resembles hypervolemic pulmonary congestion following shock and the rapid infusion of blood.[175] The mechanism of this syndrome is believed to be a neural reflex which causes pulmonary venoconstriction with resulting pulmonary capillary engorgement and alveolar collapse.

The effects of fluid overload on the right side of the heart may contribute to the production of dysrhythmias in the post-thoracotomy patient. If there is a decrease in the vascular reserve of the remaining lung due to disease, moderate fluid overload or exercise may result in rises in right heart pressures, and the resulting right atrial distension may lead to dysrhythmias.

ANESTHETIC MANAGEMENT OF SPECIAL SITUATIONS

Bronchopleural Fistula and Empyema

The presence of an abnormal external communication within the tracheobronchial tree may result in contamination of the lung, a loss of air, or the development of a tension pneumothorax during positive pressure ventilation.

A bronchopleural fistula arises most commonly following pulmonary resection for carcinoma. Other causes include traumatic rupture of a bronchus, fiberoptic bronchoscopy, open penetrating chest wound, or the spontaneous drainage into the bronchial tree of an empyema cavity or an infected pulmonary cyst (mycobacterial and mycotic). The incidence is higher following pneumonectomy than after other pulmonary resections.[176] The condition may be difficult to diagnose prior to the spontaneous drainage of fluid into the tracheobronchial tree, and the development of an air–fluid level. These patients are chronically ill and have a very high perioperative mortality. They may have undergone pulmonary resection involving a pneumonectomy or, less often, a lobectomy. A bronchopleural fistula may be suspected if the patient develops sudden postoperative hemoptysis, elevated temperature, and the collapse of a lobe, or wound breakdown following a pneumonectomy.[177] Once the fistula is established, the diagnosis may be suggested by coughing up foul sputum, often associated with changes in posture, or the persistence of bubbling via the underwater drain postoperatively.

The diagnosis may be confirmed radiologically by the instillation of radio-opaque dyes into the empyema cavity following the aspiration of fluid to outline the extent of the sinus. The appearance of a complete bronchogram demonstrates the presence of a fistula. The presence, in the pleural space, of contrast from a bronchogram also will establish the diagnosis.

As an alternative to the radiological techniques, methylene blue injected into the pleura may appear in the sputum when a fistula is present.[178] Direct visualization of the bronchial stump by fiberoptic bronchoscopy or thoracoscopy, and a fall in the fluid level in the pleural space on chest x-ray examination, can provide additional evidence of a bronchopleural fistula.[176]

The possibility of aspiration represents

the major threat in the anesthetic management of this group. Sudden drainage and aspiration of intrathoracic collections of pus cause contamination and obstruction of the healthy lung which can lead to death by asphyxia. This is analogous to the aspiration of gastric contents, and sequelae include acute respiratory failure, ARDS, lung abscess, and empyema.[179]

An additional factor to be considered is an air leak which, if the fistula is valvular, may result in a tension pneumothorax. The latter may decompress itself via the mediastinum and into the subcutaneous tissues, producing widespread surgical emphysema. When the fistula is non-valvular, the gas entering the pleural space represents dead-space ventilation. If the pleural cavity is already being drained by an underwater seal, bubbling may persist and the air leak may be so great that most of the tidal volume is lost, resulting in alveolar hypoventilation and CO_2 retention.

The first stage in the management of empyema with or without a bronchial connection is the establishment of external drainage in the most dependent part of the cavity. This is accomplished under local anesthesia with the patient sitting up and leaning towards the affected side—the antidrainage principle. The fistula is usually above the fluid level, or the communicating bronchus inclines upward and out of the fluid at a sufficient angle.[178]

In the past, a chronic cavity was allowed to develop until, following closure of the fistula, the cavity could be obliterated by a staged thoracoplasty. When the fistula occurs in the immediate postoperative period, drainage is established and an immediate thoracotomy is advocated for closure of the bronchopleural fistula.[176] The anesthetic management at this stage requires a technique which is both simple and reliable, avoiding the hazard of contamination of the healthy lung.[180] Surgery is best performed with the patient in the lateral position and the down lung isolated by the use of an en-

dobronchial tube. There is no place today for relying upon posture to contain or drain the intrathoracic collections of fluid. The postural approach is not practical and may be dangerous, since the outpouring of pus can be so overwhelming that, by the time it is sucked out, the patient is severely hypoxic.[181]

The possibility of isolating the contaminated side by the use of a bronchial blocker or by tamponading the communicating bronchus through a bronchoscope is an attractive concept. However, following a pneumonectomy there may be no bronchus to tamponade. The choice then lies between single-lumen (e.g., Gordon-Green) or double-lumen (e.g., Carlens or Robertshaw) endobronchial tubes. For the anesthesiologist who has had little experience with endobronchial tubes, the Gordon-Green tube may be easier to pass. However, it does not permit suctioning of the operative side or of any collection of pus above the endobronchial cuff on the good side. Once properly in place, it will protect the down lung from contamination (see Ch. 11).

Three approaches to isolation of the lungs by endobronchial intubation can be used: (1) awake intubation, as advocated by Dennison and Lester; (2) the use of general anesthesia with spontaneous ventilation, avoiding muscle relaxants until the patient is intubated; or (3) the use of a muscle relaxant for intubation.[180,182,183] Common to all techniques are reassurance and a full explanation of the planned procedure, particularly when patient cooperation is required for an awake intubation.

Immediately before surgery, the pleural space should be aspirated and emptied as completely as possible. Cessation of drainage is no guarantee that the cavity is empty, since empyemas are often loculated. A preoperative chest radiograph should accompany the patient to the operating room; but it should be realized that effusions of up to 500 ml may pass undetected.[184]

Premedication is kept to a minimum because of the generally poor condition of the patients and the fact that induction may be done in the sitting position. Oral diazepam to allay apprehension is generally satisfactory, if any premedication is needed.

The patient is transferred to the operating room in the sitting position, leaning towards the affected side to avoid the dangers of coughing and spill-over during transportation. Oxygen by face mask should be administered from the time of premedication and continued into the operating room. It is advisable to bronchoscope all cases before intubation in order to perform bronchial toilet and to exclude any gross abnormality of the tracheobronchial tree that might interfere with the passage of the endobronchial tube. The drainage tube must be left unclamped to avoid spillover of fluid from the pleural space during coughing bouts; and to prevent the build-up of a tension pneumothorax if a valvular mechanism exists.[180] Intra-arterial monitoring is begun prior to induction for the determination of blood gases and for continuous pressure monitoring. The use of a central venous pressure catheter is also indicated.

TECHNIQUES FOR INTUBATION

1. Awake Intubation. Where applicable, this remains the safest technique for the patient, even if not the most agreeable. It is well worth trying, as nothing has been compromised if the patient becomes too distressed and the anesthesiologist proceeds to a general anesthetic technique. The use of diazepam and neuroleptanalgesia has brought about a new dimension in the technique when local anesthesia is employed. The judicious use of small doses of diazepam (2.5 mg IV), plus 50 μg of fentanyl before the topical anesthesia, provides a much more receptive patient. The procedure must be unhurried and accompanied by constant reassurance. Oxygen by face mask should be administered after each maneuver. With the patient in the sitting position, the back of the tongue, the

epiglottis, and the larynx are sprayed successively with 4 percent lidocaine. The trachea can be anesthetized by introducing a laryngotracheal anesthetic cannula through the cords so that at the time of injection the superior surface of the larynx, as well as the trachea, will be sprayed with local anesthesia. Once the patient has settled down after breathing oxygen, the bronchoscope is passed with the endoscopist standing above and behind the patient's head. At this stage a further dose of diazepam or fentanyl may be needed. Laryngoscopy is next performed and the appropriate endobronchial tube is passed.

An endobronchial tube is selected in which the bronchial lumen will be on the side opposite the lesion. The tube is advanced gently until the tracheal cuff has passed through the larynx. As large a tube as possible provides a close fit in the trachea and helps to stabilize the tube. Gentle pressure on the reservoir bag will, if the tube is correctly placed and sealed, demonstrate chest movement on the good side only, and auscultation should confirm this. If there is spillover of air to the affected side, gases will escape up the open lumen or may appear as bubbling through the underwater drain. If more than 5 ml of air are required to obtain a seal in the bronchial cuff, it suggests that this portion of the tube might still be in the trachea and needs to be advanced. Throughout this period the patient is maintained in the sitting position breathing spontaneously (see Ch. 11).

There may be a considerable outpouring of pus from the open tracheal catheter lumen. A #10 suction catheter can be passed down the tracheal lumen to the area of the bronchial cuff and put on suction. Careful auscultation reaffirms proper tube placement and occlusion of the bronchial cuff. Vital signs are checked and an arterial blood sample is taken. If the baseline is satisfactory, general anesthesia is induced. Ventilation to the down lung is instituted with 100 percent oxygen until the results of the next blood gas measurement indicate the appropriateness of tidal volume and inspired oxygen fraction.

The likelihood of spillover is increased if the patient becomes restless during intubation under local anesthesia, and, therefore, some prefer general anesthesia from the outset, both from the points of view of patient safety and comfort.[182,183]

2. The second method involves a barbiturate induction followed by the use of oxygen and an inhalation anesthetic with the patient breathing spontaneously. When the jaw muscles are well relaxed, the patient is bronchoscoped and then the endobronchial tube is passed. Tension pneumothorax is avoided by maintaining spontaneous respiration until the tube position has been ascertained.

3. The third technique involves a ketamine or thiopental induction followed by a relaxant and a cricothyroid injection of lidocaine.[182] Following this, bronchoscopy, endobronchial intubation, and isolation of the affected side are accomplished. The time until safe inflation with oxygen can be performed may be considerable.

At the end of the procedure, the patient may again need to be bronchoscoped for adequate toilet, particularly where spillover has occurred preoperatively or is suspected intraoperatively. The patients are usually reintubated with an endotracheal tube and ventilated in the postoperative period.

Bronchiectasis and Lung Abscess

These represent similar hazards, the contamination of adjacent healthy lung. While the use of a double-lumen tube effectively contains secretions to one or the other side, it does not protect the healthy portion of the lung on the diseased side. In the past, bronchial blockers were used together with an endotracheal tube.

When dealing with an abscess in the lower lobe or a wet bronchiectasis, refractory to preoperative treatment by antibiotics and postural drainage, the patient is first bronchoscoped for tracheobronchial toilet and then the bronchus below the upper lobe orifice is tamponaded with ¼ inch gauze packing soaked in saline. The appropriate endobronchial tube is passed into the opposite bronchus and one-lung anesthesia begun with the opening of the chest. At the time of lobectomy, the packing is removed by the surgeon and the bronchus is closed. For upper lobe lesions, to avoid contamination of the lower lobe, the endobronchial tube can be introduced into the bronchus to seal the upper lobe orifice by inflation of the bronchial cuff.

Cysts of the Lung

Considerable attention has been paid to etiologic classifications of pulmonary air spaces. That of Belcher and Siddons is discussed below.[185]

The majority of pulmonary air cysts of surgical importance are bronchogenic cysts, post-infective cysts, infantile tension cysts, and anepithelial and emphysematous cysts. Lung cysts with trabeculae are regarded as anepithelial or emphysematous. They consider pedunculation a feature of anepithelial cysts, occurring often as a single lesion. By far the most common group is bullous emphysema, where the air cysts represent an exaggeration of the underlying disease process and the decision to recommend surgery is based on the relative contribution of the cyst to dyspnea, the major symptom. The type of bulla or cyst is less important than the degree to which it encroaches on adjacent lung tissue, whether or not there is a free bronchial communication, or if a valvular mechanism exists allowing for air trapping and overexpansion of the cyst. The patency of these communications may change from day to day.

The initial diagnosis is radiological. When the air cyst is a manifestation of generalized emphysema, the radiograph may demonstrate low diaphragms, wide intercostal spaces, extensive areas of radiolucency, and prominent hilar vessels with fewer peripheral vessels.[186] On a plain chest radiograph, the comparison of both inspiratory and expiratory films will demonstrate the compromise of functional lung tissue. On inspiration, the cyst becomes smaller as the surrounding parenchyma compresses it; and on expiration it assumes a greater size. This can subsequently be confirmed by ventilation/perfusion lung scans and by pulmonary angiography used to assess the functional ventilatory capacity of the compressed lung and predict its ability to expand once the cyst is removed. Re-expansion of this part of the lung depends upon the elastic recoil capacity and the condition of the vessels. Crowding of the vessels and a dense pulmonary capillary phase indicate viable parenchyma. Their absence is a sign of poor functional and expansile capacity and consequently of poor prognosis for surgical intervention.[187] Bronchospirometric studies, often difficult to do, have been largely superseded by lung scanning and tomography.[188]

In bilateral bullous diseases, the scanning techniques are of value in determining which lung is the more compromised and to estimate the extent of underlying diffuse emphysematous changes. The longer the history of bronchitis with a productive cough, the more likely it is that the changes are irreversible and the treatment symptomatic. Pulmonary function studies and blood gas estimations, while indicative of diffuse disease, are of more value in providing a baseline for subsequent objective assessment of any improvement following bullectomy. There is, however, poor correlation between subjective improvement and objective testing. In this instance the degree of clinical improvement is significantly greater than that shown by objective measurement.[189-192]

The degree of impairment of pulmonary function is related to the size of the cyst and the extent to which it communicates freely with the bronchial tree. This produces pulmonary insufficiency by ventilation of the dead space in the cyst, as well as by the compression and loss of functioning lung parenchyma. It is exacerbated by the development of a tension cyst with further encroachment on previously normal lung. The cyst, by occupying the entire hemithorax, shifting the mediastinum and interfering with venous return to the heart, may decrease cardiac output. The tension effects cause an increase in pulmonary vascular resistance with right heart strain and a cor pulmonale picture.[193]

Ventilatory evidence of diffuse obstructive emphysema may include reductions in MBC, MEFR and FEV_1/FVC, and increases in TLC and CV/FRC (see Ch. 4). Much of the air trapping and resistance to expiratory flow may be related to bronchial collapse secondary to the increase in intrathoracic pressure.[194] Following removal of the cyst, the resistance to expiratory flow can be expected to return to normal. The presence of hypoxemia or pulmonary hypertension at rest or after exercise makes a favorable outcome less likely though not an absolute contraindication to surgery.[186,195]

Other criteria for selecting patients most likely to benefit from bullectomy include: progressive dyspnea; inability to maintain a normal walking pace on level ground; bullae occupying at least 25 percent or more of one hemithorax; or bullae showing a progressive enlargement.[196] There should be radiologic evidence of compressed lung tissue that could be expected to re-expand after bullectomy. In addition to these disturbances of pulmonary function, the complications of air cysts which may require surgery are pneumothorax, infection, and hemorrhage. Surgery is also indicated where the bullae might present an occupational hazard, such as in flying personnel and submariners in whom sudden decompression could result in a massive increase in the size of the cyst.[197]

Significant improvement following surgery will depend largely on the contribution of the cyst to the disturbance of pulmonary function and the extent to which the underlying disease process is reversible.[198]

Surgery, where indicated, involves a thoracotomy for resection of the air cyst or cysts. A conservative approach is stressed by most authors with preservation of any functioning lung tissue.[199] Either local removal or plication of the walls of the air sac rather than segmental resection is recommended. Lobectomy may occasionally be indicated. Persistent postoperative air leaks have been significantly reduced by the use of a stapler. On occasion, a pleural tent is fashioned to diminish the size of the remaining pleural space. Pleurectomy, pleural poudrage, and scarification have also been recommended for obliteration of the remaining pleural space.

The anesthetic management of pulmonary air cysts must take into account whether the cysts are unilateral or bilateral, whether they are under tension, and the degree and duration of respiratory symptoms. It is usually not possible to predict which cyst will further inflate during ventilation. When the cysts are bilateral, it is useful in the preoperative evaluation to have the individual breathe oxygen with continuous positive airway pressure and observe for an increase in the size of the air cyst by fluoroscopy.

The patient may present in gross respiratory failure and be totally incapacitated with orthopnea. However, when the air cyst represents an occupational hazard only, or is a chance finding on routine x-ray examination in a patient presenting for extrathoracic surgery, the patient may be relatively symptom-free.

The main consideration in all of these situations is that IPPV may result in progressive inflation of the cyst, causing compression atelectasis, mediastinal shift, and encroachment on the sound side with both circulatory and respiratory embarrassment. In addition, a large communicating bulla could accommodate most of the tidal volume in a functional dead space. As a consequence of alveolar hypoventilation, hypoxia and hypercarbia may develop, causing severe pulmonary vasoconstriction and precipitating acute right heart failure.[193] This rapidly downhill course may terminate in a cardiac arrest unless the chest is expeditiously opened and the cyst herniates out of the cavity, thereby relieving the tension.[193, 194]

The need to avoid hyperinflation of the cyst or cysts is obvious. Where the cysts are unilateral, a single- or double-lumen endobronchial tube is placed as for a bronchopleural fistula with empyema. The situation is not strictly analogous, as there is no danger of contamination here. The choice lies between intubation under general anesthesia with a muscle relaxant technique or an awake intubation with topical analgesia and avoidance of positive pressure breathing until the hemithorax containing the cyst has been isolated. Spontaneous respiration via an endotracheal tube before the chest is opened can prove to be a hazardous procedure, as the condition of the patient, once anesthetized and in the lateral position, may deteriorate with compression of the down lung by the mediastinal shift. Where there has been respiratory embarrassment prior to induction of anesthesia, these patients may have been utilizing their accessory muscles of respiration to obtain adequate gas exchange. This mechanism will be abolished by the introduction of general anesthesia and result in hypoventilation, hypercarbia, and acidosis.

If there is no free bronchial communication, the use of nitrous oxide is contraindicated, since the volume of the cyst could rapidly increase. Nitrous oxide is able to move into the air-containing space more rapidly than the nitrogen can be eliminated, thereby expanding the cyst.[193, 200, 201] All the volatile anesthetic agents have been used in place of N_2O, although when venous return is significantly impaired by a raised intrathoracic pressure, hypotension may be refractory to fluid replacement. A neurolept technique would not be entirely acceptable, as there is the danger of awareness in the absence of N_2O. A ketamine induction is another good choice.

Once the thorax is opened, the effects of

ventilation on the involved lung may be observed. The entire tidal volume may be seen entering the compliant bullae. After bullectomy has been performed, the surgeon may ask the anesthesiologist to reinflate the lung in order to demonstrate the presence of additional bullae, an air leak, or to determine the extent to which the remaining lung is able to re-expand and fill the hemithorax. At the end of surgery, it should be possible to ventilate lobes and segments that have been atelectatic for years.

Before transferring the patient to the intensive care unit, the double-lumen tube can be replaced by an orotracheal tube. When the air leak via the underwater seal remains large, the negative suction is reduced and intermittent mandatory ventilation (IMV) is instituted. Next, spontaneous respiration is established and extubation is undertaken when possible. A considerable air leak may be expected, and the development of a tension pneumothorax must be guarded against by careful observation. The chest tube may have to be maintained for a week or longer until the air leak ceases.

Tension Cyst

When the cyst has expanded to occupy most of one hemithorax and is encroaching on the contralateral lung by herniation and mediastinal shift, the patient is severely incapacitated.[186,194] An attempt can be made to decompress the cyst immediately prior to intubation in order to return the mediastinum to a more central position and to facilitate the placement of the endobronchial tube. Cyst decompression is not always complete because of loculation within the cyst, and a bronchopleural fistula may develop, requiring a tube thoracostomy to prevent the development of a tension pneumothorax. Provided that the anesthesiologist is able to proceed immediately with isolation of the affected side, no harm will have been done. Where each hemithorax has a cyst occupying

more than ⅓ of that space, both sides will require surgical corrections; first the more severely affected side and then, at a later date, the other.

Bilateral air cysts represent a major problem because of the possible increase in size of the contralateral cysts following surgery to the up lung, and they may necessitate a bilateral thoracotomy.[194-202] Even with the aid of regional lung function studies and tomography, it is not always possible to decide which side is the more affected, nor to predict which cyst will inflate with IPPV. It has even been suggested that the left side be explored first since, in the event of a cardiac arrest, internal cardiac massage will be possible.[194]

An approach through a sternal split is now advocated more frequently for bilateral disease.[202] This may prevent the need for a tracheostomy in the postoperative period, a not uncommon occurrence when a bilateral thoracotomy is performed. In this method, the endobronchial tube is passed during spontaneous ventilation, then ventilation is assisted using 100 percent oxygen with a volatile agent. The sternotomy can be performed very rapidly and, once the thorax is decompressed, control of ventilation is instituted and a muscle relaxant administered. Each lung is then ventilated independently during the surgery.

In an extreme situation with no respiratory reserve and gross bilateral cystic disease, it may not be possible to maintain adequate oxygenation on one-lung ventilation. In such a situation, the use of an extracorporeal oxygenator primed with cystalloid may be needed. As these patients are usually polycythemic, this hemodilution is of no disadvantage. The perfusion is started after cannulation of the femoral artery and vein under local anesthesia, and results in improved blood gas tensions. The patient is stabilized on maximal flow and then is anesthetized, intubated, and one-lung anesthesia maintained with a greater margin of safety. Total body heparinization must be employed and reversed with protamine sulphate after de-cannulation.

Alternatively, this situation may be well-suited for surgery in a hyperbaric chamber. Oxygenation can be assured and the cyst, with its tamponading effect, will diminish in size. The thoracotomy may then be under-taken. The decision as to whether to proceed with the cyst on the other side has to be made at the end of the operation, unless the ap-proach has been through a median sternot-omy.

Unlike most cases of pulmonary resec-tion, these patients are left with a greater amount of functional lung than was avail-able to them preoperatively, and the me-chanics of respiration following removal of large space-occupying cysts are improved. Postoperatively, these patients are carefully watched for signs and symptoms of impend-ing respiratory failure, accumulation of se-cretions, and a tension pneumothorax. As a group they tend not to have a stormy postop-erative course and usually have a good prog-nosis.

Ectopic Hormone Production

Bronchial tumors may produce peptides which have a hormone-like action and there-fore have been termed "ectopic hormones." They represent one of the non-metastatic ef-fects of bronchial neoplasia. Symptoms re-sult from changes in distant organs and these non-metastatic symptoms account for some 14 percent of first consultations by patients with bronchial carcinoma. While the com-plete mechanism for many of these effects is still not clear, much has been discovered, and the topic has been reviewed by Nathanson and Hall.[203]

Clinical syndromes which have been re-ported due to ectopic hormone production include Cushing's syndrome, hyperpara-thyroidism, and, more rarely, hyperthy-roidism. Oat cell tumors may produce an ectopic ACTH syndrome, the adrenal hyper-plasia causing high levels of gluco- and min-eralocorticoids which in turn produce potas-sium depletion, hypertension, muscle weakness, thirst, and polyuria. Ectopic vaso-pressin (ADH) secretion results in retention of body water leading to decreased osmola-lity and possibly cerebral edema. Squamous cell tumors may secrete an ectopic hyperparathyroid hormone, resulting in hy-percalcemia, thirst, polyuria, dehydration, and weakness.

Myasthenic Syndromes

Myasthenic syndromes represent an-other non-metastatic effect of bronchial car-cinoma, and there is some recent evidence that the production of such syndromes may be humorally mediated.[204] The association of carcinoma of the bronchus with the symp-toms of myasthenia was first reported by An-derson et al.[205] They described a patient who presented at St. Thomas's Hospital in 1951 with carcinoma of the bronchus and severe muscle weakness. The weakness disappeared almost immediately following removal of the tumor. The same authors described a second patient with an oat cell tumor and progressive weakness who showed increased sensitivity to curare and succinylcholine. They noted that the responses of the patient resembled those seen in myasthenia gravis and speculated on the association between lung tumors and myasthenia (see Ch. 14).

The myasthenic syndrome associated with small cell carcinoma of the lung was described in 1956, by Lambert, Eaton, and Rooke.[206] Lambert et al described the char-acteristics of the defect of neuromuscular transmission in the "myasthenic syndrome sometimes associated with bronchogenic car-cinoma," and in subsequent studies the de-fect of neuromuscular transmission in this syndrome was shown to differ from that in myasthenia gravis.[207,208] It is a very rare disorder, and of those showing the clinical features, some 70 percent have malignant neoplasms and 50 percent have a small cell bronchogenic carcinoma. In 30 percent, no cause can be found although the syndrome may precede the discovery of the malignancy by 1 or 2 years. Associated conditions have included rectal, renal, gastric, and basal cell skin carcinomas, leukemia, reticulum cell sarcoma, and malignant thymoma.[209] It has also occurred with rheumatoid arthritis, hypothyroidism, pernicious anemia, thyrotoxicosis, Sjögrens disease, sarcoidosis, and pleural empyema.[209]

The syndrome is more common in men over 40 years of age (male:female, 4.7:1).[208] The main symptoms are weakness and easy fatigability of the proximal muscles of the limbs, especially of the thighs and pelvic girdle. Involvement of muscles supplied by cranial nerves is unusual. Unlike myasthenia gravis, where there is fatigue on exercise, there is a transient increase in strength on activity which precedes weakness. Muscle pains are common and stretch reflexes are depressed, contrary to the picture in myasthenia gravis. There is increased sensitivity to all muscle relaxants both depolarizing and non-depolarizing, whereas in myasthenia gravis there is resistance to depolarizing muscle relaxants.

In myasthenia gravis the defect of neuromuscular transmission is now known to be postsynaptic, but that in the myasthenic syndrome is presynaptic.[210] The defect in the myasthenic syndrome is like that produced by an excess of magnesium ions, botulinus toxin, or neomycin; all of which decrease the number of quanta of acetylcholine released by a nerve impulse from the motor terminal.[208]

The electrophysiologic characteristics of the myasthenic syndrome are (1) an abnormally low amplitude of muscle action potential to a single supramaximal stimulus, (2) a decremental response at low rates (2Hz) of nerve stimulation, (3) marked facilitation of the response at high rates of stimulation (50Hz) and after ten seconds of maximal contraction of the muscle, and (4) post-tetanic facilitation.

Treatment of the myasthenic syndrome differs from that of classical myasthenia gravis, since although both conditions improve with local cooling, myasthenic syndrome patients respond poorly to neostigmine.[211] The most successful therapy has been with so-called facilitatory agents which increase the release of acetylcholine from the motor nerve terminal. These agents include caffeine and calcium, guanidine and germine, and most recently 4-aminopyridine.[212-214] Treatment is not uniformly successful, however, and is usually limited by the side effects of these drugs. A more specific therapy for this syndrome may be found when the causative agent is fully isolated. Ishikawa et al described a patient with a small cell carcinoma of the bronchus and the myasthenic syndrome from whose tumor mass they were able to make an extract which produced neuromuscular transmission defects in vitro by reducing acetylcholine release from nerve endings. The chemical nature of the tumor extract was not identified, however.[204]

The possible presence of the myasthenic syndrome should always be considered when evaluating a patient with carcinoma of the bronchus for anesthesia, since the use of all muscle relaxants is contraindicated. If the condition is suspected clinically, the diagnosis can be confirmed by electromyographic studies. These patients should be managed like myasthenia gravis patients, using volatile agents to produce relaxation and avoiding all muscle relaxants.[215]

Pancoast's Syndrome

A Pancoast tumor is an apical carcinoma of the bronchus which invades the brachial plexus, producing pain in the arm by invasion and compression of the lower roots of the plexus. It is well known that muscles which are partially or totally denervated show an increased sensitivity to cholinergic nicotinic agonists. Such muscles respond to succinylcholine by developing a contracture instead of the paralysis observed in normally innervated striated muscle. Reports of the development of contracture in denervated muscle during anesthesia are scarce, but Brim described a patient with a right-sided Pancoast tumor who, in response to succinylcholine, developed fasciculation over most of the body except for the right arm, which became rigid as the rest of the body relaxed.[216] The rigidity gradually passed off within three to four minutes, at the same time that muscle power returned to the rest of the body.

It is recommended that if muscle relaxants are to be used to produce relaxation in a part of the body which has suffered peripheral nerve damage sufficient to cause nerve degeneration, depolarizing neuromuscular blockers should be avoided. Theoretically, non-depolarizing blockers should produce relaxation in these situations without inducing contractures.

REFERENCES

1. Bjork VO, Carlens E, Friberg O: Endobronchial anesthesia. Anesthesiology 14:60-72, 1953
2. Newman RW, Finer GE, Downs JE: Routine use of the Carlens double-lumen endobronchial catheter: an experimental and clinical study. J Thorac Cardiovasc Surg 42:327-336, 1961
3. Malina JR, Nordstrom SG, Sjostrand VH et al: Clinical evaluation of high-frequency positive-pressure ventilation (HFPPV) in patients scheduled for open-chest surgery. Anesth Analg 60:324-330, 1981
4. Coon RL, Kampine JP: Hypocapnic bronchoconstriction and inhalational anesthetics. Anesthesiology 43:635-641, 1975
5. Euler US von, Liljestrand G: Observations on the pulmonary arterial blood pressure in the cat. Acta Physiol Scand 12:301-320, 1946
6. Nilsson E, Slater EM, Greenberg J: The cost of the quiet lung: fluctuations in PaO_2 when the Carlens tube is used in thoracic surgery. Acta Anaesth Scand 9:49-55, 1965
7. Weinreich AI, Silvay G, Lumb PD: Continuous ketamine infusion for one-lung anesthesia. Can Anaesth Soc J 27:485-490, 1980
8. Bjertnaes LJ: Hypoxia-induced vasoconstriction in isolated perfused lungs exposed to injectable or inhalation anesthetics. Acta Anaesth Scand 21:133-147, 1977
9. Nunn JF, Freeman J: Problems of oxygenation and oxygen transport during haemorrhage. Anaesthesia 19:206-216, 1964
10. Winter PM, Hornbein TF, Smith G: Hyperbaric nitrous oxide anesthesia in man: determination of anesthetic potency (MAC) and cardiorespiratory effects. Abstracts ASA Meeting, October 1972, pp. 103-104
11. Chapman WP, Arrowood JG, Beecher HK: The anesthetic effects of low concentration of N_2O compared in man with morphine sulfate. J Clin Invest 22:871-875, 1943
12. Stoelting RK, Eger EI: Additional explanation for the second gas effect: a concentrating effect. Anesthesiology 30:273-277, 1969
13. Fink BR: Diffusion anoxia. Anesthesiology 16:511-519, 1955
14. Sheffer L, Steffenson JL, Birch AA: Nitrous oxide-induced diffusion hypoxia in patients breathing spontaneously. Anesthesiology 37:436-439, 1972
15. Grell FL, Koons RA, Denson US: Fentanyl in anesthesia. Anesth Analg (Cleve) 49:523-532, 1970
16. Sokoll MD, Hoyt JL, Gergis SD: Studies in muscle rigidity, nitrous oxide and narcotic analgesic agents. Anesth Analg (Cleve) 51:16-20, 1972
17. Freund FG, Martin WE, Wong KC et al: Abdominal muscle rigidity induced by morphine and nitrous oxide. Anesthesiology 38:358-362, 1973
18. Eckenhoff JE, Helrich M: The effect of narcotics, thiopental and nitrous oxide upon respiration and respiratory response to hypercapnia. Anesthesiology 19:240-253, 1958
19. Yacoub O, Doell D, Kryger MH et al: Depression of hypoxic ventilatory response by nitrous oxide. Anesthesiology 45:385-389, 1976

20. Munson ES: Transfer of N_2O into body air cavities. Br J Anaesth 46:202-209, 1974

21. Eger EI, Saidman LJ: Hazards of nitrous oxide anesthesia in bowel obstruction and pneumothorax. Anesthesiology 26:61-66, 1965

22. Hunter AR: Problems of anaesthesia in artificial pneumothorax. Proc Roy Soc Med 48:765-768, 1955

23. Webb SJS, Nunn JF: A comparison between the effect of nitrous oxide and nitrogen on arterial PO_2. Anesthesia 22:69-81, 1967

24. Eisele JH, Smith NT: Cardiovascular effects of 40 percent N_2O in man. Anesth Analg (Cleve) 51:956-961, 1972

25. Layzer RB, Fishman RA, Schafer JA: Neuropathy following abuse of nitrous oxide. Neurology 28:504-506, 1978

26. Amess JAL, Burman JF, Rees GM et al: Megaloblastic hemopoiesis in patients receiving nitrous oxide. Lancet 2:339-342, 1978

27. Eger EI, White AE, Brown CL et al: A test of the carcinogenicity of enflurance, isoflurane, halothane, methoxyflurane and nitrous oxide in mice. Anesth Analg (Cleve) 57:678-694, 1978

28. Koblin DD, Watson JE, Deady JE et al: Inactivation of methionine synthetase by nitrous oxide in mice. Anesthesiology 54:318-324, 1981

29. Sharp CW: It's no laughing matter. Editorial. Anesth Analg (Cleve) 58:73-75, 1979

30. Bahlman SH, Eger EI, Halsey MJ et al: The cardiovascular effects of halothane in man during spontaneous ventilation. Anesthesiology 36:494-502, 1972

31. Munson ES, Larson CP, Babad AA et al: The effects of halothane, fluroxene and cyclopropane on ventilation: a comparative study in man. Anesthesiology 27:716-728, 1966

32. Hickley RF, Fourcade HE, Eger EI et al: The effects of ether, halothane and Forane on apneic thresholds in man. Anesthesiology 35:32-37, 1971

33. Hirshman CA, Bergman NA: Halothane and enflurane protect against bronchospasm in an asthma dog model. Anesth Analg (Cleve) 57:629-633, 1978

34. Gelb AW, Knill RL: Subanaesthetic halothane: its effect on regulation of ventilation and relevance to the recovery room. Canad Anaesth Soc J 25:488-494, 1978

35. Freedman S, Campbell EJM: The ability of normal subjects to tolerate added inspiratory loads. Respir Physiol 10:213-235, 1970

36. Lehane JR, Jordan C, Jones JF: Influence of halothane and enflurane on respiratory airflow resistance and specific conductance in anaesthetized man. Br J Anaesth 52:773-780, 1980

37. Shnider SM, Papper EM: Anesthesia for the asthmatic patient. Anesthesiology 22:886-892, 1961

38. Brown D: Halothane-oxygen anesthesia for bronchoscopy. Anesthesia 14:135-137, 1959

39. Gold MI: Anesthesia for the asthmatic patient. Anesth Analg (Cleve) 49:881-888, 1970

40. Forbes AR: The influence of halothane on mucociliary clearance. ASA Abstracts of Papers 1975, pp. 253-254

41. Rodriquez R, Gold MI: Enflurane as a primary anesthetic agent for patients with COPD. Anesth Analg (Cleve) 55:806-809, 1976

42. Buckley MJ, McLaughlin JS, Fort L et al: Effects of anesthetic agents on pulmonary vascular resistance during hypoxia. Surg Forum 15:183-184, 1964

43. Sykes MK, Loh L, Seed RF et al: The effect of inhalational anaesthetics on hypoxic pulmonary vasoconstriction and pulmonary vascular resistance in the perfused lungs of the dog and cat. Brit J Anaesth 44:776-788, 1972

44. Mathers J, Benumof JL, Wahrenbrock EA: General anesthetics and regional hypoxic pulmonary vasoconstriction. Anesthesiology 46:111-114, 1977

45. Lumb PD, Silvay G, Weinreich AI et al: A comparison of the continuous ketamine infusion and halothane on oxygenation during one-lung anaesthesia in dogs. Canad Anaesth Soc J 26:394-401, 1979

46. Bjertnaes LJ: Hypoxia-induced pulmonary vasoconstriction in man: Inhibition due to diethyl ether and halothane anesthesia. Acta Anaesth Scand 22:570-588, 1978

47. Bjertnaes LJ, Mundel R: The pulmonary vasoconstrictory response to hypoxia during enflurane anesthesia. Acta Anaesth Scand 24:252-256, 1980

48. Lunding M, Fernandes A: Arterial oxygen tension and acid-base status during thoracic anaesthesia. Acta Anaesth Scand 11:43-55, 1967

49. Khanam T, Branthwaite MA: Arterial oxygenation during one-lung anaesthesia (1): a study in man. Anaesthesia 28:132-138, 1973

50. Khanam T, Branthwaite MA: Arterial oxygenation during one-lung anaesthesia (2). Anaesthesia 28:280-290, 1973

51. Tarhan S, Lundborg RO: Blood gas and pH studies during use of the Carlens catheter. Canad Anaesth Soc J 15:458-463, 1968

52. Torda TA, McCulloch CH, O'Brien HD et al: Pulmonary venous admixture during one-lung anaesthesia. Anaesthesia 29:272-279, 1974

53. Eger EI, Smith NT, Stoelting RK et al: Cardiovascular effects of halothane in man. Anesthesiology 32:396-409, 1970

54. Johnston RR, Eger EI, Wilson C: A comparative interaction of epinephrine with enflurane, isoflurane and halothane in man. Anesth Analg (Cleve) 55:709-712, 1976

55. Hug CC: Pharmacology of anesthetic drugs. In Kaplan JA, Ed: Cardiac Anesthesia, Grune & Stratton, New York, 1979, pp. 7-12

56. Strunin L: Hepatitis and halothane. Br J Anaesth 48:1035-1037, 1976

57. Cohen EN: Toxicity of inhalation anaesthetic agents. Br J Anaesth 50:665-675, 1978

58. Kerr JH, Crampton Smith A, Prys-Roberts C et al: Observations during endobronchial anaesthesia II: Oxygenation. Br J Anaesth 46:84-92, 1974

59. Virtue RW, Lund LO, Phelps M, Jr et al: Difluromethyl 1,1,2-trifluoro-2-chloroethyl ether as an anesthetic agent: results with dogs, and a preliminary note on observations with man. Canad Anaesth Soc J 13:233-241, 1966

60. Neigh JL, Garman JK, Harp JR: The electroencephalographic pattern during anesthesia with ethrane: effects of depth of anesthesia, $PaCO_2$ and nitrous oxide. Anesthesiology 35:482-487, 1971

61. Chase RE, Holaday DA, Fiserova-Bergerova V et al: The biotransformation of ethrane in man. Anesthesiology 35:262-267, 1977

62. Rehder K, Forbes J, Alter H et al: Halothane biotransformation in man: a quantitative study. Anesthesiology 28:711-715, 1967

63. Fogdall RP, Miller RD: Neuromuscular effects of enflurane, alone and combined with d-tubocurarine, pancuronium and succinylcholine in man. Anesthesiology 42:173-178, 1975

64. Calverley RK, Smith NT, Jones CW et al: Ventilatory and cardiovascular effects of enflurane anesthesia during spontaneous ventilation in man. Anesth Analg (Cleve) 57:610-618, 1978

65. Calverley RK, Smith NT, Jones CW et al: Man partially adapts to the ventilatory depressant effects of enflurane anesthesia. Abstracts of Scientific Papers, ASA Annual Meeting 1975, pp. 259-260

66. Knill RL, Manninen PH, Clement J: Ventilation and chemoreflexes during enflurane sedation and anesthesia in man. Canad Anaesth Soc J 26:353-360, 1979

67. Hirshman CA, McCullough RE, Cohen PJ et al: Depression of hypoxic ventilatory response by halothane, enflurane and isoflurane in dogs. Brit J Anaesth 49:957-962, 1977

68. Dobkin AB, Heinrich RG, Israel JS et al: Clinical and laboratory evaluation of a new inhalational agent: compound 347. Anesthesiology 29:275-287, 1968

69. Lowry CJ, Fielden BP: Bronchospasm associated with enflurane exposure: three case reports. Anaesth Intensive Care 4:254-258, 1976

70. Calverley RK, Smith NT, Prys-Roberts C et al: Cardiovascular effects of enflurane anesthesia during controlled ventilation in man. Anesth Analg (Cleve) 57:619-628, 1978

71. Smith NT, Calverley RK, Prys-Roberts C et al: Impact of nitrous oxide on the circulation during enflurane anesthesia in man. Anesthesiology 48:345-349, 1978

72. Holaday DA, Fiserova-Bergerova V, Latto IP et al: Resistance of isoflurane to biotransformation in man. Anesthesiology 43:325-332, 1975

73. Cromwell TH, Stevens WC, Eger EI et al: The cardiovascular effects of compound 469 (Forane) during spontaneous ventilation and CO_2 challenge in man. Anesthesiology 35:17-25, 1971

74. Eger EI, Dolan WM, Stevens WC et al: Surgical stimulation antagonizes the respiratory depression produced by forane. Anesthesiology 36:544-549, 1972

75. Rehder K, Mallow JE, Fibuch EE et al: The effects of isoflurane anesthesia and muscle pa-

ralysis on respiratory mechanics in normal man. Anesthesiology 41:477-485, 1974

76. Stevens WC, Cromwell TH, Halsey MJ et al: The cardiovascular effects of a new inhalational anesthetic, forane, in human volunteers at constant arterial carbon dioxide tension. Anesthesiology 35:8-16, 1971

77. Philbin DM, Lowenstein E: Lack of Beta-adrenergic activity of isoflurane in the dog: a comparison of the circulatory effects of halothane and isoflurane after propranolol administration. Br J Anaesth 48:1165-1170, 1976

78. Kopman EA, Ramirez-Inawat RC: Arterial hypoxaemia following premedication in patients with coronary artery disease. Canad Anaesth Soc J 27:132-134, 1980

79. Gravenstein JS, Anton AH: Premedication and drug interaction. Clin Anesth 3:199-219, 1969

80. Falic YS, Smilar BG: Is anticholinergic premedication necessary? Anesthesiology 43:472-473, 1975

81. Annis P, Landa J, Lichtiger M: Effects of atropine on velocity of tracheal mucus in anesthetized patients. Anesthesiology 44:74-77, 1976

82. Jones GC, Drummond GB: Effect of atropine premedication on respiratory complications. Br J Anaesth 53:441, 1981

83. Sturgess J, Reid L: An organ culture study of the effects of drugs on the secretory activity of the human bronchial submucosal gland. Clin Sci 43:533-543, 1972

84. Lopez-Vidriero MT, Costello J, Clark TJH et al: Effect of atropine on sputum production. Thorax 30:543-547, 1975

85. Ingram RHJ, Wellman JJ, McFadden ER et al: Relative contribution of large and small airways to flow limitation in normal subjects before and after atropine and isoproterenol. J Clin Invest 59:696-703, 1977

86. Nunn JF, Bergman NA: The effect of atropine on pulmonary gas exchange. Br J Anaesth 36:68-73, 1964

87. Severinghaus JW, Stupfel M: Respiratory dead space increase following atropine in man, and atropine, vagal or ganglionic blockade and hypothermia in dogs. J Appl Physiol 8:81-87, 1955

88. Smith TC, Stephen GW, Zeiger L et al: Effects of premedicant drugs on respiration and gas exchange in man. Anesthesiology 28:883-890, 1967

89. Steinberg SS, Bellville JW, Seed JC: The effect of atropine and morphine on respiration. J Pharm Exp Therap 121:71-77, 1957

90. Tomlin PJ, Conway C, Payne JP: Hypoxemia due to atropine. Lancet 1:14, 1964

91. Medrado V, Stephen CR: Effect of premedication with atropine sulfate on arterial blood gases and pH. Lancet 1:734, 1966

92. Finch JS, Zsigmond EK, DeKornfeld TJ: Arterial blood gases after atropine sulfate in healthy volunteers. Lancet 2:773, 1969

93. Butler J, Caro CG, Alcala R et al: Physiologic factors affecting airway resistance in normal subjects and in patients with COPD. J Clin Invest 39:584-591, 1960

94. Gold WM: The role of the parasympathetic nervous system in airways disease. Postgrad Med J 51 (Suppl 7):51, 1975

95. Eger EI: Atropine, scopolamine and related compounds. Anesthesiology 23:365-383, 1962

96. Andrews IC, Belonsky BL: Parasympatholytics. Clin Anesth 10/1:11-30, 1973

97. Gravenstein JS, Andersen TW, De Padua GB: Effects of atropine and scopolamine on the cardiovascular system in man. Anesthesiology 25:123-130, 1964

98. Daly WJ, Ross JC, Behnke RG: Effect of changes in the pulmonary vascular bed produced by atropine, pulmonary engorgement and positive pressure breathing. J Clin Invest 42:1085, 1963

99. Averill KH, Lamb LE: Less commonly recognized actions of atropine on cardiac rhythm. Am J Med Sci 237:304-318, 1959

100. Ramamurthy S, Ylagan LB, Winnie AP: Glycopyrrolate as a substitute for atropine. Anesth Analg (Cleve) 50:732-736, 1971

101. Wyant GM, Kao E: Glycopyrrolate methabromide. 1. Effect of salivary secretion. Canad Anaesth Soc J 21:230-241, 1974

102. Soroker D, Barzilay E, Konichezky S et al: Respiratory function following premedication with droperidol or diazepam. Anesth Analg 57:695-699, 1978

103. Utting JH, Pleuvry BJ: Benzoctamine—a study of the respiratory effects of oral doses in human volunteers and interactions with morphine in mice. Br J Anaesth 47:987-992, 1975

104. Stovner J, Endresen R: Intravenous anaesthesia with diazepam. Proceedings 2nd European Congress of Anesthesiology. Acta Anaesth Scand Suppl 24:223-227, 1966

105. Dalen JE, Evans GL, Banas JR et al: The hemodynamic and respiratory effects of diazepam. Anesthesiology 30:259-263, 1969

106. Buskop JJ, Price M, Molnar I: Untoward effect of diazepam. N Engl J Med 277:316, 1967

107. Steen SN, Weitzner SW, Amaha K et al: The effect of diazepam on the respiratory response to carbon dioxide. Canad Anaesth Soc J 13:374-377, 1966

108. Heinonen J, Muittari A: The effect of diazepam on airway resistance in asthmatics. Anaesthesia 27:37-40, 1972

109. Catchlove RFH, Kafer ER: The effects of diazepam on respiration in patients with obstructive pulmonary disease. Anesthesiology 34:14-18, 1971

110. Haslett WHK, Dundee JW: Studies of drugs given before anaesthesia XIV: Two benzodiazepine derivatives—chlordiazepoxide and diazepam. Br J Anaesth 40:250-258, 1968

111. Brandt AL, Oakes FD: Preanesthesia medication: double-blind study of a new drug, diazepam. Anesth Analg (Cleve) 44:125-129, 1965

112. Clarke PRF, Eccersley PS, Frisby JP et al: The amnesia effect of diazepam (Valium). Br J Anaesth 42:690-697, 1970

113. Straja AM, Munro DD, Gilbert RGB: Bronchoscopy with the aid of diazepam. Canad Anaesth Soc J 16:241-248, 1969

114. Cote P, Gueret P, Bourassa MG: Systemic and coronary hemodynamic effects of diazepam in patients with normal and diseased coronary arteries. Circulation 50:1210-1216, 1974

115. Kumar MS, Kothary PS, Zsigmond EK: Plasma free norepinephrine and epinephrine concentrations following diazepam-ketamine induction in patients undergoing cardiac surgery. Acta Anaesth Scand 22:593-600, 1978

116. Coppell DL, Bovill JG, Dundee JW: The taming of ketamine. Anaesthesia 28:293-296, 1973

117. Dundee JW, McGowen WAW, Lilburn JK et al: Comparison of the actions of diazepam and lorazepam. Br J Anaesth 51:439-445, 1979

118. Cormack RS, Milledge JS: Hanning CD: Respiratory effects and amnesia after premedication with morphine or lorazepam. Br J Anaesth 49:351-361, 1977

119. Denaut M, Yernault JC, De Coster A: Double-blind comparison of the respiratory effects of parenteral lorazepam and diazepam in patients with chronic obstructive lung disease. Curr Med Res Opin 2:611-615, 1975

120. Adeoshun IO, Healy TEJ, Patrick JM: Ventilatory pattern following diazepam and lorazepam. Anaesthesia 34:450-452, 1979

121. Galloon S, Gale GD, Lancee WJ: Comparison of lorazepam and diazepam as premedicants. Br J Anaesth 49:1265-1268, 1977

122. Dundee JW, Lilburn JK: Ketamine-lorazepam. Attenuation of psychic sequelae of ketamine by lorazepam. Anaesthesia 33:312-314, 1978

123. Reves JG, Corssen G, Holcomb C: Comparison of two benzodiazepines for anesthesia induction: midazolam and diazepam. Canad Anaesth Soc J 25:211-214, 1978

124. Miller R, Eisenkraft JB, Dimich I et al: Comparison of midazolam with thiopental for anesthesia induction. Anesth Review 7/12:21-27, 1980

125. Hider CF: In Shephard NW, Ed: The Application of Neuroleptanalgesia in Anesthetic and Other Practice. Pergamon Press, London, 1964

126. Whitwam JG, Russell WJ: The acute cardiovascular changes and adrenergic blockade by droperidol in man. Br J Anaesth 43:581-590, 1971

127. Graves CL, Downs NH, Browne AB: Cardiovascular effects of minimal analgesic quantities of innovar, fentanyl and droperidol in man. Anesth Analg (Cleve) 54:15-22, 1975

128. Bertolo L, Novakovic L, Penna M: Antiarrhythmic effects of droperidol. Anesthesiology 37:529-535, 1972

129. Herr GP, Conner JT, Katz RL et al: Diazepam and droperidol as I.V. premedicants. Br J Anaesth 51:537-542, 1979

130. Becsey L, Malamed S, Radnay P et al: Reduction of the psychotomimetic and circulatory side effects of ketamine by droperidol. Anesthesiology 37:536-542, 1972

131. Sadove MS, Hatano S, Zahed B et al: Clinical study of droperidol in the prevention of

the side effects of ketamine anesthesia. Anesth Analg (Cleve) 50:388-393, 1971

132. Ergbuth PH, Reiman B, Klein RL: The influence of chlorpromazine, diazepam and droperidol on emergence from ketamine. Anesth Analg (Cleve) 51:693-700, 1972

133. Prys-Roberts C, Kelman GR: The influence of drugs used in neurolept-analgesia on cardiovascular and respiratory function. Br J Anaesth 39:134-145, 1967

134. Adams AP, Pybus DA: Delayed respiratory depression after use of fentanyl during anesthesia. Br Med J 1:278-279, 1978

135. Becker LD, Paulson BA, Miller RD et al: Biphasic respiratory depression after fentanyl-droperidol or fentanyl alone used to supplement nitrous oxide anesthesia. Anesthesiology 44:291-296, 1976

136. Bjertnaes L, Hauge A, Kriz M: Hypoxia-induced pulmonary vasoconstriction. Effects of fentanyl following different routes of administration. Acta Anaesth Scand 24:53-57, 1980

137. Janis KM, Wright W: Failure to produce analgesia with ketamine in two patients with cortical disease. Anesthesiology 36:405-406, 1972

138. Coppel DL, Dundee JW: Ketamine anesthesia for cardiac catheterization. Anaesthesia 27:25-31, 1972

139. Kelly RW, Wilson RD, Traber DL et al: Effects of two new dissociative anesthetic agents, ketamine and CL 1848c, on the respiratory response to carbon dioxide. Anesth Analg (Cleve) 50:262-269, 1971

140. Savege TM, Blogg CE, Foley EI et al: The cardiorespiratory effects of althesin and ketamine. Anaesthesia 28:391-399, 1973

141. El Hawary MB, Mossad B, Abd El Wahed S et al: The effect of ketamine hydrochloride on the tracheobronchial tree. Mid East J Anaesthesiol 3:445-450, 1972

142. Corssen G, Gutierrez J, Reves JG et al: Ketamine in the anesthetic management of asthmatic patients. Anesth Analg (Cleve) 51:588-596, 1972

143. Betts EK, Parkin CE: Use of ketamine in an asthmatic child: a case report. Anesth Analg (Cleve) 50:420-421, 1971

144. Huber FC, Reves JG, Gutierrez J et al: Ketamine: its effect on airway resistance in man. South Med J 65:1176-1180, 1972

145. Baraka A, Harrison T, Kachachi T: Cate-cholamine levels after ketamine anesthesia in man. Anesth Analg 52:198-200, 1973

146. Waltemath CL, Bergman NA: Effects of ketamine and halothane on increased respiratory resistance provoked by ultrasonic aerosols. Anesthesiology 41:473-476, 1974

147. Traber DL, Wilson RD, Priano LL: The effect of alpha adrenergic blockade on the cardiopulmonary response to ketamine. Anesth Analg (Cleve) 50:737-742, 1971

148. Aviado DM: Regulation of bronchomotor tone during anesthesia. Anesthesiology 42:68-80, 1975

149. Tweed WA, Minuck M, Mymin D: Circulatory responses to ketamine anesthesia. Anesthesiology 37:613-619, 1972

150. Ivankovick AD, Miletich DJ, Reimann C et al: Cardiovascular effects of centrally administered ketamine in goats. Anesth Analg (Cleve) 53:924-931, 1974

151. Bovill JG, Dundee JW: Attempts to control the cardiostimulatory effect of ketamine in man. Anaesthesia 27:309-312, 1972

152. Nettles DC, Herrin TJ, Mullen JG: Ketamine induction in poor-risk patients. Anesth Analg (Cleve) 52:59-64, 1973

153. Waxman K, Shoemaker WC, Lippmann M: Cardiovascular effects of anesthetic induction with ketamine. Anesth Analg (Cleve) 59:355-358, 1980

154. Gooding JM, Dimick AR, Tavakoli M et al: A physiologic analysis of cardiopulmonary responses to ketamine anesthesia in noncardiac patients. Anesth Analg (Cleve) 56:813-816, 1977

155. Gassner S, Cohen M, Aygen E et al: The effect of ketamine on pulmonary artery pressure. Anaesthesia 29:141-146, 1974

156. Vaughn RW, Stephen CR: Abdominal and thoracic surgery in adults with ketamine, nitrous oxide, and d-tubocurarine. Anesth Analg (Cleve) 53:271-280, 1974

157. Wessels JV, Allen GW, Slogoff S: The effect of nitrous oxide on ketamine anesthesia. Anesthesiology 39:382-386, 1973

158. Lilburn JK, Dundee JW, Moore J: Ketamine infusions. Anaesthesia 33:315-321, 1978

159. Idvall J, Ahlgren I, Aronson KF et al: Ketamine infusions: pharmocokinetics and clinical effects. Br J Anaesth 51:1167-1172, 1979

160. Patrick RT, Faulconer AJ: Respiratory studies during anaesthesia with ether and with

pentothal sodium. Anesthesiology 13:252-274, 1952

161. Moyer CA, Beecher HK: Effects of barbiturate anesthesia (evipal and pentothal sodium) upon integration of respiratory control mechanism: a study directed towards improvement of methods for preclinical evaluation of anaesthetic agents. J Clin Invest 21:429-445, 1942

162. Lorenz W, Doenicke A, Meyer R et al: Histamine release in man by propanidid and thiopentone: pharmacological effects and clinical consequences. Br J Anaesth 44:355-369, 1972

163. Eustace BR: Suxamethonium induced bronchospasm. Anaesthesia 22:638-641, 1967

164. Jermus G, Whittingham S, Wilson P: Anaphylaxis to suxamethonium: a case report. Br J Anaesth 39:73-77, 1967

165. Johnston RR, Miller RD, Way WL: The interaction of ketamine with d-tubocurarine, pancuronium and succinylcholine in man. Anesth Analg (Cleve) 53:496-501, 1974

166. Nana A, Cardan E, Lietersdorfer T: Pancuronium bromide: its use in asthmatics and patients with liver disease. Anaesthesia 27:154-158, 1972

167. Coleman AJ, Downing JW, Leary WP et al: The immediate cardiovascular effects of pancuronium, alcuronium and tubocurarine in man. Anaesthesia 27:415-422, 1972

168. Beck-Nielsen J, Sorensen HR, Alstrup P: Atrial fibrillation following thoracotomy for noncardiac diseases, in particular cancer of the lung. Acta Med Scand 193:425-429, 1973

169. Hurt RL, Bates M: The value of quinidine in the prevention of cardiac arrhythmias after pulmonary resection. Thorax 13:39-41, 1958

170. Shields TW, Uniki GT: Digitalization for prevention of arrhythmias following pulmonary surgery. Surg Gynecol Obstet 126:743-746, 1968

171. Burman SO: The prophylactic use of digitalis before thoracotomy. Ann Thorac Surg 14:359-368, 1972

172. Silvay G, Miller R: Blood microfilters and the anesthesiologist. Anesth Rev 3/12:11-15, 1976

173. Hutchin P, Terzi RG, Hollandsworth LA et al: Pulmonary congestion following infusion of large fluid loads in thoracic surgical patients. Ann Thorac Surg 8:339-347, 1969

174. Terzi RG, Peters RM: The effect of large fluid loads on lung mechanics and work. Ann Thorac Surg 6:16-24, 1968

175. Sugg WL, Webb WR, Nakae S et al: Congestive atelectasis. Ann Surg 168:234-242, 1968

176. Young WG, Perryman RA: Complications of pneumonectomy, pp. 257-266. In Cordell AR, Ellison RG, Eds: Complications of intrathoracic surgery. Little, Brown, Boston, 1979

177. Belcher JR, Sturridge MF: Thoracic Surgical Management. 4th ed. Williams & Wilkins, Baltimore, 1969, pp. 91-95

178. Parkhouse J: Anaesthetic aspect of bronchial fistula. Br J Anaesth 29:217-227, 1957

179. Reeder GS, Gracey DR: Aspiration of intrathoracic abscess. JAMA 240:1156-1159, 1978

180. Dennison PH, Lester ER: An anesthetic technique for the repair of bronchopleural fistula. Br J Anaesth 33:655-659, 1961

181. Belcher JR, Grant I: Thoracic Surgical Management. 2nd ed. Bailliere, Tindall and Cox, London, 1955, p. 108

182. Ryder GH, Short DH, Zeitlin GL: The anaesthetic management of patients with bronchopleural fistula with the Robertshaw double-lumen tube. Br J Anaesth 37:861-865, 1965

183. Francis JG, Smith KG: An anaesthetic technique for the repair of bronchopleural fistula. Br J Anaesth 34:817-821, 1962

184. Belcher JR, Sturridge MF: Thoracic Surgical Management. 3rd ed. Bailliere, Tindall and Cox, London, 1963, p. 107

185. Belcher JR, Siddons AHM: Air-containing cysts of the lung. Thorax 9:38-42, 1954

186. Viola AR, Zuffardi EA: Physiologic and clinical aspects of pulmonary bullous disease. Am Rev Resp Dis 94:574-583, 1966

187. Chavez CM, Fain WR, Conn JH: Angiography in giant cystic disease of the lung. J Thorac Cardiovasc Surg 55:638-641, 1968

188. Garnett ES, Goddard BA, Machell ES et al: Quantitated scintillation scanning for the measurement of lung perfusion. Thorax 24:372-373, 1969

189. Billig DM, Boushy SF, Kohen R: Surgical treatment of bullous emphysema. Arch Surg 97:744-749, 1968

190. Benfield JR, Cree EM, Pellet JR et al: Cur-

rent approach to the surgical management of emphysema. Arch Surg 93:59-70, 1966

191. Tabakin BS, Adhikari PK, Miller DB: Objective longterm evaluation of the surgical treatment of diffuse obstructive emphysema. Am Rev Resp Dis 80:825-832, 1959

192. Fitzpatrick MJ, Kittle CF, Lin TK et al: Prolonged observations of patients with cor pulmonale and bullous emphysema after surgical resection. Am Rev Tuberc 77:387-399, 1958

193. Cote CJ: The anesthetic management of congenital lobar emphysema. Anesthesiology 49:296-298, 1978

194. Pierce JA, Growdon JH: Physical properties of the lungs in giant cysts. New Engl J Med 267:169-173, 1962

195. Guest JL, Yeh TJ, Ellison LT et al: Pulmonary parenchymal air space abnormalities. Ann Thorac Surg 1:102-114, 1965

196. Wesley JR, Macleod WM, Mullard KS: Evaluation and surgery of bullous emphysema. J Thorac Cardiovasc Surg 63:945-955, 1972

197. Dominy DE, Campbell DC: Surgical correctable acquired cystic disease of the lung as seen in flying personnel. Dis Chest 43:240-244, 1963

198. Dugan DJ, Samson PC: The surgical treatment of giant emphysematous blebs and pulmonary tension cysts. J Thorac Cardiovasc Surg 20:729, 1950

199. Knudsen RJ, Gaensler EA: Surgery for Emphysema. Ann Thorac Surg 1:332-362, 1965

200. Harley HRS: Otto TJ: An epithelial lung cyst. Thorax 19:343-346, 1964

201. Eger EI II: Nitrous oxide transfer to closed gas spaces. In Eger EI II, Ed: Anesthetic Uptake and Action, Ch 10. Williams & Wilkins, Baltimore, 1974

202. Goorwitch J, Weiner H: Bilateral giant subpleural blebs. Dis Chest 43:648-651, 1963

203. Nathanson L, Hall TC: Lung tumors: how they produce their syndromes. Ann NY Acad Sci 230:367-377, 1974

204. Ishikawa K, Engelhardt JK, Fujisawa T et al: A neuromuscular transmission block produced by cancer tissue extract derived from a patient with the myasthenic syndrome. Neurology 27:140-143, 1977

205. Anderson HJ, Churchill-Davidson HC, Richardson AT: Bronchial neoplasm with myasthenia: prolonged apnea after administration of succinylcholine. Lancet 2:1291-1292, 1953

206. Lambert EH, Eaton LM, Rooke ED: Defect of neuromuscular transmission associated with malignant neoplasms. (Abstr). Am J Physiol 187:612-613, 1956

207. Lambert EH, Rooke ED, Eaton LM et al: Myasthenic syndrome occasionally associated with bronchial neoplasm: Neurophysiologic studies, pp. 362-410. In Viets HR, Ed: Myasthenia gravis. The 2nd International Symposium Proceedings. Charles C. Thomas, Springfield, Ill., 1961

208. Elmqvist D, Lambert EH: Detailed analysis of neuromuscular transmission in a patient with the myasthenic syndrome sometimes associated with bronchogenic carcinoma. Mayo Clin Proc 43:689-713, 1968

209. Lauritzen M, Smith T, Fischer-Hansen B et al: Eaton-Lambert Syndrome and malignant thymoma. Neurology 30:634-638, 1980

210. Drachman DB: Myasthenia gravis. New Engl J Med 298:136-142, 1978

211. Ricker K, Hertel G, Stodieck S: The influence of local cooling on neuromuscular transmission in the myasthenic syndrome of Eaton and Lambert. J Neurol 217:95-102, 1977

212. Takamori M: Caffeine, calcium and Eaton-Lambert Syndrome. Arch Neurol 27:285-291, 1972

213. Cherington M: Guanidine and germine in Eaton-Lambert Syndrome. Neurology 26:944-946, 1976

214. Agoston S, Van Weerden T, Westra P et al: Effects of 4-Aminopyridine in Eaton-Lambert Syndrome. Br J Anaesth 50:383-385, 1978

215. Girnar DS, Weinreich AI: Anesthesia for transcervical thymectomy in myasthenia gravis. Anesth Analg (Cleve) 55:13-17, 1978

216. Brim VD: Denervation supersensitivity: The response to depolarizing muscle relaxants. Br J Anaesth 45:222-226, 1973

Roger S. Wilson, M.D.

11
Endobronchial Intubation

Endobronchial or "one-lung" anesthesia is utilized for a variety of thoracic surgical procedures when it is necessary to selectively eliminate ventilation to one portion of the lung. This chapter will consider the indications for this technique, available methods, intraoperative management, and potential complications. Although the importance of one-lung anesthesia for thoracic surgery has been recognized for several decades, the indications for use have changed and techniques have improved.[1-3] These changes have been necessitated by the nature of the lung pathology requiring surgery and the increasing complexity of the surgical procedures. Through the years there has been a notable evolution away from pulmonary pathology resulting from infection and requiring surgical drainage or resection, with an increase in numbers of operations performed for malignancy. There are three specific indications for utilizing one-lung anesthesia (see Ch. 8). One is the need for prevention of spillover of secretions or blood from one area of the lung to other noninvolved areas during the perioperative period. Although the advent of antibiotic therapy has dramatically modified the existence of the "wet" (bronchiectatic) lung and the incidence of lung in-

fections requiring surgery, patients will occasionally present with significant regional bronchiectasis. Thus, the need for isolation of an infected lung still exists today. Lung abscesses, requiring surgical excision or drainage, always pose a major problem with potential for massive intraoperative spillage and contamination of the contralateral lung. In addition, the patient with major hemoptysis requiring pulmonary resection is frequently a candidate for use of this technique.

A second indication concerns the need to maintain airway continuity in order to ensure the ability to provide positive pressure ventilation. This occurs in the presence of either an acute or chronic bronchopleural fistula or during operative techniques necessitating interruption of the airway to a lung segment, notably during a sleeve resection.

A third indication, and perhaps the most common indication for the use of this technique today, is the ability to provide better surgical exposure and operating conditions, the so-called quiet lung. In addition to these major indications used during surgery, several nonsurgical applications have been described. Endobronchial intubation has been used to provide selective positive pressure ventilation during acute respiratory failure.[4]

389

This technique is useful in ICU patients with a large chronic bronchopleural fistula or acute pulmonary disease, especially when associated with major differences in compliance between right and left lungs. In addition, the technique of bronchopulmonary lavage for alveolar proteinosis, bronchiectasis, asthma, and other pulmonary diseases requires the use of endobronchial intubation (see Ch. 8).[5]

A variety of methods have proved effective to isolate a portion of a lung or an entire lung. The choice of technique is dictated by several considerations, including the nature of the operative procedure, preexisting pulmonary pathology, urgency of the situation, anatomical considerations, and experience of the user. The methods and equipment, including advantages and disadvantages of each, are discussed below.

BRONCHIAL BLOCKERS

Intraluminal obstruction of the main bronchi or lobar divisions of the airway has been achieved with use of several devices, including gauze tampons or specially designed balloon-tip catheters, as described by several investigators.[6–9]

Although such devices are simple in design, several inherent problems have limited their use in favor of other methods. Crafoord's tampon, described in 1938, consisted of ribbon gauze which was packed into the main or lobar bronchus of the operative lung, visualized with rigid bronchoscopy.[6] Endotracheal intubation was performed with a standard endotracheal tube with resulting absorption atelectasis distal to the site of airway occlusion. The gauze was eventually removed as part of the surgical specimen. In 1936, Magill had described a similar technique using a balloon-tip bronchial blocker (Fig. 11-1).[7] The Magill blocker is a long, double-lumen rubber catheter, still manufactured today. One lumen is used to inflate a cuff on the distal end of the catheter; the sec-

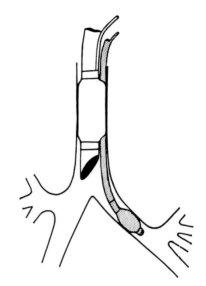

Fig. 11-1 Magill balloon-tipped bronchial blocker.

ond, to accommodate a stylet during placement and to allow suctioning and degassing of the lung distal to the catheter tip. A bronchoscope, passed with the aid of local or general anesthesia, is used to identify the bronchial segment to be blocked. The blocker is passed through the bronchoscope into position and the balloon inflated with sufficient volume to hold the catheter firmly in place. The stylet is then removed and a standard-cuffed endotracheal tube is placed with the cuff inflated to provide additional stability for the blocker. The position and function of the blocker can be confirmed by chest auscultation if a sufficient portion of the lung is nonventilated. Prior to surgical division of the bronchus, the cuff is deflated and the blocker removed from the airway.

Refinements of this technique included a larger lumen for suctioning and the addition of a woven net on the cuff to provide a firmer grip in the airway and prevent overdistention of the cuff.[8] Stephen further modified the Magill blocker with a short cuff for use in blocking the right and left upper lobe bronchi.[9] There are several reasons why these techniques are now seldom utilized in the practice of thoracic anesthesia. Positioning of the obstructing device in the desired portion of the airway requires use of the rigid bronchoscope. Thus, an additional procedure with its attendant risks and complications has to be performed. Once the blocker is placed and endotracheal intubation done, it is difficult to reconfirm the existence of the original position. Slippage of the blocker with a change in position of the patient, coughing, or surgical manipulation is not uncommon; and when the blocker inadvertently slips into the trachea, it can be associated with life-threatening obstruction. Inability to effectively suction the airway distal to the blocker is an additional disadvantage. These factors have virtually eliminated the use of this technique in favor of either single- or double-lumen endobronchial tubes.

A simplified version of this technique, using the flexible fiberoptic bronchoscope, has been recently described.[10, 11] Airway occlusion is produced by using a Fogarty catheter. This technique appears to be especially useful in selected patients when emergency pulmonary resection is necessary to control massive hemoptysis. Standard endotracheal anesthesia is associated with the potential for continued aspiration and possible asphyxiation until the bronchus of the bleeding portion of the lung can be surgically controlled. Double-lumen or single-lumen endobronchial techniques, although adequate in preventing spillage of blood to the contralateral lung, pose an additional threat of obstruction with blood in the airway owing to the narrow internal diameter of the lumens of the endobronchial tubes. Placement of a Fogarty catheter through the suction port of a fiberoptic bronchoscope has the advantage of being a safe, rapid, and effective means of controlling the bleeding by occlusion and isolation. This is done preoperatively when diagnostic bronchoscopy is performed to localize the site of bleeding. A standard endotracheal tube is placed in the airway once the bronchoscope is withdrawn over the catheter. Bronchoscopy through the endotracheal tube may be necessary to reconfirm the position of the Fogarty catheter. Once surgical control is achieved by dissecting free and cross-clamping the bronchus of the bleeding lobe or segment, the balloon catheter may be deflated and removed, which permits bilateral lung ventilation. This technique may also be of practical use for control of bleeding from a biopsy site requiring short-term tamponade and for control of hemoptysis in patients who are not candidates for pulmonary resection. In addition, Fogarty catheter occlusion may provide short-term control of a major air leak through a bronchopleural fistula. This can occur in the setting of acute pulmonary disease, where the need for mechanical ventilation may further increase air flow through the fistula and impair gas exchange.

SINGLE-LUMEN ENDOBRONCHIAL TUBES

Endobronchial anesthesia, pioneered with the design of an endobronchial tube by Gale and Waters in 1932, was intended to offer improved protection during thoracotomy by isolation of the diseased or operative lung from the contralateral lung. Numerous tubes have subsequently been designed and later improved upon in an attempt to make endobronchial anesthesia simpler and more efficient. In a recent survey conducted in the United Kingdom, only a very small percentage of anesthesiologists questioned still used single-lumen endobronchial techniques for one-lung anesthesia.[12]

In 1936, Magill introduced both a right and left endobronchial tube equipped with a single endobronchial (no tracheal) cuff.[7] This tube was later modified by Machray using a left-sided tube similar to the Magill but with a shorter bronchial cuff. Endobronchial tubes of this design required placement using an intubating bronchoscope of the Magill or modified Magill type. Intraoperative slippage from its original position, particularly with right-sided types, posed a significant

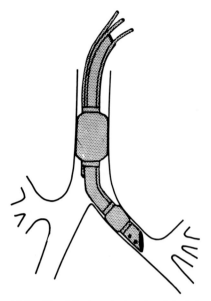

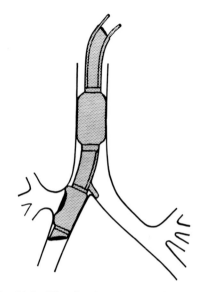

Fig. 11-2 The Macintosh-Leatherdale left-sided single-lumen endobronchial tube.

Fig. 11-3 The Gordon-Green right-sided single-lumen endobronchial tube.

risk when these tubes were used, and, hence, when combined with the need for rigid bronchoscopy for intubation, this technique has fallen into disuse.

Two existing single-lumen tubes of improved design are the Macintosh-Leatherdale (left-sided) and the Gordon-Green (right-sided), shown in Figures 11-2 and 11-3.[8, 13] The Macintosh-Leatherdale endobronchial tube, described in 1955, was designed to be used when operative procedures were performed on the right lung. Advantages of this tube are that it can be passed "blindly" (without need for bronchoscopy), its shape conforms to that of the trachea and left mainstem bronchus and therefore is not easily dislodged, and the double-cuff system allows bilateral lung ventilaton. The tube is equipped with both endobronchial and tracheal cuffs; a small pilot tube opens distally between the cuffs, near the level of the carina, and enables suctioning of the right lung or provides a means for delivery of low-flow oxygen to the right lung.

Tube insertion requires direct laryngoscopy. Tubes are available in sizes 7.5, 8.0,

9.0, and 9.5 mm internal diameter. Once the tip of the tube is passed through the cords, the laryngoscope is removed and the tube is advanced until the angle impinges on the carina, with the distal tip situated in the left mainstem bronchus just proximal to the left upper lobe bronchus. The endobronchial cuff is inflated and the position confirmed by the presence of breath sounds throughout the left chest and their absence on the right. The tracheal cuff is inflated to secure the tube in place. If ventilation to the right lung is desired, the endobronchial cuff is deflated and air entry into the right side (often limited) is confirmed by auscultation. Right lung ventilation, if not present or if limited, may be improved by slowly withdrawing the tube, which not infrequently impacts into the left bronchus, resulting in an airtight seal. The tube is withdrawn until right-sided air entry is satisfactory. Reinflation of the bronchial cuff should still permit left lung ventilation without air entry into the right side. Inadvertent intubation of the right bronchus is easily corrected by withdrawal of the tube into the trachea and attempted readvancement. A specially designed "reinforced rubber direc-

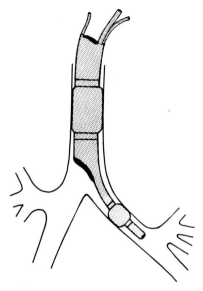

Fig. 11-4   The Macintosh-Leatherdale combined endobronchial tube and bronchial blocker used for left-sided thoracic surgery.

tor" or stylet is available to aid in the redirection from right to left bronchus. Once the surgical dissection is completed, the endobronchial cuff is deflated to allow right lung ventilation. Suctioning of the right side requires withdrawal of the tube until the distal tip is positioned in the trachea; the suction line incorporated in the side wall of the tube is generally inadequate owing to its limited diameter.

Macintosh and Leatherdale are also credited with the design of a combined endobronchial tube and bronchial blocker (Fig. 11-4) used for left thoracic surgery.[8] Available in four sizes—7.5, 8.0, 9.0, and 9.5 mm ID—this tube is introduced in the same manner as the single-lumen tube previously described. The angulated distal tip, which is a cuffed blocker with a central suction channel, enters the left bronchus. When in proper position, with bronchial and tracheal cuffs inflated, right lung ventilation is achieved through the air channel opening into the trachea just proximal to the carina. The blocker, which is hollow, can be used to supply oxygen to or to suction the left lung.

Right endobronchial intubation (for left thoracotomy) is technically more difficult than the left owing to the close proximity of the right upper lobe bronchus to the carina. It is, therefore, not possible to use a standard cuff on the bronchial limb without producing obstruction to the right upper lobe. Gordon and Green developed a right endobronchial tube with a 20 × 5 mm slot in the lateral wall for the right upper lobe.[13] As shown in Figure 11-3, this tube is designed with both bronchial and tracheal cuffs and, in addition, has a carinal hook to stabilize it, once in position. This tube, available in 8.0 and 9.0 mm ID sizes, is introduced by direct laryngoscopy. The tube is advanced until the hook impinges on the carina. The tracheal cuff is inflated to produce an airtight seal and to stabilize the tube. The bronchial cuff is next inflated until no breath sounds are present on the left. Inadvertent left endobronchial intubation is rarely encountered, owing to the angulation of the distal tip of the tube.

DOUBLE-LUMEN ENDOBRONCHIAL TUBES

The third and most popular technique involves use of double-lumen tubes, available in several designs. There are several advantages of this method when compared with those previously discussed. The ability to selectively ventilate and suction either lung and the stability of the tube once positioned are notable features. The large cross-sectional diameter of these tubes makes intubation and positioning often more difficult, a minor disadvantage of the technique. Four types of double-lumen tubes are available, designed for right or left lung surgery. These are the Carlens (left-sided intubation, right thoracotomy), White (right-sided), Bryce-Smith (right and left-sided), and Robertshaw (right and left-sided).[14-19] The general design of all such tubes is similar (Table 11-1). One lumen is long enough and appropriately angulated to reach into the mainstem bronchus

Table 11-1
Endobronchial Catheters

Tube	Date	Construction	Size	Problems
Carlens	1949	Red rubber	35, 37 39, 41	Left only; low complaint cuff
White	1960	Red rubber, molded bonded cuff, right side	37, 39, 41	Equivalent to Carlens; difficult to place
Robertshaw	1962	Red rubber, extruded bonded cuff; right cuff slotted.	small, medium, large	Low-complaint cuff; ED/ID ratio high (thick-walled)
Bronchocath (National Catheter, Corp.)	1978	Polyvinyl chloride	35, 37, 39, 41	No right-sided catheter; kink (rotate) easily; high-pressure cuff when overinflated

(usually the nonoperative dependent lung), and the second lumen is designed to terminate with its opening in the distal trachea. Separation of gas flow and isolation of foreign material from the nonoperative (dependent) lung is achieved with use of an inflatable cuff on the endobronchial limb. An airtight seal for the operative (nondependent) lung, ventilated through the tracheal lumen, is achieved with inflation of a tracheal cuff. This cuff is located in a position proximal to the endobronchial opening. Tubes designed for intubation of the right bronchus (for left thoracotomy) must incorporate a slitlike opening in the endobronchial cuff to permit ventilation of the right upper lobe. The proximal end of these tubes must be fitted with a special connector between the tube and the anesthesia system to allow diversion of gas from bilateral to unilateral ventilation, to enable each lumen and lung to be opened to atmospheric or continuous positive airway pressure, and to permit passage of suction catheters. A commonly used connector, a Cobb's suction union, is shown in Figure 11-5.

In general, it is advisable to attempt to intubate the bronchus of the nonoperative or dependent lung. Bronchial intubation of the operative lung, especially in the lateral position when the lung is in the nondependent position, can create situations in which tubes will fail to function correctly. Compression of the mediastinum or surgical manipulation can displace the bronchial limb and interrupt the isolation of the operative lung. Intermittent occlusion of the tracheal lumen against the most dependent lateral tracheal wall can create a ball-valve obstruction to gas flow. The latter situation is most common during expiration; resulting in wheezing, prolonged expiratory flow, and if severe enough, hypercarbia.

Double-lumen endobronchial tubes, although used for bronchospirometry since 1949, were not utilized for thoracic surgery until 1951. Carlens and Bjork are credited with both improvement of tube design and stimulation of interest in its application during thoracic surgery.[14,15]

The Carlens tube is manufactured of molded rubber with a latex covering (Fig. 11-6). The two lumina are D-shaped on cross section, with the endobronchial limb (left) extended as a round tube. The tip is at a 45° angle in relation to the shaft of the tube in order to enter the left bronchus. A hook is incorporated to position the tube by impinging it on the carina. Four sizes are available; 35, 37, 39, and 41 French. The smaller two

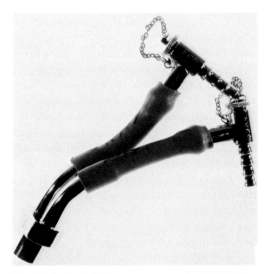

Fig. 11-5 A Cobb's connector used with double-lumen tubes. Note the suction port at the proximal end of each lumen.

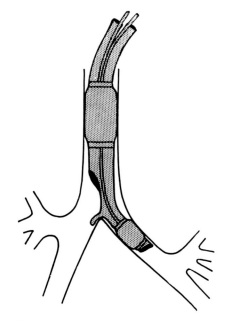

Fig. 11-6 Carlens double-lumen endobronchial tube.

sizes generally are adequate for females and adolescents, and the larger two are used for adult males.

The carinal hook, although beneficial for tube placement and stability, is a source of difficulty during intubation. In the past, techniques such as use of slip-knot silk ties to approximate the hook to the tube, or removal of the hook, have been advocated. Intubation is generally performed following induction of general anesthesia and use of muscle relaxants and topical anesthesia to the larynx and trachea. The endobronchial tip is advanced through the vocal cords following direct laryngoscopy. A Macintosh laryngoscope blade generally provides better working conditions than does a straight blade. The tube is rotated 180° to the left to allow the carinal hook to pass through the anterior commissure of the cords. Once the hook has entered the trachea, the tube is rotated 90° back to the right; the endobronchial tip is now positioned to the left and the carinal hook on the right lateral tracheal wall. The tube is slowly and gently advanced until resistance is felt as the hook engages the carina. An alternate technique is to rotate the tube 180° to the right to allow the hook to pass the cords and then to rotate it another 90° to the right (clockwise) to position the tube at the carina (Fig. 11-7). Cuff inflation techniques, although not described by Carlens, should follow a logical sequence (see Ch. 8). Inflation of the lungs with one or two positive pressure breaths is necessary to confirm (with visual inspection of chest motion) an endotracheal position. Gas flow to the tracheal lumen is occluded and the bronchial cuff inflated until left lung inflation (with manual compression of the bag) is achieved in the absence of right-sided ventilation; the latter is confirmed by visual inspection and chest auscultation. Release of the clamp on the tracheal lumen limb should permit bilateral lung ventilation. The endobronchial limb is occluded and, with positive pressure being applied, the tracheal cuff is inflated until an airtight seal is obtained. Bilateral lung ventilation is generally maintained until the pleura is opened and exposure within the thorax is required.

White has modified the Carlens tube for use in the right bronchus (Fig. 11-8).[16] This tube is also designed for blind endobronchial intubation. Made of rubber, it is molded to the shape conforming to the right mainstem bronchus with the tip at a 30° angle from the tracheal portion of the tube. As in the Carlens tube, the lumina are D-shaped at the tracheal portion, with the left lumen terminating just above the carina. A small rubber hook is designed to engage the carina. The bronchial cuff is designed with a lateral slit opening to the right upper lobe bronchus. Three sizes are available, 37, 39, and 41 French.

Intubation is accomplished by a technique similar to that described for the Carlens tube, differing only in tube manipula-

tion. The endobronchial portion of the tube is advanced through the cords; the tube is rotated 180° to position the carinal hook so it will pass through the anterior commissure. Once the hook is within the trachea, the tube is rotated 90° to the left (counterclockwise). The endobronchial tip should now point toward the right and the carinal hook toward the left. The tube is advanced until the hook engages the carina.

The cuff inflation sequence is similar to that previously decribed, with bronchial cuff inflation first. Auscultation confirms tube position but can not guarantee ideal position for right upper lobe ventilation.

In 1962, Robertshaw described a double-lumen endobronchial tube especially designed for thoracic surgery.[17] This tube is

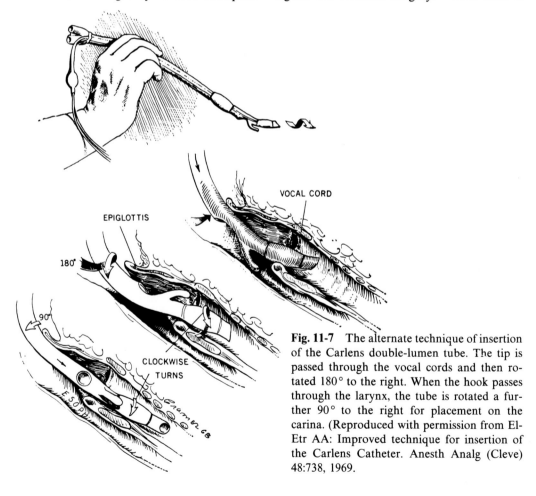

Fig. 11-7   The alternate technique of insertion of the Carlens double-lumen tube. The tip is passed through the vocal cords and then rotated 180° to the right. When the hook passes through the larynx, the tube is rotated a further 90° to the right for placement on the carina. (Reproduced with permission from El-Etr AA: Improved technique for insertion of the Carlens Catheter. Anesth Analg (Cleve) 48:738, 1969.

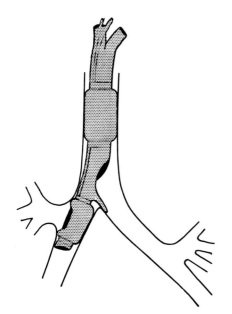

Fig. 11-8 White double-lumen endobronchial tube.

designed in both left- and right-sided versions (Fig. 11-9 A through D), and in three sizes suitable for adults and adolescents.[18] These tubes provide independent control of each lung through a double-lumen system with a larger internal cross-sectional diameter that is ovoid in shape. They are equipped with inflatable cuffs on the distal endobronchial portion and the tracheal portion. Inflating tubes for these cuffs are positioned in an anterior-posterior configuration to minimize the external cross-sectional diameter of the tubes. The advantage of this design over previous designs is that it offers a larger internal cross-sectional diameter and hence lower resistance to gas flow at equivalent external diameters.

The left-sided tube is designed to enter the left mainstem bronchus with the distal tip at an angle of 45 degrees. The right lumen terminates in the trachea just above the carina. When the left bronchial and tracheal cuffs are inflated, the right lumen communicates only with the right mainstem bronchus.

The right-sided version of this tube has a tip which is angled at 20° to enter the right mainstem bronchus. This tube follows principles described in the design incorporated by Gordon and Green. A slotted endobronchial cuff, designed to open wider with cuff inflation, allows for ventilation of the right upper lobe. The cuff is designed so that it inflates above the upper lobe slot to seal it from the trachea and the left mainstem bronchus. The tube is inserted into the larynx under direct vision by the laryngoscope techniques already described. The absence of a carinal hook makes manipulation during intubation less cumbersome than that experienced with tubes equipped with a hook. Once the double-lumen portion of the tube has passed the cords and reaches the larynx, it is advisable to withdraw the laryngoscope blade, support the jaw with the left hand, and with the right hand slowly advance the tube with the endobronchial portion directed toward the bronchus to be intubated. The appropriate position is confirmed by a firm but secure sense of impingement within the bronchus and location of the bite-block positioned between the incisors. In general, intubation with the left-sided tube, with bronchial tip angled at 45 degrees, is aided with the use of a stylet carefully placed within the left lumen. The right-sided tube, on the other hand, with an endobronchial portion directed at a 30-degree angle off-center, is easily passed without the use of a stylet. Once the tube is in appropriate position, the sequence for cuff inflation should be undertaken as described by Robertshaw (see Ch. 8).[17] One or two positive pressure breaths are required to confirm endotracheal position and adequate expansion of both lungs, generally observed with visual inspection. The tracheal lumen is clamped to eliminate fresh gas flow, and the bronchial cuff is slowly inflated (with a syringe containing a maximum of 5cc of air) until no discernible air leak is detected coming from the open port on the tracheal lumen. Visual inspection of the endobronchial side should confirm adequacy of ventilation, and proper ventilation may be reconfirmed with chest auscultation. Bilateral lung

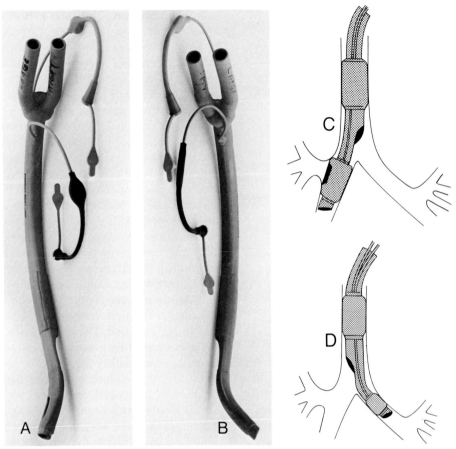

Fig. 11-9 Right and left-sided Robertshaw double-lumen endobronchial tubes are shown. A and C show a picture and a schematic of a right-sided tube and B and D a picture and schematic of a left-sided tube.

ventilation with the clamp removed ensures that overinflation of the bronchial cuff and herniation occluding the nonintubated bronchus have not occurred. Once bilateral lung ventilation is confirmed, the endobronchial limb is clamped and the tracheal cuff inflated until air no longer is detected leaking around the tracheal cuff, exiting through the oropharynx. Bilateral lung ventilation is again reconfirmed.

Selection of appropriate tube size is facilitated by the careful design and limited number of options available. This tube is manufactured in three sizes: small, medium and large, both large and medium sizes being used for adults and the small size reserved

generally for adolescents. As described by Zeitlin and colleagues, the majority of male patients will accept the large size, while most female patients will require the medium size.[18] Simpson has even shown that a large Robertshaw tube can be passed successfully via a tracheostomy stoma when needed.[19]

The advantages of the Robertshaw over other double-lumen tubes relate to the design characteristics of a large lumen, which facilitate the ease of passage of suction catheters and offer minimum resistance to gas flow. Occasionally, the tube may not be readily passed through the glottis owing to the bulk of the double-lumen portion even though the endobronchial portion is of appropriate size.

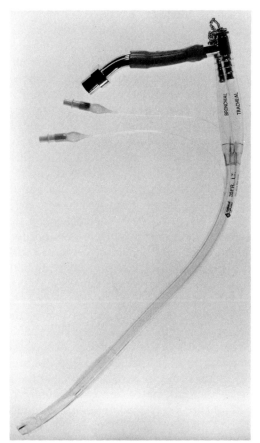

Fig. 11-10 The Bronchocath double-lumen disposable endobronchial tube with attached Cobb adapter.

Under such circumstances, it is advisable to select either a single-lumen endobronchial tube or to consider use of an ordinary endotracheal tube, depending on the surgery and the indications for lung isolation.

A disposable double-lumen tube (Broncho-cath, National Catheter Corporation) is designed for left mainstem bronchial intubation and has the features of a Robertshaw tube. The tube is manufactured of clear polyvinyl chloride with thin-walled tracheal and endobronchial cuffs (Fig. 11-10). Radiopaque markers are provided at the bottom of the tracheal cuff and at the distal tip below the bronchial cuff. Available in French sizes 35, 37, 39, and 41, these tubes are designed

for a single use. These tubes are also appropriate for use in an intensive care setting owing to the low pressure characteristics of the cuffs compared with the higher pressure ones found on the standard Robertshaw tube (see Ch. 8).

Double-lumen endobronchial tubes (right-sided) have also been designed by Bryce-Smith and Salt.[20,21] Their design features are similar to those of the right- and left-sided Robertshaw tubes, but in general these tubes are infrequently used.

Several features incorporated in the Robertshaw tube design favor its popularity and account for its being generally selected for one-lung anesthesia. Its advantages are as follows: (1) the wide lumina allow passage of large, adequate suction catheters; (2) the wide lumina provide low resistance to gas flow; (3) the absence of a carinal hook makes intubation easier and does not limit surgical resection of the bronchial stump; (4) the tubes are anatomically curved to reduce the possibility of kinking; (5) the right endobronchial tube is designed to minimize occlusion of the right upper lobe bronchus; (6) the tube is relatively inexpensive and yet offers reuse; and (7) selection of size is simplified by the limited types available.

COMPLICATIONS OF USE

Numerous complications have been reported with the use of endobronchial tubes.[22] Laryngeal and tracheal trauma and malposition of the distal tip are commonly-encountered problems. Direct laryngeal trauma, including soft tissue injury, arytenoid dislocation, and similar injuries are potentially more prone to develop, owing to the increased bulk of the double-lumen tubes, than when endotracheal tubes are used. Tracheobronchial rupture has been reported as a rare complication following intubation with Carlens and Robertshaw tubes.[23,24] The site of laceration is usually the membranous wall of the distal trachea or the mainstem bronchus. Factors leading to such complications include use of an inadequate size tube requiring overinflation of the bronchial cuff, malposition of the tip of the tube, or too-rapid inflation of the distal cuff. Insufficient ventilation, subcutaneous emphysema, airway hemorrhage, and cardiovascular instability should raise the index of suspicion for potential airway injury. Intraoperative diagnosis must generally be made by rigid or flexible bronchoscopy. Surgical repair of the tracheal laceration is essential at the time of injury.

Malpositioning of the tube in the airway with impaired gas exchange is a common problem with all types of endobronchial tubes.[22] Abnormalities of ventilation include the inability to isolate one lung so that both lungs are ventilated in spite of clamping; conditions in which neither lung is ventilated or "ball-valving" occurs, with or without air leakage around the bronchial cuff; and the inability to deflate the nonintubated lung. The most common cause for malposition appears to be the selection of a tube which is inappropriately small and thus does not advance far enough into the bronchus. Several factors often necessitate the selection of a small tube, including the inability to pass the desired size because of limitations in diameter of the upper airway, either at the laryngeal aperture or at the level of the cricoid. In addition, inability to advance the distal tip of the appropriate-size tube into the bronchus, owing to bronchial narrowing, extrinsic compression, or endobronchial pathology, may tempt intubation with a tube of smaller size. The result is that the endobronchial tip does not advance far enough into the bronchus. Thus, when the bronchial cuff inflates, it does so at or above the level of the carina, producing partial obstruction to the nonintubated bronchus. This creates a situation in which it is possible to ventilate both lungs through the endobronchial portion and impossible to ventilate with the tracheal lumen. A bronchial cuff, inflated at the carina with herniation extending to the nonintubated bronchus, often produces gas trapping and inability to deflate the nonintubated or operative lung. Abnormalities arising from such malpositioning may be detected if a carefully designed program for cuff inflation is carried out. As described above, once the tube is in position, bilateral ventilation is usually possible without inflating either cuff and is ascertained with positive pressure ventilation and direct vision or auscultation. Slow inflation of the endobronchial cuff with the tracheal limb clamped should confirm appropriate tube position in the desired bronchus. The ability to inflate both lungs when the tracheal limb is unclamped and positive pressure delivered should be confirmed with auscultation and visual inspection of both lung fields. If, during this maneuver, either poor or no breath sounds are heard over the nonintubated lung, then malposition of the cuff at or near the level of the carina should be suspected. Under such circumstances, the endobronchial cuff is deflated and the tube either advanced or withdrawn. Repositioning is then attempted and the sequence of cuff inflation is repeated. Inadvertent intubation of the opposite bronchus is detected during the second maneuver, when the endobronchial cuff is inflated. Under such circumstances, the tube is withdrawn and rotated slightly in the desired direction to obtain appropriate endobronchial intubation. Causes for intubating the opposite or wrong bronchus are generally associated with the continued use of the laryngoscope during the process of tube insertion or with an attempt by the intubator to twist or turn the tube overzealously as it is advanced down the airway. Occasionally, anatomical abnormalities within the trachea or mainstem bronchus may deviate the tube into the inappropriate lung.

A final complication relating to malpositioning may be the advancement of the tube too far down into the tracheobronchial tree. When right endobronchial tubes are used, this may produce abnormal positioning of the cuff at the takeoff of the right upper

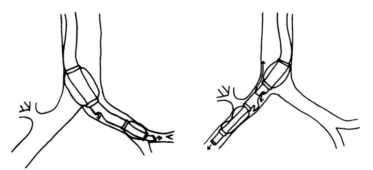

Fig. 11-11 Two examples of double-lumen endobronchial tubes passed too far down into the tracheobronchial tree. (Reproduced with permission from Stark DCC: One-lung anesthesia. Anesth Rev 7:14, 1980.

lobe bronchus, resulting in insufficient ventilation and atelectasis of the lobe. With left-sided tubes it is more difficult, owing to the length of the left mainstem bronchus, to produce left upper lobe collapse (Fig. 11-11).

The most common abnormality associated with the use of endobronchial intubation is undoubtedly hypoxemia. This subject is considered in detail in Chapter 8, which deals with the physiology of one-lung anesthesia.

REFERENCES

1. Bjork VO, Carlens E, Frieberg O: Endobronchial anesthesia. J Thorac Cardiovasc Surg 14:60-72, 1953
2. Newman RW, Finer GE, Downs JE: Routine use of the Carlens' double-lumen endobronchial catheter. J Thorac Cardiovasc Surg 42:327-333, 1961
3. Edwards EM, Hatch DJ: Experiences with double-lumen tubes. Anesthesia 20:461-467, 1965
4. Carlon GC, Ray C Jr, Klein R et al: Criteria for selective positive end-expiratory pressure and independent synchronized ventilation of each lung. Chest 74:501-507, 1978
5. Rogers RM, Tantum KR: Bronchopulmonary lavage, a "new" approach to old problems. Med Clin North Am 54:755-771, 1970
6. Crafoord C: On technique of pneumonectomy in man. Acta Chir Scand 81:1-142, 1938
7. Magill IW: Anesthetics in thoracic surgery with special reference to lobectomy. Proc Soc Med 29:643-653, 1936
8. Macintosh R, Leatherdale RAL: Bronchus tube and bronchus blocker. Br J Anaesth 27:556-557, 1955
9. Stephen EDS: Problems of "blocking" in upper lobectomies. Curr Res Anesth 31:175, 1952
10. Gottlieb LS, Hillberg R: Endobronchial tamponade therapy for intractable hemoptysis. Chest 67:482-483, 1975
11. Gourin A, Garzon AA: Control of hemorrhage in emergency pulmonary resection for massive hemoptysis. Chest 68:120-121, 1975
12. Pappin JC: The current practice of endobronchial intubation. Anesthesia 34:57-64, 1979
13. Green R, Gordon W: Right lung anesthesia. Anesthesia for left lung surgery using a new right endobronchial tube. Anesthesia 12:86-87, 1957
14. Carlens E: A new flexible double-lumen catheter for broncho-spirometry. J Thorac Cardiovasc Surg 18:742-746, 1949
15. Bjork VO, Carlens E: The prevention of spread during pulmonary resection by the use of a double-lumen catheter. J Thorac Cardiovasc Surg 20:151-157, 1951
16. White GMJ: A new double-lumen tube. Br J Anaesth 32:232-234, 1960
17. Robertshaw FL: Low resistance double-lumen endobronchial tubes. Br J Anaesth 34:576-579, 1962
18. Zeitlin GL, Short DH, Rider GH: An assess-

ment of the Robertshaw double-lumen tube. Br J Anaesth 37:858-860, 1965

19. Simpson PM: Tracheal intubation with a Robertshaw tube via a tracheostomy. Br J Anaesth 48:373-374, 1976

20. Bryce-Smith R: A double-lumen endobronchial tube. Br J Anaesth 31:274-275, 1959

21. Bryce-Smith R, Salt R: A right-sided double-lumen tube. Br J Anaesth 32:230-231, 1960

22. Black AMS, Harrison GA: Difficulties with positioning Robertshaw double-lumen tubes. Anesth Intensive Care 3:299-304, 1975

23. Guernelli N, Bragaglia RB, Briccoli A et al.: Tracheobronchial ruptures due to cuffed Carlens tubes. Ann Thorac Surg 28:66-68, 1979

24. Heiser M, Steinberg JJ, Macvaugh H et al: Bronchial rupture, a complication of use of the Robertshaw double-lumen tube. Anesthesia 51:88, 1979

DAVID D. ALFERY, M.D.
JONATHAN L. BENUMOF, M.D.
ROGER G. SPRAGG, M.D.

12
Anesthesia for Bronchopulmonary Lavage

This chapter discusses the management of patients undergoing massive bronchopulmonary lavage. In the first section the medical condition for which lung lavage is most commonly performed, pulmonary alveolar proteinosis, is described in detail, and several other conditions are discussed for which the procedure may be helpful (Table 12-1). The middle, main section of the chapter details the anesthetic management of lung lavage, including prelavage evaluation and medication, monitoring, choice of anesthesia, endotracheal tube placement, technical considerations of the lavage itself, recovery from lavage, and the immediate post-lavage period. The final section discusses several specific and especially difficult problems which may be encountered in patients severely afflicted with alveolar proteinosis undergoing lavage; in particular, the problems of hypoxemia in this patient group are addressed.

MEDICAL CONDITIONS IN WHICH BRONCHOPULMONARY LAVAGE IS BENEFICIAL

Pulmonary Alveolar Proteinosis

In 1958, Rosen et al described 27 patients who suffered from a disease of the lungs characterized by deposition within the air spaces of the lung of a granular material high in protein and lipid content.[1] The condition was called *pulmonary alveolar proteinosis* and their report described in detail the histologic, roentgenographic, and clinical features and the natural history of the condition. The etiology of the disease was and still is unknown.

The morphologic changes in this condition are confined to the lung. Grossly, the lungs are heavy and firm. Microscopically, the walls of the bronchioles and alveoli are either normal or, at most, slightly thickened

Table 12-1

Medical Conditions in Which Bronchopulmonary Lavage is Beneficial

A. Conditions of proven benefit
1. Pulmonary alveolar proteinosis
2. Radioactive dust inhalation
B. Conditions of possible benefit
1. Asthma and asthmatic bronchitis
2. Cystic fibrosis
3. Bronchiectasis

by an infiltration of lymphocytes. The alveoli are filled with a granular flocculent proteinaceous material (Fig. 12-1) that is rich in lipids and stains a deep pink by the periodic acid-Schiff (PAS) method. PAS-positive granules, probably consisting of mucopolysaccharide, may be seen in swollen type II alveolar cells. Electron microscopic studies show ultrastructurally abnormal alveolar macrophages, extracellular lamellar bodies, and myelin-like structures.[2]

Rosen et al postulated that the material

in the alveoli was derived from or excreted by the type II pneumocytes.[1] Analysis of the insoluble material obtained by pulmonary lavage of patients with alveolar proteinosis has shown that lipids constitute 55 percent of the dry weight.[3] McClenahan and colleagues analyzed proteins and lipids in material lavaged from normal subjects and from patients with alveolar proteinosis and found no quantitative differences.[4] They concluded that the alveolar material in alveolar proteinosis represented an accumulation of normal surfactant and serum rather than abnormal lipids or protein or disproportionate amounts of normal lipids. It was postulated that the accumulation of apparently normal surfactant was caused by the failure of clearance mechanisms. Work by Ramirez-R et al confirmed these findings by showing that lipid formation in the lung was not enhanced, while clearance of lipid was markedly prolonged.[5] The removal of alveolar phospholipids is impaired in this disease, and

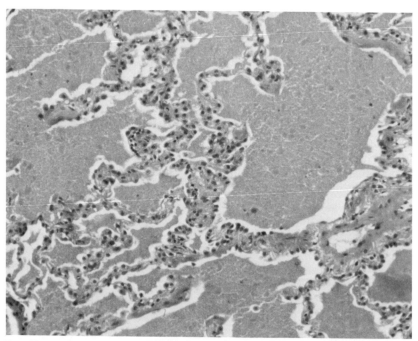

Fig. 12-1 Classical histopathologic picture of pulmonary alveolar proteinosis. The alveoli are filled with a granular proteinaceous material. The alveolar septae are only slightly widened and appear relatively normal.

other studies demonstrate a high IgG level in the lung washings of these patients.[6]

There appears to be an increased incidence of alveolar proteinosis in patients with hematologic malignancy or lymphoma.[7, 8] In addition, alveolar proteinosis has been associated with many infectious diseases, including nocardiosis, cryptococcosis, aspergillosis, histoplasmosis, and cytomegalovirus infection.[9, 10] These various infectious associations and direct in vitro demonstrations suggest that defects in cell-mediated immunity exist in these patients.[11]

Silicosis has also been linked to proteinosis.[12] McEuen et al have shown an increased content of silica-like birefringent particles in the lungs of patients with alveolar proteinosis, and chronic exposure to silica dust has been proposed as a method of producing an animal model of the disease.[13] Exposure to silica particles has the effect of diminishing macrophage function in vitro.[14] Thus, it might be suggested that altered macrophage function, caused in part by environmental factors, may be of pathogenic significance in the altered lipid clearance seen in alveolar proteinosis.

The roentgenographic pattern of alveolar proteinosis is bilateral and symmetrical; since the pathologic process is one of air space consolidation, the basic lesion is the acinar shadow. Confluence of acinar shadows is the rule, with the development of patchy, irregular, and poorly defined shadows throughout the lung (Fig. 12-2A). The hilar nodes are not enlarged. Differentiation from pulmonary edema of cardiac origin may be difficult, but the absence of other signs of pulmonary venous hypertension should help; the cardiac silhouette is not enlarged, and vessels to the upper lobes are not excessively distended. Kerly B lines may be present, presumably because of thickening of intralobular septa.[15] At times, interstitial edema may be a prominent feature. The roentgenographic picture usually parallels the course of this disease. In some cases the chest roentgenogram resolves completely

and respiratory symptoms subside, while in other patients some areas of the lung may clear while new infiltrates concurrently appear in other lung regions.

The clinical presentation and course of the illness are quite varied. Approximately one-third of cases are asymptomatic. The other two-thirds manifest a variety of symptoms. The most frequent and troublesome symptom is shortness of breath on exertion, usually progressive in severity. Cough is often persistent and is usually unproductive; less often it is associated with "chunky" gelatinous or even purulent expectoration.[1] A productive cough is more common in patients with alveolar proteinosis who are also cigarette smokers.[16] Hemoptysis may occur but is rare.[17] Fatigue, weight loss, and pleuritic pain may be present, and a low-grade fever may be found in one-half of patients.[1, 15, 17] Physical signs are usually not conspicuous, although both fine and coarse rales may be present.[1] In addition, clubbing of the digits may occur and resolve as the basic disease does.

Laboratory investigation reveals an increased incidence of polycythemia with a normal or slightly elevated white blood cell count.[1] Hyperglobulinemia is found in a minority of cases.[1, 17] Hyperlipidemia and an increase in the level of serum lactic acid dehydrogenase (LDH) have been observed in some cases.[18] The increase in LDH level may be due to an increase in both alveolar type II cells and macrophages.

Pulmonary function studies may be normal in asymptomatic patients. In most patients, however, there is a marked decrease in diffusing capacity, vital capacity, and lung compliance.[16, 19] Flow rates are usually normal but may be decreased in those patients with concurrent obstructive airway disease. Hypoxemia is due to the presence of both a low ventilation-perfusion ratio and atelectatic regions of the lung.[15, 18]

The diagnosis of alveolar proteinosis is usually made by correlating the above clinical, roentgenologic, and laboratory data with

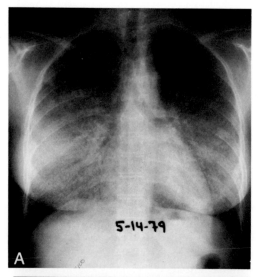

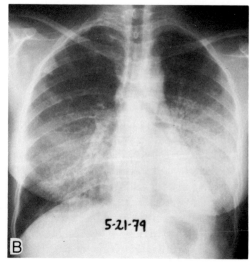

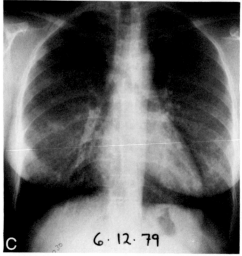

Fig. 12-2 The chest roentgenograms of a patient with biopsy-proven alveolar proteinosis. (A) Prior to lung lavage (film dated 5-14-79). (B) After right lung lavage (film dated 5-21-79). (C) After left lung lavage (film dated 6-12-79). This patient experienced dramatic improvement in subjective and objective pulmonary function following the lung lavages. A cryptococcoma is present in the right upper lobe.

the results of a lung biopsy. More recently, examination of fluid removed from the lung by either fiberoptic bronchoscopy or unilateral lung lavage has aided in making the diagnosis and occasionally has eliminated the necessity for lung biopsy.[3, 17] Once the diagnosis is made, it must be decided whether treatment is needed and, if so, what treatment to employ.

Several pharmacologic methods have been used, in general unsuccessfully, to treat alveolar proteinosis. The approaches include administration of corticosteroids, expectorants, and aerosolized acetylcysteine and trypsin.[20] It may be that the variable course

of the disease precludes any clear-cut demonstration of benefit from these pharmacologic interventions. Use of steroids may increase the risk of acquiring infection by opportunistic organisms. Aerosolized trypsin and acetylcysteine may result in cough, hoarseness, and bronchospasm.

At present, the most effective treatment for alveolar proteinosis is massive unilateral lung lavage.[15, 19, 21–25] Individuals who are asymptomatic or minimally symptomatic and do not have significant hypoxemia can be followed without treatment. Patients with an arterial oxygen tension less than 60 mmHg at rest or with hypoxemic limitation of exercise should be treated with bronchopulmonary lavage. Lavage should be performed on one lung and then repeated on the other lung after several days' rest. If the patient's condition is not significantly improved, this sequence should be repeated. If pulmonary lavage is not available, referral to a center where lung lavage is performed is indicated.

Following lung lavage there is usually significant subjective improvement within a few days. In patients who are lavaged by the method of Selecky et al, there is a clearing of the chest roentgenogram (Fig. 12-2B and C) as well as increases in vital capacity, diffusing capacity, and room air arterial blood oxygenation during rest and exercise.[26] The long-term post-lavage course, however, is not uniform. Some patients require lavage every few months, while others remain in remission for several years. Exacerbations of the disease are accompanied by increased dyspnea, reappearance of rales, and deterioration of the gas-exchange parameters noted above. Repeat lavages may reverse the clinical symptoms and physiologic abnormalities in many of the patients who have recurrences, and in many instances the disease eventually remits.

The clinical course and prognosis of alveolar proteinosis is extremely variable. Davidson et al reported on a collected series of 139 unlavaged patients, 40 of whom had complete recovery or significant improvement, while 45 died.[27] The cause of death in patients is most often respiratory failure or superimposed infection. It is very possible that improvements in lung lavage techniques will result in an improvement in the overall course of severely afflicted patients.

Radioactive Dust Inhalation

The second pathologic condition in which the performance of massive bronchopulmonary lavage is indicated is the treatment of radioactive dust inhalation. The dust may contain a wide variety of particulate radioactive materials. Lung lavage may greatly aid normal clearance mechanisms and increase the rapidity of removal of the radioactive material.

Obviously, lung lavage must be performed by persons not only experienced in the technique of pulmonary lavage but with the appropriate radiation safeguards. McClellan et al have reported the case of a worker who inhaled 450 millicuries of ^{239}Pu (plutonium-239), of which a substantial quantity was removed by sequential right and left bronchopulmonary lavage.[28]

Accumulation of Tracheobronchial Secretions

Massive lung lavage has been employed in the treatment of several other pathologic pulmonary conditions which have as a common denominator the excessive accumulation of tracheobronchial secretions. Patients with asthma, asthmatic bronchitis, cystic fibrosis, and bronchiectasis have all been subjected to bronchopulmonary lavage with varying degrees of success.[29-31] The imposition of significant airway disease in these patients makes the procedure significantly more difficult and hazardous. The small number of patients with these conditions who have undergone lung lavage makes the indications, optimal technique, and benefits of the procedure unclear.

ANESTHETIC MANAGEMENT OF BRONCHOPULMONARY LAVAGE

Massive bronchopulmonary lavage has become the accepted modality for the treatment of patients with pulmonary alveolar proteinosis. Following the pioneering work of Ramirez-R and Kylstra, the technique has been modified and improved.[25, 31, 32] It is now clear that this procedure may allow a relatively long-term symptom-free survival for many patients until such time as the disease may spontaneously remit. [16, 19, 25, 26] In this section, a technique for managing patients undergoing lung lavage is described which is a synthesis of previous anesthetic management methods with new innovations.[33–38]

Patient safety is enhanced if a relatively constant team, composed of members of the departments of anesthesia and pulmonary medicine, becomes familiar with the nuances and technique of unilateral lung lavage. Communication among the members of the team should begin when a patient with known or suspected alveolar proteinosis is admitted to the hospital, which allows ample time to evaluate the patient and schedule operating room time for the sequential lung lavage procedures. Much of the medical workup of these patients, which includes chest roentgenograms, arterial blood gas analysis during rest and exercise, and pulmonary function testing may have been accomplished on an outpatient basis. Diagnosis of the disease has usually been made previously by either analysis of lung washings obtained by fiberoptic bronchoscopy or by open-lung biopsy.

On admission to the hospital, ventilation-perfusion scans of the lung should be obtained. Ventilation can be maximized during lung lavage by performing the first lavage on the most severely affected lung, allowing the "better" lung to provide gas exchange. Thus, if the pre-lavage ventilation-perfusion scan of the lungs demonstrates one lung to be much more diseased, that is the lung which is lavaged first. If the scan indicates relatively equal involvement (as is the usual case), the left lung is lavaged first, leaving the larger right lung to support gas exchange.

In a minority of patients, most often cigarette smokers, significant reversible airway disease is superimposed on pulmonary alveolar proteinosis. In this subgroup, bronchodilators should be administered and, if aminophylline is used, serum levels of theophylline should be measured to confirm achievement of therapeutic levels.

Unilateral lung lavage must be performed in the operating room, where the appropriate amount and type of equipment and ancillary personnel are present and the location of the equipment, patient, and personnel enhance safety. These patients are usually cooperative and require only light premedication. Since many of these patients are hypoxemic at rest, they should be given oxygen by face mask following premedication and during transport to the operating room. Anticholinergic drugs are not routinely given to this group of patients.

On arrival in the operating room, the patient may be placed on a warming blanket resting on a soft spongy mattress on the operating room table. Since the procedure takes several hours to complete and lavage fluid temperature is not always precisely controlled, some patients will require external warming to maintain normal body temperature.

A peripheral intravenous cannula (18 or 16 g) is placed in the patient after arrival in the operating room. The minimal essential monitoring system consists of a blood pressure cuff, electrocardiograph, and precordial stethoscope (Table 12-2). Most anesthesiologists also use a peripheral arterial cannula (radial artery) and central venous pressure catheter (internal jugular vein) placed with use of local anesthesia prior to the induction of general anesthesia. Patients with compromised myocardial and cardiovascular function are monitored with a pul-

Table 12-2
Monitoring Patients for Pulmonary Lavage

A. Essential monitoring
  1. Esophageal stethoscope
  2. Blood pressure
  3. Electrocardiogram
  4. Temperature
  5. Peripheral nerve stimulator
  6. Arterial line and/or ear oximetry
  7. Central venous pressure (central access for emergency drugs)
  8. Airway pressure

B. Optional monitoring
  1. Pulmonary artery catheter
  2. Respiration monitor

monary artery catheter in place of the central venous catheter (See Special Problems).

After 5 to 10 minutes of preoxygenation, general anesthesia is induced with 3 to 4 mg/kg of thiopental in divided doses and inhalation of a volatile anesthetic drug in oxygen. High alveolar oxygen tensions are achievable during this time period and the alveolar/capillary oxygen gradient is thereby maximized. The volatile drug is the primary anesthetic, and halothane (0.5 to 2.5%) has been used in most cases, although enflurane (1.0 to 4%) or isoflurane (0.5 to 2.5%) could be substituted, especially in patients in whom therapeutic levels of theophylline (and the risk of dysrhythmias) are present. When a suitable level of anesthesia has been reached by administration of the chosen volatile agent, neuromuscular blockade is induced with intravenous pancuronium 0.1 mg/kg. After 3 to 5 minutes the trachea is topically anesthetized with lidocaine and intubated with the largest size left-lung double-lumen endotracheal tube that can be passed atraumatically through the glottis.

Recently, the National Catheter Corporation has introduced a left-lung Robertshaw double-lumen tube that has become the preferred tube for bronchopulmonary lavage. This tube is made of clear nontoxic plastic, has high volume–low pressure cuffs, and is disposable. This particular double-lumen tube is made only as a left-lung tube, which is a desirable circumstance since a left lung endobronchial cuff inflates symmetrically (and therefore theoretically provides a more secure seal), whereas a right lung endobronchial cuff inflates asymmetrically in order to avoid obstruction of the right upper lobe bronchial orifice. The largest size tube that can comfortably pass the glottis is used, since a relatively small double-lumen tube promotes problems related to an excessive volume of air required for a left endobronchial seal and difficulty with suctioning secretions. The use of a clear tube is helpful because it permits continuous observation of the tidal movements of respiratory moisture

as well as observation of the drainage fluid for air bubbles (see Ch. 8 and 11).

Once the double-lumen tube is thought to be in proper position, the tracheal and endobronchial cuffs are initially inflated until slight-to-moderate tension is palpated in the pilot balloon of the endotracheal tube cuff. Correct position of the double-lumen tube can be ascertained by passing a fiberoptic bronchoscope (Olympus BF2 or Machida pediatric BS 4T) down both the lumens of the endotracheal tube (Fig. 12-3). Via the left lumen separation of the lingula and left lower lobe by the bronchial carina is clearly visible. The volume of air in the left endobronchial cuff should be adjusted until the left endobronchial lumen just begins to invaginate owing to the external cuff pressure. Via the right lumen a clear, straight-ahead view of the tracheal carina as well as of the upper (cephalad) surface of the left endobronchial balloon just *below* the tracheal carina, is observed. It is important that the volume of air used to fill the left endobronchial cuff does not cause the cuff to herniate over the tracheal carina or cause the tracheal carina to deviate to the right. Both cuff herniation and deviation of the tracheal carina to the right will cause obstruction of the right mainstem bronchus orifice. Excessive left lumen constriction by the left endobronchial cuff will cause obstruction of the left airway.

The use of fiberoptic bronchoscopy alone does not provide evidence of functional separation (fluid-tight and airtight) of the two lungs. Complete separation of the two lungs by the left endobronchial cuff can be demonstrated by clamping the connecting tube to the right lung proximal to the right suction port and attaching a small tube to the open right suction port (by appropriate adapters) (Fig. 12-4). The free end of this tube is submerged in a beaker of water. When the left lung is statically inflated to 50 cm H_2O pressure and the left endobronchial cuff is *not* sealed, air will enter the left lung as well as escape from the right suction port and

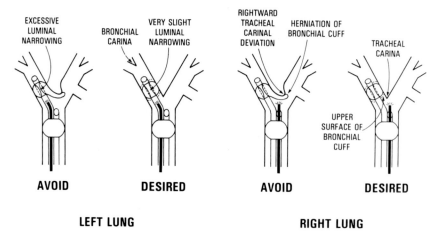

LEFT LUNG   **RIGHT LUNG**

Fig. 12-3 Use of fiberoptic bronchoscopy to determine double-lumen tube position and adequacy of cuff seal. When the bronchoscope is passed down the right lumen, a clear straight-ahead view of the tracheal carina is seen, and the upper surface of the bronchial cuff just below the tracheal carina should be apparent. Excessive pressure in the bronchial cuff as manifested by tracheal carinal deviation to the right and herniation of the bronchial cuff over the carina should be avoided. When the bronchoscope is passed down the left lumen, a very slight left luminal narrowing and a clear straight-ahead view of the bronchial carina is seen. Excessive left luminal narrowing should be avoided.

air bubbles will be observed passing through the beaker of water (right panel, Fig. 12-4). If the left endobronchial cuff is sealed, no bubbles should be observed passing through the water (left panel, Fig. 12-4). The right lung is then unclamped and ventilated, the left airway connecting tube is clamped, and the left suction port is opened to the beaker of water via the small tube. When the right lung is then statically inflated to 50 cm H_2O pressure, the absence or presence of air bubbles in the beaker of water will indicate the degree of functional separation. The prelavage absence of air flow from the nonventilated lung suction port is a very simple but sensitive indicator of functional separation of the two lungs. The use of fiberoptic bronchoscopy and this air leak detection method to correctly and precisely place the double-lumen tube and to obtain a tight but nonexcessive cuff seal are necessary because of the serious hazard of spillage during the lavage procedure.

Following positioning and checking of the endotracheal tube, additional monitoring devices are often applied (Table 12-2). Airway pressure can be electronically transduced and continuously recorded on a paper write-out; and a Wright spirometer can be placed in the expiratory limb of the anesthesia circle system in order to accurately measure tidal volume. A volume ventilator that can deliver relatively high inflation pressures is required since many of the patients to be ventilated have diseased and noncompliant lungs. Prelavage total dynamic compliance (chest wall and lung) of both lungs together and then of each lung separately should be measured. The ventilator is set to deliver a fixed measured tidal volume of 10 to 15 ml/kg and the recorded peak airway pressure is noted. A peripheral nerve stimulator should be used to ensure an adequate degree of neuromuscular blockade, since unexpected vigorous coughing during the procedure could alter double-lumen endotracheal tube position. In addition, some groups have recently used an ear oximeter to con-

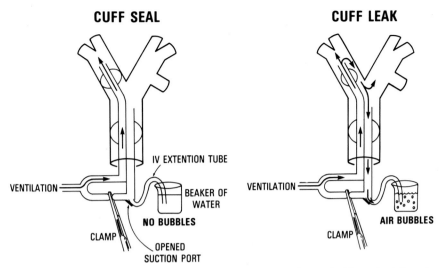

CUFF SEAL

CUFF LEAK

IV EXTENTION TUBE

VENTILATION

BEAKER OF WATER

NO BUBBLES

CLAMP

OPENED SUCTION PORT

VENTILATION

AIR BUBBLES

CLAMP

Fig. 12-4 Air bubble detection method for adequacy of cuff seal. When the left endobronchial cuff is sealed and the left lung is selectively ventilated, no air bubbles should emerege from the right open suction port (no air bubbles are observed passing through the beaker of water, left panel). When the left endobronchial cuff is not sealed (i.e., leaks) and the left lung is ventilated, air bubbles will escape from the right suction port and bubble through the beaker of water (right panel).

tinuously monitor arterial oxygen saturation. An esophageal stethoscope and temperature probe are placed and the eyes are protected with a lubricant and eye pads. Following measurement of compliance and placement of monitors and with the patient breathing 100 percent oxygen, baseline arterial blood gases should be measured.

The question of patient position during unilateral lung lavage is an important one, for there are major advantages and disadvantages related to each position. The lateral decubitus position with the lavaged lung dependent minimizes the possibility of accidental spillage of lavage fluid from the dependent lavaged lung to the nondependent ventilated lung. However, during periods of lavage fluid drainage, pulmonary blood flow, which is gravity dependent, would preferentially perfuse the nonventilated dependent lung and the right-to-left transpulmonary shunt would be maximal. The lateral decubitus position with the lavaged lung nondependent minimizes blood flow to the nonventilated lung, but, on the other hand,

increases the possibility of accidental spillage of lavage fluid from the lavaged lung to the dependent ventilated lung. As a compromise, many centers use the supine position in order to balance the risk of aspiration against the risk of hypoxemia.

The patients should be carefully preoxygenated prior to lavage for two reasons. First, as with the induction of any general anesthetic in any patient, an oxygen-filled functional residual capacity greatly minimizes the risk of hypoxemia during the apneic period required for laryngoscopy and endotracheal intubation. This procedure is especially important in those patients in whom the PaO_2 is already critically depressed. Second, and most specifically relevant to this procedure, preoxygenation denitrogenates the lung which is to be lavaged. Alveolar gas is then composed only of oxygen and carbon dioxide. During fluid filling, these gases will be absorbed, which allows the lavage fluid maximal access to the alveolar space. Failure to denitrogenate the lung prior to lavage fluid filling may leave periph-

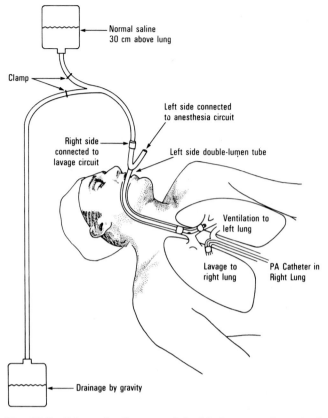

Fig. 12-5 Schematic diagram of double-lumen endotracheal tube and fluid filling and drainage set up in a patient undergoing unilateral right lung lavage for treatment of pulmonary alveolar proteinosis. A pulmonary artery catheter is located in the right main pulmonary artery.

eral nitrogen bubbles in the alveoli and thus limit the effectiveness of the lavage.

Warmed isotonic saline is used as the lavage fluid and is infused by gravity from a height of 30 cm above the midaxillary line. After the lavage fluid ceases to flow (i.e., lung filling is complete), drainage is accomplished by clamping the inflow line and unclamping the drainage line which runs to a collection bottle placed 20 cm below the midaxillary line (Fig. 12-5). The inflow and outflow fluid lines are connected to the appropriate endotracheal tube lumen by a Y adapter. The lavage fluid which is drained is typically light brown, and the sediment layers out at the bottom of the collection bottle after a short

period of time. Filling and drainage of approximately 500- to 1000-ml aliquots are repeated until the lavage effluent clears (Fig. 12-6). Volumes delivered and recovered for each tidal lavage are recorded. Total lavage fluid volumes of 10 to 20 liters are usually employed. Following the initial tidal lavage each subsequent tidal filling is accompanied by mechanical chest percussion and vibration to the lavaged hemithorax.

In one patient studied, during the tenth tidal lavage and following minimal outward traction on the double-lumen tube at the mouth level, the double-lumen tube apparently became slightly dislodged, resulting in disruption of the integrity of the bronchial

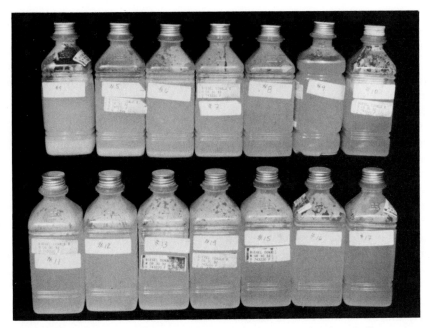

Fig. 12-6 Collection of draining lavage fluid into 1-L bottles. Sediment has layered out at the bottom of each collection bottle; bottle 4 contains the most and bottle 17 the least amount of sediment.

seal. The loss of complete lung separation *first* became apparent when small air bubbles were observed in the fluid draining the lavaged lung. In retrospect, these bubbles probably came from gas being used to ventilate the contralateral lung. During the tenth tidal filling rales were heard through the esophageal stethoscope and rhonchi were auscultated transthoracically. In addition, during this tidal lavage a small (200-ml) inequality developed between the filling and drainage volumes. Finally, arterial oxygen saturation decreased excessively during this tidal lavage, as indicated by the ear oximeter. In this patient the lavage procedure was terminated after the tenth lavage.

Based on this experience, it is probable that when a small leak around the left endobronchial cuff occurs, the following may be observed sequentially: (1) the appearance of bubbles in the lavage fluid draining from the lavaged lung; (2) rales and rhonchi in the ventilated lung; (3) a decrement between lavage volumes administered and those drained from the lavaged lung; and (4) a fall in arterial oxygen saturation. However, it should be noted that even if the anesthesiologist continuously listens with an esophageal stethoscope and the pulmonologist intermittently listens with a chest stethoscope for the appearance of new rales or rhonchi, it may be very difficult to discern *new* adventitious sounds in these very diseased lungs. Thus it is also necessary to continuously look for air bubbles in the lavage effluent as well as to record the inflow and outflow volumes of saline used for each lavage cycle.

Most patients studied have been hemodynamically stable throughout the entire lavage procedure. In particular, lavage itself has caused no significant changes in systemic and pulmonary artery pressures and cardiac output. In these patients, the arterial saturation as measured by ear oximetry has increased and decreased, with each lung filling and lung drainage, respectively. Arterial saturation increases during lung filling because blood flow to the nonventilated lung is decreased by the lavage fluid infusion pressure.[37] The opposite set of events (increased nonventilated-lung blood flow, decreased arterial oxygen saturation) occurs during drainage.[37]

After the effluent lavage fluid becomes clear the procedure is terminated. The lavaged lung is thoroughly suctioned and ventilation to it is reestablished. Since the compliance of the lavaged side will be much less than that of the ventilated side at this time, large tidal ventilations (15 to 20 ml/kg) to that side alone (with the nonlavaged side temporarily nonventilated) are necessary to reexpand alveoli. Arterial blood oxygenation may decrease precipitously during this time, but this can be minimized by clamping the opposite side after a large inspiration of 100 percent oxygen. Use of an ear oximeter is particularly helpful at this time to monitor changes in arterial oxygen saturation.

After lavage the procedure consists of repetitive periods of large tidal ventilations, suctioning and chest wall percussion to the previously lavaged side, conventional two-lung ventilation, and bilateral suctioning and postural drainage while intermittently measuring combined and individual lung dynamic compliance. As total compliance returns towards pre-lavage values, ventilation with an air-oxygen mixture may help lavaged lung alveoli with low ventilation/perfusion ratios to remain open. Just prior to periods of suctioning, it may be necessary to deepen the anesthetic in order to prevent bucking and coughing. Intravenous lidocaine (1 to 2 mg/kg) is also helpful in depressing airway reflexes during this period.

When the compliance of the hemithorax of the lavaged side returns to its pre-lavage value, the neuromuscular blockade is reversed with neostigmine and atropine. Prior to extubation, arterial blood gases and peak inspiratory force (PIF) are measured. If PIF > -20 cm H_2O and PaO_2 is significantly improved from pre-lavage values, the patient is extubated and placed on oxygen via a face mask. Should the unusual case occur in which PIF < -20 cm H_2O or PaO_2 is only minimally improved, the double-lumen endotracheal tube should be replaced with a single-lumen endotracheal tube. The patient is taken to the recovery room and placed on 5 to 10 cm H_2O positive end-expiratory pressure (PEEP) or on continuous positive airway pressure, with or without intermittent mandatory mechanical ventilation. The head of the bed is elevated for all patients in order to increase functional residual capacity. Mechanical ventilation and extubation guidelines at this point are the same as for any patient with acute respiratory failure.

In the immediate post-lavage period, deep breathing (incentive spirometry), coughing exercises, chest percussion, and postural drainage are used to remove remaining fluid and secretions and to reexpand the lavaged lung. Although most patients complain of a sore throat as a result of the endotracheal tube and chest soreness as a result of percussion during the procedure, pain medication is usually not required. After 3 to 5 days of recovery, the patient is returned to the operating room to have the opposite side lavaged. The anesthetic considerations for the second lavage are the same as for the first lavage, but it is reasonable to anticipate that oxygenation will not be nearly as severe a problem as during the first lavage.

SPECIAL PROBLEMS ENCOUNTERED WITH BRONCHOPULMONARY LAVAGE

Mechanical Problems During Lavage

The loss of complete separation of the two lungs and the development of a leak of fluid from the lavaged lung to the ventilated lung constitutes the major mechanical problem that may develop during unilateral lung lavage. The possibility of a leak occurring during lung lavage is minimized by using a large double-lumen endotracheal tube and taking care to ensure proper positioning, as discussed above. When a leak around the endobronchial cuff occurs, four abnormal events may be observed individually (and perhaps sequentially) or collectively. First, air bubbles from the ventilated lung may appear in the fluid draining the lavaged lung. Second, fluid from the lavaged lung may spill over to the ventilated lung and may be detected by new or different rales and ronchi in the ventilated lung. Third, the effluent volume may be noted to be less than the volume of lavage fluid infused. Finally, a fall in arterial oxygen saturation may occur.

If a small leak is suspected or detected by any of the above signs and the lavaged lung has been only minimally treated, the lavaged lung should be drained of all fluid and the position of the endotracheal tube and the adequacy of cuff seal and separation of the lungs rechecked. It is possible that the adequacy of the cuff seal and the integrity of the separation of the lungs may be reestablished by simply adding a little more air to the left endobronchial cuff and perhaps by gently pushing the endotracheal tube further caudad. However, if any question remains regarding the position of the endotracheal tube, there should be no hesitancy about passing the fiberoptic bronchoscope down both lumens to answer this question definitively. Before beginning the lavage procedure again, and no matter what solution to the possible leak problem has been used, the functional separation of the two lungs should be tested and found adequate by using the previously described air bubble leak detection method.

Massive spillage of fluid from the lavaged lung to the ventilated lung is not a subtle event and results in a dramatic decrease in ventilated lung compliance and a rapid and large decrease in arterial oxygen saturation. Under these circumstances the lavage procedure must be terminated no matter how much treatment has been accomplished. The patient should be moved quickly to the lateral decubitus position with the lavaged side dependent, and the operating room table placed in a head-down position in order to facilitate removal of lavage fluid. Vigorous suctioning and inflation of both lungs should be carried out. The double-lumen tube should be changed to a standard single-lumen tube and the patient additionally treated with a period of mechanical ventilatory support with PEEP. Timing of further unilateral lung lavage attempts will be dictated by the patient's subsequent clinical course and gas exchange status.

Associated Bronchopleural Fistula

A bronchopleural fistula may be present prior to lavage as a result of a previous diagnostic open-lung biopsy or due to other concurrent pathology, such as pneumonia.[19,39] Under these conditions and if there is any real question about an external air or fluid leak (to the pleural space), the side with the bronchopleural fistula should be lavaged first. It will be necessary, of course, to have a chest tube inserted into the pleural space on that side prior to lavage. The chest tube can be removed a few days after the procedure. At least four cases have been successfully managed in this way.[19,39]

Lung Lavage in Children

Lavage in the conventional manner is not possible in children (or very small adults) in whom double-lumen endotracheal tubes are too large to be inserted. This problem occurs in persons weighing less than 40 to 50 kg since the smallest double-lumen endotracheal tube made is 35 French, with each lumen being slightly less than 6 mm. In this situation, partial cardiopulmonary bypass has been successfully used to provide oxygenation during lavage. Lippman et al reported the use of this technique in two brothers aged 4 and 2½ years.[40] Both these patients underwent whole-lung lavage, during which time blood was removed from both femoral veins, oxygenated, and then returned to the left femoral artery. Both patients were eventually discharged from the hospital although they continued to require supplemental oxygen by face mask.

Alternatives to Conventional Unilateral Lung Lavage in Critically Ill Patients

Two approaches have been used for patients who are considered too ill to tolerate the physiologic trespass of unilateral lung lavage. First, extracorporeal membrane oxygenation (ECMO) has been utilized to provide support of gas exchange during standard unilateral lung lavage.[41, 42] Because of the technical problems associated with ECMO and its general lack of availability, a second approach to the patient judged too ill to undergo conventional lung lavage has been the use of lobar lavage via a fiberoptic bronchoscope under topical anesthesia.[43, 44] With this technique, a cuffed fiberoptic bronchoscope is inserted into a lobar bronchus and saline irrigation carried out. The patient remains awake and breathes high-flow oxygen delivered via a face mask. One or two lobes may be done at a time, and lobar lavages may be repeated as many times as necessary. Ventilation-perfusion scans of the lung can be used to dictate which lobes are most severely affected and should thus be lavaged first. This technique has been used successfully, and it is felt that the relative ease with which it can be done makes it a preferable alternative to the use of an ECMO support system.[43]

Adjuvants During Unilateral Lung Lavage to Increase PaO$_2$

During periods of lung filling, lavage fluid infusion pressure (the alveolar pressure of the lavaged lung) usually equals or exceeds pulmonary artery pressure, and blood flow to the nonventilated lung is diverted, in part, to the ventilated lung.[37, 45, 46] Conversely, during periods of lung drainage, pulmonary artery pressure exceeds the lavaged lung alveolar pressure (which may be atmospheric or slightly subatmospheric) and blood flow to the nonventilated lung is reestablished. Thus the degree of hypoxemia is greatest during the period of lung drainage.[34, 35, 37, 38, 45] Careful monitoring of oxygenation with ear oximetry is especially important at this time.[36] In addition, those patients with the most severe disease can be expected to have the most severe levels of hypoxemia, particularly during lavage of the *first* lung. In order to minimize hypoxemia in the first lavage procedure during periods of lung drainage, the "best" lung is ventilated first and the "worst" lung is washed first (see anesthetic management above). In addition, altering pulmonary blood flow with a pulmonary artery catheter balloon has been studied.[37, 38]

It was found that inflation of a pulmonary artery balloon in the nonventilated (lavaged) lung has caused an increase in PaO$_2$ and arterial oxygen saturation during periods of lung drainage.[37, 38] In several patients undergoing right-lung lavage, pulmonary artery catheters were inserted via the internal jugular vein under local anesthesia while the patient was awake. The position of the pulmonary artery catheter tip was ascertained by a single PA chest roentgenogram, and, as expected, all catheter tips were located in the right lung.[47] The same chest roentgenogram was used to determine how far, if necessary, to pull the catheter tip back in order to locate the tip in the right main pulmonary artery. During at least two periods of lung drainage during right lung lavage in these patients, arterial blood gases were drawn before and after inflation of the pulmonary artery catheter balloon. The pulmonary artery catheter balloon was left inflated for 5 minutes prior to measurement of PaO$_2$. Although the pulmonary artery catheter appeared to wedge with balloon inflation in these patients, it is now recommended that the balloon be carefully inflated only until the phasic pulmonary artery trace just begins to dampen (decreased pulse pressure) or until 0.7 to 1.0 cc of air has been injected. It is not advisable to wedge the catheter in view of the dangers of pulmonary hemorrhage and infarction.[48-50]

In the patients studied, inflation of the pulmonary artery catheter balloon caused no significant change in systemic arterial pressure.[38] In canine experiments utilizing similar procedures and conditions (however, with two pulmonary artery catheters), pulmonary artery catheter balloon inflation also caused no significant change in mean pulmonary artery pressure.[37] In each patient, inflation of the pulmonary artery catheter balloon during periods of lung drainage caused a significant increase in arterial oxygen saturation (Table 12-3), but during periods of lung filling caused no significant change in PaO_2 or arterial oxygen saturation. By using a two-compartment lung model (one ventilated and one nonventilated lung) and normal cardiac output, hemoglobin, and oxygen consumption, the PaO_2 change caused by pulmonary artery catheter balloon inflation was found to be compatible with a deflection of approximately 15 percent of the cardiac output away from the nonventilated to the ventilated lung. Indeed, nonocclusive inflation of the pulmonary artery catheter balloon in the lavaged canine lung has previously been shown to cause very similar changes in the electromagnetically-measured blood flow to the nonventilated lung.[37] The failure of PaO_2 to increase when the pulmonary artery catheter balloon was inflated during periods of lung filling probably indicates that blood flow to the nonventilated lung was already reduced by lavage-fluid infusion pressure.

In summary, this chapter has described the indications for, the anesthetic management of, and some particularly difficult and troublesome aspects of unilateral lung lavage. In this presentation, not only conventional aspects of lung lavage, but also a number of new methodological and procedural observations that may make the performance of unilateral lung lavage safer, have been discussed. These new methods span the entire perioperative period and include diagnostic as well as therapeutic areas. It is possible that the inclusion of some of these methods may make it possible to lavage some patients by the unilateral lung lavage method rather than by extracorporeal circulatory support.

Table 12-3[38]

Pulmonary Artery Balloon Inflation And PaO_2

Patients	Before PAB ↑*		After PAB ↑*	
	PaO_2 torr	% Sat	PaO_2 torr	% Sat
1	67	93.6	80	96.0
	81	96.5	103	97.5
2	174	98.5	305	99.5
	143	98.0	224	99.3
3	51	87.0	68	93.5
	49	86.0	69	94.0
4	62	92.0	65	93.0
	56	89.0	67	93.5
MEAN	85 ± 17	92.6 ± 1.7	123 ± 32	95.8 ± 1.0

* PAB ↑ = Pulmonary artery balloon inflation during lung drainage

REFERENCES

1. Rosen SH, Castleman B, Liebow AA: Pulmonary alveolar proteinosis. N Engl J Med 258:1123-1142, 1958
2. Hook GER, Bell DY, Gilmore LB et al: Composition of bronchoalveolar lavage effluents from patients with alveolar proteinosis. Lab Invest 39:342-357, 1978
3. Sahn S, DiAugustine RP, Lynn WS: Lipids found in the pulmonary lavage of patients with alveolar proteinosis and in rabbit lung lamellar organelles. Am Rev Respir Dis 114:117-185, 1976
4. McClenahan JB, Mussenden R: Pulmonary alveolar proteinosis. Arch Intern Med 133:284-287, 1974
5. Ramirez-R J, Harlan WJ, Jr: Pulmonary alveolar proteinosis. Nature and origin of alveolar lipid. Am J Med 45:502-512, 1968

6. Ito M, Takenchi N, Rgura T et al: Pulmonary alveolar proteinosis: analysis of pulmonary washings. Br J Dis Chest 72:313-320, 1978

7. Carnovale R, Zornoza J, Goldman AM et al: Pulmonary alveolar proteinosis: its association with hematologic malignancy and lymphoma. Radiology 122:303-306, 1977

8. Lakshminarayan S, Schwarz MI, Stanford RE: Unsuspected pulmonary alveolar proteinosis complicating acute myelogenous leukemia. Chest 69:433-435, 1976

9. Hartung M, Salfelder K: Pulmonary alveolar proteinosis and histoplasmosis: Report of three cases. Virchows Arch Pathol Anat 368:281-287, 1975

10. Ranchod M, Bissell M: Pulmonary alveolar proteinosis and cytomegalovirus infection. Arch Pathol Lab Med 103:139-142, 1979

11. Golde DW, Territo M, Finley TN, et al: Defective lung macrophages in pulmonary alveolar proteinosis. Ann Intern Med 85:304-309, 1976

12. Xipell JM, Ham KN, Price CG et al: Acute silicoproteinosis. Thorax 32:104-111, 1977

13. McEuen DD, Abraham JL: Particulate concentrations in pulmonary alveolar proteinosis. Environ Res 17:334-339, 1978

14. Gross P, deTreville RTP: Alveolar proteinosis: its experimental production in rodents. Arch Pathol 86:255-261, 1968

15. Ramarez-R J: Pulmonary alveolar proteinosis. A roentgenologic analysis. Am J Roentgenol 92:571-577, 1964

16. Rogers RM, Levin DC, Gray BA et al: Physiological effects of bronchopulmonary lavage in alveolar proteinosis. Am Rev Respir Dis 118:255-264, 1978

17. Kroeker EJ, Korfmacher S: Pulmonary alveolar proteinosis. Report of case with application of a special sputum examination as an aid to diagnosis. Am Rev Respir Dis 87:416-423, 1963

18. Martin RJ, Rogers RM, Myers NM: Pulmonary alveolar proteinosis: shunt fraction and lactic acid dehydrogenase concentration as aids to diagnosis. Am Rev Respir Dis 117:1059-1062, 1978

19. Smith LJ, Ankin MG, Katzenstein A et al: Management of pulmonary alveolar proteinosis. Chest 78:765-770, 1980

20. Covette JB, Magovern GJ, Kent EM: Alveolar proteinosis. Arch Intern Med 108:611-614, 1961

21. Ramirez-R J. Alveolar proteinosis: importance of pulmonary lavage. Am Rev Respir Dis 103:666-678, 1971

22. Ramirez-R J, Kieffer RF, Jr., Ball WC, Jr.: Bronchopulmonary lavage in man. Ann Intern Med 63:819-828, 1965

23. Wasserman K, Blank N, Fletcher G: Lung lavage (alveolar washing) in alveolar proteinosis. Am J Med 44:611-614, 1968

24. Farca A, Maher G, Miller A. Pulmonary alveolar proteinosis. JAMA 224:1283-1285, 1973

25. Kao D, Wasserman K, Costley D et al: Advances in the treatment of pulmonary alveolar proteinosis. Am Rev Respir Dis 111:361-363, 1975

26. Selecky PA, Wasserman K, Benfield JR et al: The clinical and physiological effect of whole lung lavage in pulmonary alveolar proteinosis: a ten-year experience. Ann Thorac Surg 24:451-461, 1977

27. Davidson JM, Macleod WM: Pulmonary alveolar proteinosis. Br J Dis Chest 63:13-28, 1969

28. McClellan RO, Boyd HA, Benjamin RG et al: Recovery of ^{239}Pu following bronchopulmonary lavage and DTPA treatment after an accidental inhalation exposure case. Health Phys 31:315-321, 1976

29. Rogers RM, Tatum KR: Bronchopulmonary lavage: a "new" approach to old problems. Med Clin North Am 54:755-771, 1970

30. Rausch DC, Spick A, Kylstra JA: Lung lavage in cystic fibrosis. Am Rev Respir Dis 101:1006, 1970

31. Ramirez-R J: Pulmonary alveolar proteinosis. Treatment by massive bronchopulmonary lavage. Arch Intern Med 119:147-155, 1967

32. Kylstra JA, Rausch DC, Hall KD et al: Volume controlled lung lavage in the treatment of asthma, bronchiectasis and mucoviscidosis. Am Rev Respir Dis 103:651-662, 1971

33. Lippmann M, Mok MS: Anesthetic management of pulmonary lavage in adults. Anesth Analg (Cleve) 56:661-668, 1977

34. Busque L: Pulmonary lavage in the treatment of alveolar proteinosis. Can Anaesth Soc J 24:380-389, 1977

35. Blenkarn GD, Lanning CF, Kylstra JA: Anesthetic management of volume controlled unilateral lung lavage. Can Anaesth Soc J 22:154-163, 1975

36. Bradfield HG, Maynard JP: Pulmonary la-

vage in a case of alveolar proteinosis. The value of continuous display oxygen-haemoglobin saturation using ear-oximetry. Anaesthesia 34:1032-1034, 1979

37. Alfery DD, Zamost BG, Benumof JL: Unilateral lung lavage: blood flow manipulation by ipsilateral pulmonary artery balloon inflation. Anesthesiology 55:376-381, 1981

38. Benumof JL, Spragg RG, Alfery DD: Pulmonary artery balloon manipulation of pulmonary artery blood flow during unilateral lung lavage. Anesthesiology 55:A376, 1981

39. Jenkins DW, Jr., Teichner RL, Griggs GW et al: Alveolar proteinosis. Lavage in the presence of bronchopleural fistula. JAMA 234:74-75, 1975

40. Lippmann M, Mok MS, Wasserman K: Anesthetic management for children with alveolar proteinosis using extracorporeal circulation. Report of two cases. Br J Anaesth 49:173-177, 1977

41. Altose MD, Hicks RE, Edwards MW, Jr.: Extracorporeal membrane oxygenation during bronchopulmonary lavage. Arch Surg 111:1148-1153, 1976

42. Cooper JD, Duffin J, Glynn MF et al: Combination of membrane oxygenator support and pulmonary lavage for acute respiratory failure. J Thorac Cardiovasc Surg 71:304-308, 1976

43. Brach BB, Harrell JH, Moser KM: Alveolar proteinosis. Lobar lavage by fiberoptic bronchoscopic technique. Chest 69:224-227, 1976

44. Vast C, Demonet B, Mouveroux J: Value of selective pulmonary lavage under fiberoptic control in alveolar proteinosis. Poumon Coeur 34:305-307, 1978

45. Rogers RM, Szidon JP, Shelburne J et al: Hemodynamic response of the circulation to bronchopulmonary lavage in man. N Engl J Med 296:1230-1233, 1972

46. Smith JD, Miller JE, Safer P et al: Intrathoracic pressure, pulmonary vascular pressures and gas exchange during pulmonary lavage. Anesthesiology 33:401-405, 1970

47. Benumof JL, Saidman LJ, Arkin DB, Diamant M: Where pulmonary artery catheters go: intrathoracic distribution. Anesthesiology 46:336-338, 1977

48. Katz JD, Cronau LH, Barash PG et al: Pulmonary artery flow guided catheters in perioperative period: Indications and complications. JAMA 237:2832-2834, 1977

49. Golden MS, Pinder T, Anderson WT et al: Fatal pulmonary hemorrhage complicating use of flow-directed balloon-tipped catheter in a patient receiving anticoagulant. Am J Cardiol 32:865-867, 1973

50. Paulson DM, Scott SM, Sethi GK: Pulmonary hemorrhage associated with balloon flotation catheters. J Thorac Cardiovasc Surg 80:453-458, 1980

ROGER S. WILSON, M.D.

13
Tracheostomy and Tracheal Reconstruction

TRACHEOSTOMY

General Considerations

Although tracheostomy is a commonly performed procedure and one that has been done for decades, uniformity is still lacking concerning indications and technique.[1] Indications for tracheostomy include: (1) upper airway obstruction; (2) access for tracheal toilet; (3) administration of positive pressure ventilation; and (4) airway protection from aspiration of gastric and/or pharyngeal contents. It is rare that a tracheostomy is done as a true surgical emergency; rather it should be considered an elective procedure. When done electively, the incidence of complications of tracheostomy, including hypoxia with cardiac arrest during the procedure, injury to structures immediately adjacent to the trachea, pneumothoraces, and hemorrhage, has been reduced. Tracheostomy, like any other surgical procedure, should be done in the operating room. In general, the best operating conditions are provided when an endotracheal tube has been placed and either the patient is adequately anesthetized or local anesthesia and supplemental sedation are used.

Elective tracheostomy is best carried out under "ideal" operating conditions. Such conditions are provided in a well-equipped operating suite, with adequate lighting and personnel who understand the procedure to be undertaken.

Anesthetic requirements are variable and are dictated by the state of awareness or consciousness of the patient and the nature of other systemic diseases. If necessary, the procedure can be safely done by using local infiltration, supplemented with intravenous sedative and/or narcotic drugs. The advantage of this technique, especially when used for a critically ill individual, is that it allows for the administration of high concentrations of inspired oxygen. In those patients for whom oxygenation is not a problem, additional analgesia without the use of intravenous drug therapy can be accomplished by the administration of 50 to 70% nitrous oxide and oxygen. In patients whose cardiovascular stability is not a problem, general anesthesia with any of the inhalational agents may be used with or without supplemental local infiltration.

Monitoring, including the electrocardiogram (ECG), intra-arterial pressure, and pulmonary artery pressure, is used as dictated by the complexity of the patient's overall condition. In the stable patient with normal cardiopulmonary function, the standard ECG and blood pressure cuff monitoring are adequate. The need for additional monitoring is dictated by the concomitant respiratory, cardiovascular, nervous system, or metabolic diseases.

Surgical Procedure

The patient is placed in the supine position with the neck extended, with utilization of either a rolled towel or inflatable thyroid bag placed beneath the shoulders. The head can be positioned in a "doughnut" or a head-dish for additional stability. These maneuvers provide for maximal surface exposure and in most patients bring the trachea from the intrathoracic to the cervical position. After appropriate preparation of the skin and surgical draping, the procedure is accomplished through a short horizontal incision placed at the level of the second tracheal ring (Fig. 13-1). The strap muscles are separated in the midline and the thyroid isthmus is divided and appropriately sutured to obtain hemostasis. Specific identification of the location of the tracheal rings is made by counting down from the easily palpable cricoid cartilage. The second and third rings are opened vertically in the midline for access to the trachea. The tracheostomy tube should be placed so that it will not erode the first ring and press against the cricoid cartilage. In addition, the opening should not be placed too low, or the tip of the tube and its cuff will be too close to the carina. Low placement of the tracheostomy tube is also hazardous since the innominate

artery crosses anteriorly to the trachea low in the neck, and the possibility of erosion into the vessel by either the cuff or tip of the tracheostomy tube is possible. Segments of the trachea should not be removed, since this might lead to a greater loss of tracheal wall stability and predisposes to stenosis once healing is accomplished following removal of the tube. The lateral tracheal walls are retracted with use of thyroid pole retractors, and the appropriate-size (30 or 33 FR) tracheostomy tube is inserted into the airway following slow withdrawal of the previously placed oral or nasal endotracheal tube to a more proximal position in the trachea. Once the tracheostomy tube is positioned and an adequate airway demonstrated with use of positive pressure ventilation and visual inspection of chest wall expansion, the previously placed endotracheal tube is totally removed from the trachea. The wound is appropriately closed with skin sutures, and the tracheostomy tube is secured with a skin suture through the flange and with "trachtape" or a tie around the neck.

COMPLICATIONS

Complications may occur both in the intraoperative and postoperative period. The intraoperative complications are a result of either the anesthesia, underlying disease, or surgical procedure. Surgical complications generally fall into three major categories, including hemorrhage, injury to structures adjacent to the trachea, and failure to cannulate the airway. Wound hemorrhage is usually easily controlled but may be complicated by the difficulty of exposure. Vascular structures such as the thyroid isthmus may bleed easily when divided for exposure. Injuries to adjacent structures include damage to recurrent laryngeal nerves, entrance into major vessels, and rare but possible laceration of the esophagus. Inability to cannulate the trachea is frequently due to inadequate surgical expo-

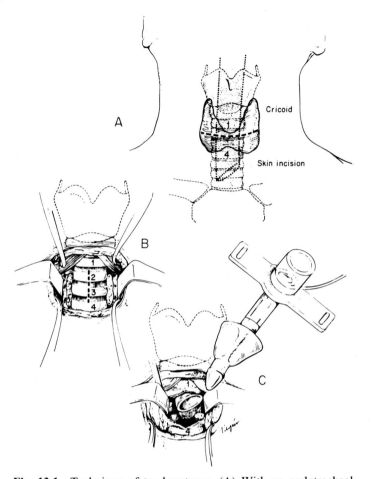

Fig. 13-1 Technique of tracheostomy. (A) With an endotracheal tube in place, a horizontal skin incision is made 1 to 2 cm below the cricoid cartilage. (B) Strap muscles are spread in the midline and the thyroid isthmus is divided. A vertical incision is made in the second and third cartilaginous rings. (C) With thyroid pole retractors holding back the cut edge of the trachea, the endotracheal tube is withdrawn and the tracheostomy tube is inserted. (Grillo HC: Congenital Lesions, Neoplasms, and Injuries of the Chest. In Sabiston DC and Spencer FC, Eds: Gibbon's Surgery of the Chest. W. B. Saunders Co., Philadelphia, 1976. Reprinted with permission of author and publisher.)

sure, inability to bring the trachea to a superficial location, or selection of a tracheostomy tube too large to fit into the tracheal stoma. Such complications can be avoided by careful planning and appropriate selection of tubes. In the presence of prior endotracheal intubation, the danger of loss of the airway is minimized. Long-term complications resulting from the use of endotracheal and tracheostomy tubes will be considered in the discussion of types of tracheostomy tubes and cuffs.

EMERGENCY TRACHEOSTOMY

An "emergency" tracheostomy is occasionally necessary. The need is dictated by the urgency of providing an airway, often due to rapidly progressing airway obstruction. This may occur following head and neck trauma, upper airway compromise due to allergic reactions, angioneurotic edema, epiglottitis, or in the postoperative period following neck surgery such as thyroidectomy, or an anterior approach for a cervical fusion. Such postoperative problems result from hemorrhage with external compression and total airway obstruction. The ability to accomplish airway control with an endotracheal tube may not be possible. Emergency procedures include needle tracheostomy, cricothyroidotomy, and formal tracheostomy. Needle tracheostomy is often of limited success since flow through the catheter or needle requires a high-pressure gas source and immediate availability of appropriate connecting devices between the gas source and the needle or catheter. With this technique, ventilation, and hence CO_2 elimination, is difficult, and thus this maneuver is potentially "life-saving" for only a limited time. Formal emergency tracheostomy in general is not technically feasible owing to the lack of adequate instruments and lighting and the time required to accomplish it before major circulatory and/or cerebral complications occur.

The technique of cricothyroidotomy has become increasingly popular and has been described in numerous publications.[1] It can be done rapidly with a minimum amount of equipment. A rolled towel is placed under the shoulders to put the neck in a hyperextended position. A small transverse incision is made through the skin into the cricothyroid membrane with a #11 scalpel blade, and the incision is spread with a surgical clamp or a knife handle or by a digital technique. A small (5.0 or 6.0 mm) pediatric endotracheal tube or tracheostomy tube is placed through the cricothyroid membrane into the trachea. This technique has the advantages of simplicity and speed and is associated with minimal bleeding. It also provides an airway sufficient for adequate gas exchange. Potential complications of this technique include injury to the cricoid or thyroid cartilages, with the potential for laryngeal stenosis, injury to the esophagus, hemorrhage from the anterior jugular vein, injury to the carotid artery or internal jugular vein, and infection at the cricothyroid incision. These complications are generally avoidable if the incision is correctly placed, a small tube is used, and the duration of use of the cricothyroidotomy is limited to a short period, i.e., hours or days. It is generally advisable to convert the cricothyroidotomy to a standard tracheostomy as soon as the patient's overall condition permits.

TRACHEOSTOMY TUBE DESIGN

The recognition that tracheal intubation with endotracheal and tracheostomy tube with cuffs may produce injury has stimulated improvement in design of both tubes and cuffs. The pathogenesis of tracheal injuries produced by cuff pressure has been well-documented.[2-6] Complications include tracheal stenosis or disruption of the tracheal wall, with the potential for development of a tracheo-esophageal fistula or a fistula into a major vessel. A number of cuff designs and techniques have been developed in the hope of minimizing tracheal injury.[7,8] Included are intermittent cuff inflation and deflation, inflation of cuffs during inspiration only, underinflation with a minimal leak technique, use of double-cuff tubes, and design of high-volume–low-pressure cuffs. The latter has proved to be the most effective way of reducing tracheal injury.[9]

The large-residual-volume, low-pressure cuff has been designed in several configurations by a variety of manufacturers. The general design of this cuff is such that it occludes the lumen of the trachea by conforming to the existing configuration of the cross-section of the trachea without deforming it. This is

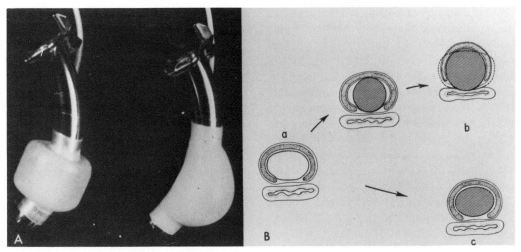

Fig. 13-2 Tracheostomy tube cuffs. (A) On the left is a large-volume, high-compliance cuff, adjacent to a partially inflated standard high-pressure cuff. (B) When the high-pressure cuff is inflated, the eccentrically shaped trachea (a) is not sealed until the airway is deformed with use of high cuff pressures (b). This is in contrast to the low-pressure cuff (c), which fills the eccentrically shaped trachea and provides occlusion without exerting significant pressure. (Grillo HC: Congenital Lesions, Neoplasms, and Injuries of the Chest. In Sabiston DC and Spencer FC, Eds: Gibbon's Surgery of the Chest. W. B. Saunders Co., Philadelphia, 1976. Reprinted with permission of author and publisher.)

depicted in Figure 13-2. Improved design of the cuff per se does not totally eliminate tracheal injury. Several precautions must be undertaken regardless of the type of cuff employed. The cuff must not be inflated beyond the minimum volume and pressure required to provide a minimal leak.

A pressure within the cuff greater than 25 mmHg will potentially increase the risk of tracheal injury. It is important that intracuff pressure be monitored and when it exceeds 25 mmHg, that appropriate measures be taken to correct it. This problem is frequently encountered when the tracheostomy tube that has been selected is too small for the cuff to completely fill the void between the tube and trachea. When this is the case, alternative measures such as an increase in tracheostomy tube size, selection of a tracheostomy tube with a larger cuff, or acceptance of a larger leak must be undertaken. In the event that increasing volumes of air are required within the cuff owing to tracheal dilatation, similar corrective measures must be undertaken.

CARE AND MAINTENANCE OF THE TRACHEOSTOMY

Adequate care must be provided to the tracheal stoma to prevent injury. The care should focus on removal of secretions from the region of the stoma and the surrounding skin. Tracheostomy dressings should be changed regularly, e.g., every 8 hours. The technique should include use of sterile gloves and cotton-tip applicators with hydrogen peroxide to cleanse the stoma site. Tracheostomy tapes, which often become soiled, should be changed on a regular basis.

Tracheostomy tubes with inner cannula are beneficial in cases in which secretions are abundant and the risk of tube obstruction exists. The advantage of this type of tube is that it allows removal of the inner cannula for cleaning without removal of the tracheostomy tube from the airway.

It is advisable to change tracheostomy tubes on a regular basis to ensure that the tube may be easily removed. Difficulty in removing tubes occurs as the stoma heals down around the shaft of the tube, the stoma size being reduced so that when the tube is partially withdrawn, the bulk of the cuff does not allow removal from the airway.[10] Elective removal and reinsertion of a new tracheostomy tube on a weekly basis obviates this problem. Elective tube changes should not be undertaken until 72 to 96 hours following placement of a new tracheostomy since inadequacy of the stomal tract during the first few days makes such changes dangerous.

The nature of the changing procedure should be explained to the patient. If mechanical ventilation is being used, 100 percent inspired oxygen should be administered for several minutes before the procedure is undertaken. A laryngoscope, endotracheal tubes, and a self-inflating manual resuscitation bag should be available. The patient is positioned flat in bed and a rolled towel placed under the shoulders to provide better visualization of the neck area. Following suctioning of the airway, the cuff is deflated and the tube withdrawn. A similar-size tracheostomy tube should be repositioned in the stoma, the cuff inflated, and adequacy of tube placement ascertained by auscultation of breath sounds, with spontaneous or positive pressure ventilation delivered through the tracheostomy tube. If the patient needs to be returned to mechanical ventilation, the adequacy of breath sounds must again be reconfirmed by use of chest auscultation after the tube is secured in place.

TRACHEAL RECONSTRUCTION

Etiology of Injuries

The etiologies of tracheal injury are numerous and are outlined in Table 13-1.

CONGENITAL LESIONS

As outlined by Grillo, congenital lesions of the trachea have been infrequently described.[11] The extent of injuries ranges from

Table 13-1
Etiology of Tracheal Lesions

I. Congenital lesions
  A. Tracheal agenesis/atresia
  B. Congenital stenosis
  C. Congenital chondromalacia
II. Neoplastic lesions
  A. Primary neoplasms
    1. Squamous-cell carcinoma
    2. Adenoid cystic carcinoma (cylindroma)
    3. Carcinoid adenoma
    4. Carcinosarcoma-chondrosarcoma
  B. Secondary neoplasms
    1. Bronchogenic carcinoma
    2. Esophageal carcinoma
    3. Tracheal carcinoma
    4. Breast carcinoma
    5. Head/neck carcinoma
III. Injuries
  A. Direct trauma
    1. Penetrating
    2. Blunt injuries
  B. Indirect trauma
IV. Infection
  A. Tubercular strictures
  B. Other
V. Postintubation injuries
  A. Laryngeal stenosis
  B. Cuff injuries
  C. Ulceration
  D. Granuloma formation
VI. Tracheostomy
  A. Cuff lesions
  B. Stoma lesions

those incompatible with life, such as tracheal agenesis or atresia, to regional segmental stenoses. Congenital tracheal stenosis may be associated with a number of other anomalies, such as an aberrant left pulmonary artery or pulmonary artery sling which produces compression of the posterior tracheal wall. This occurs when the left pulmonary artery originates from the proximal portion of the right pulmonary artery and passes behind the trachea to the left lung. Complete tracheal rings are common in this anomaly, and surgical correction of the vascular anomaly does not necessarily improve airway obstruction. In contrast, vascular ring malformations, when they compress the trachea without associated primary tracheal anomalies, are generally improved by surgical correction. Tracheal compromise of this type occurs with a double aortic arch, a right aortic arch, or a ligamentum arteriosum.

In general, surgical repair of pediatric tracheal abnormalities must be approached with caution. The small cross-sectional area of the airway, with its potential for obstruction from edema and secretions, increases the surgical risk in infancy or childhood. In addition, other increased risks of surgery and anesthesia may preclude operation at this time. If possible, it is preferable to use alternative measures, such as tracheostomy, to temporize until some later stage of life.

NEOPLASTIC LESIONS

Primary neoplastic lesions, although uncommon, may develop in the trachea. In several published series, squamous-cell carcinoma was the most common primary lesion.[11,12] Adenoid cystic carcinoma is the second most frequent, with a variety of other rare tumors having been cited in all series.

Although extensive knowledge concerning the natural history of these lesions is not clear, it is evident that both squamous-cell carcinoma and adenoid cystic carcinoma are amenable to early aggressive therapy and are potentially curable. Squamous-cell carcinoma may present as a well-localized lesion of the exophytic type or as an ulcerating lesion. Limited experience suggests that spread is first to regional lymph nodes adjacent to the trachea and then direct extension into mediastinal structures. Adenoid cystic carcinoma infiltrates the airway in a submucosal fashion, often for longer distances than is evident on gross examination. Some lesions of high malignancy have spread by direct invasion of the pleura and lungs by the time the diagnosis is made. The opportunity for complete removal of this type of tumor occurs at the initial surgery with wide resections of the margins. Currently, there is limited experience with the many other types of tumors that may invade the trachea, and thus generalizations concerning their natural history are difficult.

Primary tumors of the trachea present in several ways. Shortness of breath, especially with exertion, is often the primary symptom. As the tumor grows, this begins to worsen, producing limitations with very minimal levels of exercise. Wheezing, which is often confused and misdiagnosed as bronchial asthma, is a common feature, and stridor, with repeated attacks of respiratory obstruction due to a combination of tumor and secretions, may also occur. The patient can often give a history of position-dependent airway obstruction, especially in the case of exophytic lesions. Obstruction may occur in a specific position, such as a lateral position, and be relieved in other positions. This finding is important when a history is taken during the preanesthesia visit, since induction of anesthesia in such patients must occasionally be undertaken in a specific position to ensure initial patency of the airway. Patients can also present with episodes of unilateral and bilateral pneumonia, often unresponsive to antibiotics and physiotherapy. Hemoptysis may accompany several of the aforementioned findings or present as the sole symptom.

Secondary neoplasms may occur throughout the tracheobronchial tree. It is not uncommon for structures adjacent to the airway to involve the trachea by metastases or direct extension. Bronchogenic, laryngeal, and esophageal carcinoma can invade the trachea and main bronchi. In general, metastases of this nature are associated with far-advanced disease and obviate tracheal surgery except for palliation.

Secondary neoplasms occurring from thyroid malignancies perhaps are one area in which combined primary resection of the tumor and tracheal reconstruction is warranted. Not uncommonly, late recurrences of carcinoma originating in the thyroid have appeared in the trachea and larynx. Resection of these slow-growing late lesions has produced excellent palliation for several years.

A variety of other tumors can involve the trachea, including metastases from head and neck carcinomas, carcinoma of the breast with mediastinal involvement, and lymphoma. In general, tracheal reconstruction is not indicated in such cases.

INJURIES

Direct laryngeal and tracheal trauma can occur from both penetrating and blunt injuries to the cervical portion of the airway. The presentation of penetrating injuries such as knife wounds or gunshot wounds is dependent upon the severity of the injuries and the other vital structures, including nerves and vessels, that are involved.

Blunt injuries may severely damage the trachea and are often complicated in their presentation. Direct blows to the cervical area may be sufficient to lacerate or completely sever the trachea. Supporting tissues may hold the damaged area together, providing an airway which is adequate enough to allow the patient to reach an emergency facility. Total disruption of this airway is often produced at the time of intubation or attempts at emergency tracheostomy. If the airway is adequate, all maneuvers, such as tracheostomy and/or intubation, should be held in abeyance until clinical evaluation and diagnostic tests are performed to demonstrate the severity of the injury. Adequate facilities, ideally a well-equipped operating room, should be available for optimum management. Laryngeal fracture may occur as a primary or concomitant injury in such cases. The surgical management of such lesions, as described by Montgomery in 1968, is best undertaken after healing of the acute injury.[13]

The trachea and bronchi, like other intrathoracic organs, may also be disrupted during indirect closed-chest trauma. One area particularly susceptible to injury is the membranous wall of the trachea, which can be lacerated in a vertical direction with extension at the level of the carina into the right or left mainstem bronchus. Such injuries often present as a pneumothorax which commonly fails to respond completely to tube thoracostomy and suction. The inability to reexpand a collapsed lung or the persistence of an excessive air leak should always raise the question of tracheal or major airway disruption. Incomplete separation of the bronchi may occur and only present as a late stenosis following discharge from the hospital.

INFECTION

Although rare today, stricture of the trachea can be a complication of pulmonary tuberculosis or other infectious etiologies, including diphtheria, syphilis, and typhoid, which all have been described in the past. Rarely are chronic inflammatory conditions of the trachea involved with stenosis. Fibrosing mediastinitis and systemic diseases such as Wegener's granulomatosis or amyloidosis can produce benign strictures.

POSTINTUBATION AND TRACHEOSTOMY INJURIES

The use of endotracheal or tracheostomy tubes has been shown to produce a variety of tracheal lesions. These have been described in detail in several articles.[4-6] As shown in Figure 13-3, lesions may be produced by the cuff in any of the areas where it contacts the tracheal wall. Laryngeal injury occurs with use of either oral or nasal endotracheal tubes and at the stoma site with tracheostomy tubes.

Endotracheal intubation will produce a variety of injuries involving the nares, larynx, and trachea, with most injuries resulting from pressure necrosis.[3] At the laryngeal level, the vocal cords are a common site of injury. The extent of injury varies from edema and local irritation to more serious ulceration and erosion, often at the posterior commissure, with subsequent scar formation and/or granulomata. Although the majority

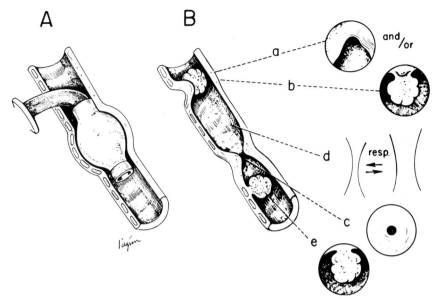

Fig. 13-3 Sites of tracheal injury. (A) A cuffed tracheostomy tube is shown in situ with dilatation of the trachea at the level of the high-pressure cuff. (B) Sites of possible tracheal injuries are shown as follows. (a) Erosion of the stoma and subsequent healing produces an anterolateral stricture. (b) Granuloma may form also at this level. (c) At the level of pressure exerted by the cuff, circumferential erosion will result in a circumferential stenosis. (d) Between the stoma and the level of the cuff, thinning of the tracheal wall with potential loss of cartilage may occur. (e) The tube tip may produce erosion and/or granulomata. (Grillo HC: Congenital Lesions, Neoplasms, and Injuries of the Chest. In Sabiston DC and Spencer FC, Eds: Gibbon's Surgery of the Chest. W. B. Saunders Co., Philadelphia, 1976. Reprinted with permission of author and publisher.)

of laryngeal lesions are reversible in time, a number require surgical correction.[13] Initial symptoms include hoarseness, sore throat, and stridor. Progression of edema with resulting airway obstruction may require reintubation, and, in a limited number of cases, tracheostomy.

Subglottic stenosis may occur as a result of mucosal erosion at the level of the cricoid cartilage. The true incidence of this lesion is unknown. Subglottic stenosis poses a difficult problem owing to limitations in surgical repair when the lesion is severe.

Cuff-related lesions with either tracheostomy or endotracheal tubes are similar. The presumed mechanism involves a force applied against the tracheal wall producing necrosis. Although many etiologic factors have been considered, including local infection and toxicity of cuff materials, it is apparent that the single most important factor is the direct pressure exerted by the inflated cuff against the tracheal mucosa.[2,5,6] The degree of injury produced depends on a number of factors, including the length of time the pressure is applied, the healing abilities of the patient, and the total amount of tissue injury produced. The extent of injury may vary from superficial ulceration with minimal sequelae to extensive erosion involving destruction of cartilage with the potential for fistula formation. The pathophysiology and visual confirmation of such lesions both in the experimental model and in patients have been extensively described.[9] The natural evolution of this injury relates to cicatrization during the healing process, which produces a circumferential stenosis (Fig. 13-3).

Tracheomalacia can also be the consequence of a cuff-related injury. This occurs at the level of the cuff, where progressive lateral force weakens a tracheal segment and local inflammation destroys the cartilage. Tracheomalacia also occurs between the level of the tracheostomy stoma and the cuff, where inflammatory changes, perhaps due to pooling of secretions and local bacterial infection, lead to thinning of cartilaginous structures without significant injury to the mucosa itself. Such segmental injuries produce a functional obstruction, particularly when a maximal respiratory effort during inspiration or expiration is produced. The tracheal stoma is a frequent site of stenosis. The mechanism is most likely related to a significant loss of anterior-lateral tracheal wall and subsequent cicatricial healing, producing an anterior-lateral stricture, as shown in Figure 13-3. Factors leading to the development of such an injury include extensive surgical resection of anterior tracheal wall, local infection of the tissue in the stomal area, and pressure necrosis created by leverage between ventilator tubing and the tracheostomy tube.

Granulation tissue can develop at several sites within the airway, including the stoma and the tip of the tracheostomy or endotracheal tube, where it impinges on the anterior tracheal wall. Such lesions produce airway obstruction which may be position-related and ball-valve in nature.

Life-threatening complications of tracheal injuries include tracheo-esophageal fistula and fistula formation between the airway and major vessels. Tracheo-esophageal fistulas are usually manifest by unexplained recurrent episodes of aspiration pneumonia, often associated with an increase or a change in the character of tracheal secretions. Presenting features during mechanical ventilation may include the presence of air in the gastrointestinal tract and/or the inability to maintain adequate tidal volume and minute ventilation. Tracheo-innominate artery fistulas manifest themselves by sudden, massive, life-threatening hemorrhage from the tracheobronchial tree or through the stoma. Such lesions are often heralded by minor episodes of bleeding from the stoma as erosion first begins to develop.

Diagnostic Evaluation

Diagnostic evaluation for patients with obstructive lesions of the airway consists of detailed history and physical examination, pulmonary function studies, roentgenographic studies, and bronchoscopy. The indications for each study and the potential benefit derived from the information are variable from patient to patient. In addition, the severity and urgency of airway compromise will often dictate the diagnostic regimen that is followed. In life-threatening situations in which there is a high index of suspicion as to the nature of the tracheal pathology, diagnosis may consist only of bronchoscopy. However, in the patient presenting for elective surgery with symptoms indicative of airway obstruction, a detailed evaluation is generally warranted.[14]

HISTORY AND PHYSICAL

The signs and symptoms produced by airway obstruction will be affected by the anatomical location, the degree of airway obstruction, and the presence of preexisting cardiopulmonary disease. The clinical symptoms generally consist of dyspnea, especially with effort, wheezing, which may present as frank stridor, difficulty in clearing secretions, and eventually airway obstruction from inability to clear mucus. Although simple and nonspecific, these symptoms are frequently misdiagnosed. It is not uncommon, especially when dealing with tracheal tumors, to find that patients have been diagnosed as having asthma. In many cases, suspicion as to some other diagnosis is aroused only when the supposed asthma fails to respond to usual treatment modalities, often including use of corticosteroids. It is essential to remember that in any patient with a history of recent intubation and/or tracheostomy the development of any of the above symptoms should be considered a result of an organic lesion until proved otherwise.

Preexisting cardiopulmonary disease will often limit exercise. In such cases, tracheal stenosis can progress to a severe stage before symptomatology is present.

Physical examination is generally of limited value. Audible stridor, either occurring at rest or provoked with a maximal expiratory effort with an open mouth, is a common finding. Chest auscultation frequently reveals diffuse inspiratory and expiratory wheezing, often difficult to differentiate from that typical of asthma. Auscultation of the upper cervical airway may reveal high-pitched inspiratory and expiratory sounds characteristic of obstruction to air flow.

PULMONARY FUNCTION STUDIES

Although standard spirometry is of limited value in diagnosing obstructive lesions, the use of flow-volume loops has been shown to be very reliable.[15] With standard spirometry, measured air flow during inspiration and expiration may be reduced. Characteristically, maximal expiratory and/or inspiratory flow is affected to a far greater degree than is the one-second forced expiratory volume (FEV_1). The ratio of peak expiratory flow to FEV_1 has been used as an index of obstruction. When this ratio is 10:1 or greater, it is suggestive of airway obstruction. The flow-volume loop is the most specific test for the diagnosis of upper airway obstruction. During a forced expiration from total lung capacity, the maximal flow achieved during the first 25 percent of the vital capacity is dependent upon effort alone. In the case of fixed airway obstruction, the peak expiratory flow is markedly reduced, producing a characteristic plateau. With fixed intra- or

extrathoracic lesions, the inspiratory flow has the same characteristic plateau. In the case of a variable obstruction, such as those seen with tracheomalacia, the maximal cutoff of inspiratory or expiratory flow will depend on the location of the lesion. Extrathoracic or cervical lesions produce a plateau during inspiration, with minimal effect on expiratory flow; while intrathoracic lesions that are variable tend to demonstrate alterations in the expiratory flow curve with minimal or no effect on inspiration. In general, stenoses that are circumferential, such as those produced by cuff lesions, are fixed in origin. Tumors and tracheomalacia frequently produce a variety of intermittent obstructions. It is often possible to estimate the functional impairment of the tracheal lesion by using a restricted orifice in the patient's mouthpiece as he undergoes the flow-volume study. When the limited orifice begins to show additional effect on the flow-volume loop, it can be assumed that the intrinsic lesion has reduced the trachea to that cross-sectional area. In general, airway obstruction must reach 5 to 6 mm in cross-sectional diameter before signs and symptoms become clinically evident. The peak expiratory flow rate decreases to approximately 80 percent of normal when the airway diameter is reduced to 10 mm.

RADIOLOGIC STUDIES

Routine and special radiologic studies will often precisely demonstrate the extent and location of the tracheal pathology (Figs. 13-4 and 13-5).[16,17] In addition to the standard posterior-anterior and lateral chest radiograph, the oblique views are often of additional benefit. The latter will often show the full extent of the trachea when mediastinal structures are rotated to the side. An anterior-posterior copper-filtered view of the trachea can be taken with the patient saying "E," which will demonstrate excellent anterior-posterior detail of the entire upper airway. Lateral cervical views are of value in demonstrating detailed laryngotracheal rela-

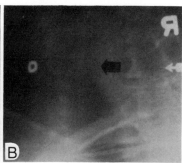

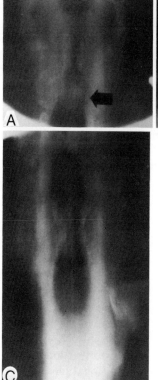

Fig. 13-4 Radiographs of benign tracheal lesions. (A) Detail of larynx and upper trachea are shown, with a large granuloma indicated by the arrow. (B) The same lesion shown in detail on a soft-tissue lateral view of the neck. The arrow indicates the granuloma within the air column. (C) Laminagram showing stomal stenosis. Above may be seen the normal upper surface of the vocal cords and the bell-shaped subglottic larynx, which terminates at the bottom of the cricoid. (Grillo HC: Congenital Lesions, Neoplasms, and Injuries of the Chest. In Sabiston DC and Spencer FC, Eds: Gibbon's Surgery of the Chest. W. B. Saunders Co., Philadelphia, 1976. Reprinted with permission of author and publisher.)

tionships and deformities impinging on the anterior or posterior tracheal walls. Whenever possible, fluoroscopy is done to determine the functional nature of the lesion and to demonstrate the presence of airway malacia. Once areas of pathology are identified, laminograms or polytome views of the trachea in both anterior-posterior and lateral projections are necessary to obtain definition and the exact position of the lesions. In general, contrast material should not be used for fear of producing airway obstruction.

Evaluation of patients with endotracheal tubes in place must be undertaken with caution, since optimal examination using radiologic techniques can only be done when the endotracheal or tracheostomy tube has been removed. Although the airway may be adequate immediately following decannulation, it is not uncommon for compromise to occur in a matter of minutes. Hence, any decannulation, especially when done in the x-ray department, must be done under the close supervision of someone trained and properly equipped to reinstitute tracheal intubation.

Bronchoscopy is the ultimate diagnostic procedure. In general, bronchoscopy is usually deferred until the time of the proposed operation in order not to precipitate airway obstruction secondary to edema or hemorrhage.

Anesthetic Management

Various approaches to the problems of airway obstruction and the maintenance of anesthesia during surgery for tracheal reconstruction have been described.[18–22] The

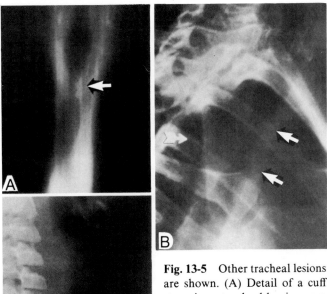

Fig. 13-5 Other tracheal lesions are shown. (A) Detail of a cuff stenosis on tracheal laminagram is shown. The bell shape of the lower larynx may be seen above with a segment of normal trachea, which tapers abruptly to a narrow stenotic segment. The trachea opens up to a normal diameter below this segment. (B) Detail from an oblique view shows the tracheal air column reaching a point of maximum narrowing between the two white arrows. (C) Ball-like anterior granuloma is shown on a lateral neck view in the lower part of a long cervical trachea. The granuloma formed at the site of anterior erosion where the tip of the tube had pressed against the tracheal wall. (Grillo HC: Congenital Lesions, Neoplasms, and Injuries of the Chest. In Sabiston DC and Spencer FC, Eds: Gibbon's Surgery of the Chest. W. B. Saunders Co., Philadelphia, 1976. Reprinted with permission of author and publisher.)

method described in this chapter is the one employed by Grillo and colleagues for several hundred patients who have undergone tracheal resection and reconstruction at the Massachusetts General Hospital since 1962.[22–26]

PREOPERATIVE ASSESSMENT

Based on the studies discussed above, preoperative workup should localize the nature, location, and extent of the trachea requiring reconstruction. The preoperative assessment from the anesthesiologist's vantage point should consider, among other things, the degree of airway limitation, the presence of preexisting disease, especially of the lungs or heart, and the potential problems in the postoperative period. The patient should be evaluated with the understanding that intraoperative difficulties associated with the airway, as well as potential problems during induction, may expose the individual to undue stresses from hypoxia, hypercarbia, and/or cardiovascular instability. The general approach to the anesthetic technique used and possible alternatives to be relied upon during the procedure must be based upon these factors as well as the surgical approach which is anticipated.

In most cases, bronchoscopy is done at the time of the contemplated surgical correction. Advantages of this approach are that: (1) only one anesthetic is required for total correction; (2) appropriate monitoring need only be undertaken once; and, (3) airway compromise following bronchoscopy, in the presence of existing pathology, should not become a life-threatening postoperative problem.

Careful detail must be undertaken to evaluate the anatomical configuration and function of the upper airway. Inspection of jaw motion, adequacy of the oral pharynx, and problems relating to mask fit must be viewed with great concern in the preoperative period, since prolonged induction with inhalation agents will rely heavily on the ability to maintain an adequate natural airway in lieu of the distal airway problems. Arterial blood gases, although possibly affected by preexisting chronic and acute parenchymal lung disease, are seldom deranged in the presence of pure upper airway stenosis. Occasionally, if obstruction is severe enough, a compensatory hypocarbia may result. Hypercarbia occurs, as with asthma, only as an extremely late event. Occasionally when severe airway compromise exists in the preoperative period, prophylactic measures may be utilized. These include use of increased inspired oxygen concentrations, increased humidity, and topical steroids or racemic epinephrine. During the course of the workup, a patient is generally admitted to an intensive care unit if his airway is felt to be extremely marginal. This provides for close and continuous observation, available monitors, and required equipment and personnel if emergency intubation should become necessary.

The type of preoperative medication is governed by the extent of airway obstruction. In patients in whom airway obstruction is minimal, the need for tranquilizers, sedatives, and/or drying agents is dictated by the usual criteria. The obvious concern when faced with airway obstruction is the avoidance of oversedation and central respiratory depression. In cases in which anxiety and emotional instability make patient management difficult, appropriate sedation with small doses of tranquilizers and/or barbiturates is relatively safe. In patients in whom airway obstruction is severe, especially when there is obvious stridor and use of accessory respiratory muscles, the administration of atropine and other drying agents should be avoided. Atropine has been reported to produce drying of secretions, creating a situation in which inspissated plugs form and become impacted in the narrow portion of the airway, creating close to total airway obstruction. When in doubt, all premedication should be withheld until the patient arrives in the operating room and is under the close supervision of the anesthesiologist and surgeon.

In those patients in whom airway obstruction exists but has been bypassed by either an endotracheal tube, tracheostomy tube, or T-tube, the use of premedication is governed by the patient's needs and the conditions compatible with safe induction of anesthesia.

MONITORING

The standard approach for monitoring the otherwise uncomplicated patient is to use an electrocardiograph, blood pressure cuff, esophageal stethoscope, and radial arterial catheter. The arterial catheter not only is useful for instantaneous monitoring of blood pressure during the intra- and postoperative periods, but is of even greater benefit in facilitating sampling of arterial blood to follow the efficiency of gas exchange. The selection of the site of cannulation is governed not only by the availability of such vessels but also by the fact that the right radial artery is often lost owing to compression or deliberate sacrifice of the innominate artery, which crosses the trachea and hence the operative field anteriorly from left to right. Thus, the left radial artery is preferred. In addition, when the approach is via a right thoracotomy and surgical exposure dictates that the right arm be prepped into the surgical field, the left radial, left brachial, dorsalis pedis, or femoral arteries are generally utilized.

A central venous catheter is appropriate when it is anticipated that vasopressor support or other intravenous medications requiring such a route will be utilized during the intraoperative period. In general, the use of central venous pressure and pulmonary artery catheters is dictated by a history of existing cardiopulmonary disease. In some cases, difficulties in interpreting these tracings occur intraoperatively with the sternum split and spontaneous ventilation, but useful information can be provided during the postoperative period. Following intubation, placement of an esophageal stethoscope not only provides useful information pertaining to breath sounds, heart tones, and rhythm, but also provides a foreign body which guides the surgeon in helping to identify the esophagus in the surgical field. Measurement of end-tidal gases, as well as transcutaneous oxygen or carbon dioxide concentrations, could also be performed during this operative procedure.

AIRWAY EQUIPMENT

In addition to a conventional anesthesia machine and appropriate monitoring, it is necessary to provide several other important pieces of equipment. It is beneficial to have an anesthesia machine with the capabilities of delivering high-flow oxygen, in excess of 20 L/min. This is particularly useful during the induction phase, when air leaks may pose problems, and during rigid bronchoscopy. In addition, appropriate equipment should be provided to facilitate laryngoscopy and topical anesthesia. The choice of a laryngoscope

blade is not as important as the individual's ability to use any given one with facility. A long bronchial sprayer, with 4 percent lidocaine, is useful for topicalization of the pharynx and tracheal mucous membranes. The most important equipment to be kept readily available is a variety of tubes for endotracheal intubation, ranging from 20 to 30 French. The optimal size to provide an adequate airway, ability to suction secretions, and enough room for surgical manipulation and suturing of the airway is 28 French. In general, the tube size is selected when visualization of the airway is accomplished during rigid bronchoscopy; and the decision is made as to whether or not it is feasible to intubate through the stenosis or rely upon a tube placed above it. These decisions are discussed below in detail in connection with the technique for bronchoscopy.

ANESTHESIA

Once the patient is positioned comfortably on the operating room table in the supine position with an appropriate intravenous catheter and monitoring in place, the induction of anesthesia commences. In patients in whom airway obstruction is of minor significance, owing to either a good natural airway or the presence of an intratracheal appliance, anesthesia may be induced with thiopental or a similar agent. When airway conditions are consistent with a high degree of obstruction, it is desirable to undertake a gentle, controlled inhalational induction with a volatile anesthetic. First the patient is denitrogenated with oxygen via a mask for an appropriate period of time, and then halothane is gradually introduced into the inspired gas. Relaxants should be avoided, with reliance placed on spontaneous ventilation and assisted breaths when possible, since the ability to intubate the larynx and provide an airway is not always guaranteed. In many cases in which airway obstruction is severe, it is impossible with mask and positive-pressure ventilation to provide adequate gas flow through a limited orifice. However, during spontaneous ventilation even in the anesthetized state, the patient is able to breathe adequately.

Anesthesia is induced until it is judged that the patient will tolerate direct laryngoscopy. Laryngoscopy is then performed and at this time topical anesthesia, generally with 4% lidocaine, is applied to the oral pharynx and glottis.

The mask is reapplied, halothane-oxygen administered, and a judgment made as to whether or not the patient has responded unfavorably to this procedure. If conventional signs, including tachycardia, hypertension, tearing, or any other manifestations of light anesthesia are evident, then continued induction with halothane is carried out for an adequate period of time. When conditions again are favorable, a second laryngoscopy is undertaken and an attempt is made to topicalize the trachea by inserting the tracheal spray immediately below the cords. When an adequate depth of anesthesia is present, bronchoscopy can be undertaken.

During bronchoscopy, it is critical for the anesthesiologist to visually inspect the status of the airway with regard to the nature and extent of the lesion. This is important in terms of appreciating the difficulty of endotracheal tube placement and selection of the appropriate-size tube. There are several potential problems which must be considered at this time. Lesions involving the upper third of the trachea, especially those in the subglottic area, pose special problems with placement owing to cuff position. A lesion that is located high in the airway, where the tube cannot be passed through the lesion because of the limited orifice, will not allow the cuff to pass below the cords and results in inability to attain a complete seal of the airway. Selection of a tube which is small enough to pass through the lesion with the cuff below it produces additional problems due to decreased internal diameter, especially where 20 to 24 French tubes are utilized, and creates problems of potential airway obstruction with secretions and blood

during the operative procedure. Lesions located in the mid and lower thirds of the trachea are less problematic with respect to position but must be considered in view of the need to pass the tube through the lesion itself to maintain adequacy of ventilation until the trachea is transected, and/or the need to dilate the lesion at the time of bronchoscopy in order to provide adequacy of the airway. Dilatation must be considered with great caution owing to the risk of significant airway damage, complicated by bleeding or perforation into other structures such as the esophagus or great vessels. Grillo's approach has been to dilate strictures if the airway measures less than 5 mm in diameter.[22,23] Dilatation is done under direct vision with several rigid pediatric ventilating bronchoscopes. Dilators passed through a large bronchoscope may easily perforate the tracheobronchial wall, especially if the stricture is in the distal trachea. If the airway measures more than 5 mm, an endotracheal tube is generally passed to a point above the stricture in lesions of the mid to lower trachea and passed through it in lesions of the upper trachea. Caution must be exercised when tumors are present in the airway because of the potential for direct trauma if passage of the endotracheal tube results in obstruction from a dislodged piece of tumor with or without serious hemorrhage in the airway. Strictures of the anterior tracheal wall or stoma strictures are generally easily dealt with, since the mobile posterior membranous tracheal wall usually allows passage of an endotracheal tube or gas flow if the tube is positioned above the lesion.

Once bronchoscopy is completed, endotracheal intubation with the appropriate-size endotracheal tube is performed. This procedure is done in the usual manner by employing the sniffing position and direct laryngoscopy. As the tube is advanced down the airway, passage of the tube through the area of stricture can often be felt. Once the tube is thought to be in the appropriate position, the chest is auscultated in standard fashion to ensure bilateral lung ventilation. The tube is then secured, the eyes taped, and an esophageal stethoscope passed. Anesthesia is maintained with halothane-oxygen or, in cases in which normal pulmonary function exists and an adequate airway is present, with a combination of nitrous oxide and oxygen to supplement the halothane. Relaxants are avoided, and ventilation is generally accomplished by hand.

SURGICAL POSITIONING

As shown in Figure 13-6, several approaches are used depending upon the extent and location of the tracheal lesion. For most lesions located in the upper half of the trachea, an anterior collar incision is used with or without a vertical partial sternal split. For this incision, the patient is positioned supine with a thyroid bag or bolster placed under the shoulders and the head on a supporting doughnut. The back of the table is elevated approximately 10 to 15 degrees to position the cervical and sternal area parallel to the floor when the head is in the fully extended position. The arms are either left at the side or extended on arm boards at 90-degree angles. Exploration of the lesion is done through the anterior collar incision, and the sternum is divided later on if this is deemed necessary for surgical exposure.

Lesions of the lower half of the trachea

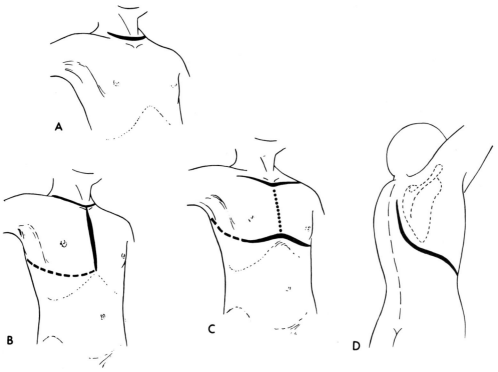

Fig. 13-6 Incisions for tracheal resection. (A) Standard collar incision for the majority of benign strictures and neoplastic lesions of the upper trachea. (B) Sternotomy extension: the dotted line shows an extension which may be carried through the fourth interspace to provide total exposure of the trachea from cricoid to carina. (C) Technique for raising a large bipedicle flap for total exposure and use in cases in which mediastinal tracheostomy is required. (D) Posterolateral thoracotomy, carried through the bed of the fourth rib or the fourth interspace for exposure of the lower half of the trachea. (Grillo HC: Congenital Lesions, Neoplasms, and Injuries of the Chest. In Sabiston DC and Spencer FC, Eds: Gibbon's Surgery of the Chest. W. B. Saunders Co., Philadelphia, 1976. Reprinted with permission of author and publisher.)

are approached through a right posterior lateral thoracotomy incision in the fourth interspace or in the bed of the fourth rib. The position for this incision is a standard left lateral decubitus with the right arm draped and prepared so that it can be moved into the field for easier access to the neck. In this position, it is necesasry to have intravenous and monitoring catheters in the left upper or lower extremities. In this position, a thoracotomy can be done and a collar incision added to free the trachea if there is need to perform a laryngeal release. In special cases of extensive or unusual lesions involving a greater area of the trachea, a vertical incision can be extended into the right and left fourth intercostal spaces from the sternal incision, as shown in Figure 13-6.

RECONSTRUCTION OF THE UPPER TRACHEA

For lesions of the upper half of the trachea the surgical approach is shown in Figure 13-7. A low, short collar incision is made across the neck and a T-incision is extended vertically over the sternum. Anterior dissec-

tion of the trachea is carried from the cricoid cartilage to the carina, with care taken not to injure the innominate artery or other structures adjacent to the trachea. Dissection around the back of the trachea is done at a point inferior to the lesion. If the patient has not been intubated through the stricture, caution must be undertaken during this dissection, since it is possible with release of the external supporting structure of the trachea to produce progressive, and eventually complete, airway obstruction.

During this portion of the cervical procedure, anesthesia is maintained through a previously placed oral endotracheal tube. At the point at which it is anticipated that the trachea will be divided, nitrous oxide is eliminated from the anesthetic gas mixture and anesthesia is maintained with halothane-oxygen alone. At this point, a tape is placed around the trachea below the lesion, and lateral traction sutures are placed through the full thickness of the tracheal wall in the midline on either side at a point no more than 2 cm below the point of division of the trachea. It is important to anticipate the placement of these sutures so that the cuff on the endotra-

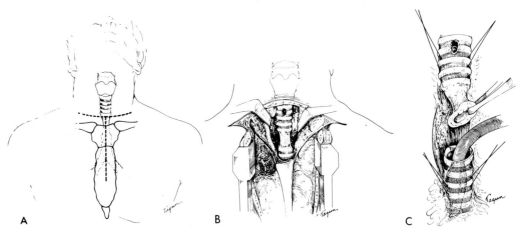

Fig. 13-7 Reconstruction of the upper trachea. (A) Collar incision and extension for upper sternotomy. (B) Dissection is carried down to isolate the damaged segment. (C) Circumferential dissection is carried out immediately beneath the lower level of pathology. Traction sutures are in place and the distal airway intubated via the operating field. (Grillo HC: Congenital Lesions, Neoplasms, and Injuries of the Chest. In Sabiston DC and Spencer FC, Eds: Gibbon's Surgery of the Chest. W. B. Saunders Co., Philadelphia, 1976. Reprinted with permission of author and publisher.)

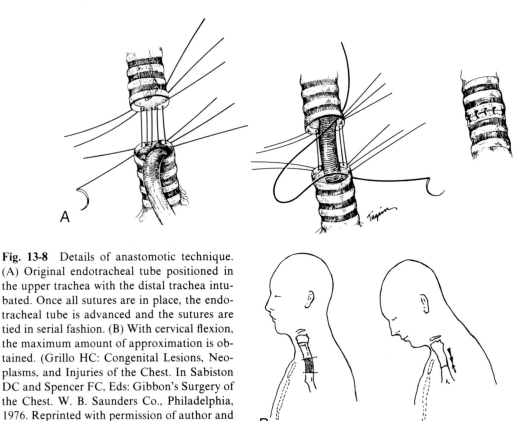

Fig. 13-8 Details of anastomotic technique. (A) Original endotracheal tube positioned in the upper trachea with the distal trachea intubated. Once all sutures are in place, the endotracheal tube is advanced and the sutures are tied in serial fashion. (B) With cervical flexion, the maximum amount of approximation is obtained. (Grillo HC: Congenital Lesions, Neoplasms, and Injuries of the Chest. In Sabiston DC and Spencer FC, Eds: Gibbon's Surgery of the Chest. W. B. Saunders Co., Philadelphia, 1976. Reprinted with permission of author and publisher.)

cheal tube may be deflated to prevent it from being injured by the suture needle. The trachea is then transsected below the lesion, as demonstrated in Figure 13-7C, and the distal trachea is intubated across the operative field with a flexible armored tube. The necessary sterile connecting equipment, consisting of corrugated tubings and Y-piece, are then passed to the anesthesiologist for connection to the anesthesia machine. The ability to ventilate the lungs is then assessed by use of positive pressure. The surgical dissection continues in order to free and excise the injured portion of the trachea.

Once adequacy of the tracheal lumen and extent of the tracheal resection have been determined, an attempt is made to approximate the two free ends of the trachea. This is accomplished by use of the traction sutures with the anesthesiologist flexing the

neck by grasping the head from above. When it is deemed possible to directly reanastomose the tracheal ends, intermittent sutures are placed through and through the trachea, with anesthesia continuing through the distal portion. In cases where it is not possible to bring the ends together owing to undue tension, a laryngeal release is performed. Once all sutures have been placed, the distal armored tube is removed and the oral endotracheal tube, which has remained in the proximal portion of the trachea, is advanced through the anastomosis into the distal trachea under direct vision (Fig. 13-8). Care must be taken at this point not to pass the tube too far distally in the trachea, since subsequent flexion of the neck for surgical foreshortening of the trachea will potentiate right mainstem bronchial intubation. Prior to this exchange, the airway is suctioned to remove aspirated blood. Anesthesia is then administered through the oral endotracheal tube into the distal trachea as the sutures are tied down to produce an airtight anastomosis. After all sutures have been placed, the patient's neck is flexed and the head supported in the position shown in Figure 13-8E.

At the completion of the operation, the patient should be breathing spontaneously, and extubation should be anticipated either under awake conditions or under moderately deep anesthesia. The selection of this technique, which is designed to afford a good airway, must be balanced against the occasional need to reintubate the patient if laryngeal difficulty and/or other aspects of unresected tracheal disease promote airway obstruction. In most cases, it is prudent to extubate patients in a deeper level of anesthesia and maintain the airway, thus avoiding the potential for struggling, bucking, and excessive neck motion which could injure the suture line. In patients in whom intubation was difficult because of upper airway pathology, it is prudent to allow the patient to awaken, supporting the head and neck during the excitement phase to avoid excessive motion. It is generally preferable to attempt extubation in the operating room, where the quality of airway patency may be quickly evaluated. Under such controlled circumstances, reintubation or diagnostic bronchoscopy can be done more easily and safely than in the recovery room or intensive care unit. Once the airway and ventilation are judged to be adequate, the patient can be safely transported, with supplemental oxygen, to the recovery room or intensive care unit.

RECONSTRUCTION OF THE LOWER
TRACHEA

The basic incision and surgical approach for the lower trachea has been described above. The general principles concerning intubation and early maintenance of anesthesia are similar to those described for the upper trachea with the exception of tube selection. In dealing with lower tracheal, and especially carinal, lesions it is advantageous to have a tube which is adequate in length to enter either mainstem bronchus. For this purpose an armored tube with an added extension of some 4 to 5 inches on the proximal portion is used to provide both flexibility at the distal end and adequate length for bronchial intubation. This tube is generally passed with aid of a stylet and positioned according to the anatomical location and extent of the lesion.

During the thoracotomy and surgical resection of the trachea, positive pressure ventilation is used while maintaining the ability of the patient to ventilate spontaneously, which is often needed during periods of discontinuity of the airway when positive pressure ventilation is not possible. Although ventilation is impaired with the open thorax, adequate gas exchange has been maintained with high-flow insufflation of oxygen and anesthetic agent while relying upon the dependent lung for the bulk of ventilation.

In general, resection involving the distal trachea and carina is carried out with the endotracheal tube in a position that is proximal to the lesion. Surgical exposure and resection is much the same as previously described for upper tracheal lesions. Once the trachea is divided, it is not infrequent to find that the distal tracheal stump is too short to hold the endotracheal tube and cuff. Under these circumstances, it is not convenient or possible to adequately ventilate both lungs. Generally, the left mainstem bronchus is intubated through the operative field and ventilation and anesthesia are carried out entirely via the left lung while the diseased segment is excised. Although it is theoretically possible temporarily to eliminate perfusion to the right lung with pulmonary artery clamping, this is often technically very difficult and entails the potential hazard of injury to the right pulmonary artery. In cases in which adequate oxygenation and ventilation are not attainable with one lung, an easy approach is to advance a second tube into the

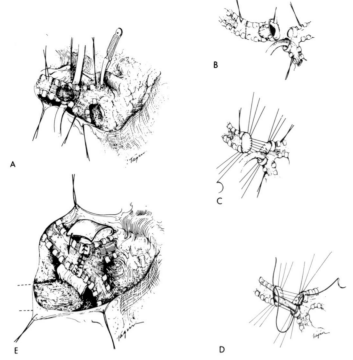

Fig. 13-9   Transthoracic approach. (A) The lesion in the distal trachea has been isolated and the right pulmonary artery is shown to be clamped, although this is not done routinely. (B) The trachea has been divided above the carina and the left main bronchus intubated. (C) Anastomotic sutures are placed by a procedure similar to that used in the upper trachea. (D) The endotracheal tube has been advanced through the anastomosis and the remaining sutures appropriately placed. (E) Anastomosis completed with a pedicle pleural flap secured for additional support. (Grillo HC: Congenital Lesions, Neoplasms, and Injuries of the Chest. In Sabiston DC and Spencer FC, Eds: Gibbon's Surgery of the Chest. W. B. Saunders Co., Philadelphia, 1976. Reprinted with permission of author and publisher.)

right mainstem bronchus, preferably in the bronchus intermedius. A second anesthesia machine and sterile tubings are used to maintain continuous positive airway pressure (5 cm water) with oxygen to the up lung, while ventilation is carried out in the dependent left lung. With lesions of the distal trachea not involving the carina, anastomosis and tube positioning are carried out in much the same way as for the upper tracheal lesions. This is depicted in Figure 13-9. Once the anastomosis is complete, it is prudent to withdraw the endotracheal tube back into the proximal trachea so that ventilation goes through the area of anastomosis.

In resections involving the carina in which end-to-end and end-to-side anastomosis between trachea and right and left mainstem bronchi must be carried out, a variety of tube manipulations and combinations of the previously considered maneuvers must be undertaken (Fig. 13-10). Generally, the right mainstem bronchus is anastomosed to the distal trachea and the left bronchus reim-

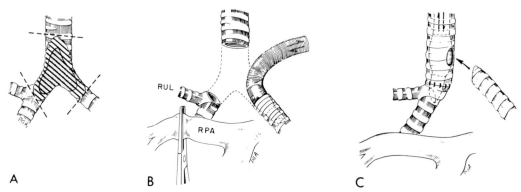

Fig. 13-10 Resection and reconstruction of the carina. (A) Tumor position is outlined by stippled area. (B) With the tube positioned in the left main bronchus, the right lung is mobilized and the stump of the right mainstem bronchus sutured into the trachea. (C) The left main bronchus is anastomosed in end-to-side fashion into the trachea. (Grillo HC: Congenital Lesions, Neoplasms, and Injuries of the Chest. In Sabiston DC and Spencer FC, Eds: Gibbon's Surgery of the Chest. W. B. Saunders Co., Philadelphia, 1976. Reprinted with permission of author and publisher.)

planted in end-to-side fashion into the bronchus intermedius or the distal trachea. It is not uncommon during such procedures to have significant periods of one-lung anesthesia, with the need to insufflate the second lung dictated by the level of arterial oxygenation.

Once all the anastomoses have been completed and adequacy of ventilation is assured by quality of breath sounds and visual inspection of chest wall expansion, closure of the surgical wound is undertaken in standard fashion.

When a right thoracotomy has been employed for surgical dissection, the decision as to whether or not to extubate the airway is of major importance. The potential for inadequacy of ventilation and pulmonary toilet must be balanced against the problems of continued intubation, potential infection, and direct trauma to the suture line. Providing that no significant parenchymal lung disease was present preoperatively, it is generally possible to extubate patients following thoracotomy and major carinal reconstruction without undue consequences. Exceptions are generally those patients in whom bilateral thoracotomy has been undertaken and significant postoperative pain is ex-

pected to limit cough and ventilation. These patients require tracheal intubation and some amount of mechanical ventilatory support. Following thoracotomy, the procedures for extubation are similar to those described for the upper airway approach. An exception is that the patient is generally taken out of the lateral position and placed supine prior to extubation to facilitate adequate exposure if reintubation is deemed necessary. The patient is transported to the recovery area once stability of circulation and adequacy of ventilation are achieved.

POSTOPERATIVE CARE

Postoperative patients are admitted to the intensive care unit for a minimum period of 24 hours. Patients are monitored by using ECG, arterial pressure, and serial arterial blood gases. A radiograph of the chest is obtained shortly following admission to ensure that a pneumothorax is not present. Sufficient oxygen is administered with a high-flow humidified system via a face mask to provide adequate arterial oxygenation and thinning of secretions. The head is maintained in the flexed position by a number of firm pillows placed behind the occiput and sutures located from the chin to the anterior chest. Chest physical therapy and routine nursing procedures are dictated by the nature of other underlying diseases and the ability to effectively maintain gas exchange and pulmonary toilet. Blind nasotracheal suctioning is undertaken with caution in those patients whose cough is inadequate to raise secretions. This is best done by physicians, chest physical therapists, or nurses trained specifically in this procedure. Potential complications include perforation of the anastomotic site and tracheal irritation with subsequent edema and airway obstruction, which may induce vomiting and aspiration. In cases in which abundant secretions are a problem, frequent transoral flexible fiberoptic bronchoscopy can be used to provide pulmonary toilet. This is especially true in cases in which the carina has been resected and secretions tend to pool in major bronchi without being propelled by normal mechanisms into the trachea. The need for emergency intubation because of hemorrhage, airway obstruction, or dehiscence of the anastomosis has arisen extremely rarely.

In cases of inadequate ventilation, with increasing levels of carbon dioxide and/or deterioration of oxygenation, endotracheal intubation is undertaken. This procedure must be done with caution, generally with the aid of sedation and topical anesthesia; the tube is placed either nasally or orally with direct visualization of the larynx. This can be accomplished with the patient maintained in the flexed position without producing undue stress on the suture line. Following intubation, the need for ventilation is reassessed after pulmonary toilet has been achieved, and therapy is directed at minimizing both positive pressure on the airway and the time for which the intubation is maintained. The latter is especially true in cases in which the endotracheal tube passes through the anastomosis (high tracheal reconstructions) because of the potential for dehiscence in an early stage of recovery. When prolonged intubation, generally con-

sidered more than 2 to 3 days, is anticipated, elective tracheostomy should be seriously considered. The hazards of the tracheostomy are dictated by body habitus, the location of the anastomosis, and the ability to safely dissect and position the tracheostomy tube following the reconstructive surgery.

Upper airway obstruction, secondary to laryngeal edema, is an infrequent complication. It has most commonly occurred when there has been a high anastomosis or previous history of laryngeal disease. When there is a history of cord paralysis and/or recurrent episodes of laryngeal edema or when the trachea is anastomosed directly to the larynx at the cricoid cartilage, prophylactic measures are taken to avoid laryngeal edema. This therapy includes use of high humidity and inhalation of topical steroids and racemic epinephrine. Dexamethasone and racemic epinephrine, 0.5 ml of a 1:200 dilution in 2.5 ml water, are administered with a nebulizer every 4 hours. Schedules are arranged so that inhalation of one or the other drug is achieved every 2 hours. This regimen is continued for a minimum of 24 hours, or longer if laryngeal edema, as evidenced by stridor and hoarseness, persists.

Patients should be kept in the intensive care unit for a period of one or more days until it is deemed safe to return them to a general surgical floor. This is dictated by the ability to discontinue cardiovascular monitoring, the need for repeated measurement of arterial blood gases, and the quality of nursing care. In most cases in which the procedure has been uncomplicated, patients are able to sit out of bed in a chair on the day following surgery and are often able to begin taking clear liquids and/or soft solids by the first postoperative day.

Summary of Results

Primary resection and reconstruction of the trachea and carina have been utilized for tumor surgery only since 1962. Primary tracheal tumors that are potentially removable, even by existing techniques, are extremely rare and hence the experience in any given institution is limited. From 1962 to 1977, 36 patients with primary or secondary tumors in the trachea underwent isolated tracheal resection and reconstruction at the Massachusetts General Hospital. In total, 56 patients were seen during this period and considered for resection of either primary or secondary airway tumors. Of the 56 patients, 10 had tumors involving the larynx that were too extensive for partial laryngectomy. In these cases, combined laryngotracheal resections were done with varying amounts of adjacent tissue removed to attempt cure. Ten additional patients, two with primary squamous-cell carcinomas of the trachea, five with very extensive adenoid cystic carcinomas, one with a granular cell tumor, and two with invasion by thyroid carcinomas could not have primary reconstruction. Excluding these 20 patients, there were 36 who successfully underwent resection of tumors with primary reconstruction.

In general, the experience and time course is too limited to make any conclusive statements regarding long-term outcome. Adenoid cystic carcinoma, in particular, may require 10 to 15 years, owing to its natural history, to fully evaluate the outcome of surgical therapy. Although the series of patients treated by primary resection and reconstruction for primary tumors is small, the results are encouraging.[11] If a patient is amenable to resection, the operation must be carefully planned and executed in an initial and definitive procedure with cure as the goal. Resection and primary reconstruction is the treatment of choice since secondary procedures almost never succeed. Results of treatment of benign strictures have, in general, been quite satisfactory. Grillo et al reported on the first 100 patients with end-to-end reconstruction of the trachea, a series completed in 1972.[26] In that series, 84 patients underwent resection and reconstruction for stenosis from a variety of causes. Seventy-three patients ob-

tained excellent functional results, with good to excellent anatomic reconstruction as judged radiologically. Four patients were listed as satisfactory and able to accomplish daily tasks without difficulty but with varying degrees of postoperative narrowing at the anastomotic site. Four failures occurred, and there were three deaths in the stenotic group.

Complications, as noted in that series, were quite varied: there were two cases of partial suture line separation with recovery; eight of granulomas at the suture line requiring removal with bronchoscopy; and five of late narrowing sufficient to be considered as partial restenosis. A variety of other infrequent problems such as wound infection, innominate artery bleeding, and partial vocal cord dysfunction are potential complications which have been seen in other series.

The majority of technical problems relating to tracheal reconstruction have been solved. It is clear that approximately half of the human trachea can be resected and reconstructed by the techniques described. In cases in which extensive amounts of trachea have been destroyed or involved with tumor, reconstruction is still not possible, since a satisfactory technique using prosthetic materials has not been devised.

REFERENCES

1. Meade JM: Tracheostomy in the management of respiratory problems. N Engl J Med 264:587-591, 1961
2. Andrews MJ, Pearson FG: Incidence and pathogenesis of tracheal injury following cuffed tube tracheostomy with assisted ventilation; analysis of a two-year prospective study. Ann Surg 173:249-263, 1971
3. Lindholm CE: Prolonged endotracheal intubation. Acta Anesthesiol Scand, suppl, 33:1969
4. Stauffer JL, Olson DE, Petty TL: Complications and consequences of endotracheal intubation and tracheostomy. A prospective study of 150 critically ill adult patients. Am J Med 70:65-76, 1981

5. Ching NPH, Ayres SM, Spina RC, et al: Endotracheal damage during continuous ventilatory support. Ann Surg 179:123-127, 1974

6. Cooper JD, Grillo HC: The evolution of tracheal injury due to ventilatory assistance through cuffed tubes. A pathologic study. Ann Surg 169:334-348, 1969

7. Carroll RG, McGinnis GF, Grenvik A: Performance characteristics of tracheal cuffs. Int Anesthesiol Clin 12:111-135, 1974

8. Crawley BE, Cross DE: Tracheal cuffs. A review in dynamic pressure study. Anesthesia 30:4-11, 1975

9. Cooper JD, Grillo HC: Experimental production and prevention of injury due to cuffed tracheal tubes. Surg Gynecol Obstet 129:1235-1241, 1969

10. Pavlin EG, Nelson E, Pulliam J: Difficulty in removal of tracheostomy tubes. Anesthesiology 44:69-70, 1976

11. Grillo HC: Congenital lesions, neoplasms and injuries of the trachea, pp. 256-293. In: Surgery of the Chest, W.B. Saunders, Philadelphia, 1976

12. Grillo HC: Tracheal tumors: surgical management. Ann Thorac Surg 26:112-125, 1978

13. Montgomery WW: The surgical management of supraglottic and subglottic stenosis. Ann Otol Rhinol Laryngol 77:534-546, 1968

14. Kryger M, Bode F, Antic R, et al: Diagnosis of obstruction of the upper and central airways. Am J Med 85-93, 1976

15. Hyatt RE, Black LF: The flow-volume curve. A current perspective. Am Rev Respir Dis 107:191-199, 1973

16. MacMillan AS, James AE Jr, Stitik FP, et al: Radiologic evaluation of post-tracheostomy lesions. Thorax 26:696-703, 1971

17. Pearson FG, Andrews MJ: Detection and management of tracheal stenosis following cuffed tube tracheostomy. Ann Thorac Surg 12:359-374, 1971

18. Lee P, English ICW: Management of anesthesia during tracheal resection. Anesthesia 29:305-306, 1974

19. Clarkson WB, Davies JR: Anesthesia for carinal resection. Anesthesia 33:815-819, 1978

20. Ellis RH, Hinds CJ, Gadd LT: Management of anesthesia during tracheal resection. Anesthesia 31:1076-1080, 1976

21. Geffin B, Bland J, Grillo HC: Anesthetic management of tracheal resection and reconstruction. Anesth Analg (Cleve) 48:884-894, 1969

22. Grillo HC: Circumferential resection and reconstruction of mediastinal and cervical trachea. Ann Surg 162:374, 1965

23. Grillo HC: Terminal or mural tracheostomy in the anterior mediastinum. J Thorac Cardiovasc Surg 51:422-427, 1966

24. Grillo HC: The management of tracheal stenosis following assisted respiration. J Thorac Cardiovasc Surg 57:521-71, 1969

25. Grillo HC: Surgical approaches to the trachea. Surg Gynecol Obstet 129:347-352, 1969.

26. Grillo HC: Reconstruction of the trachea. Experience in 100 consecutive cases. Thorax 28:667-679, 1973

TADIKONDA L.K. RAO, M.D.
ADEL A. EL-ETR, M.D.

14
Esophageal and Mediastinal Surgery

This chapter deals with the perioperative management of patients undergoing esophageal and other mediastinal surgery, excluding operations on the heart and the great vessels. For the safe anesthetic management of patients undergoing esophageal or mediastinal surgery, it is crucial for the anesthesiologist to understand the systemic effects produced by these lesions. After evaluation of these effects, the preoperative preparation, monitoring, intraoperative anesthetic course, and postoperative problems will be discussed.

ESOPHAGEAL SURGERY

The growth of esophageal surgery was limited by the developments in thoracic anesthesia. Various techniques to evaluate the functional status of the esophagus (radiologic studies, endoscopy, manometry, potential difference determination, acid perfusion test, pH reflux test, and esophageal motility studies) have been recently developed and perfected, allowing for the diagnosis of various surgical disorders of the esophagus.[1,2] Common conditions of the esophagus which are ameliorated by surgery include achalasia, stricture due to ingestion of caustics, especially in children, reflux esophagitis, and tumors.

Preoperative Evaluation

Assessment of the patient's physical status and correction of the biochemical abnormalities prior to surgery are of paramount importance in patients undergoing transthoracic esophageal surgery. Patients with optimized nutritional status have lower morbidity and mortality and decreased incidence of wound sepsis.[3,4]

NUTRITIONAL STATUS

Patients with esophageal strictures or tumors present with dysphagia. Initially, the dysphagia is to solid foods, but as the disease

447

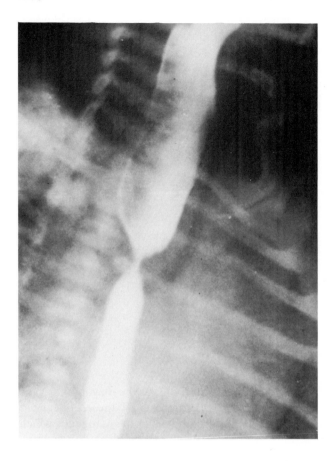

Fig. 14-1   Cancer in the upper third of the esophagus. The esophageal lumen is almost occluded by the tumor and the proximal esophagus is distended, forming a pouch.

progresses and the esophageal lumen narrows, the patients develop dysphagia to liquids. As a result, they may regurgitate the liquid food material. In a debilitated or a geriatric patient in whom the laryngeal reflexes are not intact, the regurgitant liquid may be aspirated into the tracheobronchial tree, resulting in atelectasis and/or pneumonia.[5] It may take many hours for the esophagus above the stricture to empty, and having the patient fast overnight prior to surgery does not guarantee an empty pouch above the stricture or obstruction (Figs. 14-1 and 14-2). Therefore, regurgitation and aspiration during induction of anesthesia is of great concern. Poor nutrition leads to secondary metabolic and functional consequences. The metabolic changes that are of special interest to anesthesiologists are summarized below.

1. Dehydration and depletion of body fluids are present. Administration of potent intravenous or inhalational drugs to hypovolemic patients may result in severe hypotension and cardiac arrest.

2. Hypoalbuminemia commonly occurs as a result of greatly reduced protein intake, and albumin values lower than 1 gm% may be seen. Most of the drugs used in anesthetic practice, including thiopental, muscle relaxants, and local anesthetics, are highly protein-bound (the protein-bound moiety is inactive). Since hypoalbuminemic patients have very low albumin values, these drugs may not find enough albumin sites to bind. With an increase in the unbound drug in the plasma, an exaggerated response may result.[6] When local anes-

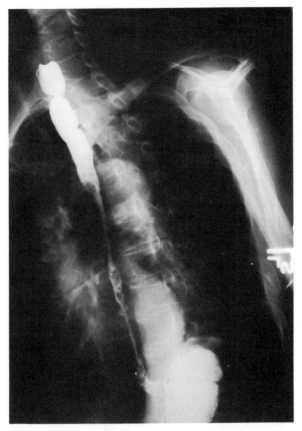

Fig. 14-2 Twenty-four hours following a barium swallow, contrast material can still be seen in the esophagus.

thetics are used, unbound drug in the plasma may reach toxic threshold values and ordinary doses may result in convulsions or cardiovascular depression. In addition, albumin plays a key role in the Starling forces in the lung, which tend to keep the alveoli dry. Further reduction in the oncotic pressure secondary to crystalloid administration during surgery, or an increase in pulmonary intravascular pressure due to either fluid overload or early left ventricular dysfunction, can easily precipitate fulminant pulmonary edema.

3. Low levels of hemoglobin, due either to poor iron intake or to chronic bleeding from the site of the tumor, are frequently seen. If the anemia develops over a period of time, these patients may compensate by increased cardiac output and a shift of the oxyhemoglobin dissociation curve to the right. Potent anesthetic drugs may depress the increased cardiac output, resulting in tissue hypoperfusion. Hyperventilation or overzealous alkalinization may negate the right-sided shift of the oxyhemoglobin dissociation curve. Thus, drugs causing myocardial depression should be used carefully, and mechanical ventilation should aim for normocarbia.

4. Electrolytes may be altered secondary to starvation, commonly producing either hypokalemia or hypomagnesemia. Hy-

pokalemia may be accentuated by unintentional hyperventilation or alkalinization, leading to cardiac dysrhythmias, especially in a digitalized patient. Low levels of magnesium may cause alterations in the electrocardiogram and in neuromuscular transmission.

5. Prerenal failure as manifested by decreased urine output and increased BUN and creatinine may be seen secondary to limited fluid intake. Prerenal azotemia should be evaluated and corrected prior to surgical intervention.

6. Malnutrition suppresses the immune response and impedes wound healing.[7] These two abnormalities may increase the risk of wound infection. Malnutrition also decreases muscle power, and a poorly nourished patient is more likely to develop postoperative respiratory complications.

All the above-mentioned metabolic abnormalities and functional consequences could be corrected by parenteral nutrition. In the past 25 years, researchers in this country and in Europe have developed and refined fat and nitrogen sources, which when combined with hypertonic glucose solutions provide the essential caloric and macronutrient requirements. Trace minerals and other micronutrients such as vitamins can be incorporated in these solutions. Administration of these parenteral solutions through an intravenous infusion for 2 to 3 weeks can greatly improve the nutritional status of these patients prior to surgery.[8]

Total parenteral nutrition can be defined as the intravenous administration of nitrogen, caloric sources, and other essential nutrients in amounts sufficient to achieve tissue synthesis and anabolism in patients with normal or excessive nutritional needs. The concept of intravenous therapy is not new. In 1968, Dudrick et al published work outlining how six beagle puppies were fed entirely by the intravenous route for periods ranging from 72 to 256 days, after which they were compared with their orally fed littermates.[9] In all cases, they not only exceeded the controls in weight gain but also matched them in skeletal growth, development, and activity. In 1969, the same authors demonstrated the successful use of total parenteral nutrition in over 300 patients with diseases that totally precluded nourishment by the gastrointestinal tract.[10] These reports opened the floodgates to the techniques of prolonged intravenous feeding as the sole means of nutritional support.

Indications for parenteral nutrition in patients with dysphagia include: (1) inability to swallow any food; (2) greater than 10 percent decrease in ideal body weight; (3) serum albumin < 3 gm %; (4) anergy; (5) total lymphocyte count < 1000 cells per mm,[3] and (6) serum transferrin < 180 mg %.

The solution should supply the complete nutritional needs, including caloric requirements, nitrogen, minerals, vitamins, fatty acids, and water (Table 14-1).[11,12] Daily caloric requirements are about 30 kcal/kg for normal ambulatory patients, but following elective surgery this may increase to 40 kcal/kg. In hypermetabolic states such as severe sepsis, extensive burns, and maximum stress, the caloric requirements may have to be increased to as much as 80 kcal/kg. Concentrated dextrose solution is the caloric

Table 14-1
Parenteral Nutrient Intake Daily Dose Range in Adults

Nutrient	Amount
Water	2,500–3,500 ml
Calories	2,500–3,500 kcal
Glucose	600–900 gm
Protein equivalent, as amino acids or protein hydrolysates	60–130 gm
Sodium	70–180 mEq
Potassium	90–150 mEq
Calcium	4–10 mEq
Magnesium	12–24 mEq
Phosphate	20–30 mEq

Vitamin, trace minerals, and essential fatty acid allowances as required.

source in the nutrient. Normal adults tolerate 0.5 g/kg per hour of glucose without significant urinary loss. Since these solutions are extremely hypertonic (2,000 mOsm/L), they must be administered into a high-flow venous system to permit rapid dilution and minimal vascular damage. This can be achieved by delivering the solution to the superior vena cava by either the subclavian route or the internal jugular venous route.

Recently, fat emulsions have been introduced for intravenous administration (Intralipid).[13] This contains 10 percent soybean oil and egg yolk phospholipid and provides 1.1 kcal/ml in an isotonic neutral form. Since the solution is isotonic, it can be administered through a peripheral vein. Parenteral administration of fat emulsions is contraindicated in patients with liver disease, pathologic hyperlipedemic conditions, or bleeding diathesis.

Complications due to parenteral nutrition may be secondary to solution preparation, catheter placement and organ injury, fungal infections, and metabolic derangements[14,15] (Table 14-2). However, the use of total parenteral nutrition in these dysphagic patients with esophageal lesions can bring them back to optimal nutritional status preoperatively.

Anesthesia and surgery in patients receiving parenteral nutrition pose special problems. The risk of intraoperative hypoglycemia is of special importance in these patients.[16] The islet cells of the pancreas are stimulated during the infusion of dextrose-rich solutions and the patients have high levels of endogenous insulin. If the infusion is stopped, the islet cells continue to secrete insulin when the patient arrives in the operating room, and intraoperative hypoglycemia may develop within 45 to 60 minutes. If the hypoglycemic episode is prolonged, it may result in delayed awakening or coma in the postoperative period. This problem can be avoided either by infusing the parenteral nutrition solution throughout the intraopera-

Table 14-2

Complications Secondary to Total Parenteral Nutrition

Metabolic complications secondary to infusate
Overhydration
Dehydration
Hyperosmolar coma
Hypoglycemia or hyperglycemia
Additive incompatabilities
Allergic reaction
Pyrogenic reaction
Specific deficiency
Specific excess
Hepatic encephalopathy
Metabolic acidosis
Hypermetabolism
Hypercapnia
Mechanical system complications
Sepsis
Trauma
Thrombosis
Embolism
Psychologic adjustment

tive period at half the presurgical flow rate or by substituting 10 percent dextrose in water at the same infusion rate. Either technique prevents the intraoperative hypoglycemia, but monitoring of the blood sugar in the perioperative period is still indicated.

The administration of glucose-rich parenteral nutritional solutions in excess of what is required results in lipogenesis.[17] Oxidation of glucose for energy purposes results in a nonprotein respiratory quotient (RQ) of 1.0; but when excess solution is administered, glucose is converted to lipids. This lipogenesis requires a certain amount of energy expenditure and results in a small increase in oxygen consumption together with a nonprotein RQ which rises above 1.0, resulting in an increased production of carbon dioxide.

Patients breathing spontaneously increase their ventilation to get rid of excess CO_2 produced. However, when these patients are paralyzed and mechanically ventilated intraoperatively, the use of normal minute ventilation may result in severe hypercarbia. This can be prevented by hyperventilation, sometimes in excess of twice the normal minute ventilation. Postoperatively, the increase in CO_2 production may be a critical factor inhibiting the weaning of a patient from mechanical ventilatory support. Decreasing the glucose load or changing to fat emulsions with an RQ of 0.7 may be useful in these circumstances.[17]

PULMONARY STATUS

Immediately following thoracotomy, the functional residual capacity decreases up to 60 percent of the preoperative value.[18] Pulmonary reserve should be carefully evaluated in the preoperative period since patients undergoing esophageal surgery for hiatal hernia may have altered respiratory function. Respiratory changes associated with a hiatus hernia are a reduction in maximum voluntary ventilation and an increase in residual lung volume. Examination of a group of patients by ^{133}Xe radiospirometry in the supine position revealed a significant reduction in the regional ventilation, perfusion, and lung volume.[19,20]

Patients with esophageal cancer and obstruction may develop chronic regurgitation and aspiration resulting in pneumonic consolidation. Chronic smokers should be advised to refrain from smoking for at least 2 weeks prior to surgery, and deep breathing exercises and postural drainage should be used to clear up secretions. Pulmonary changes may occur secondary to chemotherapeutic drugs and will be discussed under preoperative chemotherapy.

CARDIAC STATUS

Controversy still exists regarding preoperative prophylactic digitalization of patients with no history of congestive failure undergoing thoracic surgery.[21–23] Thoracotomy and manipulation of the lungs, heart, and mediastinum are associated with a high incidence of supraventricular tachydysrhythmias either intraoperatively or postoperatively.

Preoperative digitalization has been shown to decrease both the incidence of these dysrhythmias and the mortality from postoperative congestive heart failure.[24] However, others have warned that the hazards of digitalis toxicity may outweigh the beneficial effects of prophylactic digitalization, since during prophylactic digitalization there is no clinical endpoint to which the drug can be titrated, i.e., tachycardia, increased jugular venous pulse, dyspnea, or edema.[25] Thus, in patients receiving digitalis prophylactically, intraoperative digitalis toxicity may occur.

INFLUENCE OF OLD AGE

Most of the patients undergoing esophageal cancer surgery are in the geriatric age group, which adds the problems of: (1) low cardiopulmonary reserve requiring mechanical ventilatory assistance in the immediate postoperative period; (2) cardiovascular and cerebrovascular accidents in the perioperative period; (3) prostatic enlargement; and (4) poor mental adjustment.[26]

PREOPERATIVE CHEMOTHERAPY

Patients with esophageal cancer are often treated with chemotherapeutic drugs prior to surgery. These drugs affect not only the cancer cells but also rapidly growing normal cells (erythropoiesis, leukocyte and platelet production, and gastrointestinal tract lining). Commonly used chemotherapeutic drugs in carcinoma of the esophagus belong to the antibiotic group, which includes adriamycin, bleomycin, and mitomycin C. The anticancer effect of these antibiotics is produced by formation of relatively stable complexes with DNA, which inhibits DNA and/or RNA synthesis or both.[27]

Toxicity secondary to adriamycin includes severe cardiomyopathy, seen in 1.8 percent of patients treated. When cardiomyopathy develops, it has been shown to be irreversible in 60 percent of the patients, with death occurring within 3 weeks of the onset of the symptoms.[28] Prior history of heart disease or ECG abnormality increases the risk of cardiomyopathy.

The left ventricular failure that occurs with adriamycin is refractory to inotropic drugs. Other cardiac abnormalities associated with adriamycin toxicity include ECG abnormalities such as supraventricular tachydysrhythmias, premature ventricular and supraventricular contractions, abnormal conduction patterns, and a variety of nonspecific ST-T wave changes. These ECG abnormalities resolve 1 to 2 months after cessation of therapy.[29]

Bleomycin's action is similar to the effect of radiation, and bleomycin and radiation may act synergistically during simultaneous therapy.[30] It rarely causes bone marrow depression, but pulmonary toxicity is the most life-threatening drug-limiting effect, reported in 15 to 25 percent of patients.[31,32] Predisposing factors include age greater than 20 years, dose greater than 400 units, underlying pulmonary disease, and prior radiation therapy. Signs and symptoms of pulmonary toxicity are cough, dyspnea, and basal rales. The disease may manifest itself with minimal radiologic changes and normal resting PaO_2, or it may progress to severe hypoxemia at rest, with radiological changes similar to severe adult respiratory distress syndrome. A factor that predisposes patients to pulmonary toxicity is the administration of oxygen in higher concentrations. Thus, they are at a high risk of developing pulmonary toxicity in the perioperative period, when they may receive high concentrations of supplemental oxygen, either intraoperatively or postoperatively.[33] This risk can be decreased by reduction in FIO_2 both during surgery and in the immediate postoperative period.

Mitomycin C is also highly toxic and can cause pulmonary fibrosis and nephrotoxicity.[34] Thus, patients receiving mitomycin C should have their pulmonary and renal status fully evaluated in the preoperative period.

Monitoring

Consideration should be given to the patient's associated systemic diseases, the duration of surgery, and the anesthetic technique used. Monitoring includes standard sphygmomanometry, electrocardiography, temperature probe, radial artery cannulation, central venous catheterization, and urinary output measurement. A pulmonary artery catheter may be inserted prior to anesthetic induction if there is an indication to monitor left atrial filling pressure, as in patients with a history of previous myocardial infarction or in patients with minimal cardiovascular reserve. Careful and close monitoring of the cardiovascular system and immediate correction of any hemodynamic aberration in patients with unstable hemodynamics or a recent myocardial infarction have been associated with a very low incidence of perioperative reinfarction.[35] Blood sugar and arterial PO_2 should be frequently monitored depending on the clinical situation.

Airway Consideration

PROXIMAL POUCH

Emphasis should be given to the presence of liquid or solid food particles above the esophageal obstruction in patients with a history of dysphagia. The esophageal pouch proximal to obstruction should be emptied by passing a large nasogastric tube and suctioning prior to induction of anesthesia. In spite of these attempts, this pouch may not be completely empty, and these patients should be considered to have a full stomach.

TRACHEAL COMPRESSION

Another important consideration is that following anesthetic induction the trachea may be compressed by large mediastinal lymph nodes; in which case, the patient may

Table 14-3
Drugs and Esophageal Function

	Increase Tone	Decrease Tone	No Effect
Upper esophagus	Decamethonium	Curare	Atropine
Body of esophagus	Propranolol Metoclopromide	Atropine Isoproterenol Trimethaphan	Epinephrine Phenoxybenzamine Phentolamine

Lower esophageal sphincter	Methacholine
	Bethanechol
	Norepinephrine
	Metoclopramide
	Cyclizine
	Prostaglandin F_2
	Atropine 1.2 mg and
	     neostigmine 5 mg
		Atropine
		Morphine
		Meperidine
		Diazepam
		Droperidol
		Phentolamine
		Isoproterenol
		Hexamethonium
		Amyl nitrite
		Prostaglandin E_1
		Volatile anesthetic
		     agents
			Propranolol
			Phenylephrine
			Atropine 1.2 mg and
			     neostigmine 2.5 mg

Adapted from: Owitz et al., Anesthesiol Rev 8:21–25, 1981.

not be able to be ventilated by bag and mask. This airway obstruction can be relieved only by passing an endotracheal tube distal to the tracheal compression.

LOWER ESOPHAGEAL SPHINCTER

Patients with a hiatal hernia have an obliterated esophagogastric angle and physiologically incompetent or dysfunctioning lower esophageal sphincter.[36] They are thus prone to regurgitation and aspiration during induction of anesthesia. Many drugs affect esophageal function (Table 14-3). With all these considerations, intubation should be performed either in an awake patient with sedation and topical anesthesia or by rapid-sequence induction.

AWAKE INTUBATION

To alleviate apprehension and discomfort, the patient can be sedated with small incremental doses of either diazepam or Innovar. The oropharynx and laryngopharynx are topically anesthetized with a local anesthetic spray. Once the patient tolerates laryngoscopy, the trachea is intubated, and after the airway has been secured the patient can be anesthetized with thiopental.

RAPID-SEQUENCE INDUCTION

The patient is preoxygenated for 5 minutes for denitrogenation purposes. If succinylcholine is to be used for muscle relaxation for intubation, pretreatment with a small dose of a nondepolarizing muscle relaxant is recommended to prevent fasciculations and the subsequent rise in intragastric pressure, especially in patients with a hiatus hernia. A sleep dose of thiopental is rapidly administered and a skilled assistant provides cricoid pressure (Sellick's maneuver) to occlude the esophagus. The trachea is intubated 30 to 60 seconds following the administration of succinylcholine, during which time no positive pressure ventilation is applied. Again, once the airway is secured and sealed, the maintenance anesthetics are started.

Careful positioning during induction of anesthesia, intubation, and operation is important. In patients with a hiatus hernia, who may also be obese, the supine position during induction of anesthesia and intubation may precipitate regurgitation and aspiration. Induction and intubation may be safely done in these patients with a head-up position, which reduces the incidence of regurgitation. In patients with an esophageal stricture secondary to cancer and an empty proximal esophageal pouch, anesthetic induction and intubation can be done in the supine position.

SELECTION OF ENDOTRACHEAL TUBES

The upper third of the esophagus can be approached from a cervical incision and the lower third of the esophagus can be approached through a laparotomy and splitting of the diaphragm. In these instances, a regular endotracheal tube can be satisfactorily used. The midthoracic esophagus is approached via a thoracotomy, either left-sided or right-sided.[26] Advantages of a left thoracotomy include the ability to split open the left diaphragm, mobilize the stomach, and bring it up into the chest without having to change the patient's position. The disadvantages of a right thoracotomy are that the position of the patient must be changed after the abdominal part of the operation is completed. In addition, after an extensive procedure in the abdomen and opening of the chest, the lesion may be found to be nonresectable. However, a right thoracotomy has the advantage of allowing the surgeon to perform a bypass between the esophagus and the fundus of the stomach with complete relief from dysphagia in the presence of an unresectable lesion. Also, if the azygos vein is infiltrated by tumor, it is safer to dissect it from the right.

Whether the thoracotomy is on the right or left side, use of one-lung anesthesia during the dissection of the midthoracic portion of the esophagus provides a quiet operating field for the surgeon and may facilitate the operation. Any of the available double-lumen tubes can be used; since its purpose is only to collapse the nondependent lung, providing easy access to the posterior mediastinum.

Following intubation, the patient is placed in either the right or left lateral position for the thoracotomy. Care should be taken regarding the function of intravenous infusion catheters, patency of the arterial catheter, venous return from the lower extremities, pressure on the nerves of the upper extremities and the eyes, and position of the endotracheal tube. If a standard endotracheal tube is used, breath sounds must be checked over both lung fields to avoid accidental endobronchial intubation during the movement of the patient. If an endobronchial tube is used and was satisfactorily placed in the supine position, the same maneuvers should be made after lateral positioning to ensure proper positioning of the endobronchial tube.

The major disadvantage of one-lung anesthesia is hypoxemia due to the persistent perfusion of the collapsed, nondependent lung despite the effect of gravity diverting most of the pulmonary circulation to the ventilated, dependent lung.[37] When one-lung anesthesia is instituted in pulmonary surgery, usually the nondependent, collapsed lung is diseased with decreased blood supply and so the magnitude of hypoxemia is less.[38] If the pulmonary artery to this lung is ligated, the arterial oxygen tension significantly increases. In nonpulmonary surgery, such as esophageal surgery, the lung is not diseased and the pulmonary artery is never ligated. The hypoxemia that occurs in these situations is of greater magnitude and persists as long as the lung is collapsed.[39]

Normally, decreased regional alveolar PO_2 leads to regional pulmonary vasoconstriction known as *hypoxic pulmonary vasoconstriction*.[40] This diverts the pulmonary blood flow from hypoventilated or nonventilated lung to the ventilated areas of the lung. The mechanism of the hypoxic pulmonary vasoconstriction response is not well understood. Commonly used inhalation anesthetic drugs have been shown to abolish this reflex, resulting in increased true intrapulmonary shunt.[41] However, intravenous anesthetic drugs such as ketamine and fentanyl do not inhibit this reflex[42] (Ch. 8).

Intrapulmonary shunt during one-lung anesthesia could worsen when high airway pressure is used. When the alveolar pressure exceeds the intravascular pressure, flow through the dependent ventilated lung is shifted to the nondependent, nonventilated lung. This could be minimized by utilizing lower airway pressures, attained by small tidal volumes and increased respiratory rates.

Intraoperative Considerations

Maintenance of anesthesia can be readily achieved with inhalational drugs in oxygen. If hypoxemia worsens because of abolition of hypoxic pulmonary vasoconstriction, the inhalational drug can be stopped and anesthesia maintained with intravenous supplementation of either ketamine or fentanyl.

The following intraoperative problems can occur during esophageal surgery.[43] The carotid sinus reflex may be stimulated during neck dissection, resulting in bradycardia and hypotension, which can be easily reversed with 0.4 to 0.6 mg atropine sulfate administered intravenously.

Hypotension may also be secondary to hypovolemia from intraoperative blood loss or from inferior vena caval obstruction during the dissection of the lower end of the esophagus. Injury to major veins or arteries during dissection of the tumor may lead to sudden hemorrhage.

Deliberate hypotensive anesthesia can be used during esophageal surgery to decrease the blood loss and improve the surgical field. However, many of these patients may be medically unsuited for the deliberate hypotensive anesthesia technique. It may also be desirable to maintain the arterial pressure at near normal levels to ensure adequate perfusion of the graft in a colon interposition.

Rupture of the trachea can occur during the dissection of the middle third of the esophagus. When an endobronchial tube is used for intubation purposes, the tracheal lumen is clamped, and one lung can be satisfactorily ventilated and protected through the endobronchial lumen until the trachea is repaired. If an endotracheal tube is used, it should be pushed down the trachea until an endobronchial intubation occurs, following which one lung could be safely ventilated until the trachea is repaired.

During cervical exploration of the esophagus, with movement of the neck and with the anesthesiologist removed from close proximity to the head, anesthetic circuit disconnection is a potential hazard. The connection between the endotracheal tube adapter and the Y-connector is particularly vulnerable. Care must be taken regarding a tight fit of all the system connections.

Postoperative Complications

Immediate complications include hypotension secondary to hypovolemia or bleeding, pneumothorax, and atelectasis.

Delayed awakening or inability to regain consciousness can occur in the immediate postoperative period. This may be due to an intraoperative cerebrovascular accident, to prolonged hypoglycemia in a patient who was on parenteral nutrition therapy which was discontinued during the operation, or to hyperosmolar coma in a patient who received excessive volumes of parenteral nutrition fluid. Hypoglycemia can be avoided by monitoring blood glucose values frequently during the intraoperative period and treating with dextrose solutions if needed. Hyperosmolar coma can be prevented by reducing the rate of fluid infusion and supplementing the total fluid intake with intravenous 5 percent dextrose in water.[16]

Delayed complications include bilateral or unilateral pleural effusion, sepsis, leak from the anastomotic site resulting in mediastinitis, or hydro- or pyothorax.[43]

Hypoxemia and atelectasis secondary to hypoventilation due to incisional pain is a common immediate postoperative problem.[44] The incisional pain can be relieved either by parenteral analgesics, intercostal nerve blocks, epidural block using either local anesthetics or narcotics, or intrathecal narcotics. When parenteral analgesics are administered in the immediate postoperative period, the $PaCO_2$ remains in the normal range, but it is associated with a significant decrease in PaO_2 due to an increase in venous admixture and a low V/Q ratio. Parenteral narcotics also abolish occasional spontaneous deep breathing. Their inhibitory effect on the gastrointestinal motility, which causes bowel distention, results in chest roentgenograms with a "high diaphragm".[45] This high diaphragm interferes with respiratory mechanics, further decreasing functional residual capacity and causing significant airway closure, which results in increased venous admixture.

When unilateral intercostal nerve blocks are used for pain relief, the pulmonary functions significantly improve in the postoperative period.[46] Epidural block with local anesthetics leads to a normal respiratory rate with larger tidal volumes and preservation of spontaneous deep breaths.[47] Epidural blockade also results in stimulation of gastric propulsion due to sympathetic blockade and increased vagal tone, which avoids a high diaphragm and its respiratory consequences. However, the sympathetic block produced by epidural analgesia may produce unwarranted hypotension in the immediate postoperative period. This can be avoided by using the recently introduced epidural or intrathecal narcotics. Good analgesia with no sympathetic or motor block can be produced in these patients either by epidural meperidine or fentanyl or by intrathecal morphine.[48]

Because of the low lipid solubility of morphine, it does not cross the dura mater easily. Thus epidural morphine produces minimal analgesia compared with intrathecal morphine. However, meperidine and fentanyl are more lipid-soluble than morphine and can easily cross the dura mater and produce analgesia. When fentanyl or meperidine are used for epidural analgesia, either 50 to 100 μg of fentanyl in 5 ml of normal saline or 30 to 50 mg of meperidine in 5 ml of normal saline can be used every 8 hours. Morphine in doses of 1 to 3 mg administered intrathecally produces excellent analgesia for postoperative pain. Epidural and intrathecal narcotic administration for pain relief is associated with very few side effects. However, when large quantities of narcotics are administered either epidurally or intrathecally, small concentrations may reach the floor of the fourth ventricle and can cause respiratory arrest.

MEDIASTINAL SURGERY

The mediastinum is an extremely important and complex portion of the thorax extending from the superior aperture to the diaphragm and bound laterally by the mediastinal pleura and posteriorly by the vertebral bodies. It contains important anatomic structures and organs, and it is the site of numerous primary and secondary disorders. The most commonly found tumors of the mediastinum in descending order of occurrence are: neurogenic tumors (neurilemmoma, neurofibroma, neurosarcoma, ganglioneuroma, neuroblastoma, sympathicoblastoma, paraganglioma, and pheochromocytoma), cysts (bronchogenic, pericardial, enteric, and nonspecific), teratodermoids, lymphomas, thymomas, and miscellaneous tumors, which include parathyroid adenomas, retrosternal thyroid tumors, and others[49] (see Fig. 14-3).

The plethora of symptoms associated with mediastinal disorders vary widely. Two-thirds of the lesions are associated with symptoms which include chest pain, cough, recurrent respiratory infections, dysphagia,

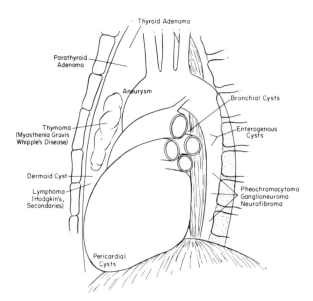

Fig. 14-3   Commonly occurring mediastinal tumors.

and dyspnea. There is a positive correlation between malignancy of the mediastinal mass and the presence of symptoms. The common mediastinal lesions and their associated perioperative problems are discussed below.

Thymoma and Myasthenia Gravis

SYSTEMIC EVALUATION

Thymoma

Thymoma is the most common neoplasm originating in the anterior mediastinum. Thymic tumors occur with equal frequency in both sexes, with a peak incidence between the fourth and sixth decades. Seventy percent of the patients with a thymic tumor have an associated systemic syndrome. Myasthenia gravis is the most commonly associated disease, occurring in 10 to 50 percent of patients with a thymoma. Other systemic diseases associated with thymomas are red-cell aplasia, hypogammaglobulinemia, collagen vascular diseases, megaesophagus, myocarditis, and nonthymic malignancies.

Myasthenia Gravis

Myasthenia gravis (MG) is a chronic disorder of neuromuscular synaptic transmission caused by an autoimmune response to acetylcholine receptors (AChR) of the postsynaptic muscle membrane. It is characterized by easy fatigability and weakness of skeletal muscles.

More than 85 percent of patients with myasthenia gravis have a thymic abnormality: 15 percent of the patients have thymomas, and more than 70 percent have thymic hyperplasia. The germinal centers in this hyperplastic thymus have an abnormal number of B cells.

Myasthenia gravis is classified into the three types characterized below.[50]

Neonatal MG occurs in the newborns of myasthenic mothers and is self-limiting. It is due to the passive transfer of AChR antibodies from the mother to the fetus. Improvement of MG symptoms in the infant is associated with a declining antibody titer, which may take from 1 to 8 weeks.

Ocular MG comprises a group involving only ocular muscles. The symptoms include ptosis and diplopia. These patients show good response to prednisone therapy and there is no increased incidence of mortality with this form of the disease.

Generalized MG can be further subdivided into four types.

In *mild* generalized MG, ocular manifestations are frequent. The disease gradually spreads to skeletal and bulbar muscles, but respiratory muscles are not involved. Patients with mild generalized MG show a good response to prednisone therapy.

In *moderate* generalized MG, ocular muscles are initially involved, with gradual onset in skeletal and bulbar muscles. This may be associated with dysarthria, dysphagia, and masticatory problems. Respiratory muscles are not involved, but the response to prednisone therapy is only fair. The general activity of patients with this form is restricted, but again is associated with low mortality.

In the *acute fulminating* form, the symptoms have a rapid onset, with severe skeletal and bulbar muscle involvement, and the respiratory muscles are involved early in the course of the disease. A high percentage of these patients have associated thymomas. The response to prednisone therapy is fair to poor, but plasmaphoresis may alleviate the symptoms. Patients with acute fulminating MG have restricted activity, but the disease is associated with low mortality.

The *late severe* form occurs in patients who have a mild or moderate MG but who develop severe symptoms about 2 years after the onset of the disease. These patients usually do not respond to drug therapy, and mortality among them is high.

Etiology of Myasthenia Gravis. The etiology and pathogenesis of MG are still not completely understood. However, diverse and extensive studies of this disease have shown that the defect in the neuromuscular transmission in MG is localized to the motor end-plate of striated muscles, which shows morphological, electrophysiological, and biochemical abnormalities.[51-54] These changes may be due to the presence of humoral antibodies, detected in the serum of most patients with MG, that bind to the nicotinic acetylcholine receptors.[55,56]

Both humoral and cellular immune responses, but mainly humoral AChR antibodies, are directed against AChR in most patients with MG. These antibodies lead to a decreased concentration of functional AChR in the motor end-plate of skeletal muscles. This may be due to: (1) AChR antibodies blocking the access of acetylcholine to AChR; (2) bound antibodies stimulating the lysis of the postsynaptic membrane; (3) accelerated AChR degradation; (4) inhibition of AChR synthesis; or (5) alteration in AChR ion conductance interactions[57] (see Fig. 14-4).

There is much evidence to substantiate the importance of AChR antibodies in clinical MG, but various host factors can modify the individual response to the antibody, for example, as follows: (1) A patient with MG may have a high titer of circulating AChR antibody and be clinically normal, or may have severe manifestations of the disease with undetectable antibody titer.[58] (2) Identical AChR antibodies have produced different degrees of clinical symptoms of weakness in different individuals.[57] (3) AChR antibody-binding specificity with the AChR can be a factor in determining the clinical state of patients with myasthenia gravis.[59] The reason for the initiation of the immune response to the patient's own antigen (AChR) in MG is unknown at the present time, but genetic and environmental factors both may play a role in determining the occurrence of the autoimmune response.

Diagnosis. Moderately severe and severe MG can be easily diagnosed by history

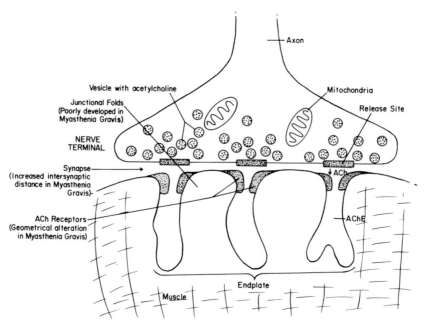

Fig. 14-4   Neuromuscular junction in patients with myasthenia gravis.

and physical examination alone. Mild cases of MG have to be differentiated from other central nervous system diseases, including poliomyelitis, amyotrophic lateral sclerosis, pseudobulbar paralysis, encephalitis, multiple sclerosis, and psychiatric fatigue as seen in severe neurasthenia and conversion hysteria.[60] Various tests that can be performed to help in the diagnosis of MG are listed below.

Dynamometry gives information on the maximal performance of a group of skeletal muscles during tetanic contraction. In patients with MG, early fatigue will be seen.[61]

Ergography provides semiquantitative assessment of the tension output of a single voluntary muscle twitch and that of fatigability. Ergography is primarily used for hand muscles.[62]

Electromyography is performed by repetitive supramaximal percutaneous electric stimulation of ulnar and median nerves at the wrist. Evoked potentials are recorded from the abductor pollicis brevis and abductor digiti minimi.[63] Responses are considered to be diagnostic of MG if the amplitudes of the second through sixth evoked potentials show a gradual decrement and if the decrement of any of these potentials is greater than 10 percent when compared with the first.[64] Similar patterns may be found in patients with poliomyelitis and amyotrophic lateral sclerosis, which are associated with degeneration of the anterior horn cells of the spinal cord. When electromyography is combined with the regional curare test, 90 percent of MG patients can be diagnosed by their abnormal response to repetitive supramaximal stimulation.[63]

Pharmacological tests can be performed with use of either provocative (d-tubocurarine) or corrective (edrophonium) drugs. Although the edrophonium test is safer, its administration is associated with both muscarinic (salivation) and nicotinic (twitching of extraocular muscles) side effects, recognizable by the patients, and this makes a true "double blind" test with a placebo almost impossible. The intravenous curare test is useful in the diagnosis of patients with an equivocal edrophonium test. However, this test is potentially dangerous and the presence during its performance of personnel trained in respiratory resuscitation is mandatory.

Edrophonium test: Following cessation of at least 12 hours of anticholinesterase medication, 1 to 4 mg of edrophonium (Tensilon) is administered intravenously. The performance of skeletal muscle is assessed both subjectively and objectively by dynamometry, ergometry, and vital capacity before and 60 to 90 seconds following the edrophonium administration. Definite muscular function improvement is pathognomonic of MG.[65]

Curare test: As emphasized earlier, during the performance of this test either an anesthesiologist or a person knowledgeable in respiratory resuscitation should be present. Depending on the patient's degree of weakness, d-tubocurarine is administered in incremental doses of 0.2 mg, up to a maximum of 4 mg over a period of 1 to 3 minutes. Muscle performance is assessed 5 minutes after each incremental dose, and a significant decrease in skeletal muscle performance is diagnostic of MG.[66] An occasional patient may develop significant muscular weakness requiring airway protection and mechanical ventilation.

Regional intravenous curare test: The advantages of this test over the curare test are the elimination of the systemic effects and the use of the noninjected extremity as a control in a true double blind fashion.[67] Following the regional intravenous curare administration, muscle strength can be ascertained either by measuring grip strength or by recording the potential amplitude of evoked muscle action from the abductor digital minimi. After control measurements of both hands are made, the arms are raised vertically for 30 seconds, after which cuffs applied to the forearms are inflated to 50 mm Hg above the systemic pressure. The arms are laid down and 0.125 mg of d-tubocurarine diluted in 20 ml normal saline is injected through a catheter placed in a dorsal vein of the hand over a period of 60 seconds. Twenty milliliters of normal saline is injected into the control arm. Ischemia is maintained for another 4½ minutes, and after release of the cuffs, a further minute is allowed before neuromuscular stimulation or measurement of handgrip strength is commenced. Despite the documented safety of the test, following the release of the tourniquet systemic weakness and respiratory failure requiring assisted ventilation have been reported, even with doses as small as 0.125 mg.[68]

Drug Therapy. The therapeutic implications of MG stem from the localization of the defect in neuromuscular transmission to two causes: a deficiency in AChR and an apparent autoimmune etiology.

The mainstay in the treatment of patients with MG are oral anticholinesterases such as pyridostigmine (Mestinon). Commonly used anticholinesterases are shown in Table 14-4. Anticholinesterases maintain the local concentration of acetylcholine at the motor end-plate and increase the chance of acetylcholine binding to an AChR. Occasional patients with MG may not respond to anticholinesterase drug therapy, which may be due to complete absence of postsynaptic AChR so that the acetylcholine present in

Table 14-4

Equivalent Doses and Therapeutic Efficacy of Commonly Used Anticholinesterase Drugs

	Dose (mg)			
Drug	Intravenous	Intramuscular	Oral	Efficacy
Neostigmine (Prostigmine)	0.5	0.7–1.0	15.0	1
Pyridostigmine (Mestinon)	2.0	3.0–4.0	10.0	0.25
Ambenonium (Mytalase)	Not available	Not available	6.0	2.5

increased concentration has no place to act.[57] Also, myasthenics on prolonged chronic anticholinesterase drug therapy may show decreased sensitivity to the drug. This may be due to alteration of the geometry of the neuromuscular junction such that the widened synaptic cleft permits the increased acetylcholine to diffuse out and be hydrolyzed before it can act on the available receptor sites.[69]

The therapeutic benefits of steroids and thymectomy are due to MG being an autoimmune disease.[70] However, complete explanation of why these therapies are useful is far from clear. Steroid therapy and thymectomy may alter the immune response against AChR and thus benefit neuromuscular function. Shortly after thymectomy or institution of steroid therapy, the AChR antibody titer may not change for several weeks but clinical improvement of symptoms may occur. These therapeutic maneuvers may repair the widened intersynaptic cleft in an unknown fashion and affect the geometry of the neuromuscular junction as much as they affect the immune attack on the AChR.

Plasmaphoresis. Recently, plasmaphoresis has been introduced as an alternate therapy for MG in patients not improving with standard drug therapy.[71] The demonstration of circulating AChR antibodies in the plasma as the etiologic factor of MG has provided the rationale for plasmaphoresis. During plasmaphoresis, continuous flow plasma exchange is done until the total plasma volume is replaced. These serial plasma exchanges are performed over extended periods of time. Although the AChR antibody titers decrease below 25 percent of their original values, the clinical improvement may not correlate to the same degree as changes in the antibody titer. The clinical improvement of symptoms of MG following plasmaphoresis may be due to: (1) a decrease of AChR antibody; (2) removal of immune activating factors; or (3) addition of immune-suppressing factors such as anti-idiotype antibody present in the normal replacement plasma.

SURGICAL APPROACH FOR THYMECTOMY

Controversy exists regarding the approach for removal of the thymus. Proponents of the transcervical approach claim a lower postoperative morbidity and mortality and a shorter hospital stay.[72] However, thymic tissue may be difficult to approach from the neck and it has been confirmed that islands of thymic tissue that are present in the mediastinum are not readily accessible by this route.

In many institutions, a median sternotomy which involves splitting only the upper one-third of the sternum, is utilized for thymectomies. This technique provides excellent exposure to perform a complete thymectomy, and current methods of preparing patients for thymectomy have almost completely eliminated the morbidity and mortality of the sternal splitting approach.

Patients with MG may undergo elective thymectomy or other major elective or emergency operations. Since these patients have associated respiratory muscle impairment, poor nutritional status, emotional instability, altered response to drugs used in the perioperative period, and increased susceptibility to infection, the perioperative management of myasthenic patients poses serious problems.

Patients with MG should be admitted to the hospital several days before the scheduled elective operation, and elective surgery, including thymectomy, should not be performed until the patient is in optimum physical condition. Perioperative care of patients with MG includes the aspects discussed below.

Physical Examination and Laboratory Workup

Physical examination should include airway evaluation and tests of muscle strength and the ability to chew and swallow. Vital capacity and maximum breathing capacity should be recorded and a chest roentgenogram reviewed to assess the size of the thymic tumor. Myasthenic patients may also have associated myocardial degenerative changes, which makes a preoperative electrocardiogram necessary. Thyroid abnormalities may be associated with MG, and patients need to be evaluated clinically and by laboratory tests for evidence of hypo- or hyperthyroidism. In patients with bulbar involvement, nutritional status can be evaluated by the measurement of serum electrolytes, albumin, globulin, and hemoglobin. Patients with impaired respiratory function need complete pulmonary function tests performed, including analysis of arterial blood gases.

Optimizing the Physical Status

Following the assessment of physical status, measures should be taken to correct nutritional deficiencies, dehydration, and electrolyte imbalances, if present. Patients with severe bulbar involvement may have to be fed with a nasogastric tube. Infections, especially of the respiratory tract, should be treated with appropriate antibiotics, with consideration of the fact that some antibiotics, especially the aminoglycoside group, may precipitate muscle weakness. Associated thyroid abnormalities may have to be treated to bring the patient into a euthyroid status. Patients with myocardial degeneration may have their cardiac status improved by prophylactic digitalization. Plasmaphoresis is commonly used in the preoperative period to optimize the patient's physical status.

Drug Therapy

At present it is recommended that anticholinesterase therapy at regular dose be continued until the day of surgery.[73] On the day of surgery, in mild cases half the amount of the morning dose of pyridostigmine is suggested, while in severe cases the full morning dose is prescribed. In patients receiving systemic steroids, suppression of the pituitary-thalamicoadrenal axis should be considered and their regular dose of steroid given until the day of surgery. Genkins recommends that on the day of surgery 100 mg of hydrocortisone be administered intramuscularly in the morning, followed by 100 mg in 1,000 ml of electrolyte solution every 8 hours. Then the cortisone administration may be tapered from the second postoperative day, and on the fourth or fifth postoperative day the patient may be returned to regular maintenance doses.[73]

Premedication

Emotional instability is often present to a greater extent in these patients than in patients with other chronic diseases, and because of the influence of anxiety and fear on the severity of myasthenic symptoms, special attention must be paid to the psychological preparation of these patients. Premedication may include a barbiturate or minor tranquilizer for sedative purposes, but narcotics should be avoided as they suppress the cough reflex and promote collection of secretions in the airway. Belladonna drugs are often given, but it should be remembered that they can mask a cholinergic crisis produced by an overdose of anticholinergics and can also cause thickening of tracheobronchial secretions.

Choice of Anesthesia

Regional anesthesia should be considered, if adequate anesthesia can be provided for the particular operation. However, it should be remembered that anticholinesterase administration not only inhibits true cholinesterase at the synaptic folds but also inhibits plasma pseudocholinesterase present in the blood.[74] Therefore, administration of the usual dose of an ester-type local anesthetic, which is metabolized by pseudocholinesterase, may precipitate toxic reactions.

In patients requiring general anesthesia, induction can be achieved by a sleep dose of thiopental followed by the administration of either halothane or enflurane in 50 percent nitrous oxide and 50 percent oxygen. If intubation is required for protection of the airway or for prolonged intermittent positive pressure ventilation, this can be achieved under deep halothane or enflurane anesthesia plus topical anesthesia without resorting to muscle relaxants. During thymectomy, there is no need for muscle relaxation and the endotracheal tube can be inserted under deep inhalational anesthesia. However, in patients maintained on full doses of anticholinesterase therapy until the day of surgery, intubation might be difficult without the aid of muscle relaxants. In addition, when MG patients are undergoing abdominal surgery, muscle relaxation may be required. In these situations, muscle activity should be monitored by a nerve stimulator and very small doses of nondepolarizing muscle relaxants administered. It should be remembered that these patients are very sensitive to nondepolarizing relaxants, and adequate muscle relaxation can be achieved by 0.5 to 2 mg of d-tubocurarine or 0.1 to 0.4 mg of pancuronium. The time course of the neuromuscular blockade after these small doses of nondepolarizing muscle relaxants is similar to that observed after larger doses in normal subjects, and at the end of the operation the residual effects of the muscle relaxant can be effectively antagonized by neostigmine. In patients who are to be mechanically ventilated in the postoperative period, the nondepolarizing neuromuscular block need not be reversed with neostigmine. An alternative to the use of muscle relaxants is the use of lower thoracic or lumbar epidural anesthesia for abdominal muscular relaxation.

Postoperative Care

Following surgery, the myasthenic patient should be closely observed in the recovery room or in an intensive care unit. The important question that arises in the immediate postoperative period is whether to extubate the trachea or to mechanically ventilate the patient. In the past, multiple risk factors have been taken into consideration when making the decision as to whether to extubate the patient, but no combination of factors has worked satisfactorily. Recently, Leventhal et al studied 24 patients in whom they collected 21 variables for each patient undergoing thymectomy and subjected the variables to multivariate discriminant analysis based on the stepwise addition of variables

Table 14-5
Risk Factors Predicting the Need for Mechanical Ventilation in Myasthenic Patients

Preoperative Factor	Points
Duration of MG $\geq$ 6 Years	12
History of chronic respiratory disease	10
Pyridostigmine dose > 750 mg/day	8
Vital capacity < 2.9 L	4
Total	34

Total score < 10: trachea readily extubatable
  10 to 12: borderline
  13 to 34: needs ventilation

Adapted from: Leventhal et al., Anesthesiology 53:26–30, 1980.

according to their predictive ability.[75] This analysis identified four risk factors that had a statistically significant correlation with the need for postoperative ventilation: (1) duration of myasthenia of 6 years of more; (2) history of other chronic respiratory disease; (3) pyridostigmine dosage 48 hours preoperatively of more than 750 mg/day; and (4) preoperative vital capacity of less than 2.9 L. No other variable or combination of variables was found to add to the predictive power. Table 14-5 lists these four risk factors and their assigned clinical "point" value; by using these points a total score was obtained for each patient. If the total score was less than 10, these patients could be extubated readily with no consequences. However, if the score was 13 to 34, the patients needed mechanical ventilatory support. The zone of 10 to 12 points may be considered as a borderline area between those needing and those not needing ventilatory support. Few centers now perform prophylactic tracheostomy in patients with MG following any surgery, including thymectomy.

Postoperative Pain Relief

Following intrathoracic or upper abdominal surgery, pain may interfere with adequate respiratory gas exchange. This pain can be alleviated by small doses of the commonly used narcotics; however, it should be remembered that morphine and probably other narcotics are potentiated by anticholinesterases.

Postoperative Resumption of Anticholinesterases

Surgery and anesthesia may alter requirements for the anticholinesterase drugs in the immediate postoperative period, both increased and decreased needs for anticholinesterases having been reported.[73,76] The aim of the immediate postoperative anticholinesterase therapy is the maintenance of adequate spontaneous respiratory exchange. If the spontaneous ventilation is adequate or if mechanical ventilation is instituted, the anticholinergics are not required in the postoperative period. However, if spontaneous respiratory exchange is not adequate, half the regular dose of anticholinesterase may be administered during the first three postoperative days. On the fourth postoperative day, regular doses of anticholinesterases may be started. If the patient cannot take oral medications, parenteral administration of anticholinesterase may be carried out until the patient can tolerate oral feedings when the oral medication is adjusted to obtain optimal strength.

Neurogenic Tumors

Neurogenic tumors are the most common mediastinal tumors in many of the reported series, constituting about 24 percent of all mediastinal tumors.[49] Most of the neurogenic tumors occur in the posterior mediastinum along the paravertebral gutter, and only rarely in the anterior mediastinum. Several histologic types of tumors occur, including neurilemmoma, neurofibroma, neurosarcoma, ganglioneuroma, neuroblastoma, sympathicoblastoma, paraganglionoma, and pheochromocytoma. These tumors can occur at any age and most often are benign in adults, but in children they tend to be malignant.

Most of the symptoms associated with neurogenic tumors are produced by pressure on the surrounding areas. Pressure on the esophagus may cause dysphagia, while pressure on the trachea may produce cough, shortness of breath, and airway obstruction. In addition to the symptoms produced by pressure, some of these tumors may exhibit hormonal activity, and symptoms may occur secondary to the high levels of circulating hormones. Tumors such as ganglioneuromas, neuroblastomas, and pheochromocytomas may be chromaffin-positive and are capable of secreting catecholamines and producing diarrhea, abdominal distention, flushing, increased sweating, and paroxysmal hypertension.

PERIOPERATIVE MANAGEMENT OF
HORMONALLY ACTIVE NEUROGENIC
TUMORS

Preoperative Evaluation

Hormonally active neurogenic tumors of the posterior mediastinum include pheochromocytomas, neuroblastomas, and ganglioneuromas, and of these the most common tumor is the pheochromocytoma.[77] Though pheochromocytomas mostly occur in the adrenal gland, about 10 percent are multiple in origin and are found in other sites, with about 3 percent occurring in the posterior mediastinum. Regardless of their histological origin, once they secrete catecholamines they all behave in a similar fashion, causing similar symptoms and similar problems in the perioperative period.

Symptoms include headache, excessive sweating, palpitations, anxiety, tremors, chest pain, nausea, fatigue, weight loss, and dizziness.[78] Paroxysmal hypertension, or hypertension precipitated by exercise or postural change, may be an important diagnostic sign in these patients.

Abnormalities of the laboratory data include hyperglycemia, impaired glucose tolerance, glycosuria, hypermetabolism, and increased free fatty acids. Biochemical tests that confirm or exclude the diagnosis of hormonally active tumors include estimation of 24-hour urinary epinephrine, norepinephrine, dopamine, metanephrine, normetanephrine, and vanillylmandelic acid. Normal values are shown in Table 14-6.

Pharmacologic Tests

With the refinement of quantitative chemical methods for accurate measurement of catecholamines or their metabolites in both urine and blood, pharmacologic tests are rarely used now to confirm the diagnosis of pheochromocytoma. The most common provocative test utilizes an intravenous histamine injection to provoke a pressor crisis.[79] The basic principle of this test is that patients with hormonally active neurogenic tumors have a tendency to develop a significant increase in arterial blood pressure following the intravenous administration of histamine in doses of 25 to 50 μg. The criteria for a positive test is a rise in arterial pressure in excess of 60/40 mm Hg above the control pressure. Disadvantages of this test include a significant number (25 percent) of false

Table 14-6
Normal Concentrations of Urinary Catecholamines and Metabolites*

Catecholamines	
Epinephrine	0.02
Norepinephrine	0.08
Dopamine	0.20
Metanephrines	
Metanephrine	0.4
Normetanephrine	0.9
Vanillylmandelic acid	6.5

* Upper limits of normal in adults, mg per 24 hours

positive and false negative responses, and patients may experience severe side effects, including flushing, headaches, and occasionally an extreme pressor crisis.

Another pharmacologic test is the phentolamine (Regitine) test.[80] This is performed by the injection of 1 to 5 mg of phentolamine intravenously. A positive response occurs in 2 to 3 minutes, resulting in a fall in arterial pressure of at least 35/25 mm Hg which lasts for more than 10 minutes. Though false negative responses are rare, false positive responses frequently occur. Other pharmacologic tests include intravenous injection of 1 mg of tyramine or glucagon, resulting in an increase in blood pressure of more than 20 mm Hg.[81,82]

Preoperative Preparation

Since surgical removal is the only curative therapy, expertise and teamwork are essential to the successful management of these intrathoracic, hormonally active, neurogenic chromaffin tumors. The therapeutic objective in patients with these tumors is to prevent the physiological and metabolic consequences of the excess catecholamine production of the tumor. Thus pharmacological therapy is mandatory in all these patients prior to surgery to minimize serious, potentially fatal intraoperative cardiovascular complications.

Effective pharmacological therapy commonly used in these patients to block the alpha-adrenergic effect of catecholamines includes phenoxybenzamine (Dibenzyline) and phentolamine (Regitine). Phentolamine (1 to 5 mg intravenous) is a rapidly acting drug with a short duration of action (2 to 10 minutes) and is primarily used to control the blood pressure intraoperatively. For preoperative preparation of these patients, phenoxybenzamine has proved to be an excellent drug to block the pressor effects of the hormones.[81] Because of its long duration of action, the drug is administered once daily in doses ranging from 20 to 100 mg/day. Most patients require about 40 to 60 mg/day and

this dose should be attained gradually, starting with 10 mg per day and increasing the dose by 5 to 10 mg every other day.

Preoperative beta-adrenergic blockade with propranolol has considerably enhanced the ability to provide pharmacological control in these patients. Beta-blockers are extremely useful in patients with a persistent tachycardia or multiple ventricular tachydysrhythmias. Oral doses of 5 to 10 mg four times a day usually suppress undesirable cardiac dysrhythmias. However, beta-blockers should not be given to these patients without first obtaining alpha-adrenergic blockade since beta-blockade even in the presence of alpha-blockade may significantly increase the blood pressure. This is especially true in patients whose neurogenic tumor predominantly synthesizes and secretes epinephrine. A paradoxical hypertensive crisis following beta-adrenergic blockade may occur since the beta-vasodilating effects of epinephrine are blocked by the beta-blocker while the alpha-vasoconstrictor effect is not blocked. This results in the pharmacological conversion of epinephrine into primarily an alpha-adrenergic catecholamine such as norepinephrine or phenylephrine. Under these circumstances it is not uncommon that increased doses of alpha-adrenergic blockers may be required to control blood pressure after the addition of beta-blocker therapy.[83]

Another drug that may be useful in controlling or reducing the secretion of catecholamines by these tumors is α-methyltyrosine in oral doses of 1 to 4 gm daily, since the rate-limiting step in catecholamine synthesis is the conversion of tyrosine to dopa by the enzyme tyrosine hydroxylase. α-Methyltyrosine is an inhibitor of tyrosine hydroxylase and its administration results in a striking decrease in tissue levels of norepinephrine concomitant with the reduction in catecholamine production.[84] Following its administration, patients have normalization of blood pressure and reversal of most of the signs and symptoms attributable to the tumor.

Hemodynamic monitoring with a pulmonary artery catheter is valuable during the perioperative management of patients undergoing resection of these tumors.[85] Preoperatively, excessive catecholamine output in these patients leads to a chronically constricted blood volume, producing a disparity between the circulating blood volume and the capacity of the vascular system. Following alpha-blockade the vascular system expands, requiring blood and/or crystalloid therapy to fill the expanded system, and this can be safely accomplished by measuring left atrial filling pressure by a pulmonary artery catheter in the preoperative period.

Certain drugs such as morphine and the phenothiazines should be avoided as premedicants in these patients since they may precipitate either a hypertensive crisis or hypotension.

Intraoperative Management

Careful monitoring of the ECG, arterial pressure, right and left heart filling pressures, and urine output is crucial to the successful intraoperative management of these patients. Drugs that should be readily available include phentolamine (1 mg/ml), lidocaine (20 mg/ml), a sodium nitroprusside infusion (50 mg in 250 ml), a neosynephrine infusion (10 mg in 250 ml), and a norepinephrine infusion (4 mg in 250 ml).

Anesthetic induction can be achieved with thiopental, and muscle relaxation for intubation can be obtained with metocurine, which has minimal effect on heart rate and blood pressure. Following induction of anesthesia, the patient should be well-anesthetized with an inhalation drug prior to laryngoscopy and intubation in order to obtund laryngeal and tracheal reflexes. The use of enflurane has been associated with minimal cardiac dysrhythmias and hemodynamic changes, and recently fentanyl in doses of 150 to 200 μg/kg has been used for the induction and maintenance of anesthesia with good hemodynamic stability. The trachea can be intubated with either an endotracheal tube or an endobronchial tube for better exposure of the operative field by collapsing the nondependent lung.

During dissection and manipulation of the tumor, catecholamine release can cause hypertension, which may have to be controlled either with phentolamine or sodium nitroprusside. Dysrhythmias, mostly ventricular, may occur and can be treated with lidocaine or propranolol. Following ligation of the vascular supply of the tumor, the circulating catecholamine level decreases rapidly, often resulting in hypotension. This can be avoided by monitoring the left atrial filling pressure and maintaining it at an optimal level with fluid infusions. If the blood pressure does not remain at normal levels with fluid therapy alone, either a neosynephrine or norepinephrine infusion can be started and titrated to obtain precise blood pressure control.

Postoperative Care

These patients do not require routine mechanical ventilation postoperatively. At the end of the operation, any residual neuromuscular block can be reversed with atropine and neostigmine, and extubation of the trachea can be performed when the patient meets the criteria for extubation. Monitoring and close observation should be continued postoperatively until the patient's condition is stable. In addition to the withdrawal of high circulating levels of catecholamines, bleeding at the operative site may be the cause of immediate postoperative hypotension. Postoperative hypertension may be due to fluid overload, pain, or residual active neurogenic tumor.

Other Common Mediastinal Lesions and Related Anesthetic problems

LYMPHOMAS

Following dissemination, all types of lymphomas commonly metastasize to the mediastinum. Hodgkin's disease, lymphosarcoma, and lymphoblastoma may occur in the mediastinum as primary lesions, where they usually are present in the anterior mediastinum. Surgical excision is indicated when these lesions are localized. When the patients are anesthetized, chest roentgenograms should be carefully reviewed for the signs of a widened mediastinum, since following the induction of anesthesia in patients with a widened mediastinum, the anterior mediastinal mass can compress the vena cava, pulmonary vessels, heart, and bronchi, producing acute cardiovascular collapse.[86] Thus, general anesthesia is potentially dangerous in patients with a widened anterior mediastinum, and if these patients have to be anesthetized, they should be treated with about 1,000 rad to the mediastinum 1 week prior to the anticipated time of surgery in order to reduce the size of the mediastinal mass and to avoid compression of the heart and great vessels.

THYROID

A substernal goiter in the anterior superior mediastinum is very common and is usually an extension of a thyroid enlargement from the neck. Occasionally, the thyroid may be present in the mediastinum without any continuity from the neck. These patients should be brought to a euthyroid state prior to surgery. Anesthetic problems associated with a substernal thyroid include airway obstruction after induction of anesthesia, which can be relieved by passing an endotracheal tube beyond the tumor. In patients with a long-standing thyroid tumor, pressure from the tumor over the tracheal rings may cause degeneration of these rings, resulting in tracheomalacia. Prior to the removal of the tumor the trachea is kept patent by the attachments of the trachea to the tumor; however, following excision of the tumor when the trachea is extubated, it can collapse, causing acute airway obstruction. These patients require immediate reintubation and a tracheostomy. Care should be taken that the distal end of the tracheal tube

is beyond the collapsed trachea and this should be confirmed radiographically.

FIRST RIB RESECTION FOR THORACIC OUTLET SYNDROME

The thoracic outlet syndrome is one of the most controversial subjects in thoracic surgery. Not only is there a lack of agreement among physicians as to the diagnosis and treatment, but some even question the existence of this syndrome.[87] The reason for this is that there are no objective tests or signs with which to establish the diagnosis, and a syndrome is recognized only by history and a few subjective physical findings.

Etiology and Symptoms

The thoracic outlet syndrome may be caused either by a first rib or by the scalene muscles. Patients with a first rib may have a history of clavicular or first rib fracture with callous formation which narrows the costoclavicular space, producing symptoms in the arm and hand.[88] Compression of the subclavian vein in the costoclavicular space can lead to intermittent occlusion or thrombosis of this vein, and compression of the subclavian artery may cause vascular insufficiency. Also, compression of the brachial plexus in this space can cause symptoms of nerve compression in the hand and arm.

In patients in whom the syndrome is caused by the scalene muscles, there is usually a history of a hyperextension nerve injury.[89] The injured muscle swells and causes neck pain referred to the occiput. Later on, the muscle may scar and tighten, pressing on the brachial plexus and causing arm and hand parasthesias.

Diagnostic tests to help in the diagnosis of the thoracic outlet syndrome include plethysmography, subclavian arteriography and venography, ulnar nerve conduction velocity studies, and scalene muscle blocks. Definitive treatment for this syndrome includes first rib resection with or without scalenectomy.[87]

Table 14-7
Complications of First Rib Resection

Pneumothorax without need for a chest tube
Brachial intercostal neuralgia
Temporary phrenic nerve palsy
Pleural effusion requiring tap
Subclavian vein injury
Pneumothorax requiring tube
Partial transection of the T_1 nerve root
Winged scapula
Phrenic nerve palsy—temporary
Empyema requiring thoracotomy
Subclavian artery injury

Anesthetic Management

Anesthetic management is very similar to that used in any other surgical procedure, depending on the patient's physical status. If arterial cannulation for pressure recording is required because of the patient's physical status, the artery on the opposite side of surgery should be cannulated. Intravenous infusion also should be started on the opposite side of surgery.

Perioperative complications following first rib resection and scalenectomy are shown in Table 14-7 in order of decreasing incidence. Since pneumothorax is a common occurrence during resection of a first rib, a chest roentgenogram must be obtained immediately after arrival in the recovery room and checked to rule out pneumothorax.

REFERENCES

1. Fisher RS, Cohen S: Disorders of the lower esophageal sphincter. Ann Rev Med 26:373-398, 1975
2. Cohen S: Recent advances in the management of gastroesophageal reflux. Postgrad Med 57:97-110, 1975
3. Moghissi K, Hornshaw J, Teasdale PR, et al: Parenteral nutrition in carcinoma of the esophagus treated by surgery: nitrogen balance and clinical studies. Br J Surg 64:125-128, 1977
4. Heatley RV, Williams RHP, Lewis MH: Preoperative intravenous feeding—a controlled trial. Postgrad Med J 55:541-545, 1979
5. Pontoppidan H, Beecher HK: Progressive loss of protective reflexes in the airway with the advance of age. JAMA 174:2209-2213, 1960
6. Ghoneim MM, Pandya H: Plasma protein binding of thiopental in patients with impaired renal or hepatic function. Anesthesiology 42:545-549, 1975
7. Law DK, Dudrick SJ, Abdou N: Immunocompetence of patients with protein-calorie malnutrition: the effect of nutritional repletion. Ann Intern Med 79:545-551, 1973
8. Ruberg RL, Dudrick SJ: Intravenous hyperalimentation in head and neck tumor surgery: Indications and precautions. Br J Plast Surg 30:151-153, 1977
9. Dudrick SJ, Wilmore DW, Vars HM, et al: Long-term total parenteral nutrition with growth, development and positive nitrogen balance. Surgery 64:134-141, 1968
10. Dudrick SJ, Wilmore DW, Vars HM et al: Can intravenous feeding as the sole means of nutrition support growth in the child and restore weight loss in the adult? An affirmative answer. Ann Surg 169:976-982, 1969
11. Meng HC, Law DH: International symposium on parenteral nutrition. Charles C. Thomas, Springfield, Ill., 1970
12. White PL, Nagy ME, Eds.: Total Parenteral Nutrition. Acton Publishing Sciences Group, 1974
13. Hanson LM, Hardie WR, Hidalgo J: Fat emulsion for intravenous administration. Ann Surg 184:80-88, 1976
14. Law DH: Total parenteral nutrition. Adv Intern Med 18:389-410, 1972
15. Fleming CR, McGill DB, Hoffman HN II et al: Total parenteral nutrition. Mayo Clin Proc 51:187-199, 1976
16. Reinhardt GF, DeOrio AJ, Kaminski MV Jr: Total parenteral nutrition. Surg Clin North Am 57:1283-1301, 1977
17. Askanazi J, Carpentier YA, Elwyn DH et al: Influence of total parenteral nutrition on fuel utilization in injury and sepsis. Ann Surg 191:40-46, 1980
18. Benedixen HH, Hedley-White J, Layer MB: Impaired oxygenation in surgical patients during general anesthesia with controlled ventilation. N Engl J Med 269:991-998, 1963
19. Semyk J, Arborelius M Jr, Lilja B, et al: Respiratory function in esophageal hiatus hernia. I. Spirometry, gas distribution and arte-

rial blood gases. Respiration 32:93-102, 1975

20. Semyk J, Arborelius Jr M, Lilja B: Respiratory function in esophageal hiatus hernia. II. Regional lung function. Respiration 32:103-111, 1975

21. Deutsch S, Dalen JE: Indications for prophylactic digitalization. Anesthesiology 30:648-653, 1969

22. Goldberg AH, Maling HM, Gallney TE: The value of prophylactic digitalization in halothane anesthesia. Anesthesiology 23:207-211, 1962

23. Selzer A, Cohn KE: Some thoughts concerning the prophylactic use of digitalis. Am J Cardiol 26:214-219, 1970

24. Bille-Brahe NE, Engell HC, Sorensen MB: Acute postoperative digitalization of patients with arteriosclerotic heart disease after major surgery. A randomized hemodynamic study and proposal for therapy. Acta Anaesthesiol Scand 24:501-506, 1980

25. Juler GL, Stemmer EA, Connolly JE: Complications of prophylactic digitalization in thoracic surgical patients. J Thorac Cardiovasc Surg 68:352-358, 1969

26. McKeown KC: Carcinoma of the esophagus. Proc R Soc Med 67:389-395, 1974

27. Umezawa H: Principles of antitumor antibiotic therapy, pp. 817-826. In Holland JF, Frei R III, Eds: Cancer Medicine. Lea and Febiger, Philadelphia, 1973

28. Gottlieb JA, Lefrak EA, O'Bryan RM et al: Fatal adriamycin cardiomyopathy: prevention by dose limitation. Proc Am Assoc Cancer Res 14:88-97, 1973

29. Lefrak EA, Pitha J, Rosenheim S et al: Adriamycin (NSC - 12317) cardiomyopathy. Cancer Chemother Rep 6:203-208, 1975

30. Jorgensen SJ: Time-dose relationships in combined bleomycin therapy and radiotherapy. Eur J Cancer 8:531-534, 1972

31. Samuels MS, Johnson DE, Holoye PY et al: Large-dose bleomycin therapy and pulmonary toxicity: a possible role of prior radiotherapy. JAMA 235:1117-1120, 1976

32. Rudders RA, Mensley GT: Bleomycin pulmonary toxicity Chest 63:626-628, 1976

33. Goldiner PL, Carlon G, Cvitkovic E et al: Factors influencing postoperative morbidity and mortality in patients treated with bleomycin. Br Med J 1:1664-1667, 1978

34. Selvin BL: Cancer chemotherapy: implications for the anesthesiologist. Anesth Analg (Cleve) 60:425-434, 1981

35. Rao TLK, EL-Etr AA: Myocardial reinfarction following anesthesia in patients with recent infarction. Anesth Analg (Cleve) 60:271-272, 1981

36. Lowery BD, Vaccaro P, Anderson E, et al: The operative management of symptomatic esophageal reflux. Ohio State Med J 28:446-450, 1980

37. Rehder K, Hatch DJ, Sessler AD et al: The function of each lung of anesthetized and paralyzed man during mechanical ventilation. Anesthesiology 37:16-24, 1972

38. Torda TA, McCulloch CH, O'Brien HD et al: Pulmonary venous admixture during one-lung anesthesia. Anaesthesia 29:272-279, 1974

39. Hatch D: Ventilation and arterial oxygenation during thoracic anesthesia. Thorax 21:310-314, 1966

40. Euler USV, Liljestrand G: Observations on the pulmonary blood pressure in the cat. Acta Physiol Scand 12:301-305, 1946

41. Bjertnaes LF, Mundal R: The pulmonary vasoconstrictor response to hypoxia during enflurane anesthesia. Acta Anaesthesiol Scand 24:252-256, 1980

42. Weinreich AI, Silvay G, Lumb PD: Continuous ketamine infusion for one-lung anesthesia. Can Anaesth Soc J 27:485-490, 1980

43. Condon HA: Anaesthesia for pharyngo-laryngo-esophagectomy with pharyngo-gastrostomy. Br J Anaesth 43:1061-1065, 1971

44. Kaplan JA, Miller ED, Gallagher EG: Postoperative analgesia for thoracotomy patients. Anesth Analg (Cleve) 54:773-777, 1975

45. Modig J: Lumbar epidural blockade versus parenteral analgesics. Acta Anaesthesiol Scand 70:30-35, 1978

46. Enberg G: Relief of postoperative pain with intercostal blockade compared with the use of narcotic drugs. Acta Anaesthesiol Scand 70:36-38, 1978

47. Renck H: Thoracic epidural analgesia in the relief of postoperative pain. Acta Anaesthesiol Scand 70:42-46, 1978

48. Behar M, Magora F, Olshwang D, et al: Epidural morphine in treatment of pain. Lancet 1:527-528, 1979

49. Wychulis AR, Payne WS, Clagett OT, et al: Surgical treatment of mediastinal tumors. A 40-year experience. J Thorac Cardiovasc Surg 62:379-388, 1971

50. Osserman KE, Genkins G: Studies in myasthenia gravis: Review of a twenty year experience in over 1200 patients. Mt Sinai J Med (NY) 38:497-537, 1972

51. Engel AG, Santa T: Histometric analysis of the ultrastructure of the neuromuscular junction in myasthenia gravis and in the myasthenic syndrome. Ann NY Acad Sci 183:35-58, 1971

52. Albuquerque EX, Rash JE, Mayer RF et al: An electrophysiological and morphological study on the neuromuscular junction in patients with myasthenia gravis. Exp Neurol 51:536-563, 1976

53. Elias SB, Appel SH: Acetylcholine receptor in myasthenia gravis: increased affinity of alpha bungarotoxin. Ann Neurol 4:250-252, 1978

54. Fambrough DM, Drachman DB, Satrjamurti S: Neuromuscular junction in myasthenia gravis: decreased acetylcholine receptors. Science, 182:293-295, 1973

55. Almon RR, Andrew CB, Appel SH: Serum globulin in myasthenia gravis: inhibition of alpha bungarotoxin binding to acetylcholine receptors. Science 186:55-57, 1974

56. Appel SH, Almon RR, Levy N: Acetylcholine receptor antibodies in myasthenia gravis. N Engl J Med 293:760-761, 1975

57. Elias SB, Appel SH: Current concepts of pathogenesis and treatment of myasthenia gravis. Med Clin North Am 63:745-757, 1979

58. Lindstrom JM, Seybold MF, Lennon VA et al: Antibody to acetylcholine receptor in myasthenia gravis: prevalence, clinical correlates and diagnostic value. Neurology 26:1054-1059, 1976

59. Mitty T, Kornfeld P, Tormay H et al: Detection of antiacetylcholine receptor antibodies in myasthenia gravis. N Engl J Med 293:760-761, 1975

60. Simpson JA: Myasthenia gravis: A new hypothesis. Scott Med J 5:419-421, 1960

61. Greene R, Rideout PF, Shaw ML: Ergometry in the diagnosis of myasthenia gravis. Lancet 2:281, 1961

62. Schwab RS, Watkins AL, Brazier MAB: Quantitation of muscular function in cases of poliomyelitis and other motor nerve lesions; electrical excitability tests and electromyographic and ergographic studies. Arch Neurol Psychiatr 50:538-547, 1943

63. Horowitz SH, Genkins G, Kornfeld P, et al: Electrophysiologic diagnosis of myasthenia gravis and the regional curare test. Neurology 26:410-417, 1976

64. Desmedt JE: The neuromuscular disorder in myasthenia gravis: Electrical and mechanical nerve stimulation in hand muscles, p. 241. In Desmedt JE, Ed: New Developments in Electromyography and Clinical Neurophysiology. Vol 1. S. Karger, Basel, 1973

65. Osserman KE, Kaplan LI: Rapid diagnostic test for myasthenia gravis: increased muscle strength without fasciculations after intravenous administration of edrophonium (Tensilon) chloride. JAMA 150:265-267, 1952

66. Bennett AE, Cash PT: Myasthenia gravis. Curare sensitivity: a new diagnostic test and approach to causation. Arch Neurol Psychiatr 49:537-541, 1943

67. Foldes FF, Klonymus DH, Maisel W, et al: A new curare test for the diagnosis of myasthenia gravis. JAMA 203:133-137, 1968

68. Brown JC, Charlton JE: A study of sensitivity to curare in myasthenic disorders using a regional technique. J Neurol Neurosurg Psychiatry 38:27-33, 1975

69. Engel AG, Lambert EH, Santa T: Study of long-term anticholinesterase therapy: effects on neuromuscular transmission and on motor end plate fine structure. Neurology (Minneap) 23:1273-1281, 1973

70. Jenkins RB: Treatment of myasthenia gravis with prednisone. Lancet 1:765-767, 1972

71. Dau PS, Lindstrom JM, Cassel CK et al: Plasmaphoresis and immunosuppressive drug therapy in myasthenia gravis. N Engl J Med 297:1134-1140, 1977

72. Papatestas AE, Genkins G, Kornfeld P et al: Transcervical thymectomy in myasthenia gravis. Surg Gynecol Obstet 140:535-540, 1975

73. Genkins G, Kreel I, Jacobson E et al: Studies in myasthenia gravis: technical care of the thymectomy patient. Bull NY Acad Med 30:826-835, 1960

74. Foldes FF, Smith JC: The interaction of human cholinesterases used in the therapy of myasthenia gravis. Ann NY Acad Sci 135:287-293, 1966

75. Leventhal SR, Orkin FK, Hirsh RA: Prediction of the need for postoperative mechanical ventilation in myasthenia gravis. Anesthesiology 53:26-30, 1980

76. Matthews WA, Derrick WS: Anesthesia in patients with myasthenia gravis. Anesthesiology 18:443-448, 1957

77. Winkler H, Smith AD: Pheochromocytomas

and other catecholamine-producing tumors, pp. 900-933. In Blaschko H, Muscholl E, Eds: Springer-Verlag, New York, 1972

78. Manger WM, Gifford Jr RW: Current concepts of pheochromocytoma. Cardiovasc Med 3:289-309, 1978

79. Roth GM, Kvale WF: A tentative test for pheochromocytoma. Am J Med Sci 210:653-700, 1945

80. Grimson KS, Longino FH, Kernade E et al: Treatment of a patient with a pheochromocytoma. JAMA 140:1273-1274, 1949

81. Engleman K, Sjoerdsma A: A new test for pheochromocytoma JAMA 189:81-86, 1964

82. Lawrence AM: Glucagon provocative test for pheochromocytoma. Ann Intern Med 66:1091-1096, 1967

83. Engleman K: Phaeochromocytoma. Clin Endocrinol Metab 6:769-797, 1977

84. Spector S, Sjoerdsma A, Udenfriend S: Blockade of endogenous norepinephrine synthesis by alpha methyltyrosine, an inhibitor of tyrosine hydroxylase. J Pharmacol Exp Ther 147:86-95, 1965

85. Rao TLK, Mathru M, Rao TRM: Perioperative hemodynamic monitoring during resection of pheochromocytoma. Anesthesiol Rev 5:15-18, 1978

86. Piro AJ, Weiss DR, Hellman S: Mediastinal Hodgkin's disease: A possible danger for intubation anesthesia. Int J Radiat Oncol Biol Phys 1:415-419, 1976

87. Sanders RJ, Monsour JW, Gerber WF et al: Scalenectomy versus first rib resection for treatment of the thoracic outlet syndrome. Surgery 85:109-121, 1979

88. Wright JS: The neurovascular syndrome produced by hyperabduction of the arms. Am Heart J 29:1-19, 1945

89. Ochsner A, Gage M, DeBakey M: Scalenus anticus (Naffziger) syndrome. An J Surg 28:669-695, 1935

BRENDAN T. FINUCANE, M.D.

15
Thoracic Trauma

When sorrows come, they come not single spies, but in battalions.

Act 4, Scene 5, *Hamlet*

This quotation from Shakespeare perhaps aptly describes thoracic injuries, which are rarely single and are often associated with severe pain and, in many cases, death.

In 1896 Paget was quite pessimistic when he wrote: "Surgery of the heart has probably reached the limits set by nature".[1] In that same year Rehn successfully sutured the myocardium of a patient who had sustained a penetrating wound to the heart.[2] Trauma is a very serious public health problem in the United States today. It is the third most common cause of death in the first three decades of life, only exceeded in incidence by cardiovascular disease and cancer. The magnitude of this problem is even more startling in pediatrics, where it accounts for approximately 50 percent of all deaths in children of school age.[3] Excluding wartime, the majority of injuries involving the thoracic cage and its contents are secondary to motor vehicle accidents and violence. There are about 50,000 traffic fatalities in this country each year.[4] In recent years there has been a tremendous surge in the incidence of violence in the poverty-stricken areas of our cities. This, coupled with the ready availability of handguns, has resulted in a vast increase in the number of murders. The murder rate in the United States has increased from about 8,500 in 1960 to approximately 21,000 in 1978. When the death rate among teenagers and young adults in this country is compared with those in Sweden, the United Kingdom, and Japan, the incidence is about 50 percent higher in the United States. About 25 percent of all adult deaths from trauma occur primarily as a result of chest trauma.[5] This percentage may be somewhat higher in children.[6] Approximately 72 percent of patients who die at the scene of an accident have sustained a major chest injury. Many of these deaths are due to asphyxia. A recognizable percentage of these patients can be sustained by basic cardiopulmonary resuscitation (CPR) until the better-equipped emergency medical technicians arrive.

In 1977 it was estimated that 12 million Americans had been instructed in the techniques of basic CPR.[7] If this interest continues, a decrease in mortality from asphyxial deaths at the scene of accidents can be expected. The development of emergency medicine as a specialty has also focused much more attention on trauma, both at the scene of the accident and in emergency rooms. With the aid of sophisticated audio-visual communications and telemetry, decision-making by physicians can be brought to the scene of the accident very rapidly. One of the major corrective actions required to improve the care of the seriously injured patient is regionalization of trauma care. Not every hospital has the equipment or personnel to deal with these patients; therefore, this activity should be confined to those hospitals that do. This simple measure would result in a significant reduction in mortality among trauma victims, not to mention the monetary benefits to the community.

TYPES OF INJURY

Thoracic injuries are classified as penetrating and nonpenetrating (Table 15-1).

Penetrating Injuries

Penetrating injuries to the chest are usually the result of gunshot wounds or stab-

Table 15-1
Classification of Thoracic Injuries

1. Penetrating injuries
a. Gunshot
b. Stab
2. Nonpenetrating injuries
a. Blunt
b. Deceleration
c. Blast

bings. The amount of destruction occurring secondary to a gunshot wound is related to the kinetic energy transmitted to the tissues on impact and can be expressed mathematically as:

$$KE = \frac{WV^2}{2G}$$

$$W = \text{weight}$$
$$V = \text{velocity}$$
$$G = \text{acceleration of gravity}$$

In simpler language, tissue destruction following gunshot wounds is related to the muzzle velocity of the weapon and the weight of the bullet discharged. Soft bullets, which fragment on impact, cause much more local destruction than hard bullets, which traverse the tissues cleanly. Rifles generally cause more destruction because of the higher velocity and greater mass of the bullet. Close-range shotgun blasts usually cause severe tissue destruction over a wide area.[8] When evaluating patients with gunshot wounds, some of these facts may be helpful in the overall assessment of the injury (Table 15-2). Stabbings, on the other hand, are less complex. The damage inflicted is usually confined to the structures directly underlying the point of contact. These wounds are far less likely to be fatal than gunshot wounds to the chest and indeed are far easier to treat.

Nonpenetrating Injuries

The vast majority of chest injuries seen in practice today are a result of blunt trauma to the chest. Injuries may range from simple rib fractures to severe destruction of tissues, such as rupture of thoracic viscera. The more serious the injury, the greater the likelihood of rib fractures.[9] Furthermore, fractures of the upper five ribs are usually associated with more serious injuries. Because of the greater flexibility of the thoracic cage in children, it requires greater force to produce fractures. The exact mechanisms producing visceral injury within the thoracic cavity fol-

Table 15-2
Kinetic Energy Calculated for Bullets Commonly
Used in the United States

Type Cartridge	Weight Bullet (Grain)	Velocity (ft/sec)	Kinetic Energy (ft-lb)
.218 Bee	45	2,860	818
M16 (AR-15)	55	3,250	1,290
.22 Savage	70	2,750	1,175
.243 Winchester	100	3,000	1,998
.257 Roberts	117	2,630	1,797
.270 Winchester	130	3,140	2,846
30/06 Springfield	150	2,750	2,519
.30.30 Winchester	150	2,380	1,887
.300 Savage	180	2,380	2,264
.300 H and H Magnum	220	2,610	3,328
.338 Winchester Magnum	250	2,650	3,899
.375 H and H Magnum	300	2,540	4,298

(Reprinted from Shepard GH: High-energy, low-velocity close-range shotgun wounds. J Trauma 20:1066, 1980, with permission of author and publisher)

lowing blunt or decelerating injuries are poorly understood, but generally the extent of injury depends on the mass of the offending object, the physical characteristics of the resulting shock wave, and the ability of the target tissue or tissues to dissipate this shock wave. Deceleration injuries can be divided into *impact* and *momentum* injuries. The impact injury usually results in fractures to the sternum and ribs, with minimal damage to underlying structures. Momentum injuries occur to those organs which are suspended within the thoracic cage, such as the heart, lungs, and aorta. When the body is suddenly brought to a grinding halt on impact, these structures continue to move. The amount of destruction is proportional to the shearing forces imparted to the organ involved. Rupture of the descending aorta, at the isthmus, commonly occurs in severe deceleration injuries.[10] Other serious injuries that occur following blunt trauma include cardiac contusions and rupture, tracheal and bronchial tears, lung contusions, and diaphragmatic and esophageal injuries.

Injuries to the thoracic cage are among the most common encountered in practice today. The injury may range from a simple fracture of one or two ribs to the more complex flail chest injury. The one factor common to all rib fractures, simple or complex, is that they cause a disproportionate degree of pain. To the young, healthy adult this is usually of no consequence, but to the inveterate smoker, with advanced chronic obstructive pulmonary disease, there may be serious consequences. In the conscious patient the diagnosis can be made clinically. Patients can usually pinpoint, with great accuracy, the exact location of the fracture or fractures. A chest radiograph should always be performed, not necessarily to confirm the diagnosis but rather to rule out pneumothorax or atelectasis.

The range of treatments used to manage patients with rib fractures include immobilization, narcotic and non-narcotic analgesics, intercostal nerve blocks, and epidural blocks. Immobilization techniques are mentioned only for completeness. This method is obsolete in the modern practice of medicine and encourages atelectasis and further splinting in predisposed patients. In order to achieve adequate relief for this condition, large doses of analgesics are required, often resulting in hypoventilation. Faust compared the effects of meperidine and intercostal nerve block on pulmonary function in patients following thoracic procedures and found that there was a significant improvement in vital capacity in those patients who had intercostal nerve blocks.[11] Intercostal nerve block is probably the most satisfactory method of managing pain secondary to rib fractures.[12] With the recent introduction of the longer-acting local anesthetic agents bupivacaine and etidocaine, pain relief can be provided for periods varying between 6 and 12 hours.[13] There is little difference between bupivacaine 0.5 percent and etidocaine 0.5 percent in terms of duration of analgesia; however, epinephrine, 1:200,000, should be added to both solutions to reduce peak blood levels and prolong the duration of action.[14,15]

Kaplan et al have suggested that the addition of dextran solutions to bupivacaine may prolong the duration of action of intercostal nerve blocks.[16] However, the use of dextran still remains controversial.[17] Studies have indicated that the highest blood levels of local anesthetics are achieved following intercostal nerve block (Fig. 15-1).[18,19] The reasons for this are unclear but are probably related to the large vascular surface area exposed when performing this block. The technique itself is quite simple, however painful to the patient, especially when multiple blocks are performed. Careful attention should be paid to the total dose of local anesthetic used. The risk of pneumothorax is a real one. Moore reports an incidence of 0.7 percent in 10,961 patients; however, other investigators report a much higher incidence.[20,21]

If, as a result of trauma, a patient requires a general anesthetic, intercostal blocks should be performed while the patient is anesthetized. When a thoracotomy is performed, intercostal nerves may be blocked by the surgeon under direct vision. A full description of the technique of intercostal block is beyond the scope of this chapter. It should

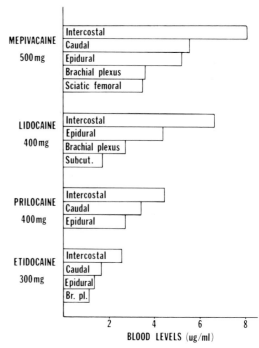

Fig. 15-1 Intercostal nerve blocks produced the highest blood levels with all four anesthetic agents shown. (Reprinted from Covino BG, Vassallo HG: Local Anesthetics: Mechanisms of Action and Clinical Use by permission of Grune & Stratton, New York, 1976, p 97.)

be sufficient to say that it is a simple block, and with careful attention to anatomical landmarks and the total dose of medication, it can be performed with minimal risk to patients.

DIAGNOSIS AND MANAGEMENT OF SPECIFIC INJURIES

Flail Chest

Flail chest may be defined as an abnormal movement of the chest wall occurring as a result of fractures of three or more ribs in two places on the same side. On inspiration the injured segment tends to encroach upon the lung, leading to impairment of ventilation and oxygenation. This injury is most commonly associated with blunt trauma to the chest wall and involves the anterolateral aspect of the chest. The posterior wall is heavily fortified with muscle and therefore is rarely involved. Injury to the upper ribs usually signifies serious trauma. The flail chest injury is rarely isolated and is usually an ominous sign, indicating serious underlying injuries to intrathoracic and/or intraabdominal organs. The thoracic cage in older age groups is more calcified and brittle and therefore more susceptible to flail and other serious injuries. In contrast, the thoracic cage in pediatric patients is extremely elastic and resilient, affording much greater protection to underlying structures.[22]

The diagnosis should always be suspected in patients presenting with a history of blunt trauma to the chest or upper abdomen. This condition may go unnoticed for hours, and in some cases even days, and is sometimes overshadowed by more overt injuries. The diagnosis is particularly difficult when the upper thoracic cage is involved. Chest radiography may not reveal fractures unless films are overpenetrated and oblique views are taken.[23] Radiologic signs of parenchymal damage to the lung may not be evident in the early stages; however, the presence of mediastinal air may signify bronchial or tracheal injury. Serial blood gas measurements can be very helpful in establishing the diagnosis. Repetitive clinical assessment of patients with blunt trauma is the key to early detection of flail chest.

For many years now, the major cause of respiratory dysfunction associated with flail chest has been attributed to the *pendelluft phenomenon,* which is a to-and-fro movement of air from the damaged to the normal lung. Recent reports indicate that this theory is no longer tenable.[24,25] In fact, one investigator demonstrated that there was an increase in ventilation and improved gas exchange on the injured side.[26] It is likely that serious damage to the chest wall will lead to disturbances of ventilation. Coupled with parenchymal damage to the underlying lung, this can very readily cause respiratory failure. The primary pathophysiologic defect associated with flail chest injury is inadequate oxygenation (see Ch. 20).

The management of this condition is controversial. The goals of treatment are directed towards stabilization of the injured segment, maintenance of adequate ventilation, and effective pain relief. All patients with a flail chest should be admitted to a surgical intensive care unit. Temporary stabilization of the flail segment should be carried out as soon as possible by using either sandbags or pillows until a decision about definitive treatment has been made. The treatment varies with the severity of the injury, ranging from simple supportive therapy, such as oxygen enrichment, physical therapy, and pain management, to full ventilatory support. The latter is now considered to be the most effective treatment for patients who develop respiratory failure. Another treatment that has been used is external stabilization of the flail segment by traction on the injured segment.[27] Currently there are few indications for this mode of treatment. Moore and his colleagues stabilize the chest wall in selective cases by intramedullary pinning of fractured ribs.[28]

Which patients need endotracheal intubation and ventilatory support? This decision is usually determined by clinical observation, sequential arterial blood gas analysis, and assessment of the vital capacity and inspiratory force over a period of time (Table 15-3). These criteria should only serve as a guide to therapy. Any one alone may not be sufficient grounds for committing a patient to ventilation, but certainly two or more in any one patient would make a strong case for

Table 15-3
Criteria for Intubation

$PaO_2 < 70$ mmHg with O_2 enrichment
$PaCO_2 > 50$ mmHg
ph < 7.25
Tachypnea > 30/min
Vital capacity < 15 ml/kg
Negative inspiratory force < -20 cm H_2O

doing so. When a decision has been made to institute mechanical support of ventilation, an endotracheal tube is inserted, with use of sedation and topical anesthesia. Nasal intubation is probably more comfortable for the patient; however, some investigators have indicated that nasal intubation causes maxillary sinus infections and for that reason opt for the oral route.

When is tracheostomy indicated? Historically, patients with flail chest injury needing ventilation were subjected to tracheostomy at the commencement of therapy. Clinicians are now convinced that tracheostomy can be a serious source of morbidity and mortality and therefore make every effort to avoid it if possible.[29] Unless there is extreme difficulty in clearing secretions, tracheostomy is deferred for up to 2 weeks. There is considerable disagreement among anesthesiologists and surgeons about this issue. The Lanz tracheostomy or endotracheal tube offers certain advantages over conventional tubes, especially when long-term ventilation is anticipated.[30] The cuff of this tube is fitted with a special pressure-relieving valve, which prevents the application of excessive pressures to the tracheal wall. All gases delivered to patients should be humidified, as inhalation of dry gases for lengthy periods causes serious disruption of the tracheal mucosa and encourages the formation of mucus plugs and erosions.[31] In the initial stages of treatment, patients are placed on intermittent mandatory ventilation (IMV). The rate per minute is determined by the arterial carbon dioxide tension and the patient's intrinsic rate. An IMV rate of about 6 per minute is usually adequate initially. About 5 cm H_2O of distending airway pressure is also selected in these patients. The inspired oxygen tension is determined by that concentration of oxygen which maintains the arterial oxygen tension around 80 mmHg. Weaning is attempted when the arterial blood gases are in an acceptable range, the vital capacity approaches 15 ml/kg, and the inspiratory force is about −20 cm H_2O.

Extubation can be carried out when the patient is capable of maintaining normal blood gases on room air, is capable of generating a negative inspiratory force between −30 and −40 cm H_2O; and has a vital capacity greater than 20 ml/kg of body weight (see Ch. 20).

How should these patients be monitored? Because this condition is associated with such a poor prognosis, extensive monitoring, including continuous monitoring of the electrocardiogram, is recommended. Chest injuries sufficient to fracture several ribs are often associated with cardiac contusions; therefore dysrhythmias may be a problem. The need for frequent arterial blood gas and other laboratory data certainly justifies arterial catheterization. The inspired oxygen tension should be monitored with an oxygen analyzer. Pulmonary artery pressure monitoring is extremely useful in this situation, allowing the clinician to calculate the degree of pulmonary shunting, as well as numerous cardiovascular parameters.[32]

Adequate pain relief should be instituted as soon as possible after the injury to the cardiorespiratory systems. In the early stages of treatment small increments of morphine (3 to 4 mg per 70 kg) may be given every 2 to 3 hours. In order to facilitate the weaning process, other methods of pain relief, such as intercostal nerve blocks and continuous epidurals, are preferable. The former method has the serious limitation of requiring repeated injections. Continuous thoracic epidural anesthesia, although not widely practiced, is probably the method of choice in respiratory failure secondary to chest injury. Recent reports from Europe have suggested the use of continuous infusions of 0.25 percent bupivacaine with epinephrine for the control of postoperative pain in patients undergoing upper abdominal surgery.[33] The use of continuous lumbar epidural anesthesia, on the other hand, has the serious limitation that much larger volumes of local anesthetic would be required to achieve adequate pain relief. The resulting sympathetic block may not be desirable in patients with unstable cardiovascular systems.

There seems to be general agreement about the use of prophylactic antibiotics in these patients. However, frequent cultures should be performed and the appropriate antibiotic commenced when indicated. Are steroids indicated in these patients? Large doses of steroid are recommended by some clinicians in the initial stages of therapy, but no data are available to support this therapy.

Flail chest injury is associated with significant morbidity and mortality. Shackford performed a prospective study in 36 patients who presented with this injury.[35] Of those patients 30 percent required mechanical ventilation; 69 percent developed pneumonia; and about 30 percent developed adult respiratory distress syndrome. The mean duration of ventilation was 10.5 days. The mortality rate in this group was about 10 percent. Depending upon the series, the mortality rate may vary between 6 and 50 percent.[36,37]

Pneumothorax

Pneumothorax occurs secondary to blunt or penetrating trauma to the chest wall. Open pneumothorax is often associated with shotgun wounds to the chest wall at close range. In this situation, intrapleural pressure equalizes with the atmosphere, resulting in a diminished movement of air on the affected side. Venous return is impaired by positive pressure and mediastinal shift. The diagnosis of the sucking chest wound is fairly obvious from clinical observation, and the immediate treatment of this condition is to occlude the defect. Definitive treatment involves insertion of a chest tube and repair of the defect. Less obvious pneumothoraces occur as a result of penetration of the chest wall and lung by sharp objects, such as bullets, knives, ice picks, or rib fragments. The presence of surgical emphysema should signal the possibility of pneumothorax.

Pneumothoraces of less than 20 percent are usually not detectable clinically. Patients usually complain of chest pain, which is accentuated by deep breathing. Cyanosis may be evident, and the trachea may be deviated with larger pneumothoraces. Percussion of the chest reveals a tympanitic sound and breath sounds may be diminished or absent. Conditions that may mimic pneumothorax include hemothorax or atelectasis. Radiologic examination is the best diagnostic aid available, and all films should be taken during expiration. The presence of rib fractures or surgical emphysema should provide a clue to the diagnosis. Pneumothoraces with a volume greater than 10 percent should be treated by tube thoracostomy in trauma patients.

Tension pneumothorax occurs when air enters the pleural cavity during inspiration but, owing to a ball-valve action, cannot escape during expiration. In conscious patients, rapid deterioration is noted. Breath sounds are barely perceptible and the trachea is markedly deviated. Cyanosis and cardiovascular collapse are noted (Table 15-4). This condition can be easily confused with pericardial tamponade. During general anesthesia, a dramatic decrease in compliance should alert the anesthesiologist to the problem. Nitrous oxide should be discontinued as soon as possible, as it accentuates the size of the pneumothorax.[38]

As soon as a tension pneumothorax is suspected, a large-bore needle should be inserted into the pleural cavity, allowing air to drain freely. If the diagnosis is correct, a rapid improvement is noted. This is a surgical emergency and valuable time should not be wasted seeking radiologic confirmation. Figure 15-2A shows a portable radiograph of

Table 15-4
Cardinal Signs of Tension Pneumothorax

1. Cyanosis
2. Marked decrease in pulmonary compliance
3. Rapid deterioration in vital signs
4. Diminished or absent breath sounds

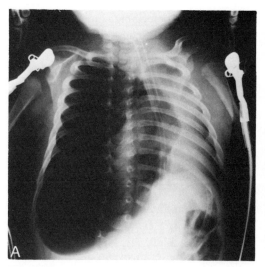

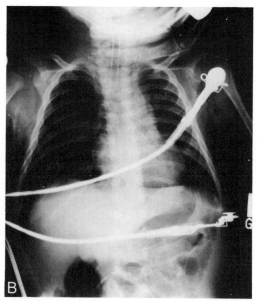

Fig. 15-2 (A) Tension pneumothorax in a 2-month-old child. (B) Supine chest film 20 minutes later.

a 2-month-old infant with a large tension pneumothorax. At the time of the diagnosis, the child was moribund. The arterial blood gases on 100 percent O_2 were as follows: PaO_2 = 19 mmHg, $PaCO_2$ = 75 mmHg, pH = 6.94, and a base deficit of −18 mEq/L. The repeat radiograph in 20 minutes was much-improved and the blood gases on 100 percent oxygen were: PaO_2 = 85 mmHg, $PaCO_2$ = 47 mmHg, pH = 7.21, and base deficit of −9 mEq/L. A radiograph was taken in this instance after initial attempts to decompress the pleural cavity were unsuccessful. This example demonstrates the dramatic reversibility of this potentially-lethal condition (Fig. 15-2B).

The incidence of pneumothorax associated with subclavian puncture even in capable hands is about 2 percent.[39] Despite this fact, in many centers the subclavian vein is one of the first vessels selected for cannulation in trauma patients. Large antecubital veins are more than adequate for rapid infusion of fluids. If central venous pressure monitoring is warranted, cannulation of the internal jugular vein is an excellent alternative to the subclavian and is associated with fewer serious complications.[40] Hemothorax

and hydrothorax are other recognizable complications of subclavian cannulation. The position of the cannula should be verified by aspirating for blood intermittently. The waveform may also be studied with the appropriate electronic equipment. Radiologic confirmation of the catheter tip is not always feasible initially but should be carried out when time permits.

Acute Traumatic Hemothorax

Hemothorax occurs in about 70 percent of all major chest injuries. Gay and McCabe classify penetrating injuries of the chest into three categories based on severity.[41] Those in category one are patients who are moribund on arrival in the hospital and need immediate treatment. The second category comprises those patients who present in shock, but for whom there is sufficient time to evaluate the injury. The third category comprises those patients who are stable on arrival in the hospital; therefore, a thorough evaluation of the injury can be carried out.

The diagnosis of hemothorax is made on the basis of history and clinical examination of the chest. When a significant quantity of blood has accumulated in a chest cavity, the trachea may be deviated, the chest wall is dull to percussion, and breath sounds are diminished on auscultation. A chest radiograph and an ECG should be obtained on all patients except those presenting in extremis. About 500 ml of blood must accumulate in the chest cavity before it is detectable radiologically. Upright chest films are preferable, if possible. Hypovolemia from blood loss is the most common presenting problem in patients with significant chest injury. Therefore, the immediate treatment should be directed towards restoring blood volume.

Two large-bore intravenous cannulae should be inserted as soon as possible. Central venous pressure monitoring is invaluable in both the diagnosis and management of patients with hemothorax. Oxygen therapy is mandatory in these patients who have mechanical interference with ventilation. A chest tube should be inserted as soon as possible in the sixth intercostal space in the midaxillary line on the injured side and connected to suction at a negative pressure of about -15 cmH$_2$O. Tube thoracostomy is invaluable in suspected hemothorax because it allows immediate confirmation of the diagnosis. Furthermore, it provides an accurate assessment of the cumulative blood loss and of ongoing losses, facilitates re-expansion of the lung, and finally, simplifies the technique of autotransfusion when major bleeding is encountered. Concurrent pneumothoraces are frequently present. Thoracostomy tube insertion alone is the only surgical treatment required in more than 80 percent of patients presenting with hemothorax.[42] In the majority of cases, the source of bleeding is the pulmonary vessels, which normally have low perfusion pressures. On the other hand, bleeding from systemic vessels or the heart is usually more persistent and voluminous and may require thoracotomy (Table 15-5).

In most situations, there is sufficient time to allow the thoracotomy to be performed in the relative comfort of an operating room. Emergency room thoracotomy may be indicated in those patients who present in extremis. Baker et al presented their experience with this mode of therapy in 168 patients over a 5-year period.[43] In this series, optimal results were achieved in patients presenting with penetrating wounds of the chest. The poorest results were obtained in those patients presenting with multiple blunt trauma. The overall survival rate was 19.6 percent. The authors concluded that emergency room thoracotomy was a productive exercise both in terms of patient care and cost effectiveness. Therefore, it appears that this mode of therapy may be life-saving in selected cases. The rationale behind this treatment is to relieve cardiac tamponade if present and to control arterial bleeding by clamping the aorta above the site of bleeding. The patient is then transported to the operating room for definitive treatment.

The anesthetic requirements of moribund patients undergoing thoracotomy are minimal. An endotracheal tube should be inserted as soon as possible, 100 percent oxygen should be administered, and the thoracotomy should be performed while using controlled ventilation. If and when adequate perfusion pressures are restored, an appropriate level of anesthesia can be provided by using small doses of ketamine or narcotics.

Tracheal and Bronchial Injuries

Tracheal and bronchial injuries are among the more serious encountered in thoracic surgery. Most penetrating wounds to these structures result from gunshot wounds

Table 15-5

Indications for Thoracotomy

1. Persistent hypotension despite aggressive volume replacement
2. Bleeding greater than 300 ml/hour for 4 hours
3. Massive continuing hemorrhage > 2,000 ml
4. Left hemothorax in the presence of widened mediastinum

and stabs. These injuries also occur following blunt trauma. Lloyd suggests that when the elastic capability of the lungs has been exceeded as a result of the impact, tears occur, mainly in the vicinity of the carina.[44] A more serious tear results if the impact is delivered during glottic closure. This injury should be suspected in any patient presenting with subcutaneous emphysema, cough, or hemoptysis associated with blunt or penetrating trauma to the neck or upper chest. Tension pneumothorax may occur, especially if the tracheal wound communicates with the pleural cavity. In some cases a massive air leak may be evident on attempting to ventilate the patient. All patients with suspected tracheal or bronchial injury require diagnostic bronchoscopy as soon as they are stable.

Small tracheal wounds with good apposition may be treated by endotracheal intubation, with the cuff of the endotracheal tube placed below the wound site. The tracheal wound should heal within 48 hours.[45] Other clinicians recommend tracheostomy in this situation. Tracheostomy is indicated when there is extensive injury to the larynx and the cervical trachea or when endotracheal intubation cannot be performed. More extensive injuries involving complete separation of the trachea or bronchi require open surgical treatment. The long-term sequelae of these injuries are bronchial and subglottic stenosis.

Tracheal and bronchial surgery, to be successful, require close cooperation between the surgeon and anesthesiologist at all times.

Traumatic Rupture of the Diaphragm

Traumatic rupture of the diaphragm usually occurs secondary to blunt trauma to the chest and abdomen. The majority of ruptures occur on the left side in the posterior central area; however, avulsion of the diaphragm from the rib cage has been described.[46,47] In most circumstances, the intra-abdominal pressure exceeds that of the thoracic cavity. This pressure difference is greater during inspiration; therefore, when a deficit occurs in the diaphragm, there is a tendency for abdominal viscera to enter the thoracic cavity. Herniation of abdominal contents does not always take place immediately. Incarceration and strangulation are more likely to occur with small tears.

A patient with this injury may be asymptomatic or may present with respiratory distress. Patients with chronic rupture usually present with symptoms of intestinal obstruction. This injury must be suspected in all patients presenting with blunt trauma. In overt cases, in which viscera have entered the chest, the diagnosis may be obvious on clinical grounds. If the diagnosis is suspected, it can be confirmed by chest radiography and by performing a diagnostic pneumoperitoneum. In Brooks' series of 42 cases, about 70 percent were recognized immediately, and 17 percent were diagnosed after a delay varying between 4 and 47 days.[46]

The anesthesiologist should be aware of this condition, which must be suspected when unexplained changes in compliance occur intraoperatively in patients who have sustained serious chest injury. Patients with significant migration of viscera into the chest cavity would appear to be at greater risk from aspiration pneumonitis also. Diaphragmatic injuries are quite often associated with fractured ribs and flail chest and therefore frequently require mechanical ventilation for several days. The treatment of this condition, once diagnosed, is operative as soon as the patient's condition permits. The optimal approach to repair this injury is through the thoracic cavity.[48,49]

Penetrating Cardiac Injuries

Penetrating cardiac injuries occur as a result of gunshot or knife wounds to the neck, precordium, or upper abdomen. Gunshot wounds are usually more devastating, causing destruction of one or more cham-

Table 15-6
Site of 54 Penetrating Wounds of the Heart

Wound Site	RV	LV	RA	LA
Stab	24	7	4	0
Bullet	3	11	3	2
Percent of total	50	33.3	12.9	3.7

(Reprinted, with permission of author and publisher, from Symbas PN, Harlaftis N, Waldo WJ: Penetrating cardiac wounds: a comparison of different therapeutic methods. Ann Surg 183:379, 1976.

bers. Knife wounds, on the other hand, are usually singular and less destructive. Numerous reports support the fact that about 50 percent of all victims of penetrating cardiac wounds die at the scene of the accident.[50]

The right ventricle, which occupies the largest area beneath the precordium, is most commonly penetrated (Table 15-6). Symbas' experience with penetrating wounds of the heart at Grady Memorial Hospital revealed an *overall* mortality rate of 18.4 percent in 102 patients.[51] When these data were broken down further, 11.1 percent of the deaths resulted from stab wounds, whereas 27.3 percent occurred as a result of bullet wounds. Several serious effects may result from penetrating cardiac injuries, the most common being cardiac tamponade.

Cardiac Tamponade

The normal heart is surrounded by a fibrous, poorly compliant membrane, which in the adult contains about 60 ml of serous fluid. Rapid accumulation of 100 to 200 ml of fluid in this closed space limits the degree of dilatation of the heart during diastole. The pericardial sac can accommodate as much as 2 L of fluid if the fluid is allowed to accumulate slowly.

Cardiac tamponade should always be suspected in patients with wounds in the vicinity of the neck, precordium, or upper abdomen. Patients may appear restless, cyanotic, or clearly shocked. The symptomatology may be misleading in intoxicated patients.[52] Beck's triad, consisting of venous distention of the neck veins, hypotension, and muffled heart sounds, is present in only 41 percent of cases with penetrating cardiac wounds.[53-55] Pulsus paradoxus, which is a decline in systolic blood pressure of 10 mmHg or more on inspiration, is also of limited value in these patients unless continuous arterial pressure monitoring is used.[56] Paradoxical filling of neck veins on inspiration may be too subtle to detect in uncooperative, struggling patients. Since a number of these patients deteriorate rapidly, there is usually insufficient time to carry out investigations such as echocardiography, which is very accurate diagnostically. The electrocardiogram is usually not helpful; however, occasionally a patient will show electrical alternans, which is usually diagnostic of tamponade (Fig. 15-3). Usually the ECG shows nonspecific ST-segment or T wave abnormalities, but it may appear normal. Chest radiographs are also of limited value; occasionally air may be seen in the pericardial sac. Heavy reliance is placed on clinical impressions in patients with cardiac tamponade. Elevation of central venous pressure in the face of shock or hypotension is clear evidence of the diagnosis and should be acted upon immediately.

Experts in the field of thoracic surgery feel that the definitive treatment of this condition is surgery as soon as possible.[57,58] Pericardiocentesis may be used to relieve the tamponade in rapidly deteriorating patients. Aspiration of nonclotting blood from the pericardial sac is diagnostic, but the converse is not true.[59]

Pericardiocentesis should be carried out in a semi-sitting position. A 16- or 18-gauge metal needle is inserted in the subxiphoid region at an angle of 35° and advanced toward the left shoulder. The hub of the needle can be connected to the V-lead of the electrocardiograph and ECG monitoring can be carried out while the needle is advanced toward the pericardial sac. Accidental encroachment of the needle on the ventricular wall will be

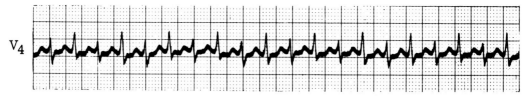

Fig. 15-3   Electrical alternans is demonstrated in a patient with cardiac tamponade. (Reprinted, with permission of author and publisher, from Goldman MJ: Principles of Clinical Electrocardiography. 10th ed. Lange Medical Publications, Los Altos, 1979, p 299.)

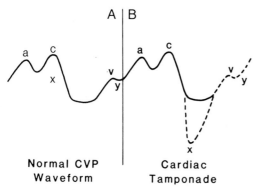

Fig. 15-4   (A) Normal A, C, and V waves, with the X and Y descents. (B) Pronounced X descent seen with cardiac tamponade.

evident as ST elevation. Removal of 30 to 60 ml of blood may result in dramatic improvement. If a plastic catheter is used for aspiration, it should be secured to allow frequent use.

Time will dictate the degree of monitoring carried out on patients with cardiac tamponade. In many situations, basic monitoring techniques are used. Whenever possible, central venous pressure (CVP) should be monitored electronically, allowing the anesthesiologist to study the wave form and providing continuous readings. The normal CVP has three waves: the A wave, which coincides with atrial contraction; the C wave, which is due to bulging of the atrioventricular (A-V) valves during isometric contraction; and the V wave, which is due to atrial filling when the A-V valves are closed (Fig. 15-4A). On each side of the V wave there are two pronounced depressions, referred to as X and Y, which are used to identify the V

wave. In pericardial tamponade or effusion there is a pronounced systolic X dip with minimal diastolic Y dip (Fig. 15-4B).

Central venous pressure monitoring not only is useful in the diagnosis but also may be used as a guide to volume replacement. High central venous pressures, in the vicinity of 15 cm H_2O should be maintained until the tamponade is relieved.

ANESTHETIC MANAGEMENT

The patient should be prepped and draped while conscious and the incision should be made as rapidly as possible after anesthesia is induced. The classic incision for this lesion is a horizontal cut in the fourth or fifth left intercostal space. The administration of a general anesthetic to a patient with a significant tamponade is potentially lethal.[60,61] Almost any maneuver, other than administration of 100 percent O_2 which is carried out by the anesthesiologist, including positive pressure ventilation, causes deterioration.[62,63] It is for this reason that experts in the field of anesthesiology recommend local anesthesia for this procedure.[64-66] This may be a satisfactory approach in a moribund, lifeless patient or in patients with large, chronic pericardial effusions, but it is less than optimal in struggling, uncooperative patients with serious penetrating wounds of the heart. The surgeon needs good access in order to find the source of bleeding. It is for this reason that general anesthesia is preferable in most patients with pericardial tamponade secondary to trauma.

What are the choices of general anesthesia under these circumstances? Inhalation agents or thiopental cause further cardiac depression and impairment of diastolic filling. Peripheral vasodilatation associated with these agents further impairs filling. The anesthesiologist can effectively manage these patients by maintaining an elevated central venous pressure (> 15 cm H_2O) and by avoiding myocardial depressants (see Table 15-7). Ketamine, which is a phencylidine derivative, is ideal for this purpose. It causes cardiac depression in the isolated heart, but in the intact heart it has a biphasic action—the initial negative inotropic effect is immediately followed by a positive inotropic effect.[67,68] Tweed studied the effects of ketamine on contractility in four normal subjects and found a consistent increase (Fig. 15-5).[69]

Table 15-7
Ideal Anesthetic Agent in the Presence of Cardiac Tamponade

1. Positive inotropic and chronotropic action
2. Peripheral vasoconstriction
3. Antidysrhythmic action
4. Anesthetic properties

Ketamine has some other features that are beneficial in this situation: (1) it causes dissociative anesthesia; (2) it also has excellent analgesic properties so that supplementation with other anesthetic agents is unnecessary; (3) high inspired oxygen concentrations can be delivered; and (4) cardiac tamponade is frequently associated with ventricular dysrhythmias, and Corssen and others have indicated that ketamine has antidysrhythmic properties.[70-72] These findings further substantiate the use of ketamine for patients with pericardial tamponade. The recommended dose for patients with diminished cardiac output is 0.25 to 0.50 mg/kg. Despite careful anesthetic management, patients may deteriorate before the tamponade is relieved. Isoproterenol in a dose of 0.1 to 0.5 μg/kg/min is the drug of choice in this situation.[73] When the pericardium is decompressed, the vital signs usually improve instantaneously. Conservative anesthetic management must prevail even after the tamponade has been relieved to allow the myocardium time to recover from this serious insult.

Myocardial Contracticity After Ketamine

Pat No.	dp/dt $\triangle$ CPIP	per * cent	$\triangle$ LVEDP+
1	+12		−7
2	+26		−6
3	+45		−2
4	+21		+5
Mean	+26% $p < 0.05$		−2.5

* Per cent change in the ratio $\frac{dp/dt}{CPIP}$ after Ketamine

+ Change in absolute value of LVEDP after Ketamine

Fig. 15-5 Ketamine increased $\frac{dp/dt}{CPIP}$ by 26 percent while decreasing LVEDP by 2.5 mmHg in four normal subjects. CPIP = common peak intraventricular pressure; LVEDP = left ventricular end diastolic pressure. (Reprinted, with permission of author and publisher, from Tweed WA: Ketamine and the cardiovascular system, Ketalar. Edited by Parke, Davis and Company Ltd., Parke, Davis and Company, Montreal, 1971, p 41.)

Coronary Artery Injuries

The incidence of coronary artery laceration following penetrating cardiac wounds is in the region of 4 percent.[74] Division of a coronary artery invariably leads to hemorrhage and tamponade and, depending upon the size of the vessel, may cause myocardial infarction. Most injuries involve the left coronary artery or its branches. The right coronary artery is protected by the sternum. These injuries are usually discovered at the time of surgery and lacerations of larger arteries are re-anastomosed if possible. Saphenous vein grafts from the aorta to a coronary artery distal to the injury have been described.[75,76] Blunt injuries may result in occlusion of a coronary artery, eventually leading to myocardial infarction. From an anesthetic standpoint, these patients should be managed similarly to patients with acute myocardial infarctions.

Cardiac Contusions

Blunt trauma to the chest wall resulting in cardiac contusions can occur in a variety of ways. Rapid deceleration injuries as a result of motor vehicle accidents are the most common cause of cardiac contusions, simply because the heart is suspended by the great vessels in the thoracic cavity. On sudden impact the heart strikes the inner aspect of the chest wall with great force, often resulting in cardiac contusion and more serious injuries (Table 15-8).

Rhythm disturbances are among the

Table 15-8
Cardiac Injuries Resulting from Blunt Trauma

Cardiac contusion
Rupture of a chamber
Tears of valves and connecting structures
Coronary artery injuries
Rupture of pericardium
Left ventricular aneurysm

most common presenting signs in patients with cardiac contusion.[77] Conduction disturbances are more commonly associated with injuries to the right atrium and ventricle.[78]

All patients presenting with blunt or penetrating injuries to the chest should have an ECG as soon as possible after admission. Typical signs of injury may not appear for several hours afterwards. There should be a high index of suspicion in patients presenting with rhythm or conduction disturbances. The ECG changes may be nonspecific or they may reveal an obvious infarction. Enzyme studies are of little help.[79] Cardiac scanning and echocardiography have been carried out in animals with excellent success.[80] These methods need to be evaluated clinically and clearly have excellent diagnostic potential in the future. Patients with these injuries should be handled in the same manner as patients with myocardial infarctions. Many patients with cardiac contusions need immediate surgery for other reasons. Subsequent management may play a major role in the outcome for patients presenting with cardiac trauma.

Injuries to the Great Vessels

The intrathoracic aorta can be injured as a result of penetrating or blunt trauma to the chest. The resulting hemorrhage is usually devastating, allowing only about 15 percent of patients to reach a medical facility alive.[81]

The vast majority of aortic ruptures occur as a result of motor vehicle accidents.[82] The most frequent site of aortic rupture is at the isthmus[83] (Table 15-9). The three most common presenting signs are mediastinal widening, hemothorax, and tracheal deviation. Injuries to other major intrathoracic arterial vessels may present with hemorrhagic shock, hemothorax, or tamponade.[84] Caval injuries are among the most difficult to deal with surgically and are associated with an extremely high mortality.[85]

Table 15-9
Site of Aortic Rupture

Site	Early	Chronic	Total
Ascending aorta	3	2	5
Aortic arch	1	2	3
Aortic isthmus	82	114	196
Distal descending aorta	2	2	4
Unspecified	2	—	2

(Reprinted, with permission of author and publisher, from Symbas PN, Tyras DH, Ware RE et al: Traumatic rupture of the aorta. Ann Surg 178:9, 1973.

The foremost goal of the anesthesiologist when dealing with major thoracic vessel injuries is simply to maintain an adequate blood volume, allowing the surgeon time to find the source of bleeding and if possible to repair the injured vessel. It is only very rarely that cardiopulmonary bypass is needed in major thoracic injuries; however, the perfusionist must be ready at a moment's notice to go on bypass if necessary.

Hemorrhagic Shock

Hemorrhagic shock may be defined as inadequate perfusion of the tissues with oxygen and substrate and failure to remove the end products of metabolism. The syndrome may be divided into three distinct stages depending upon the overall blood loss and the rate at which blood is lost. Mild shock is present when up to 20 percent of the blood volume is lost and is usually manifested by anxiety and restlessness. The blood pressure may be normal or even slightly increased and a slight tachycardia may be evident. Shenkin has shown that adults in the supine position may lose up to 1,000 ml of blood with little change in the pulse rate.[86] When patients lose more than 20 percent of their blood volume without treatment, they are in a moderate state of shock, which is characterized by hypotension and tachycardia. The pulse usually feels thready and the extremities feel cool to touch. At this stage, patients appear apathetic and complain of thirst. Patients who have lost 50 percent of their blood volume or more are in a severe state of shock. They usually appear obtunded and may be comatose. Their systolic blood pressure is usually less than 60 mmHg; there is a marked tachycardia; the extremities appear distinctly cold; the skin appears mottled and cyanotic; and the urine output declines to the point of anuria.

The organism invokes a number of responses to blood loss if given sufficient time. The most important compensatory mechanism is a redistribution of blood from the skin, muscle, and splanchnic vessels to the heart and brain. Normally about 70 percent of the total blood volume is harbored in the venous capacitance vessels. This blood is rapidly redistributed to vital organs. This redistribution of blood is brought about by an elevation in serum catecholamines. Fluid migrates from the interstitial space to the intravascular space as a result of decline in hydrostatic pressure in the capillaries; serum lactate levels increase in response to the change to anaerobic metabolism. In the final stages of untreated shock, cardiac decompensation occurs. This may be related to the release of a specific myocardial depressant factor or to an increased pulmonary vascular resistance. Animal studies suggest that cardiac decompensation does occur in hemorrhagic shock but that it is a late event.

MANAGEMENT

Hemorrhagic shock is managed initially by inserting large-bore intravenous cannulae. Antecubital veins are suitable for this purpose. At the same time, blood can be drawn for type and cross-match. In patients who are hypovolemic, 1,000 ml of Ringer's lactate solution should be infused as rapidly as possible. One liter of Ringer's lactate can be infused in less than 5 minutes by using a blood pump. A central venous pressure line may be inserted in the internal jugular vein quite safely with minimal risk of pneumo-

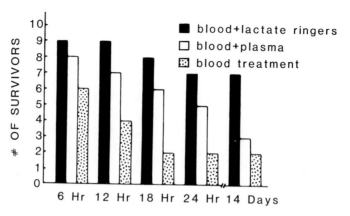

Fig. 15-6 Survival of acutely bled dogs was greatest when they were treated with a combination of blood and crystalloid solution. Colloid treatment alone was not as successful. (Reprinted, by permission of author and publisher, from Carrico CJ: Fluid resuscitation following injury: rationale for the use of balanced salt solutions. Crit Care Med 4:48, 1976.)

thorax. However, many physicians still select the subclavian route, despite the risk of pneumothorax; it is a reasonable choice in patients who already have a chest tube in place. A urinary catheter should be inserted as soon as possible after the diagnosis of shock has been made. The optimal treatment of patients in hemorrhagic shock is a combination of blood and Ringer's lactate. Shires measured the plasma volume, red cell mass, and extracellular fluid volume in dogs using the triple isotope determination.[87] He exsanguinated these animals to the point of severe shock and demonstrated that there was a large deficit in the interstitial space. He concluded that this loss of fluid was shared by both the intravascular and the intracellular space. Furthermore, he demonstrated that the most effective method of correcting volume deficits secondary to hemorrhagic shock is the use of combinations of whole blood and a balanced salt solution, which in this case was Ringer's lactate. Animals which had received combinations of whole blood and plasma had lower survival rates (Fig. 15-6). The findings in this paper have been corroborated by numerous clinicians dealing with patients in hemorrhagic shock.

Infusions of large volumes of balanced salt solutions without protein supplementation must interfere with the colloid osmotic pressure. When the hydrostatic pressure in the pulmonary capillaries exceeds the colloid osmotic pressure, pulmonary edema occurs. Virgilio measured pulmonary capillary wedge pressures and colloid osmotic pressures in patients receiving both colloid and crystalloid solutions and found that pulmonary edema occurred only when the pulmonary capillary wedge pressure was elevated.[88] If the wedge pressure remained within normal limits, pulmonary edema did not develop regardless of the colloid osmotic pressure. This is thought to be due to an increased rate of pulmonary lymph removal. There are other studies which support the view that when the colloid osmotic pressure in the pulmonary capillaries is less than the hydrostatic pressure, pulmonary edema occurs; that is, even when the pulmonary capillary wedge pressure is within normal limits.[89,90] It would appear that balanced salt solutions should be used in combination with whole blood in the early treatment of hemorrhagic shock and that caution should be exercised when the colloid osmotic pressure is exceeded by the pulmonary capillary wedge pressure.

There seems to be some concern about elevating serum lactate levels in patients with hemorrhagic shock by administering large volumes of Ringer's lactate. Studies performed in both animals and humans do not support this finding.[91,92] In fact, studies have shown that the combination of blood and Ringer's lactate results in a more rapid return to normal acid-base balance.[93]

A number of blood substitutes can be used in the absence of blood; they include plasma, dextrans, and hetastarch, an artificial starch with a mean molecular weight of 70,000. It is currently being used as a plasma expander in the presence of shock. A 6 percent solution has osmotic properties similar to those of human albumin, about 40 percent being excreted in 24 hours. Hetastarch is less likely to cause anaphylaxis or a coagulopathy than Dextran 40. Dextran 40 may be used as a plasma expander in the presence of shock, since it remains within the intravascular space for about 12 hours. Hypersensitivity reactions to this agent have been reported. It may cause an increased bleeding time by interfering with platelet function when more than 1 L is infused. Dextran causes rouleau formation and therefore may interfere with crossmatching techniques.

There comes a point at which red cells are needed in order to maintain adequate oxygenation to the tissues. It usually requires 45 minutes to perform satisfactory typing and crossmatching of blood. In massive hemorrhage involving the heart or great vessels, type-specific blood or O negative blood may be used. Occasionally a patient is encountered who, for religious reasons, refuses blood transfusion. However, some patients with these convictions will settle for autotransfusion. Therefore, it is important to remember this compromise when faced with this dilemma.

Autotransfusion

This technique involves the collection of blood from a body cavity which, after appropriate preparation and filtration, is returned to the donor. It is particularly indicated in massive bleeding into the chest cavity.[94] It may also be indicated when significant bleeding occurs into the abdominal cavity, as following ruptured ectopic pregnancy. It may be used in elective surgery of the liver or great vessels when massive bleeding is anticipated, and it may also be used in those patients with rare blood groups. Autotransfusion should not be used when the blood is soiled by fecal material. Various devices are used to achieve autotransfusion. The Bentley apparatus is equipped with a roller pump, which aspirates blood from the field and forces it through a reservoir, where it is primed with a balanced saline solution[95] (Fig. 15-7). It is then filtered before it is reinfused back into the patient. Various methods of anticoagulation are used, including citrate-phosphate-dextrose (CPD) preservative or systemic heparinization. Heparinization should not be used in patients with suspected intracranial bleeding. Symbas has shown that it is not necessary to add anticoagulants to defibrinated blood aspirated from the chest.[96] Autotransfusion is frequently associated with damage to the various blood components, which may result in a decreased red cell mass, elevated bilirubin level, and hemoglobinuria. When massive quantities of blood are autotransfused (>5,000 ml) coagulopathies frequently develop. Air embolism is a real risk when the equipment is run by untrained personnel.

Blood Replacement and Massive Blood Transfusion

Enormous strides have been made in blood transfusion technology and rheology in recent years. Currently, blood is combined with the anticoagulant citrate-phosphate-dextrose and adenine (CPD-A), the addition

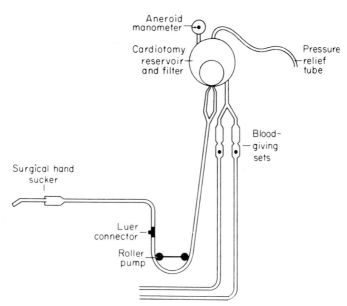

Fig. 15-7 The Bentley autotransfusion apparatus. (Reprinted with permission of author and publisher, from Johnston B, Kamath BSK, McLennan I: An autotransfusion apparatus. Anaesthesia 32:1020, 1977.)

of which extends the shelf life of the blood to 35 days. Certain serious hazards are associated with the administration of blood to patients, some of the most serious complications resulting from administration of a mismatched unit. Data from the Food and Drug Administration during a 3-year period in the 1970s revealed that 69 deaths occurred directly as a result of blood transfusion reactions; approximately one-third of these were due to acute hemolytic reactions, all of which resulted from mismatched transfusions secondary to human error.[97] The majority of mistakes were due to incorrect identification of blood or of the patient. It must be reemphasized that the simple act of administering a unit of blood to a patient carries with it grave responsibility. Therefore, methodical scrutiny of the necessary documentation, including patient identity, are absolutely necessary on each occasion.

Since the discovery of the Australia antigen and its definite association with serum hepatitis, there has been a 25 percent reduc-

tion in the incidence of this serious disease associated with blood transfusion.[98] Cytomegalic virus has also been implicated as a cause of post-transfusion hepatitis. Investigators have shown that the addition of gammaglobulin to stored blood can provide passive immunity to patients receiving blood.[99] Patients receiving pooled plasma are at the greatest risk from serum hepatitis; therefore, this component should be avoided, if at all possible. All blood should be warmed during administration. This becomes increasingly important during massive blood replacement, when temperature may decline to dangerous levels. Certain substances precipitate when mixed with blood; these include bicarbonate, calcium, and lactated Ringer's and dextrose solutions.

There is clear evidence that large quantities of unwanted debris accumulate in stored blood.[100] Therefore, there is general agreement among practitioners that all stored blood should be filtered during transfusion. There is usually considerable debate about the optimal pore size which is most beneficial. Although 20- and 40-μm filters are in general use, there are no objective data to support this practice. In fact, Virgilio has compared the incidence of pulmonary dysfunction in patients receiving extensive transfusions using standard (170-μm) and fine filters and could find no significant difference between them.[101] In emergency situations, when rapid transfusion is required, fine filters offer considerable impedance to the flow of packed red blood cells. This problem can be easily remedied by the addition of a small quantity of normal saline.

These are some of the problems associated with routine administration of small quantities of blood. Additional complications can be expected when massive blood replacement is required.

Massive blood transfusion may be defined as replacement of at least 1½ times a patient's blood volume in a short period of time. Does massive transfusion predispose patients to pulmonary insufficiency? Simmons et al found a significant correlation between massive transfusion and postoperative hypoxemia.[102] On the other hand, Collins found no such relationship.[103] The most definitive information on this topic is also provided by this author, who demonstrated that patients with peripheral injuries receiving massive blood transfusion did not develop respiratory failure postoperatively.[104] Conversely, patients with serious thoracic and abdominal injuries showed a high incidence of respiratory failure in association with massive transfusion. It appears likely that respiratory failure in these cases is related to pulmonary damage rather than to massive transfusion. The other possible causes of postoperative pulmonary insufficiency in these patients are left ventricular failure, microemboli, and denatured proteins. Disseminated intravascular coagulation is often overlooked as a possible etiologic factor.[105]

Dilutional thrombocytopenia is usually the most common cause of coagulopathy in patients receiving massive blood transfusion.[106,107] When the platelet count declines to less than 65,000, spontaneous hemorrhage becomes evident.[108] Three units of platelets should be administered for every ten units of stored blood that have been transfused. It has been estimated that one unit of platelet concentrate will raise the platelet count by 10,000. Although factors V and VIII are markedly reduced in stored blood, these deficiencies rarely lead to coagulopathies by themselves. When the levels of these factors fall to less than 20 percent of normal, they add to the primary deficiency, however. In order to maintain sufficient levels of these two factors, some recommend administering 2 units of fresh frozen plasma for every 10 units of stored blood transfused.[109] Other authorities question the value of giving fresh frozen plasma prophylactically. Disseminated intravascular coagulation (DIC) must be included in the differential diagnosis in any patient presenting with a bleeding diathesis. This is a rather bizarre coagulopathy occurring in patients with trauma and shock and those receiving large quantities of stored blood.[110] It is characterized by an initial tendency toward coagulation, which is rapidly followed by deficiencies in the clotting mechanism.

The following approach should be used in all patients receiving large quantities of stored blood. When 10 units of blood have been administered to an adult patient, blood should be drawn for a platelet count. A specimen of blood should also be drawn for subsequent evaluation of the clot. At this time, two units of fresh frozen plasma and three units of platelet concentrate should be administered. This routine should be followed for every 10 units of blood given. Should spontaneous bleeding occur from intravenous sites, an estimation of the platelet count, partial thromboplastin time (PTT), and plasma fibrinogen must be made as soon as possible, and the clot should be examined for evidence of lysis within 2 hours. If the PTT is elevated but the clot remains intact, bleeding is probably due to deficiency of fac-

Table 15-10

DIC	Dilutional Thrombocytopenia
Thrombocytopenia	Thrombocytopenia
Hypofibrinogenemia	Normal or slightly reduced fibrinogen
Clot lysis (after 2/hours)	Intact clot (after 2/hours)

tors V and VIII and can be readily treated with fresh frozen plasma. If, on the other hand, thrombocytopenia, hypofibrinogenemia, and clot lysis occur, DIC is likely[111] (Table 15-10). The definitive diagnosis is made by a determination of the fibrin split products, which distinguishes between primary and secondary fibrinolysis. When serious coagulation disturbances occur, the expertise of a pathologist well-versed in the subject is strongly advised. However, the anesthesiologist is expected to closely monitor the coagulation status of patients receiving large quantities of stored blood and to treat the more common disturbances.

Citrate, when infused intravascularly, binds with calcium. With normal rates of infusion, changes in the ionized calcium level are minimal; however, when infusion rates exceed 1.5 ml/kg of body weight per minute, symptoms and signs of hypocalcemia appear. These include hypotension, elevation of central venous pressure, and tetany. The electrocardiogram may show evidence of a prolonged QT interval. Normally, citrate is metabolized in the Krebs cycle. Therefore, any factor interfering with metabolism, such as hypothermia or hepatic disease, may lead to elevated citrate levels. Hyperventilation causes a decrease in ionized calcium levels and therefore should be carefully avoided during rapid infusions of stored blood. Should calcium salts be given prophylactically under these circumstances? Most authorities are opposed to the use of prophylactic calcium because it is extremely difficult to predict the associated changes in ionized calcium levels. It is generally felt that rhythm disturbances associated with hy-

percalcemia may be more immediately life-threatening than hypocalcemia.[112] Anesthetic agents which are known to cause cardiac depression should be avoided during rapid infusions of stored blood. Measurements of serum ionized calcium levels are readily available in most critical care laboratories and are certainly recommended during massive blood replacement, but calcium therapy should be carried out with caution.

Stored blood contains anywhere between 4 and 23 mEq per liter of potassium and, therefore, hyperkalemia is usually not a problem during normal rates of infusion. Even during rapid infusions, potassium from stored blood enters donor cells or is excreted by the kidneys. Hyperkalemia occurs in adults only when the rates of infusion exceed 120 ml/min; however, it appears that infants and children are more prone to this problem than are adults.[113,114]

There appears to be no general agreement about changes in hydrogen ion concentration during massive transfusion. These changes are extremely variable; therefore, bicarbonate should not be given prophylactically.[115] Approximately 14 millimoles of hydrogen ions are generated in each unit of stored blood; however, these ions are buffered by the plasma bicarbonate and red cells during infusion.

Quantities of 2, 3 DPG decline in stored blood in proportion to the duration of storage.[116] This is associated with increased binding of oxygen with hemoglobin and a shift to the left of the oxygen-hemoglobin dissociation curve. The significance of increased oxygen affinity in patients receiving large quantities of stored blood is not clear. Theoretically, at least, this may be important in patients who have lost the ability to regulate regional blood flow to organs, such as the heart, through disease.

Hypothermia is a common occurrence in patients receiving large quantities of stored blood.[117] Every effort should be made to keep the body temperature above 35 °C.

In summary, the transfusion of massive

quantities of blood induces several biochemical, physiologic, and metabolic changes, which if not corrected may cause serious morbidity and mortality.

Inotropes and Vasodilators in Shock

Vasopressors have no logical place in the long-term treatment of shock due to hemorrhage. The primary pathophysiologic defect is inadequate tissue perfusion secondary to blood loss; therefore, the primary treatment should be directed towards replenishing fluid and blood losses. Occasionally it will be necessary to use vasopressors such as epinephrine in patients presenting in extremis. Vasopressor support is of vital importance in this situation. Those drugs with predominant alpha-stimulating properties appear to be the most beneficial, and drugs with predominant beta-stimulating effects the least. Dopamine, a precursor of norepinephrine, has been used in clinical practice for about 6 years and has some interesting properties. In low doses (1 to 6 μg/kg/min) it acts on the β-adrenergic and dopaminergic receptors. The latter, when stimulated, dilate the renal and splanchnic blood vessels, redirecting blood to the corresponding organs. Therefore, this vasopressor may be of some definite benefit to patients in shock. However, it is important to replace blood and fluid losses while attempting this therapy. In the terminal stages of shock, dopamine may provide some inotropic support also. Dopamine should always be infused through a central vein. Digitalis is not recommended routinely for patients in hemorrhagic shock. However, it may be of value in older debilitated patients who have been subjected to this insult.

Is there a place for vasodilators in the presence of hemorrhagic shock? There seems to be a better case for this mode of therapy than for vasopressors. A number of animal studies showed increased survival rates when vasodilators were used to treat shock.[118,119] Chlorpromazine, which has alpha-blocking properties, has been used in humans for this purpose.[120] It appears that vasodilator therapy now has a firm place in the therapy of cardiogenic shock, but most clinicians are still reluctant to use it in patients with hemorrhagic shock. Again, adequate volume replacement must be achieved before attempting this form of therapy.

Renal Failure

A discussion of thoracic trauma would be incomplete without some reference to renal failure. Although post-traumatic renal failure is quite rare, with an incidence of about 3 percent, it is associated with a 60 percent mortality rate.[121] The etiology of renal failure in the trauma setting is predominantly secondary to acute tubular necrosis. Intense renal vasoconstriction accompanying hypovolemic shock accounts for the majority of cases of renal failure in trauma victims. Patients with serious muscle injuries may also develop renal failure secondary to myoglobulinuria. Finally, some patients develop renal failure secondary to drug toxicity in the course of treatment. Aminoglycosides and cephalosporins are known nephrotoxic substances, and radiographic contrast materials are also nephrotoxic.[122,123] It has been clearly established that enflurane and methoxyflurane may cause high-output renal failure in association with the production of elevated levels of the fluoride ion.[124,125] Therefore, it would be prudent to avoid these agents in a setting in which renal failure is likely to occur. Furosemide has also been shown to be a cause of renal failure despite the fact that it is frequently used to treat the condition.[126–128]

Oliguria, defined as a volume of less than 400 ml of urine in 24 hours, is the most common sign of renal failure following major trauma. The cause of oliguria is uncertain but may involve renal tubular obstruction, passive backflow of the glomerular filtrate, or intense prerenal vasoconstriction. The predominant effects of filtration failure are the retention of creatinine, urea, and some electrolytes. In complete failure the serum creatinine will rise by about 1.5 mg% per day. However, these biochemical changes in blood or urine are of minimal help to the anesthesiologist during surgery. It is mandatory to measure the urine output in all patients presenting with significant blood loss or blunt trauma, and the urine output should be recorded on an hourly basis. The most likely cause of oliguria in the surgical setting is inadequate fluid or blood replacement. Should oliguria occur in the course of a surgical procedure, the most rational approach to the problem is to first rule out any technical problems with the catheter. Then patients should be given a fluid challenge, but this maneuver should be used cautiously in patients with cardiac disease. Measurement of the central venous pressure is an invaluable tool in the assessment of the volume status of traumatized patients. Infusion of 500 ml of a balanced salt solution or free water is recommended, and if there is no response to this approach after about 30 minutes, 50 to 100 ml of 25% mannitol should be infused over 20 minutes. Mannitol alters the distribution of blood in the renal parenchyma, promoting urine flow.[126] Furosemide has also been recommended in this situation although a firm basis for its use has not been established.[127,128] The recommended dose of furosemide is 0.5 to 1 mg/kg initially, and this dose is doubled every 30 minutes until diuresis is evident or up to 400 mg has been administered. Dopamine is the only vasopressor recommended in renal failure, and the dose should be carefully monitored. Doses in the range of 1 to 5 μg/kg/min have a favorable effect on the dopaminergic receptors in the renal vessels causing dilatation. Acute renal failure is an important entity occurring in patients with serious trauma, and the anesthesiologist, who is usually first in line to detect the onset of this condition, must treat oliguria in these patients aggressively.

BASIC ANESTHETIC REQUIREMENTS FOR MAJOR TRAUMA

Certain basic arrangements must exist in a hospital for optimal care of the seriously injured patient. A trauma team consisting of surgeons at every level of training should be available on a 24-hour basis. This team must have access to a consultant surgeon with expertise in the area of trauma. An anesthesiologist, although not an integral member of the team, must be available in the house with similar support on a 24-hour basis. Seriously injured patients are best handled in facilities with tertiary care capabilities. Other necessary services for optimal patient care include capable blood bank facilities, a critical care laboratory, and intensive care facilities. Nursing and ancillary personnel familiar with the management of trauma patients are also highly desirable (Table 15-11).

Preoperative Preparation and Evaluation of the Trauma Patient

The anesthesiologist usually does not become involved in the management of trauma victims unless they present with airway problems or are candidates for surgery. The initial resuscitation is carried out by surgeons or emergency medicine physicians. When patients are scheduled for surgery, the anesthesiologist is called to evaluate the patient. In some very urgent situations minimal information is obtainable. If time permits, a rapid but comprehensive history and physical examination should be carried out. Pa-

Table 15-11
Basic Requirements for Major Trauma

---
1. Trauma center
2. Trauma team
3. Blood bank (24-hour availability)
4. Critical care laboratory
5. Intensive care facilities
6. Tertiary care facilities
---

tients presenting with chest trauma frequently are in a state of flux, and within minutes the situation may change drastically.

The history should include information about recent food or alcohol ingestion. It is important, both from a medical and medicolegal point of view, to know what the approximate blood alcohol level of these patients is. Occasionally, poor behavior on behalf of the patients is blamed on excessive ingestion of alcohol when serious intracranial injury may be responsible. Furthermore, levels of alcohol above 250 mg % may be sufficient to cause cardiac depression in the presence of anesthesia.[129] It is important to record symptoms of cardiovascular, respiratory, hepatic, and renal disease. Is the patient a diabetic? What medications is she or he currently taking? When examining the patient, some baseline information should be obtained about the state of consciousness, the pupil size and reactivity, and the presence or absence of motor activity. The airway should be carefully evaluated and the trachea examined for evidence of deviation, which might indicate hemothorax or pneumothorax. Tracheal injuries should be suspected in patients presenting with hoarseness, surgical emphysema, or hemoptysis. Cervical spine fractures should be suspected in those patients with trauma to the head or face. The chest wall should receive a careful evaluation, including inspection, palpation, percussion, and auscultation.

What investigations are necessary before induction of anesthesia? Each patient presenting with significant chest trauma should have a chest radiograph and ECG performed preoperatively. Blood should be drawn for typing and crossmatching as well as for a blood count and SMA 6; however, the results may not be available prior to surgery. Arterial blood gases and hematocrit should be estimated before induction of anesthesia.

The extent of monitoring will depend on the urgency of the situation; in dire emergencies basic monitoring techniques are used. If time permits, direct arterial and central venous pressure monitoring should be established and recorded electronically. The radial artery is usually chosen for arterial monitoring. Femoral artery cannulation is probably best avoided, particularly if major arterial bleeding is suspected, since aortic occlusion is frequently used to control bleeding in these patients. A CVP is usually inserted during the initial resuscitation attempts; if not, the internal jugular vein can be readily cannulated with minimal risk to the patient. Pulmonary artery monitoring is rarely necessary during the early management of trauma patients. Because time is such an important element in the survival of a number of patients with thoracic trauma, it is important to be prepared in advance. Ideally, an operating room should be set aside each day for the sole purpose of dealing with trauma victims. In it, monitoring equipment should be calibrated and ready for immediate use; all necessary medications, including emergency cardiac drugs, should be prepared and labeled; blood pumps and blood warming equipment should be available; and a functioning defibrillator must be present.

INDUCTION

Unconscious, moribund patients are intubated immediately and surgery is performed without anesthesia until vital signs or state of consciousness indicate a need for anesthesia. Conscious, combative patients, often smelling of alcohol, can be particularly difficult to handle. Patients who are in a state of shock are particularly susceptible to the thiobarbiturates; therefore, these drugs should be strictly avoided in these situations. Halford, referring to his experiences with thiopental at Pearl Harbor, wrote that it was the "ideal form of euthanasia when used in the presence of shock."[130] As in the case of pericardial tamponade, ketamine in small doses (0.25 to 0.75 mg/kg) is a satisfactory agent to use in the presence of hypovolemia. In hypovolemic patients, only fractions of the usual doses of medications are necessary owing to a significant reduction in the volume of distribution. This is particularly relevant in shocked patients, in whom the greater part of the cardiac output is distributed to the heart and brain at the expense of other less vital structures. Shocked patients, who are deprived of an adequate hepatic and renal blood flow, may also respond differently from normovolemic patients in terms of metabolism and excretion of drugs. Although acute blood loss is not associated with significant hypoproteinemia, replacement of blood loss with large volumes of crystalloid may lead to a relative hypoproteinemia and subsequent pharmacokinetic disturbances.[131] Finally, acid-base and temperature disturbances in these patients may give rise to further pharmacokinetic aberrations.

With the majority of patients, the anesthesiologist will have had sufficient time to replace intravascular fluid deficits and thiobarbiturates can be used safely. Trauma is frequently associated with a decrease in gastric emptying, which places these patients at greater risk from aspiration pneumonitis, so that a rapid-sequence induction is indicated. This is accomplished by intravenous administration of 3 mg d-tubocurarine to prevent excessive muscle fasciculation caused by succinylcholine, followed by preoxygenation of the patient for about 3 minutes. Following the induction dose of thiopental and succinylcholine, cricoid pressure is applied and maintained until the trachea has been intubated and the cuff inflated. In stable patients, maintenance of anesthesia is left to the discretion of the anesthesiologist. If major blood loss is anticipated, it is probably advisable to use nitrous oxide, oxygen, muscle relaxants, and intermittent doses of narcotic; otherwise there is no contraindication to the use of inhalation agents. Mechanical ventilation of the lungs is useful, especially when limited assistance is available, and acid-base

balance should be monitored closely. Intraoperative calcium, potassium, and glucose determinations should be carried out on an hourly basis. Every effort should be made to maintain normothermia. Other medications that can be used for induction of anesthesia in the presence of hypovolemia include the benzodiazepine derivatives diazepam, lorazepam, and midazolam. These agents have recognizable amnesic properties which may be valuable in this situation. Fentanyl may also be useful in hypovolemic patients, because even in the presence of hypovolemia there is minimal suppression of vascular reflexes.

MAINTENANCE

During surgery for major trauma the anesthesiologist has the responsibility for providing good operating conditions for the surgeon; and he must clinically observe the major organ systems for the development of new signs and treat them appropriately. Successful resuscitation of patients with major chest trauma requires teamwork; blood and fluid replacement must be prompt and given in appropriate quantities. After the surgeon has entered the chest cavity, compression of the aorta above the site of bleeding may provide valuable time to restore blood volume. Little, if any, anesthesia is required in shocked patients; however, when the blood volume is restored, consciousness rapidly returns. At this point, anesthesia can be maintained with nitrous oxide, oxygen, and pancuronium. On recovery, these patients rarely recall any unpleasant experiences associated with surgery or anesthesia.

What special precautions are necessary when using neuromuscular blocking drugs in the presence of serious trauma? Succinylcholine, a rapid-acting, depolarizing neuromuscular blocking drug, is usually chosen to facilitate excellent conditions for the rapid-sequence induction. However, caution should be exercised when patients present with extensive muscular damage since potassium levels may rise dangerously in this situation.[132] There are numerous nondepolarizing drugs to choose from during the maintenance of anesthesia. Pancuronium is probably the most popular drug in this group since it stimulates the heart and peripheral circulation, but its mechanism of action is poorly understood.[133] It also has minimal histamine-releasing properties, while d-tubocurarine has quite significant ganglion-blocking and histamine-releasing properties. There has been some renewed interest recently in metocurine, which does not exhibit these undesirable properties. Gallamine, also a nondepolarizing muscle relaxant, is excreted via the kidneys and is probably best avoided in patients with serious trauma, which is often associated with renal failure.[134] Finally, these drugs are subject to aberrant behavior in the presence of changing acid-base status and altered metabolism and excretion. Also, interactions with certain antibiotics are clearly documented. For these reasons, intelligent monitoring of neuromuscular function is mandatory.

In summary, trauma is the penalty modern society pays for high-speed travel. It is interesting to note that the mortality rate from motor vehicle accidents has declined dramatically since the speed limit was reduced to 55 miles per hour. It is difficult to believe that legislators in some states are lobbying to increase it again! The anesthesiologist plays a very important role in the management of patients with serious thoracic trauma. In the majority of cases, the anesthesiologist is confronted with patients who are seriously hypovolemic from blood loss. Whenever possible, the blood volume must be replaced before the patients are subjected to anesthesia. Occasionally, time will not permit adequate restoration of blood volume, especially when major arterial bleeding occurs. In this situation, the anesthesiologist is expected to proceed with minimal information about the patient. Central venous pressure monitoring is extremely valuable in these patients because it helps distinguish between hypovolemia and cardiac tamponade. Ketamine in small doses combined with muscle relaxants provides excellent anesthetic conditions to surgically explore moribund patients with minimal depression of the heart and peripheral circulation.

REFERENCES

1. Paget S: Surgery of the Chest. Wright, London, 1896, p. 121
2. Rehn L: Ueber penetrirende herzuden und herznaht. Arch Klin Chir 55:315, 1897
3. Holler JA, Talbert JL, Shermeta DW: Trauma and the child, pp. 731-754. In Zuidema GD, Rutherford RB, Ballinger WF, Eds: The Management of Trauma. W.B. Saunders Company, Philadelphia, 1979
4. National Safety Council. Accidents facts, 1976 edition. National Safety Council, Chicago, 1976
5. Ebert PA: In Textbook of Surgery. Sabiston DC Jr, Ed: Thoracic trauma. pp. 2063-2073. W.B. Saunders Company, Philadelphia, 1977
6. Mayer T, Walker ML, Johnson DG et al: Causes of morbidity and mortality in severe pediatric trauma. JAMA 245:719-721, 1981
7. National Conference of Cardiopulmonary resuscitation and Emergency Cardiac Care. Standards and guidelines for cardiopulmonary resuscitation and emergency cardiac care. JAMA 244:453-508, 1979
8. Shepard GH: High-energy, low-velocity close-range shotgun wounds. J Trauma 20:1065-1067, 1980
9. Attar S, Kirby WH: The forces producing certain types of thoracic trauma, p. 4. In Daughtry DC, Ed: Thoracic Trauma. Little, Brown & Company, Boston, 1980
10. Ibid., p. 7
11. Faust RJ, Nauss LA: Post-thoracotomy intercostal block: comparison of its effects on pulmonary function with those of intramuscular meperidine. Anesth Analg (Cleve) 55:542-546, 1976
12. Moore DC: Intercostal nerve block for postoperative somatic pain following surgery of thorax and upper abdomen. Br J Anaesth 47:284-288, 1975
13. Willdeck-Lund G, Edstrom H: Etidocaine in

intercostal nerve block for pain relief after thoracotomy; a comparison with bupivacaine. Acta Anesthesiol Scand, suppl, 160:33-38, 1975

14. Buckley FP, Simpson, BR: Acute traumatic and postoperative pain management, pp. 588-589. In Cousins MJ, Bridenbaugh PO, Eds: Neural Blockade. J.B. Lippincott Company, Philadelphia, 1980

15. Cottrell WM, Shick LM, Perkins HM et al: Hemodynamic changes after intercostal nerve block with bupivacaine-epinephrine solution. Anesth Analg (Cleve) 57:492-495, 1978

16. Kaplan JA, Miller ED, Gallagher EG: Postoperative analgesia for thoracotomy patients. Anesth Analg (Cleve) 54:773-777, 1975

17. Bridenbaugh LD: Does the addition of low molecular weight dextran prolong the duration of action of bupivacaine? Reg Anesth 3:6, 1978

18. Tucker GT, Moore DC, Bridenbaugh PO et al: Systemic absorption of mepivacaine in commonly used regional block procedures. Anesthesiology 37:277-287, 1972

19. Scott DB, Jebson PJR, Braid DP et al: Factors affecting plasma levels of lignocaine and prilocaine. Br J Anaesth 44:1040-1049, 1972

20. Moore DC: Intercostal nerve block for postoperative somatic pain following surgery of thorax and upper abdomen. Br J Anaesth 47:284-288, 1975

21. Ablondi MA, Ryan JF, O'Connell CT et al: Continuous intercostal nerve blocks for postoperative pain relief. Anesth Analg (Cleve) 45:185-190, 1966

22. Bloomer WE: Chest trauma as affected by age and preexisting disease, p. 201. In Daughtry DC, Ed: Thoracic Trauma. Little, Brown & Company, Boston, 1980

23. Gay WA, McCabe JC: Trauma to the Chest, p. 263. In Shires CT, Ed: Care of the Trauma Patient. McGraw-Hill, New York, 1979

24. Maloney JV Jr, Schmutzer KJ, Raschke E: Paradoxical respiration and "pendulluft." J Thorac Cardiovasc Surg 41:291-298, 1961

25. Sarnoff SJ, Gaensler EA, Maloney JV: Electrophrenic respiration. The effectiveness of contralateral ventilation during activity of one phrenic nerve. J Thorac Cardiovasc Surg 19:929-937, 1950

26. Duff JH, Goldstein M, McLean APH et al:

Flail chest: a clinical review and physiological study. J Trauma 8:63-74, 1968

27. Jones TB, Richardson EP: Traction on the sternum in the treatment of multiple fractured ribs. Surg Gynecol Obstet 42:283, 1926

28. Moore BP: Operative stabilization of nonpenetrating chest injuries. J Thorac Cardiovasc Surg 70:619-630, 1975

29. Dane TEB, King EG: A prospective study of complications after tracheostomy for assisted ventilation. Chest 67:398-404, 1975

30. King K, Mandava B, Kamen JM: Tracheal tube cuffs and tracheal dilatation. Chest 67:458-462, 1975

31. Chalon J, Loew DAY, Malebranche J: Effects of dry anesthetic gases on tracheobronchial ciliated epithelium. Anesthesiology 37:338-343, 1972

32. Swan HJC, Ganz W, Forrester J et al: Catheterization of the heart in man with use of a flow-directed balloon tipped catheter. N Engl J Med 283:447-451, 1970

33. Gibbons J, James O, Quail A: Relief of pain in chest injury. Br J Anaesth 45:1136-1138, 1973

34. Gay WA, McCabe JC: Trauma to the chest, p. 267. In Shires GT, Ed: Care of the Trauma Patient. McGraw-Hill, 1979

35. Shackford SR, Virgilio RW: Selective use of ventilator therapy in flail chest injury. J Thorac Cardiovasc Surg 81:194-201, 1981

36. Sankaran S, Wilson RF: Factors affecting prognosis in patients with flail chest. J Thorac Cardiovasc Surg 60:402-410, 1970

37. Thomas AN, Baisdell FW, Lewis FR et al: Operative stabilization for flail chest after blunt trauma. J Thorac Cardiovasc Surg 75:793-801, 1978

38. Eger EI II, Saidman LJ: Hazards of nitrous oxide anesthesia in bowel obstruction and pneumothorax. Anesthesiology 26:61-66, 1965

39. Defalque RJ: Subclavian venipuncture: a review. Anesth Analg (Cleve) 47:677-682, 1968

40. Defalque RJ: Percutaneous catheterization of the internal jugular vein. Anesth Analg (Cleve) 53:116-121, 1974

41. Gay WA, McCabe JC: Trauma to the chest, pp. 275-276. In Shires GT, Ed: Care of the Trauma Patient. McGraw-Hill, New York, 1979

42. Symbas PN: Acute traumatic hemothorax. Ann Thorac Surg 26:195-196, 1978

43. Baker CC, Thomas AN, Trunkey DD: The role of emergency room thoracotomy in trauma. J Trauma 20:848-855, 1980

44. Lloyd JR, Heydinger DK, Klassen KP et al: Rupture of the main bronchi in closed chest injury. Arch Surg 77:597, 1958

45. Symbas PN, Hatcher CR, Boehm GA: Acute penetrating tracheal trauma. Ann Thorac Surg 22:473-477, 1976

46. Brooks JW: Blunt traumatic rupture of the diaphragm. Ann Thorac Surg 26:199-203, 1978

47. Hood RM: Traumatic diaphragmatic hernia. Ann Thorac Surg 12:311-324, 1971

48. Brooks JW, Seiler HH: Traumatic hernia of the diaphragm, pp. 175-193. In Daughtry DC, Ed: Thoracic Trauma. Little, Brown & Company, Boston, 1980

49. Ebert PA: Physiologic principles in the management of the crushed-chest syndrome. Monogr Surg Sci 4:69-94, 1967

50. Parmley LF, Mattingly TW, Manion WC: Penetrating wounds of the heart and aorta. Circulation 17:953-973, 1958

51. Symbas PN, Harlaftis N, Waldo WJ: Penetrating cardiac wounds: a comparison of different therapeutic methods. Ann Surg 183:377-381, 1976

52. Symbas PN: Traumatic Injuries of the Heart and Great Vessels. Charles C Thomas, Springfield, Ill. 1972, p. 13

53. Beck CS: Two cardiac compression triads. JAMA 104:714-716, 1935

54. Asfaw I, Arbulu A: Penetrating wounds of the pericardium and heart, pp. 37-48. In Walt AJ, Ed: Symposium on Trauma. Surg Clin North Am. WB Saunders Co., Philadelphia, Feb. 1977

55. Yao ST, Vanecko RM, Printen K et al: Penetrating wounds of the heart: a review of 80 cases. Ann Surg 168:67-78, 1968

56. Trinkle JK, Marcos J, Grover FL et al: Management of the wounded heart. Ann Thorac Surg 17:230-236, 1973

57. Beach PM Jr, Bognolo D, Hutchinson JE: Penetrating cardiac trauma. Am J Surg 131:411-414, 1976

58. Lemos PCP, Okumura M, Acevedo AC et al: Cardiac wounds: experience based on a series

59. Warburg E: Myocardial and pericardial lesions due to nonpenetrating injury. Br Heart J 2:271-280, 1940

60. Cassell P, Cullum P: The management of cardiac tamponade: drainage of pericardial effusions. Br J Surg 54:620-626, 1967

61. Proudfit WL, Effler DB: Diagnosis and treatment of cardiac pericarditis by pericardial biopsy. JAMA 161:188-192, 1956

62. Guntheroth WG, Morgan BC, Mullins GL: Effect of respiration on venous return and stroke volume in cardiac tamponade: mechanism of pulsus paradoxus. Circ Res 20:381-390, 1967

63. Morgan BC, Guntheroth WG, Dillard DH: Relationship of pericardial to pleural pressure during quiet respiration and cardiac tamponade. Circ Res 16:493-498, 1965

64. Stanley TH, Weidauer HE: Anesthesia for the patient with cardiac tamponade. Anesth Analg (Cleve) 52:110-114, 1973

65. Kaplan JA: Pericardial diseases, p. 495. In Kaplan, JA, Ed: Cardiac Anesthesia. Grune & Stratton, New York, 1979

66. Kaplan JA, Bland JW Jr, Dunbar RW: The perioperative management of pericardial tamponade. South Med J 69:417-419, 1976

67. Dowdy EG, Kaya K: Studies of the mechanism of cardiovascular responses to CI-581. Anesthesiology 29:931, 1968

68. Traber DL, Wilson RD, Priano LL: Differentiation of the cardiovascular effects of CI-581. Anesth Analg (Cleve) 47:769-778, 1968

69. Tweed WA: Ketamine and the cardiovascular system, Ketalar. pp. 37-43. Edited by Parke, Davis and Company, Ltd. Parke, Davis and Company, Montreal, 1971

70. Williams C, Soutter L: Pericardial tamponade. Arch Intern Med 94:571-584, 1954

71. Corssen G, Allarde R, Brosch F et al: Ketamine as the sole anesthetic in open-heart surgery—a preliminary report. Anesth Analg (Cleve) 49:1025-1031, 1970

72. Dowdy EG, Kaya K: Studies of the mechanism of cardiovascular responses to CI-581. Anesthesiology 29:931, 1968

73. Fowler NO, Holmes JC: Hemodynamic effects of isoproterenol and norepinephrine in

acute cardiac tamponade. J Clin Invest
48:502, 1969

74. Rea WJ, Sugg WL, Wilson LC et al: Coronary artery lacerations—an analysis of 22 patients. Ann Thorac Surg 7:518-528, 1969

75. Tector AJ, Reuben CF, Hoffman JF et al: Coronary artery wounds treated with saphenous vein bypass grafts. JAMA 225:282-284, 1973

76. Levitsky, S: New insights in cardiac trauma. pp. 43-55. In Nyhus LM, Ed: Symposium on New Skills in Surgery. Surg Clin North Am. WB Saunders Company, Philadelphia, 1975

77. Kissane RW: Traumatic heart diseases, especially myocardial contusion. Postgrad Med 15:114-119, 1954

78. Moseley RV, Vernick JJ, Doty DB: Response to blunt chest injury: a new experimental model. J. Trauma 10:673-683, 1970

79. Watson JH, Bartholomae WM: Cardiac injury due to nonpenetrating chest trauma. Ann Intern Med 52:871-880, 1960

80. Coleman J, Gonzalez A, Harlaftis N et al: Myocardial contusion: diagnostic value of cardiac scanning and echocardiography. Surg Forum 27:293-294, 1976

81. Parmley LF, Mattingly TW, Marion WC: Nonpenetrating traumatic injury of the aorta. Circulation 17:1086-1101, 1958

82. Greendyke RM: Traumatic rupture of aorta: special reference to automobile accidents. JAMA 195:527-530, 1966

83. Symbas PN, Tyras DH, Ware RE et al: Traumatic rupture of the aorta. Ann Surg 178:6-12, 1973

84. Symbas PN, Kourias E, Tyras DH et al: Penetrating wounds of great vessels. Ann Surg 179:757-762, 1974

85. Bricker DL, Morton JR, Okies JE et al: Surgical management of injuries to the vena cava: changing patterns of injury and newer techniques of repair. J Trauma 11:725-735, 1971

86. Shenkin HA, Cheney RH, Govons SR et al: On the diagnosis of hemorrhage in man—a study of volunteers bled large amounts. Am J Med Sci 208:421-436, 1944

87. Shires T, Coln D, Carrico J et al: Fluid therapy in hemorrhagic shock. Arch Surg 88:688-693, 1964

88. Virgilio RW, Smith DE, Rice CL et al: Effect of colloid osmotic pressure and pulmonary

capillary wedge pressure on intrapulmonary shunt. Surg Forum 27:168-173, 1976

89. Stein L, Berand J, Morissette M et al: Pulmonary edema during volume infusion. Circulation 52:483-489, 1975

90. Stein L, Berand J, Cavanilles J et al: Pulmonary edema during fluid infusion in the absence of heart failure. JAMA 229:65-68, 1974

91. Baue AE, Tragus ET, Wolfson SK et al: Hemodynamic and metabolic effect of Ringer's lactate solution in hemorrhagic shock. Ann Surg 166:29-38, 1967

92. Trinkle JK, Rush BF, Eiseman B: Metabolism of lactate following major blood loss. Surgery 63:782-787, 1968

93. McClelland RN, Shires GT, Baxter CR: Balanced salt solution in the treatment of hemorrhagic shock. JAMA 199:830-834, 1967

94. Stehling LC, Zauder HL, Rogers W: Intraoperative autotransfusion. Anesthesiology 43:337-345, 1975

95. Reul GJ, Solis RT, Greenberg SD et al: Experience with autotransfusion in the surgical management of trauma. Surgery 76:546-555, 1974

96. Symbas PN, Levin JM, Ferrier FL et al: A study on autotransfusion from hemothorax. South Med J 62:671-674, 1969

97. Schmidt PJ: Transfusion mortality; with special reference to surgical and intensive care facilities. J Fla Med Assoc 67:151-153, 1980

98. Gocke, DJ: A prospective study of post-transfusion hepatitis; the role of Australia antigen. JAMA 219:1165-1170, 1972

99. Katz R, Rodriguez J, Ward R: Post-transfusion hepatitis—effect of modified gamma-globulin added to blood in vitro. N Engl J Med 285:925-932, 1971

100. Solis RT, Goldfinger D, Gibbs MB et al: Physical characteristics of microaggregates in stored blood. Transfusion 14:538-550, 1974

101. Virgilio RW: Blood filters and post-operative pulmonary dysfunction. Weekly Anaesthesiology Update 2: Lesson 14, pp. 2-8, 1979

102. Simmons RL, Heisterkamp CA, Collins JA et al: Respiratory insufficiency in combat casualties. Ann Surg 170:53-62, 1969

103. Collins JA, Gordon WC, Hudson TL et al: Inapparent hypoxemia in casualties with wounded limbs: pulmonary fat embolism? Ann Surg 167:511-520, 1968

104. Collins JA: Massive transfusion: what is current and important? pp. 1-16. In Nusbacher J. Ed: Massive Transfusion 1978. American Association of Blood Banks, Washington, 1978

105. Ibid, p. 3

106. Miller RD, Robbins TO, Tong MJ et al: Coagulation defects associated with massive blood transfusions. Ann Surg 174:794-801, 1971

107. Krevans JR, Jackson DP: Hemorrhagic disorder following massive whole blood transfusions. JAMA 159:171-177, 1955

108. Miller RD: Complications of massive blood transfusions. Anesthesiology 39:82-93, 1973

109. Gill W, Champion HR: Volume resuscitation in critical major trauma. pp. 77-105. In Dawson RB, Ed: American Association of Blood Banks, Technical Workshop, Transfusion Therapy. Gunthrop-Warren Printing Co., Chicago, 1974

110. Rodriguez-Erdmann F: Bleeding due to increased intravascular blood coagulation. N Engl J Med 273:1370-1378, 1965

111. Deykin D: The clinical challenge of disseminated intravascular coagulation. N Engl J Med 283:636-644, 1970

112. Bunker JP: Metabolic effects of blood transfusion. Anesthesiology 27:446-455, 1966

113. Taylor WC, Grisdole LC, Steward AG: Unexplained death from exchange transfusion. J Pediatr 52:694-700, 1958

114. Bolande RP, Traisman HS, Philipsborn HF: Electrolyte considerations in exchange transfusions for erythroblastosis fetalis. J Pediatr 49:401-406, 1956

115. Miller RD, Tong MJ, Robbins TO: Effects of massive transfusion of blood on acid-base balance. JAMA 216:1762-1765, 1971

116. Bunn HF, May MH, Kocholaty WF et al: Hemoglobin function in stored blood. J Clin Invest 48:311-321, 1969

117. Boyan CP, Howland WS: Blood temperature: a critical factor in massive transfusion. Anesthesiology 22:559-563, 1961

118. Wiggers HC, Ingraham RC, Roehild F et al: Vasoconstriction and the development of irreversible hemorrhagic shock. Am J Physiol 153:511-520, 1948

119. Baez S, Zweifach BW, Shorr E: Protective action of Dibenamine against the fatal outcome of hemorrhagic and traumatic shock in rats. Fed Proc 11:7, 1952

120. Collins VJ, Jaffee R, Zahony I: Anesthesia conference; shock—a different approach to therapy. IMJ 121, 122:350-353, 1962

121. Baek S, Makabali GG, Shoemaker WC: Clinical determinants of survival from postoperative renal failure. Surg Gynecol Obstet 140:685-689, 1975

122. Silverblatt FJ: Antibiotic nephrotoxicity—a review of pathogenesis and prevention. pp. 557-567. In Cox CE, Ed: Symposium on Urinary Tract Disease. Urol Clin North Am. W.B. Saunders Co., Philadelphia, Oct. 1975

123. Ansari Z, Baldwin DS: Acute renal failure due to radiocontrast agents. Nephron 17:28-40, 1976

124. Cousins MJ, Mazze RI, Barr GA et al: A comparison of the renal effects of isoflurane and methoxyflurane in fischer 344 rats. Anesthesiology 38:557-563, 1973

125. Cousins MJ, Greenstein LR, Hitt BA et al: Metabolism and renal effects of enflurane in man. Anesthesiology 44:44-53, 1976

126. Loughridge L: Anaesthesia and the kidneys. p. 321. In Scurr C, Feldman S, Eds: Scientific Foundations of Anaesthesia. William Heinemann Medical Books Ltd., London, 1974

127. Baek SM, Brown RS, Shoemaker WC: Early prediction of acute renal failure and recovery: renal function response to furosemide. Ann Surg 178:605-608, 1973

128. Epstein M, Schneider NS, Befeler B: Effect of intrarenal furosemide on renal function and intrarenal hemodynamics in acute renal failure. Am J Med 58:510-516, 1975

129. Lee JF, Giesecke AH, Jenkins MT: Anesthetic management of trauma: influence of alcohol ingestion. South Med J 60:1240, 1967

130. Dundee JW, Wyant GM: pp. 3-4. In Intravenous Anesthesia. London, Churchill Livingston, Edinburgh and London, 1974

131. Cloutier CT, Lowery BD, Carey LC: The effect of hemodilutional resuscitation on

serum protein levels in humans in hemorrhagic shock. J Trauma 9:514-521, 1969

132. Mazze RI, Escue HM, Houston JB: Hyperkalemia and cardiovascular collapse following administration of succinylcholine to the traumatized patient. Anesthesiology 31:540-547, 1969

133. Coleman AJ, Downing JW, Leary WP et al: The immediate cardiovascular effects of pancuronium, alcuronium and tubocurarine in man. Anaesthesia 27:415-422, 1972

134. Feldman SDA, Levi JA: Prolonged paresis following gallamine. Br J Anaesth 35:804-806, 1963

James W. Bland, Jr., M.D.
John C. Reedy, M.D.
Willis H. Williams, M.D.

16
Pediatric and Neonatal Thoracic Surgery

Remarkable advances in medicine and allied sciences have occurred during the last half-century. Nowhere is this fact more dramatically illustrated than in the amazing progress made in treating pediatric surgical conditions. The rapid progress in the surgical management of infants and children has gone hand-in-hand with equally significant advances in pediatric anesthesiology and intensive care, pediatric cardiology, neonatology, nutritional support measures, and antimicrobial therapy. Specific examples of advances which have greatly enhanced the field of pediatric anesthesiology and intensive care include: greater understanding of the physiology of the neonate; the development of nonflammable anesthetic agents and safe muscle relaxants in infants and children; improved monitoring systems and techniques; improved technology and understanding of intensive respiratory support; and the development of ultramicro-techniques for analysis of blood for pH, blood

gas tensions, and other biochemical parameters.

Downes and Raphaely state that good pediatric anesthesia demands adequate analgesia, life support, intensive surveillance, and appropriate operating conditions for the surgical team.[1] Anesthesia for thoracic operations in infants and children is especially demanding and requires the utmost cooperation and close communication among anesthesiologists, surgeons, intensivists, and nursing personnel. All must understand and respect the problems faced by the other members of the "team" if optimal results are to be achieved.

UNIQUENESS OF THE PEDIATRIC PATIENT

Physiologic, anatomic, and neuropsychiatric developmental variables require that children *not* be treated simply as "small adults." Even within the pediatric age group there are significant differences among the preterm infant, the normal newborn, the young child, and the adolescent. Some of these important differences are summarized in Table 16-1. In order to assure the efficient conduct of a safe surgical procedure, the pediatric anesthesiologist must carefully consider these age- and size-related variables, as well as factors related to the specific disease process being treated, the operation being performed, the level of postoperative care available, and the preferences of the individual surgeon. Indeed, the anesthetic management of the premature infant is virtually a specialty in itself, requiring a high degree of coordination among the anesthesiologist and the many other members of the team caring for the high-risk newborn. As the child grows, matures, and passes into an "age of awareness," psychological factors play an increasingly important role in anesthetic management, if the trauma associated with hospitalization, fear, pain, and separation of child and parents is to be minimized.

Changes Related to Birth

The fetus has intrauterine renal, hepatic, endocrine, hematopoietic, and neural function. Maternal organ systems may assist fetal function to some extent by placental exchange, but, for the most part, these systems are functional at birth, requiring no great transition. The gastrointestinal and neuromuscular systems certainly continue to develop after birth, but they are usually capable of meeting the infant's needs immediately. The greatest changes required in adapting to extrauterine life involve the cardiovascular and respiratory systems.

FETAL RESPIRATION

Fetal respiration takes place at the capillary interfaces of the placenta. Maternal oxygen diffuses across the placenta to the fetal blood because of the gradient which exists between the mother's arterial blood (PO_2 90-100 mmHg) and that of the fetus (PO_2 30-35 mmHg). Fetal carbon dioxide diffuses similarly by a reverse gradient into maternal blood. Oxygen and carbon dioxide transfer are optimized by the Haldane and Bohr effects, respectively.[2] Obviously, fetal lungs contain no air; circulation of blood to the lungs is thus much less than normal prior to birth, since the lungs are performing no ventilatory function.

FETAL CIRCULATION

During intrauterine life, the fetus depends upon three communications or "shunts" not normally present after birth—the ductus arteriosus, foramen ovale, and ductus venosus. Each of these communications plays a vital role in maintaining efficient fetal circulation *in utero*, allowing the fetal blood to bypass the nonaerated lungs, and in making a gradual transition to the normal adult-like extrauterine circulation as the lungs inflate and the pulmonary vascular resistance falls after birth.

Relatively oxygenated placental blood having a PO_2 of 60 mmHg flows from the low-pressure side of the placenta via the fetal umbilical vein to the fetal liver through which it enters the inferior vena cava via the ductus venosus. This oxygenated blood mixes with fetal inferior vena caval blood; and, to a lesser degree, superior vena caval blood, resulting in blood with a PO_2 of about 35-40 mmHg which flows into the right atrium. The anatomical characteristics of the atrial septum with the "trap-door" flap of the foramen ovale direct most of this oxygen-rich blood across to the left atrium. The higher pressure in the right atrium keeps the foramen ovale open prior to birth; reversal of this pressure gradient at birth allows functional closure of the foramen ovale even though it may not anatomically close for many years. Left atrial blood then mixes with the small amount of pulmonary venous

Table 16-1
Normal Valves

	Age	Heart Rate (BPM)	Blood Pressure (mmHg)	Respiratory Rate (Breaths/min)	Hematocrit (%)	Blood Volume (cc/kg)	Maintenance Fluids (cc/kg/24 hr)	Caloric Requirements (cal/kg/24 hr)
Premature (< 2000 g)	Preterm	140–160	50/30	40–60	40–50	100	100–120	120
Neonate	0–28 day	120–140	60/40	40–60	40–60	100	80–100	100
Infant	28 days–1 yr.	80–120	$\frac{60-90}{40-60}$	30–50	30–40	80	80	80–100
Child	1–10 yrs.	80–100	$\frac{80-120}{40-70}$	20–30	30–40	70	60–80	40–80
Young Adult	11–16 yrs.	60–90	$\frac{90-140}{50-80}$	10–20	35–45	60–70	60	40–60

blood, crosses the mitral valve into the left ventricle, and is pumped into the aorta and systemic circulation. The brachiocephalic and coronary vessels receive the relatively well saturated arterial blood.

Venous blood from the superior vena cava enters the right atrium, mixing minimally with blood from the inferior vena cava and placenta before crossing the tricuspid valve into the right ventricle. A small percentage of the blood ejected by the right ventricle goes to the lungs. The lower PO_2 of this blood results in pulmonary vasoconstriction and elevation of the pulmonary vascular resistance. This small fraction of right ventricular output that goes to the lungs mixes with blood from the bronchial arteries and drains into the left atrium. The remaining blood pumped from the right ventricle follows the path of least resistance, passing from the pulmonary artery into the aorta via the ductus arteriosus to perfuse the lower portion of the systemic vascular bed, and the fetal portion of the placenta via the two umbilical arteries. Because of streaming of caval blood in the right atrium, the blood in the lower body is not as well oxygenated as that of the aortic arch and brachiocephalic vessels.

In contrast to the extrauterine circulation, the arterial side of the fetal circulation is the low pressure—low resistance circuit due to the runoff into the low resistance placenta. Pulmonary vascular resistance greatly exceeds systemic vascular resistance until the first breath is taken and the umbilical cord is clamped. These two actions cause a simultaneous decrease in pulmonary vascular resistance and an increase in systemic vascular resistance. As the arterial PO_2 rises, pulmonary vascular resistance falls further and left-to-right (aortic-to-pulmonary arterial) shunting may occur across the still-patent ductus arteriosus. With further increases in PO_2, the ductus begins to close and systemic vascular resistance rises, effectively closing the foramen ovale by increasing the left atrial pressure. Pulmonary vascular resistance continues to fall over a period of approximately seven days, but normal values for pulmonary vascular resistance may not be achieved for several weeks after birth as the pulmonary vessels thin out and become more compliant.[3]

TRANSITIONAL CIRCULATION

The foregoing discussion of the adaptation from the fetal to adult circulation is somewhat simplified. The changes are not immediate and are essentially reversible for about 72 hours. This period of a "transitional circulation" has important anesthetic implications. Stress to the newborn infant such as hypoxia, hypercarbia, acidosis, hypoglycemia, anemia, sepsis, and hypothermia can interrupt the normal progress of circulatory adaptation. The pulmonary vasculature is sensitive to the partial pressure of oxygen and may constrict under conditions of hypoxemia. The ductus arteriosus responds in a reciprocal manner to hypoxemia and may reopen, resulting in decreased pulmonary flow and right-to-left shunting from the pulmonary artery to aorta. Right atrial pressure rises as pulmonary vascular resistance increases, making the foramen ovale the potential site of a paradoxical embolus should air enter the venous circulation. For this reason, it is essential to exclude all air from intravenous fluid administration sets.

Under conditions of right-to-left shunting due to increased pulmonary vascular resistance, drugs should not be administered which will reduce systemic vascular resistance and further increase shunting. In addition, inhalational anesthetics have a decreased uptake and elimination under such conditions of decreased pulmonary blood flow, and should be used with caution.

The extreme example of extrauterine right-to-left shunting through the patent ductus arteriosus and patent foramen ovale is called "persistence of the fetal circulation" (PFC). This syndrome is usually associated with infection, polycythemia, diaphragmatic hernia, hypoglycemia, hypocalcemia, meconium aspiration, fetal asphyxia, or central nervous system abnormalities. There is, however, an idiopathic form with no apparent cause. Differentiation of PFC from congenital heart disease may be quite difficult without the use of echocardiography; and, in some cases, cardiac catheterization and cineangiography. Therapeutic intervention may require careful titration of vasodilating medications into the pulmonary artery. The vascular bed remains labile, however, and careful attention is required to prevent stressful situations which may increase pulmonary vascular resistance.

NEONATAL HEPATIC FUNCTION

Neonatal hepatic function is, for all practical purposes, intact at birth. The capacity of the neonate's liver to metabolize bilirubin, however, is almost equal to the normal load of hemoglobin presented. The result is that any stress which may impede metabolism or increase hemolysis may exceed the liver's capacity to conjugate bilirubin, with resultant hyperbilirubinemia. The glucuronyl transferase system requires a period of six to seven days to reach full functional capacity.[4] Elevated levels of unconjugated bilirubin may result in bilirubin encephalopathy (kernicterus). When bound to albumin, unconjugated bilirubin tends not to enter the CNS; therefore, any condition which increases the presence of unbound bilirubin increases the possibility of permanent brain damage from kernicterus. Those conditions most commonly seen and most preventable are hypoalbuminemia, acidosis, hypoglycemia, hypoxia, hypothermia, and competition for or displacement from albumin binding sites by drugs such as sulfisoxazole and salicylates. Less preventable are sepsis and hemolysis.

Vitamin K_1 is usually given to newborn infants in the United States to prevent hemorrhagic disease of the newborn. The synthesis of coagulation factors II, VI, IX, and XI is dependent on the presence of Vitamin K_1 of which the newborn may be deficient. Therefore, Vitamin K_1 (0.5 – 1.0 mg intramuscularly or subcutaneously) should be given prior to surgery during the newborn period, especially if the child has never been fed.

Carbohydrate, fat, protein, and drug metabolism are less influenced by hepatic immaturity, but may become important during periods of stress (see hypoglycemia below).

NEONATAL RENAL FUNCTION

The neonatal kidney is functionally suited for antenatal life and shares responsibility with the placenta and the mother's kidneys for removal of metabolites. After birth there is a period of maturation as the kidney assumes greater functional capacity and growth by the increased workload. Glomerular filtration rate doubles soon after birth, continues to rise, and quadruples when fully mature. Unlike the liver, the period of renal maturation is much longer; but, by the age of one year, it is nearly complete.[5] Traditionally, the neonatal kidney has been thought to be unable to excrete sodium loads or to concentrate urine to a significant degree. More recently, this theory has been modified to state that because of the higher extracellular fluid volume in the neonatal period and reduced solute loads, e.g., urea and sodium, the neonatal kidney *appears* not to concentrate.[6] For the normal neonate, unstressed and not undergoing surgery, the large extracellular fluid volume provides the necessary electrolytes to maintain normal serum sodium concentrations in the first week of life, while the excess extracellular fluid is passed as dilute urine. It is for this reason that salt-free fluids are frequently given to the newborn. However, the neonatal surgical candidate may translocate fluids the same as any other patient and needs electrolyte replacement. Therefore, salt-containing fluids should be given and electrolytes measured regularly.

FLUID, ELECTROLYTE AND CALORIC
REQUIREMENTS

Maintenance requirements for fluids and calories are summarized in Table 16-1. Sodium, potassium and chloride requirements are all similar to adults at 1 to 3 mEq/kg/24 hr. It must be stressed that these are accepted maintenance requirements and should be used only as a guideline. Adjustments should be made for third space losses, the presence of congestive heart failure, existing deficits, changes in insensible losses, and drainage losses during surgery. Babies under phototherapy for hyperbilirubinemia, or under infrared warmers for temperature maintenance, may have as much as a 20 percent increase in fluid requirements because of increased evaporative losses.[7]

Glucose requirements are 2 to 6 mg/kg/min under normal circumstances and may be reduced under anesthesia. The basic glucose requirement is fulfilled by using 5 percent dextrose in H_2O. Caution must be exercised in conditions where large volumes of fluid are administered (e.g., replacement of intraoperative volume loss) not to administer an excess of glucose, since hyperosmolarity will result. Hyperosmolarity secondary to hyperglycemia or hypernatremia may play a part in the pathogenesis of intraventricular hemorrhage in neonates.[8,9] It cannot be overemphasized that premature infants, term newborns, and infants undergoing major thoracic procedures need careful monitoring of glucose, sodium, potassium, and calcium, as well as monitoring of their blood pressure, heart rate, and blood gases.

AIRWAY ANATOMY

Anatomically, the child, and especially the infant, is different enough from the adult to make intubation more difficult (Table 16-2 and Fig. 16-1). The head is larger in proportion to the rest of the body, sometimes making it less stable; however, this disparity, particularly of the occiput, can be used to advantage during intubation by affording a natural "sniffing" position. In a normal newborn infant the neck is short in comparison to the adult. The tongue, like the head, is relatively larger in children than in adults, and may cause obstruction during induction and ventilation by mask. The larynx is more

Table 16-2

Unique Features of Infant Airway Anatomy (See Fig. 16-1)

1. Relatively large head (occiput more prominent)
2. Short neck
3. Relatively large tongue
4. Small nares easily obstructed by secretions. Infants are obligate nose breathers until approximately 2 months of age and will not open mouth to breathe even if nares are totally obstructed for any reason (e.g. secretions, edema, choanal atresia).
5. The infant's larynx is located more cephalad than that of the older child or adult. At term, the larynx has descended somewhat so that the lower border of the cricoid cartilage is located opposite the middle of the 6th cervical vertebra. In the adult, the lower border of the cricoid cartilage lies opposite the lower border of C_6
6. Narrowest portion of the infant's airway is the subglottic area at the level of the cricoid cartilage. Edema at that level greatly diminishes the cross-sectional diameter of the airway and can result in stridor or varying degrees of airway obstruction.
7. Epiglottis is relatively long and usually rather stiff. It is omega-shaped and extends from the base of the tongue at 45 degrees posterior and cephalad.
8. Trachea is short (approximately 4 cm); thus carina is more cephalad making endobronchial intubation more likely if careful placement of endotracheal tube is not carried out. In adults, carina at level of T_5. In infants, carina at level of T_3.
9. The angles formed by the main bronchi with the trachea vary considerably in infants: 10–35 degrees on the right and 30–50 degrees on the left.
10. Thorax is relatively small; sternum soft, ribs are horizontally placed; diaphragms relatively high; accessory muscles of respiration weak.

cephalad in the child, lying approximately at the level of C_{2-3} as compared to C_5 in adults. It is not, however, more anterior, though it may seem so due to its cephalad placement and the large tongue. Beyond the larynx, the trachea-to-carina distance is only 4 cm in the infant. Extreme caution must be taken in passing the endotracheal tube past the cords by only 1.5 to 2.0 cm in order to avoid bron-

ANATOMY

HEAD SIZE

SHORT NECK

LARGE TONGUE

LARYNX — C2-4 (ADULT C5)

        — NOT MORE ANTERIOR

LARYNX TO CARINA DISTANCE 4 cm VS. "12 – 15"

EPIGLOTTIS – 45° ∠ FROM ANTERIOR WALL – MORE VERTICAL

SMALL AIRWAYS

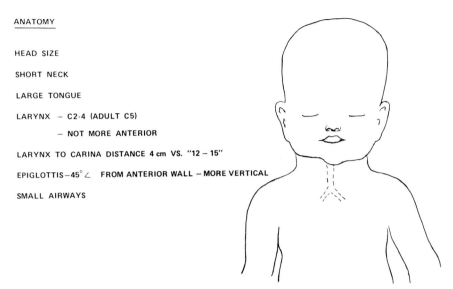

Fig. 16-1 Infant airway anatomy.

chial intubation. The epiglottis projects cephalad at approximately 45 degrees from the
anterior wall of the larynx. This often makes
the epiglottis easier to visualize, but more
difficult to displace to allow intubation. Finally, the air passages themselves, the nose,
nasopharynx, and trachea, must be considered. Being small, but not out of proportion
to the infant, they may be easily obstructed
due, for example, to mucus, edema, nasogastric tubes, tape, or endotracheal tubes. Care
to prevent inadvertent obstruction must be
exercised at all times.

The Premature Infant

Premature infants are unique and deserve separate consideration. They demand
understanding and special attention during
anesthesia and surgery. Not having had the
opportunity to fully develop prior to birth,
they are dependent upon good care and support while they mature. Morbidity and mortality figures increase dramatically in neonates weighing less than 2000 grams and of
less than 37 weeks gestation.[10] Reducing
these figures and providing a better quality

of life for those who survive are the aims of
the neonatal intensivists. Consequently, the
appearance of "prematures" in the operating
room has become more frequent, requiring
anesthetic expertise which gives consideration to their unique problems.

Most evident is size. A term infant may
weigh 2500 g or more; while a 30-week premature may not exceed 1000 grams. There is
less subcutaneous fat, accounting for some of
the weight difference, but premature infants
are generally small in all aspects and require
appropriately small equipment. The use of a
O Miller laryngoscope blade and 2.5 mm ID
endotracheal tube may sometimes seem inappropriately large. Once the premature infant is ready for surgery, the anesthesiologist
must accept the fact that he will have little, if
any, access to the patient because of the surgical positioning and draping. It is, then, of
the utmost importance that every aspect of
monitoring, venous cannulation, and securing of airway be complete prior to draping.

RESPIRATORY DISTRESS SYNDROME

Until the advent of continuous positive
airway pressure (CPAP), premature infants

succumbed most frequently to hyaline membrane disease or respiratory distress syndrome of the newborn (RDS). Advances in neonatal respiratory care and equipment have reduced the deaths from RDS, but other causes of death such as intraventricular hemorrhage, necrotizing enterocolitis, and sepsis have increased in numbers due to the longer survival of premature infants.

Respiratory distress syndrome is a disease of atelectasis based on the deficiency of surfactant normally secreted by the type II alveolar cells. Surfactant acts to reduce surface tension in the alveolus, allowing for expansion during respiration. When surfactant is absent or reduced in quantity, atelectasis and ventilation/perfusion (V/Q) abnormalities develop. The primary aim of the intensivist in treatment of RDS is to open those atelectatic alveoli, using increasing peak airway pressures, but avoiding barotrauma and circulatory disturbances, and then to keep the alveoli open using CPAP or positive end-expiratory pressure (PEEP). Intermittent mandatory ventilation (IMV) is used as required to maintain normocarbia, and the inspired oxygen is adjusted to keep the arterial PO_2 in the range of 60 to 80 mmHg (Fig. 16-2).

The anesthetic considerations for a child with RDS are critical. Casual removal of CPAP or PEEP may result in a profound alveolar collapse and the development of marked hypoxia, acidosis, and hypercarbia. It is highly desirable, if not absolutely necessary, to continue all ventilatory support measures during the operative period in babies with RDS. If there is no means available to deliver CPAP or PEEP in the operating room, the infant's own ventilator should be brought to the operating room and used during surgery.

Respiratory distress syndrome is not a contraindication to the use of inhalational agents, although the reduced uptake, distribution, and pulmonary excretion of these agents secondary to the primary disease should be considered.

RETROLENTAL FIBROPLASIA

Oxygen sensitivity is another unique feature of the premature newborn and is a consideration until they reach 40 to 44 weeks gestational age. Unlike adult RDS patients, the usual neonate with RDS is premature and subject to retrolental fibroplasia if the retinal arteries are exposed to high partial pressures of oxygen. The degree of damage is mostly influenced by the maturity and vascularization of the retina itself when the hyperoxygenation takes place.[11] The anesthesiologist's responsibility is to maintain the PO_2 of the arterial blood between 60 to 80 mmHg, if possible. Use of nitrous oxide as a diluting gas or an air/oxygen blender is recommended. Arterial blood gases or transcutaneous PO_2 monitoring is necessary, and oxygen tension should be measured frequently during surgery, especially during thoracic procedures, to ensure adequate oxygenation, but not hyperoxygenation.

PERIODIC BREATHING AND APNEA

Typical of the premature infant is a breathing pattern of 10 to 15 seconds of normal breathing interrupted by 5 to 10 seconds of no respiratory efforts. This pattern of breathing is not associated with hypoxemia or bradycardia and may respond to minimal increases (2-3%) in FiO_2. Periodic breathing is so common as to be called normal in the premature age group. Apnea is characterized by episodes of not breathing which *are* associated with hypoxemia and bradycardia, and is definitely abnormal. Duration of true apneic episodes are greater than 15 seconds, and stimulation is usually required to terminate them. Various mechanical devices have been used to stimulate infants periodically, and drug therapy using low doses of theophylline has been effective in reducing the incidence of the apneic episodes.[12] From the anesthesiologist's standpoint, the significance of apnea is obvious. In the operating room where the patient is intubated and mechanical ventilation is available, there is little to do

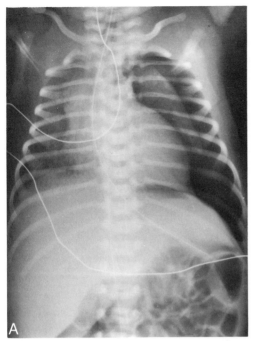 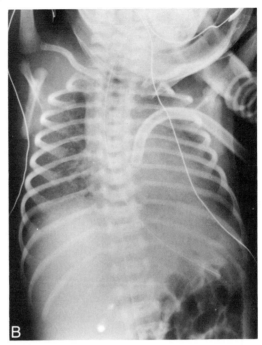

Fig. 16-2 Newborn premature infant with respiratory distress syndrome and tension pneumothorax. (A) Pre-treatment chest radiograph shows collapse of left lung with shift of heart and mediastinum to right. Note also widening of intercostal spaces on the left and depression of left hemidiaphragm. (B) Repeat film following insertion of thoracotomy tube shows re-expansion of left lung and return of mediastinal structures to normal position.*

other than to recognize apnea. In preparation for extubation after surgery, premature infants should be carefully observed for apneic episodes, the presence of which is a contraindication to removal of the endotracheal tube. Apnea monitors are available and may be quite useful postoperatively in the recovery room or intensive care unit.

Apnea in the premature infant or newborn may be associated with hypothermia, sepsis, intraventricular hemorrhage, hypoglycemia, pneumonia, and meningitis, and may be the first evidence of such conditions. Careful evaluation of the child with apnea is, therefore, required.

---

* Radiographs in this chapter are courtesy of Turner Ball, Jr., M.D. and Brit Gay, M.D., Department of Radiology, Henrietta Egleston Hospital for Children, Emory University School of Medicine, Atlanta, Georgia.

HYPOGLYCEMIA

The occurrence of hypoglycemia in the newborn period is quite common. In small-for-gestational age infants, it is the most common form of morbidity, approaching 67 percent.[13] Lower values of blood sugar are accepted as normal in infants, and hypoglycemia is defined as a blood sugar of less than 30 mg% during the first 72 hours of life, and less than 40 mg% after 72 hours. In low-birth-weight infants, i.e., term infants less than 2500 grams, hypoglycemia is defined as a blood sugar of less than 20 mg%.

Prior to delivery, both the fetal and the maternal pancreas regulate the blood sugar with some degree of placental crossover. At birth, the interruption of this interdependence may manifest itself as a delayed assumption of normal glucose metabolism in the newborn. The most common example is that of the infant of a diabetic mother. Fetal insulin production is quite high, in an attempt to make up for maternal hypoinsulinism and hyperglycemia. At birth, insulin output is still quite high, or at least the response to increases in blood sugar is greater than normal, resulting in severe hypoglycemia.

Other conditions which contribute to the incidence of hypoglycemia in the newborn period are perinatal distress of any kind, toxemia, twinning, erythroblastosis fetalis, sepsis, asphyxia, CNS defects, hypothermia, hypocalcemia, congenital heart disease, maternal medications, endocrine deficiency (hypothyroidism), adrenal hemorrhage, polycythemia, hyperbilirubinemia, and abrupt withdrawal of glucose. The history of any of these conditions should make the anesthesiologist aware of the possibility of hypoglycemia and the need to determine blood glucose levels in the perioperative period. Normal sugar requirements for prematures and other newborns are 2 to 6 mg/kg/min and may need to be three times that much to prevent hyperglycemia. If hypoglycemia is present prior to anesthesia, the occurrence of hypoglycemia and the dangers of hyperosmolarity must be prevented once the child is anesthetized, since anesthesia may reduce glucose requirements. It may become necessary to stop glucose therapy during anesthesia or change to solutions of lower glucose concentration.

HYPOCALCEMIA

While hypocalcemia may be seen in all newborns, it is most prevalent in stressed infants and prematures. Usually hypocalcemia, defined as less than 7 mg%, presents as jitteriness or a high-pitched cry, but may present with frank tetany. Since it is frequently seen with hypoglycemia, the first sign may be a convulsion. Hypocalcemia occurs most commonly in prematurity, infants of diabetic mothers, sepsis, asphyxiated infants, and infants with respiratory distress syndrome. As with hypoglycemia, awareness on the part of

the anesthesiologist should be the rule, and treatment should be available. A rapid infusion of 10 mg/kg of calcium chloride or 30 mg/kg of calcium gluconate is usually effective in reversing tetany. Maintenance therapy should start at 250 mg/kg/24 hrs of calcium chloride or 750 mg/kg/24 hrs of calcium gluconate. Signs of hypoglycemia and hypocalcemia may be masked during anesthesia when muscle relaxants are used with artificial ventilation.

Neonatal hypocalcemia is related to low parathyroid hormone activity and decreased stores of available calcium.[14] Parathyroid hormone activity is normal after about three days in the term infant, but may not be normal for up to several weeks in the premature.[15,16]

THERMOREGULATION

Hypothermia in the newborn and small child undergoing surgery continues to be a problem, particularly in major surgery of the chest where a large surface area is exposed to the air, allowing high evaporative and convective heat loss. Both anesthesiologist and surgeon should attempt to *prevent* the heat loss rather than try to correct it after it occurs. The consequences of unintentional hypothermia in the newborn have been reported since 1900, when Budin reported 90 percent mortality in newborns whose temperatures were allowed to fall to 32° C.[17] It has been shown that not only the degree of hypothermia but the frequency of deviation from normothermia, even without extreme temperature changes, contributes significantly to morbidity and mortality in the newborn period.[18] It is, therefore, the responsibility of those caring for the premature infant and newborn undergoing surgery to prevent unintentional hypothermia, which results in acidosis and cardiovascular depression, and to minimize fluctuations of temperature. Thermoneutrality is a delicate balance between heat production and heat conservation. The newborn and small child have a limited ability to produce heat, mostly through the metabolism of brown fat. Premature infants have reduced stores of brown fat. In order to maintain thermoneutrality, the premature infant, newborn, and small child must depend heavily on heat conservation. Because of a higher alveolar ventilation, the rate of heat lost to unheated, dry anesthetic gases by an infant is greater than that of an adult, and the development of hypothermia may be quite rapid. Anesthesia ablates the body's response to cold stress, making heat conservation in the operating room essential if the morbidity of hypothermia is to be avoided. Accepted techniques include raising the ambient temperature of the operating room, warming and humidifying anesthetic gases, using only warm scrub and irrigating solutions, using swaddling and other insulation and protection from wetting, non-ionizing heat lamps, thermal mattresses, and warming of all intravenous fluids. The importance of using as many of these heat conservation methods as possible cannot be overemphasized if thermoneutrality is to be preserved. In children, oxygen consumption has been shown to double in the immediate postoperative period if the child is allowed to emerge from anesthesia in a hypothermic state.[19] If respiratory function is even mildly depressed by narcotics, relaxants, or intrinsic disease, the child may not be able to meet his oxygen demands and can deteriorate rapidly. If unintentional hypothermia does occur during surgery, it must be corrected prior to removal of respiratory support. Equally important is maintenance of temperature during transport to and from the operating room. Portable heated Isolettes and open beds equipped with warming lights or radiant heaters are available for this purpose.

PREOPERATIVE ASSESSMENT

All too often the amount of preoperative information available to the anesthesiologist is inversely related to the severity of the disease being treated. The critically ill, cyanotic newborn may be transferred from another facility and must be evaluated quickly by the receiving physicians in order to establish a diagnosis. Investigative procedures such as radiographs, cardiac catheterization, and laboratory evaluation must be accomplished quickly so that life-saving measures may be taken.

Evaluation of the cyanotic newborn infant poses special problems, since there are multiple causes resulting in arterial desaturation. Congenital heart defects must be considered, but other causes of hypoxemia include congenital diaphragmatic hernia, tracheo-esophageal fistula with aspiration pneumonia, other forms of pneumonia, sepsis, pneumothorax, congenital pulmonary-space-occupying defects, and upper airway obstruction. (Table 16-3 and Figs. 16-3 to 16-5).[20]

Older children scheduled for elective thoracic operations are usually hospitalized one to several days prior to the planned surgery, during which time necessary consultations may be obtained from physicians such as pulmonologists, cardiologists, hematologists, and other specialists as indicated. Appropriate laboratory data can be obtained and the child observed by the medical and nursing staff for evidence of upper respiratory infections, contagious childhood diseases, febrile episodes, or gastrointestinal symptoms.

When dealing with congenital anomalies such as tracheo-esophageal fistula or certain forms of congenital heart disease, the anesthesiologist should always be aware that other associated anomalies may be present.[21-23] Such defects should be discussed with the parents, and their expected influence on the immediate and late outcome of the proposed operation considered. Nutritional status should be evaluated by the history and the anesthesiologist's physical examination. The upper airway and mobility of the mandible and the cervical spine are examined. Pulmonary function may be evaluated by careful auscultation of the lungs, observation of the child's breathing pattern, the results of arterial or capillary blood gases

Table 16-3
Mnemonics for Differential Diagnosis of the Cyanotic Infant

"C" Cardiac Disease	"O" Obstruction of the airway	"P" Pulmonary Parenchymal Disease	"S" Space-occupying Lesion
The 5 "T's"	Choanal atresia	Respiratory distress	Diaphragmatic hernia
Tetralogy of Fallot	Pierre-Robin syn-	syndrome	Pneumothorax
Transposition of	drome	Persistence of the fetal	Hemothorax
great vessels	Laryngeal web	circulation	Lung cysts
Tricuspid atresia	Macroglossia	Pneumonia	Chylothorax
Total anomalous	Laryngotracheal mala-	Meconium aspiration	Eventration of dia-
pulmonary ve-	cia	Hyaline membrane	phragm
nous return	Subglottic heman-	disease	
Truncus arteriosus	gioma		
The 2 "AT's"			
Aortic atresia			
Pulmonary atresia			

(COPS = Causes of Cyanosis; 5 T's and 2 AT's = Cardiac Causes of Cyanosis).

and the chest radiograph, as well as any indicated pulmonary function tests. The need for ventilatory support following thoracic operations can often be determined during the preoperative visit.

Cardiac function can be estimated from details in the history and physical examination recorded by referring physicians, as well as the anesthesiologist's own examination of the precordium, peripheral pulses, color, and general habitus of the patient. Hepatic and renal function may well be affected by the presence or absence of cardiac dysfunction. Palpation of the liver edge and a careful review of significant laboratory data including blood urea nitrogen, creatinine, and liver enzymes may help elucidate the status of these organs.

Whenever possible, a patient's previous anesthetic history should be evaluated by noting his response during previous hospitalizations if surgery was performed, and by discussing the patient's past history with the parents. Important also is the determination of any family history suggesting problems associated with anesthesia, including such entities as malignant hyperthermia or pseudocholinesterase deficiency.

An understanding of the details of the planned surgical procedure is essential for the anesthesiologist caring for any patient. In thoracic operations these are frequently complex, and information is best obtained by direct communication with the attending surgeon. It is also helpful to ascertain the status of the opposite lung in cases involving a thoracotomy. This information can frequently be obtained in discussions with the surgeons and other physicians involved in the care of the patient.

The preoperative visit by the anesthesiologist to the patient and his family is extremely important in the overall management of patients requiring any operation, but especially those which involve thoracic surgery. Besides obtaining the needed information about the patient and his condition, the anesthesiologist's preoperative visit is helpful in allowing the parents to ask questions, express fears and anxieties, and to more clearly understand what is planned for their child. An explanation is made to the parents as to the plan for premedication drugs, induction techniques, expected time for surgery, and the need for intensive care unit or respiratory support postoperatively.

Preoperative Orders and Premedication

It is unnecessary, and may indeed be harmful, to withhold oral feedings for long periods before operation. This is especially true in the young infant or the cyanotic,

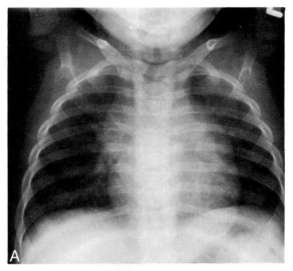

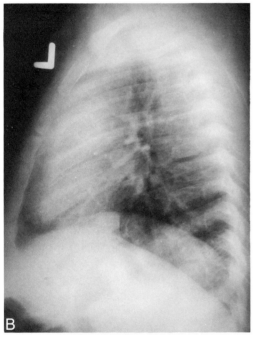

Fig. 16-3 (A) Normal infant's chest radiograph showing widening of mediastinum due to normal thymic shadow, horizontal ribs, and relatively high diaphragm. The buckling of the trachea toward the right is normal with expiration. (B) The lateral radiograph shows retrosternal fullness also due to normal thymic shadow.

polycythemic child. Except in the very ill patient, gastric emptying time is sufficiently rapid to allow oral intake of glucose-containing clear liquids up to three or four hours prior to induction of anesthesia. Breast-fed babies may be breast-fed with the last feeding being completed four hours prior to induction, since the curd of breast milk is more quickly digested in the infant's stomach.[24] Newborn infants requiring surgery usually

are not being fed due to the condition prompting the operation (e.g., tracheo-esophageal fistula, diaphragmatic hernia, cyanotic congenital heart defects), but will usually be nourished with parenteral glucose-containing fluids.

Steward states that premedication for children should be effective for the purpose—an adequate dose of appropriate drug(s), not a routine regimen, and as pain-

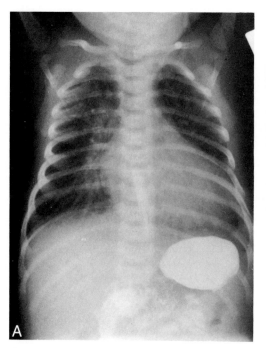
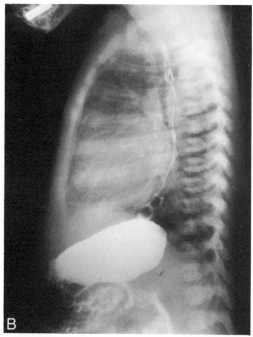

Fig. 16-4 6-week-old female infant with transposition of the great arteries and ventricular septal defect. (A) Chest radiograph showing large transverse cardiac silhouette with narrow base ("egg-on-a-string" configuration) related to superimposition of aorta and pulmonary artery shadows in the A-P view; absence of thymic shadow; increased pulmonary blood flow and mild interstitial pulmonary edema. (B) In lateral view, note increase in heart size.

less as possible.[25] Certainly all children do not require premedication. Some children respond to certain preanesthetic drugs with significant dysphoria, and many are willing to accept a skillfully performed intravenous induction through a small-bore needle rather than undergo the pain of intramuscular injections. However, many authors believe that children undergoing most thoracic surgical procedures, including open heart surgery, should be relatively heavily premedicated using a combination of a sedative or tranquilizer, usually administered orally, and a narcotic and anticholinergic agent administered intravenously or intramuscularly.[26-30] The anticholinergic agents are often omitted in patients with asthma or cystic fibrosis, or those with a relatively fixed cardiac output (e.g., aortic stenosis, pulmonary stenosis, or mitral stenosis) in whom a significant increase in heart rate is undesirable. Infants

beyond the newborn period undergoing intrathoracic procedures during the first year of life are usually premedicated with morphine sulfate (0.2 mg/kg) and atropine sulfate (0.015 mg/kg) given intramuscularly 45 minutes prior to arrival in the operating area. Children over one year of age are usually premedicated with a sedative or tranquilizer administered by mouth, as well as morphine and atropine, or morphine and scopolamine (0.01 mg/kg). In the older child, it may be advantageous to add diazepam (0.1 mg/kg), or lorazepam (0.05 mg/kg, maximum dose 3 mg) the night prior to the proposed operation and two hours prior to the administration of the morphine and anticholinergic medication (Table 16-4).

Patients with certain forms of congenital heart disease may present unique premedication problems. Children with tetralogy of Fallot may experience intermittent hyper-

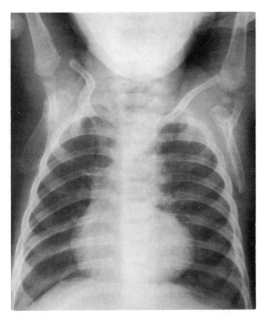

Fig. 16-5 4-month-old male with tetralogy of Fallot. A-P chest radiograph shows "boot shaped heart" (coeur en sabot) with upturned apex: concave pulmonary artery segment; decreased pulmonary vascular markings; right aortic arch proven at catheterization.

cyanotic episodes ("spells") due to an increase in right ventricular outflow tract obstruction and an increase in the right-to-left shunt. These "spells" may be precipitated by agitation, anger, and trauma; or they may occur without any apparent cause. They are usually treated with morphine and oxygen, and by placing the infant or child in the knee-chest position, thus increasing venous return and allowing more blood to flow to the lungs. Morphine is theoretically a desirable premedicant drug for patients demonstrating these "spells." Some patients with tetralogy of Fallot who experience hypercyanotic spells take propranolol to ameliorate the severity and frequency of these dangerous episodes.[31-33] Propranolol has been effective in terminating the acute infundibular spasm that sets off these attacks, and such patients are frequently receiving propranolol on a chronic basis. If these patients present as candidates for palliation or for thoracic surgical procedures other than correction, it is preferable not to discontinue this drug prior to anesthesia if signs of ex-

Table 16-4
Anesthetic Premedication

Drug	Dose	Route
Anticholinergics		
Atropine	.01 mg/kg	IV, IM
Scopolamine	.005 mg/kg	IV, IM
Glycopyrrolate (Robinul)	.005 mg/kg	IV, IM
Narcotics and narcotic like drugs		
Morphine	.1 mg/kg	IV, IM
Meperidine (Demerol)	2 mg/kg	PO
Pentazocine (Talwin)	1 mg/kg	IV, IM
Hypnotics		
Pentobarbital (Nembutal)	1–2 mg/kg	PO, IV, IM, PR
Secobarbital (Seconal)	1–2 mg/kg	PO, IV, IM, PR
Thiopental (Pentothal)	10–15 mg/kg	PR
Methohexital (Brevital)	15 mg/kg	PR
Chloral Hydrate	50 mg/kg	PO, PR
Tranquilizers		
Promethazine (Phenergan)	0.3 mg/kg	PO, IV, IM, PR
Hydroxyzine (Vistaril)	2 mg/kg	PO, IM
Diazepam (Valium)	0.2 mg/kg	PO, IV, IM
Flurazepam (Ativan)	.05 mg/kg	PO, IM
Droperidol (Inapsine)	0.1 mg/kg	IV, IM

cessive beta-blockade are absent. In addition, propranolol diluted to 0.1 mg/ml should be available. If a "spell" occurs as evidenced by increasing cyanosis, developing acidosis, or the disappearance of the systolic ejection murmur indicating infundibular spasm, propranolol should be given intravenously (0.01 mg/kg up to a total dose of 1 mg). Other methods of managing hypercyanotic episodes include the administration of morphine, an increase in FIO_2 to 100 percent, volume expansion, and/or the administration of a pure alpha-adrenergic agonist to increase peripheral resistance.[34]

Atropine effectively blocks the action of the cardiac vagus nerve and may obviate the fall in cardiac output seen with induction doses of the potent anesthetic agents halothane, enflurane, and isoflurane.[35,36] Atropine probably should always be administered prior to the administration of succinylcholine, even in patients with asthma or cystic fibrosis, as well as to patients who receive ketamine for induction of anesthesia. It probably should not be given to children who have a history of a recent significant elevation of body temperature. In patients undergoing insertion of permanent pacemakers, atropine may theoretically cloud the issue of pacemaker capture if the heart rate is faster than the desired rate of the pacemaker being inserted. However, this is not usually a problem, since most pacemakers used in children are placed to treat congenital complete heart block which does not respond to atropine.

ANESTHETIC MANAGEMENT

In general, the pathological condition prompting the need for surgery, as well as the physical status of the patient, determines the choice of the anesthetic technique to be used.

Infants and children requiring thoracic operations may fall into ASA Physical Status I or II (e.g., an asymptomatic patent ductus arteriosus); but more often than not, young patients for thoracic operations will fall into ASA Physical Status III or IV. Sicker patients will usually come to the operating room with intravenous catheters and monitoring devices in place. This often facilitates the induction of anesthesia, since the administration of narcotics and muscle relaxants can be titrated to the desired effect.

If no direct monitoring devices are in place, the essential monitoring instruments are applied before induction is begun. These include:

1. The *precordial stethoscope* applied so that both heart sounds and breath sounds are audible;
2. A *blood pressure cuff* (usually either a Doppler-principle device (Arteriosonde or Infrasonde) or oscillometric type (Dinemapp); and,
3. The oscillographic display of the *electrocardiogram.*

Induction of anesthesia is then begun by one of several methods depending on the overall anesthetic plan and the condition being treated.

Induction Techniques

In the very sick patient, preoxygenation is desirable before any drugs are administered. If the presence of the mask is disturbing to the child, holding the mask a few inches above the face between cupped hands and giving a high flow of oxygen from the anesthesia machine will suffice. If no intravenous is established, a large-bore cannula can be inserted during pre-oxygenation after appropriate local anesthesia of the skin. An alternative method of intravenous induction, especially useful in older healthier children, is to give the induction medications (usually thiopental and atropine) via a very small bore needle (27 gauge) followed by succinylcholine (from a separate non-Luer-Lok syringe). This needle is removed after induction is complete and the trachea intubated; a large-bore intravenous cannula is then inserted with the patient asleep.

Thiopental is rarely used in patients classified ASA IV because of its direct depressant effect on the heart. Rather, a combination of a narcotic such as fentanyl and diazepam is titrated to loss of the lid reflex.

For the cyanotic patient, ketamine, given either intramuscularly (up to 5 mg/kg) or intravenously (up to 2 mg/kg) is often employed. The theoretical disadvantage of ketamine is its sympathomimetic action which produces an increase in heart rate and in systemic and pulmonary artery pressure. In the patient with tetralogy of Fallot physiology (i.e., some form of right ventricular outflow obstruction, and a ventricular-septal defect with a right-to-left shunt), ketamine might increase the right-to-left shunt by precipitating infundibular "spasm" as is seen in the previously described "spells." In addition, ketamine produces dose-related myocardial depression in the isolated heart preparation.[37,38] However, if the sympathetic nervous system is intact or only slightly depressed, ketamine appears to result in an increase in cardiac output and can be used safely as an induction agent in patients with tetralogy physiology.[39] It is important that propranolol be available and ready for administration should a hypercyanotic episode occur during induction of ketamine anesthesia in these patients.

In spite of the theoretical disadvantages of ketamine as an induction agent, it has been found to be quite safe and effective in many cyanotic patients. Such patients should be adequately premedicated with morphine (0.2 mg/kg). Inadequate premedication may result in fright and agitation; excessive doses of sedatives or tranquilizers may result in hypoventilation, hypoxemia, and hypercarbia which can produce an increase in sympathomimetic activity and make a hypercyanotic episode more likely. In addition, hypercyanotic spells appear more likely to occur during manipulation of the heart than during the induction process, probably due to changes in venous return resulting in relative or actual hypovolemia.

If an inhalation induction is selected for a relatively healthy patient, the child is allowed to breathe nitrous oxide and oxygen for several minutes after the initial monitoring devices are applied. The patient is talked to during this period in a quiet and reassuring manner. Then, halothane, enflurane, or isoflurane is begun using low concentrations, with a gradual increase in dose every four or five breaths. Systemic blood pressure, heart sounds, and peripheral pulse volume are monitored. After the patient is asleep, intravenous catheters are inserted, other drugs are administered, and further monitoring established.

Monitoring During Thoracic Operations

The monitoring selected by the anesthesiologist depends on several factors: (1) the physical status of the patient, (2) the operation anticipated, and (3) the expected postoperative course. Even the simplest operation in the very sick infant or child may warrant extensive monitoring. Many children undergoing thoracic surgery require accurate and reliable monitoring in the operating room and intensive care unit.

No matter how many physiologic parameters are measured, no monitoring scheme is infallible. Correct interpretation by the anesthesiologist of the data provided is essential. Each additional monitoring technique must be evaluated from the standpoint of (1) its ease of application, (2) the risk/benefit ratio, and (3) the cost/benefit ratio.[40]

Even the most sophisticated monitoring systems available today fail to tell what is really necessary to know: the presence of pain, the accurate assessment of regional perfusion, and the metabolic changes occurring within the cell.[41] The anesthesiologist is the "ultimate" monitor; the instruments employed, either simple or complex, are only data-collecting devices which enable him to

Table 16-5
Monitoring of the Pediatric Thoracic Surgical Patient

1. Pre-induction
   a. Precordial stethoscope
   b. Blood pressure cuff (usually Doppler or oscillometric device)[a]
   c. Electrocardiogram (ECG)
   d. Neuromuscular blockade monitor electrodes
   e. Temperature (usually axillary probe or cutaneous strip)
2. Post-induction, prior to start of operation
   a. Intra-arterial catheter[a]
   b. Central venous pressure catheter[b]
   c. Urinary bladder catheter
   d. Rectal temperature thermistor probe (or esophageal or nasopharyngeal)[c]
   e. Esophageal stethoscope[c]
   f. Neuromuscular blockade monitor (determine twitch, tetanus, and train-of-four responses BEFORE administering neuromuscular agents.)
3. Before closure
   a. Pacing wires (atrial and/or ventricular)[d]
   b. Atrial pressure catheters (left and/or right)[d]
   c. Pulmonary artery catheters (for pressure measurements and administration of medications directly into the pulmonary circulation.)[d]
   d. Pulmonary artery thermistor catheter (for cardiac output determination.)[d]

[a] Blood pressure cuffs and intra-arterial lines are placed on the contralateral side of a previous or proposed Blalock-Taussig shunt or on the right side during repair of coarctation of the aorta.
[b] Usually via the right internal jugular vein placed percutaneously or via the external jugular vein using a J-wire; occasionally, via either antebrachial vein.
[c] Esophageal stethoscopes and temperature probes should be avoided during operations involving the esophagus. If used, the surgeon should *always* be informed of the presence of such devices.
[d] Utilized in selected patients.

receive, process, assimilate, and appropriately respond.

Table 16-5 lists the monitoring devices which should be considered for use in patients undergoing thoracic operations (see Ch. 6). Such an outline is useful for monitoring most patients, but additional measurements may be indicated in *specific* patients.

ELECTROCARDIOGRAPHY

The use of the electrocardiogram (ECG) as a monitoring device in the operating room has been a relatively late development, coming during the early 1960s.[42,43] Leads should be placed to clearly demonstrate atrial depolarization (P wave), ventricular depolarization (QRS), and the repolarization complex (T wave), so that dysrhythmias arising from atrium or ventricle, and changes in repolarization due to drug effect or electrolytes (K^+ or Ca^{++}) can be appreciated. While the electrocardiogram is a valuable source of information about the cardiovascular system, it must be remembered that it is only an *electrical* signal, and gives no information as to the actual *function* of the heart.

The infant or child's resting heart rate is normally more rapid than that of the adult. Therefore, the definitions of significant tachycardia and bradycardia are different.[44] In infants, a heart rate greater than 180 beats per minute or less than 100 beats per minute should be carefully evaluated.

ARTERIAL BLOOD PRESSURE

The systemic arterial pressure is determined by blood volume, cardiac output, peripheral resistance, elasticity of the arterial wall, proximal patency of the artery, and the characteristics of the recording system. Systemic arterial pressure and organ perfusion are related through vascular resistance. Blood flow to any given organ may be adequate even when there is relative hypotension; conversely, organ flow may be inadequate when the blood pressure is normal or even elevated. Nevertheless, the accurate measurement and recording of systemic blood pressure, either directly or indirectly using oscillometric or Doppler devices, are important in assessing adequacy of cardiac function.

Most, but not all, thoracic operations require the insertion of intra-arterial catheters for direct pressure measurement. If intra-arterial pressure measurement is not considered necessary, an oscillometric system (e.g., Dinamapp) can be used in cases where blood pressure measurement is needed frequently throughout the surgery. The cuff should be placed on an extremity opposite that in which intravenous infusions are being given, since the time for inflations and deflations of the cuff interfere with fluid and drug administration. If intra-arterial monitoring is utilized, the cannula is placed in a location convenient to the anesthesiologist to allow frequent arterial blood sampling for measurements of blood gases, hematocrit, serum electrolytes, blood glucose, and other necessary parameters The radial artery is usually selected for percutaneous catheterization just proximal to the volar carpal ligament. Stopcocks should *not* be used at the hub of the 22-gauge one-inch plastic cannula. A T-connector with a rubber diaphragm should be used instead of a stopcock in order to reduce the risk of inadvertent injection of air, frequent motion and arterial trauma produced by turning the stopcock handle, and bacterial contamination from the open end of the stopcock. The rubber diaphragm of the T-connector can be used for sampling by puncturing it with a small-bore needle and allowing a few drops of blood to drip out to clear the cannula of flush solution. Little or no negative pressure need be applied to the syringe during sampling, since it will fill from the force of the intra-arterial pressure. Negative pressure tends to collapse the very small vessel and leads to thrombogenic trauma, spasm, and early loss of the monitoring catheter.

The indwelling arterial cannula is connected to a pressure transducer and the wave form displayed on an oscilloscope. The cannula should be continuously flushed with a solution of normal saline containing 1000 units of heparin per 100 cc fluid at a rate of 2 cc/hour. The arterial cannula, cannulation site, and T-connector should be conspicuously labeled to avoid inadvertent injection of medications or air into the artery.

When the radial artery on either side is not patent or otherwise not available, alternative sites of cannulation must be considered. The left radial artery should *not* be used for monitoring during operations for repair of coarctation of the aorta or vascular rings, since the left subclavian artery will be clamped during the repair and the radial artery trace lost. When a Blalock-Taussig shunt has been or is being done, the radial artery on the ipsilateral side cannot be used, since the subclavian artery is utilized to construct the shunt. For the best accessibility for the anesthesiologist, the superficial temporal artery may be used as an alternative site for cannulation. Direct femoral arterial cannulation may be necessary in cases where radial and temporal arteries have already been used, but this is quite inconvenient since blood sampling must be done from the leg. Umbilical arterial lines are useful if present in the neonate presenting for intrathoracic operation. However, in repair of a coarctation, an arterial line proximal to the coarctation must also be inserted. Blood sampling for blood gases from an umbilical arterial line, in the presence of increased pulmonary vascular resistance and a patent ductus arteriosus, may be misleading. In this case, blood shunted right-to-left through the ductus will cause the PaO_2 below the ductus to be falsely low. Blood leaving the heart and perfusing the retinal arteries may have a dangerously high PaO_2, placing the susceptible patient at risk for retrolental fibroplasia.[45–47]

CENTRAL VENOUS PRESSURE

Central venous pressure (CVP) measurement is indicated when the volume status of the child is unstable or likely to change rapidly, as would be expected when massive blood or third space loss is anticipated. Monitoring catheters for CVP can be inserted percutaneously through the brachial vein in older children, and sometimes in younger ones undergoing thoracic operations. This relatively large-bore catheter also provides a useful route for the injection of irritating medications such as calcium, vasopressors, or blood products.

Central venous catheters can also be inserted by the external jugular veins in children. An 18-gauge 1¼-inch intravenous catheter is introduced into an external jugular vein through which a J-wire is passed and manipulated into the chest. The CVP catheter is then placed over the J-wire and advanced into the central circulation. Percutaneous internal jugular vein catheterization is often utilized in pediatric patients having thoracic operations. A low incidence of complications is reported by advocates of this technique.[48-50] A high approach to the internal jugular vein is advisable in children to avoid the lung.[51]

Extreme caution must be exercised in the care of centrally placed catheters, indeed, *all* venous catheters in children with cyanotic congenital heart disease. Even very small air bubbles in any intravenous catheter, tubing, or connectors pose potentially lethal hazards due to the possibility of an air embolus to the brain, coronary arteries, or other vital organs. In the acyanotic child, air in the venous system may also reach the systemic circulation through either a patent foramen ovale, atrial or ventricular septal defect, or patent ductus arteriosus during coughing, a Valsalva maneuver, or positive pressure ventilation.

Transthoracic right and left atrial catheters are used in lieu of CVP catheters in some cardiac surgical procedures not requiring cardiopulmonary bypass (CPB), and in most cases in which CPB is used. The catheters are passed through the chest wall, secured to the skin, and kept patent using a constant infusion of saline and heparin. When no longer needed, these catheters are withdrawn through the chest wall, and, surprisingly, the incidence of complications (bleeding, catheter entrapment, sepsis, thrombosis) is very low.

TEMPERATURE

The importance of monitoring and maintaining body temperature near normal in children during surgery and anesthesia is well-documented.[52-57] Changes in body temperature during anesthesia may result from exposure to a cold environment, reaction to anesthetic drugs, infusion of cold intravenous fluids or blood, and vasoconstriction or vasodilatation. Uncontrolled hypothermia in any patient is undesirable, but in the neonate and premature infant produces metabolic acidosis and myocardial and respiratory depression. Hyperthermia is also dangerous, since oxygen consumption increases significantly.[52,58] For this reason, significant hyperthermia is especially detrimental in patients with cyanotic forms of congenital heart disease.

Temperature should be monitored in every pediatric patient by use of a thermistor probe placed in the nasopharynx, or orally into the upper esophagus. During bronchoscopy or esophagoscopy, axillary or rectal temperature should be measured.

URINARY OUTPUT

Continuous monitoring of urine output during surgery is one of the most reliable signs of adequate hydration, blood volume, and cardiac output. Almost all patients undergoing cardiovascular surgery or other complex intrathoracic procedures should have a urinary bladder catheter placed for accurate timed measurements of urine volume, and, at times, specific gravity and osmolarity. In short procedures such as ligation of a patent ductus, urinary catheters are often safely omitted. The urethral meatus of the newborn or premature infant may be too small to accept even the smallest Foley catheter. If this is the case, a small infant feeding tube (8 Fr) can be inserted just beyond the point of first urine drainage, and fixed in place to the skin either with a suture or using benzoin and adhesive tape. Adequate urine production is considered to be 1 cc/kg body weight/hour.[27,28,59,60]

NEUROMUSCULAR BLOCKADE

Muscle relaxants are used as anesthetic adjuncts in many thoracic operations. Like other drugs, they should be administered in a safe and controlled manner. For neuromuscular blockade monitoring, two ECG electrodes are attached over the ulnar aspect of the wrist in which the arterial catheter is placed. Muscle twitch, tetanus, and train-of-four responses are determined *prior to* the administration of any muscle relaxants and checked periodically throughout the operation; additional muscle relaxants are given as needed based on frequently observed responses. If postoperative mechanical ventilation is not needed, nondepolarizing muscle relaxants are reversed at the end of operation and the blockade monitor used as one indicator of adequacy of reversal.

ARTERIAL BLOOD GASES,
ELECTROLYTES, HEMOGLOBIN, AND
GLUCOSE

Blood obtained from the arterial cannula is periodically analyzed for blood gases, sodium, potassium, hemoglobin/hematocrit, glucose, and ionized calcium. No particular interval between these samples is recommended, the frequency being determined by the hemodynamic stability of the patient and, to some extent, by the experience of the anesthesiologist. It is important to make some or all of these determinations shortly after induction of anesthesia to determine acid-base status, adequacy of ventilation, and baseline serum electrolytes and glucose.

ASSESSMENT OF BLOOD LOSS

Accurate estimation of blood loss is difficult, at best; but careful attention must be paid to this aspect of thoracic operations in patients of all ages, especially in the very young infant. This is best accomplished by:

1. Close observation of the operative field.
2. Careful monitoring of pulse rate, estimation of pulse volume, and frequent measurement of blood pressure. The systolic blood pressure is probably the most reliable indicator of blood volume in the infant.[61]
3. Weighing of all sponges and laps *before* they begin to dry out, and subtracting known dry weight from weight of bloody sponges or laps.
4. Measuring of blood suctioned from the surgical field in low-volume graduated suction bottles easily visible or accessible to the anesthesiologist.
5. Keeping an accurate record of irrigation used in the surgical field to avoid confusion with actual blood loss on sponges or in suction containers.
6. Estimation of blood on drapes.

A running total of estimated blood loss should be recorded on the anesthesia record at appropriate intervals, and the final total as well as the amount replaced reported to the surgeon and to the nurse receiving the patient postoperatively.

Intubation of the Trachea

For children undergoing intrathoracic surgical procedures the choice of nasal vs. oral intubation is relatively easy. Any child who is expected to need postoperative ventilatory support should be given the advantages of a nasal intubation. A nasotracheal tube may be placed initially in some patients, or an orotracheal tube may be replaced by a nasal tube after the surgical procedure is completed. Nasal tubes are easier to secure, tolerated better with less chewing and gagging, and the need for an uncomfortable oral airway is eliminated. If heparin is going to be used during surgery, caution must be exercised during insertion of the nasotracheal tube in order to avoid bleeding from the nasal mucosa.

In preparation for intubation all needed equipment should be tested and at hand. The low oxygen reserves of the premature newborn allow little enough time for intubation without having to stop and obtain equipment. The choice of laryngoscope blades depends upon personal preference. Anatomic considerations, i.e., the short neck and bulky tongue, make the use of straight blades generally more desirable in the newborn and small child. Most prematures and small-for-gestational-age infants require a Miller O, or Guedel 1 blade; the Miller 1 is more suitable for term infants. Beyond the age of two years, curved blades become an equally acceptable choice. In all cases, more than one size of blade should be on hand should the primary choice be unsuitable.

Choice of appropriate tube size and type should be based on the patient's age and size (Table 16-6). Other considerations such as a previous recent intubation, history of prolonged intubation, or previous surgery may modify the selection of the expected tube size. Cuffed tubes less than 5.0 mm I.D. are not recommended, even though available.

The presence of the cuff occupies vital space, increasing resistance and possibly hampering adequate ventilation. If prolonged intubation in older children is anticipated, the high volume, low pressure (Lanz type) cuffs are recommended. The Cole type, or tapered tubes, are not recommended for long term use in neonates. Double-lumen tubes are not available in pediatric sizes, but selective mainstem intubation and bronchial blockade using a Fogarty catheter have been employed to achieve one-lung ventilation.[62]

Tradition has held that newborns should be intubated awake. This attitude is a carry-over from the days of ether anesthesia and should be modified to accommodate today's anesthetic techniques. There are surgical indications for awake intubation without relaxation or assisted ventilation, e.g., tracheo-esophageal fistula, where gas introduced under pressure might pass from the trachea into the distal esophagus and distend the stomach; and there are airway indications in which muscle relaxants are relatively contraindicated, e.g., severe Pierre-Robin syndrome, where management of the airway may become difficult or impossible if the patient is paralyzed. Just as an awake intubation in an older child or adult would not be considered without some form of sedation

Table 16-6
Selection of Endotracheal Tubes

A. Guidelines for selection of endotracheal tube, measured in millimeters of internal diameter

Premature or small for gestational age:	2.5–3.0 mm
Normal term newborn:	3.5 mm
6 months to 2 years:	4.0–4.5 mm
Greater than 2 years:	$\dfrac{age + 18}{4}$ = mm I.D.

B. Guidelines for proper depth of insertion of endotracheal tubes, approximate

	Oral	Nasal
Newborn:	9.5 cm	Crown-heel length × .21 cm
6 months:	10.5–11 cm	Crown-heel length × 0.16 + 2.5 cm
Greater than 1 year:	$\dfrac{age + 12}{2}$ cm	Crown-heel length × 0.16 + 2.5 cm

(except in the "full stomach" situation), the use of small amounts of sedation is often indicated before intubation in children.

Pre-oxygenation plays a critical role in the safety of intubation in the infant and small child. These patients are already at a disadvantage by having increased oxygen demands (4 ml/kg/min) and proportionately less alveolar surface through which to absorb oxygen. Their alveolar ventilation is normally twice that of an adult. Thus, it is understandable why the time elapsed between loss of oxygen supply or alveolar ventilation and the onset of hypoxemia is very short. When other pathology exists, such as congestive heart failure, pneumonia, or respiratory distress of the newborn, borderline hypoxemia may already exist and can be dangerously exaggerated during intubation if pre-oxygenation is not employed. Pre-oxygenation prior to intubation should be done in most children using 100 percent oxygen. An exception to this is in the premature infant who is at risk for developing retrolental fibroplasia in whom an oxygen concentration no more than 10 percent greater than that which is the therapeutic level prior to surgery should be used for pre-oxygenation.

Intubation technique should include the following points:

1. *Stabilize the head.* The prominent occiput and relatively large head size make the infant's head roll easily on the table. The use of a foam rubber "doughnut" or similar device is useful in stabilizing the head and placing the head in the "sniffing" position.
2. *Identify both esophagus and trachea.* The newborn and small child's vocal apparatus does not resemble that of the adult. Care is required to avoid inadvertent esophageal intubation. The placement of a suction catheter or nasogastric tube into the esophagus may aid in identifying airway structures.
3. *Visually assess endotracheal tube passage beyond the cords.* The short distance (4-6 cm) between the vocal apparatus and carina makes accidental passage into the right or left mainstem bronchus relatively easy, but can be prevented by careful observation of the endotracheal tube as it is inserted. The formulas for depth of insertion shown in Table 16-6 are only guidelines. Immediate auscultation after intubation should be done to determine that breath sounds are equal bilaterally. Radiographic confirmation should be used when needed.

4. *Avoid excessive manipulation of the vocal cord structures.* Multiple attempts at intubation result in tissue edema and bleeding, both of which can complicate extubation. Of all the causes of post-intubation croup, multiple attempts at intubation has been cited as one of the most important.[63] The small airways of the infant and small child are extremely susceptible to obstruction secondary to edema.

5. *Do not prolong attempts to intubate.* Infants and small children do not have the oxygen reserves present in older children and adults. The first sign of hypoxemia is usually bradycardia. If the heart rate slows during attempts to intubate, the anesthesiologist should stop immediately, re-oxygenate, and then proceed. Vagal stimulation may also decrease the heart rate and should be blocked with atropine (0.01 mg/kg intravenously).

Proper anchoring of the endotracheal tube is essential, since the patient may be virtually inaccessible during thoracic surgery. Nasal intubation requires anchoring which will prevent in-and-out motion of the tube and avoid compression of the nares. Oral intubation requires both lateral stabilization and prevention of in-and-out motion. Tincture of benzoin can be applied to the face and to the tube prior to taping, since saliva will dissolve most adhesives. If the patient will be positioned so that secretions will drain out of the mouth onto the endotracheal tube, a bite block made of an absorbent material may be placed in the mouth to prevent secretions from reaching the tape. Newborn infants have a waxy layer of material on the skin known as vernix caseosa. This material may interfere with adhesives (e.g., tape, ECG and grounding pads), and should be removed with mild soap or alcohol prior to surgery. After the endotracheal tube is well anchored, the stomach should be aspirated to remove any air or other material contents.

The complications of intubation in infants and children are the same as in adults. Hypoxia is the most common, followed by soft tissue damage and tooth dislocation. Perforation of the trachea or esophagus is, fortunately, a rare complication, but does occur. The use of stylets on a routine basis is discouraged for this reason.

The minimum criteria for extubation are listed in Table 16-7. A post-extubation chest radiograph is usually indicated after any thoracic surgical procedure, since right upper lobe atelectasis is quite common after prolonged intubation in children. Competency of the glottic structures to prevent aspiration may not be regained for as long as eight hours after extubation; therefore, cautious feedings of clear liquids should be given initially and progressed only as tolerated (see appendix).[64]

Maintenance of Anesthesia

After induction of anesthesia has been accomplished, intravenous and monitoring lines established, the trachea intubated and the endotracheal tube secured, the appropriate level of anesthesia is usually maintained with a combination of nitrous oxide/oxygen and halothane, enflurane, or isoflurane in low concentrations along with a nondepolarizing muscle relaxant. In higher risk patients, the potent anesthetics are omitted and a narcotic substituted.

In most pediatric thoracic operations, a sump-type nasogastric tube is inserted into

Table 16-7
Minimum Criteria for Extubation

1. Inspired oxygen $\leq 40\%$
2. IMV ≤ 2
3. CPAP or PEEP ≤ 4 cm H_2O
4. Stable blood gases
   PaO_2 80–100 mmHg
   $PaCO_2$ 35–45 mmHg
   pH 7.30–7.40
5. Cardiovascular stability—no vasopressors
6. Metabolism or reversal of muscle relaxants and respiratory depressants
7. CNS stability—no active seizure disorder or progressive coma
8. Electrolyte balance—including glucose and calcium

the stomach to avoid gastric distention intraoperatively from swallowed air or from anesthetic gases which may leak around the endotracheal tube. Gastric distention may interfere with the surgical exposure, especially during operations in the left hemithorax, and can cause reflex bradycardia and hypotension. An esophageal stethoscope is placed with its tip in the mid-esophagus to monitor heart sounds and breath sounds during surgery. In thoracic procedures, the surgeon should *always* be informed of the presence of an esophageal stethoscope, since palpation of the instrument in the esophagus may cause the surgeon to believe the esophagus is the trachea (see discussion of tracheoesophageal fistula below).

It is important that the anesthesiologist have a clear view of the operative field in order to keep up with the progress of the operation and to be able to correlate hemodynamic changes with surgical manipulations. He can assist the surgeon with the intrathoracic exposure by hypoventilating during crucial maneuvers and ventilating adequately when these measures are accomplished. Ventilation should be decreased or stopped during placement of pericostal sutures to prevent puncture or laceration of the lung parenchyma. In perhaps no other type of surgery is such close cooperation between the surgeon and anesthesiologist as vital as in operations within the chest, since what each does profoundly affects the other. Close observation of the surgical field by the anesthesiologist, as well as an appreciation of anesthesia problems by the surgeon are imperative for a successful outcome.

The maintenance of a patent airway (endotracheal tube) during thoracic operations is the primary responsibility of the anesthesiologist. The use of humidified anesthetic gases decreases the likelihood of obstruction due to secretions or small amounts of blood which can enter the tracheobronchial tree during surgery. The judicious use of small amounts of normal saline as irrigation (0.5-2.0 cc) followed by gentle suctioning at an appropriate point in the operation may prevent catastrophic obstruction of the airway. Mechanical ventilation is used in some patients during thoracic operations (rarely, if ever, in the newborn or very small patient), but *manual* ventilation is necessary for the detection of subtle or gross changes in compliance.

Termination of Operation, Immediate Postoperative Measures, and Transport to Intensive Care Unit

Once the planned operation is complete, and before chest closure, an attempt should be made to correct any atelectasis which may have occurred due to lung compression. This should be done gently and gradually, and under direct vision, so that excessive pressures are not applied to the airways which could result in a pneumothorax on the contralateral side. During the placement of chest tubes, and especially during the puncture of the pleura, ventilation should be temporarily interrupted. If the chest tube is to be removed in the operating room and not left in place during the immediate postoperative period (as with an uncomplicated patent ductus arteriosus ligation), it is usually placed directly through the incision and the pericostal sutures pulled together tightly around it. It can safely be removed after several positive pressure breaths are given. A chest radiograph in the operating room is taken to confirm re-expansion of the lung on the affected side.

The use of intercostal nerve blocks from within the chest just before closure may be used to alleviate some of the immediate postoperative pain in patients older than five or six months. The surgeon injects the local anesthetic as far posteriorly as possible at the level of the incision, as well as one or two segments above and below. Bupivicaine (0.25%), maximum total dose of 2 mg/kg body weight, is usually selected due to its long duration of action. This is especially helpful in patients who undergo early extubation, since it minimizes the splinting often encountered in the immediate postextubation period.

The need for postoperative ventilatory support should be anticipated preoperatively, discussed with the parents, and explained to the patient if of an appropriate age. It is based on the preoperative condition of the patient, the specific operation planned, the anesthetic technique utilized, and the expected postoperative course. In very small infants and in almost all newborn babies undergoing thoracic operations, the endotracheal tube is left in place and mechanical ventilation employed for several hours to days, depending on the general condition of the patient. Weaning is begun as soon as hemodynamic and respiratory parameters appear stable.

It is important that a well-defined system for transfer of the patient to the care of the ICU nurses from that of the anesthesia personnel be clearly understood by both to ensure a safe and effective transition. In critically ill children, a battery-powered monitor should be used to display the arterial pressure and ECG during transport. Upon arrival, the arterial pressure monitoring system is transferred to the ICU equipment from the transport monitor. The venous or atrial monitoring catheters are then connected to the appropriate transducers. While

this is being done, the anesthesiologist or respiratory therapist should continue to ventilate the patient by hand, and not until after
the pressure monitors are connected and displayed should hand ventilation be discontinued and the patient placed on mechanical
ventilation. The ventilator settings can be
preset by the respiratory therapist before the
patient arrives in the ICU, after communication with the anesthesia personnel in the
operating room. Examination by the anesthesiologist and respiratory therapist after
institution of mechanical ventilation should
be done to ensure adequate chest expansion,
presence of bilateral breath sounds, the need
for suctioning of the endotracheal tube, and
the rate of actual ventilation. Blood gas
values should be obtained to determine the
adequacy of ventilation shortly after arrival
in the ICU.

A detailed report by the anesthesiologist
to the ICU nurse responsible for the patient
should be given as soon as both feel the patient is stable. This report should include the
procedure performed, anesthetic technique
used, total amount of drugs, fluids, and blood
administered, drugs reversed at the end of
surgery (e.g., muscle relaxants, heparin),
problems encountered during the case, urine
output, and any anticipated postoperative
difficulties.

Management of Postoperative Complications

Infants and children undergoing thoracic surgical procedures are subject to several postoperative complications involving
the lungs, airway, heart, great vessels, upper
gastrointestinal tract, and lymphatic system
(see Ch. 18). Most of them can be prevented
by meticulous attention to intraoperative detail by both surgeon and anesthesiologist.
Morbidity and mortality from intrathoracic
operations can be further reduced by systematic postoperative assessment and the application of a few simple principles of general
postoperative support.

PNEUMOTHORAX

Pneumothorax is an accumulation of air
outside the lung, but within the pleural cavity and/or mediastinum, which occupies
space needed for full lung inflation and cardiac filling. Air may remain in the chest following any intrathoracic operation, or it may
accumulate postoperatively from an air leak
in the lung or tracheobronchial tree. A rubber or plastic tube is usually left in the
pleural cavity following thoracotomy or in
the mediastinum when a median sternotomy
incision is used. This tube is connected to a
collection and drainage system which allows
air, blood, and fluid to escape while preventing air from entering the chest. Most drainage systems employ the "water-seal" principle. However, some surgeons prefer not to
leave a chest tube in place following relatively simple intrathoracic procedures in
which the lung itself has not been incised and
bleeding is negligible. In that case, air is
evacuated from the chest as the ribs and
muscle are approximated, and positive
pressure is maintained on the airways by the
anesthesiologist until the chest is completely
closed. A radiograph is obtained immediately following completion of the operation
to be sure that no more air remains. A small
residual pneumothorax will usually resolve
spontaneously in a few hours without causing difficulty, but careful followup is required.

Two specific problems related to pneumothorax deserve special consideration.
First, the development of a tension pneumothorax in which air continues to leak from
the lung or tracheobronchial tree into the
undrained pleural space or mediastinum requires the immediate insertion of a chest
tube to prevent compression of the lung, shift
of the mediastinum, and life-threatening hypoxia, hypercarbia, and low cardiac output.
A tension pneumothorax can occur from the
rupture of the lung surface or rupture of a
small bleb due to excessive positive pressure,
coughing, intraoperative trauma, or agitation
in a patient receiving mechanical ventilation.

It is diagnosed by clinical deterioration in the patient's vital signs (hypertension followed by hypotension, tachycardia followed by bradycardia, and respiratory distress), acute reduction in breath sounds, decreased pulmonary compliance, displacement of the cardiac point of maximal impulse, and by hypoxemia, hypercarbia, and acidosis as reflected in the arterial blood gases. A chest radiograph can be used to confirm the diagnosis (Fig. 16-2).

The second important problem relates to the development of a pneumothorax in the unoperated pleural cavity where a chest tube is not likely to be in place. This problem is dangerous and so likely to be overlooked that some surgeons open and drain both pleural cavities in addition to the mediastinum in critically ill patients undergoing certain intrathoracic operations, particularly when a median sternotomy is done. Chest tubes are left in place for 24 to 48 hours postoperatively, or until drainage of blood and fluid ceases. They are "stripped" frequently to avoid the accumulation of a blood clot which might prevent adequate drainage of air and blood. The tubes are not removed if there is evidence of a continued air leak within the chest. At the time of removal, precautions need to be taken to avoid entry of air into the chest through the opening in the chest wall or through the holes in the tubes themselves. A chest radiograph is obtained shortly after removal of the tubes to confirm that no pneumothorax remains, and the patient is observed carefully for the next few hours for signs of respiratory distress or deterioration in vital signs suggestive of a recurrent pneumothorax. Occlusive dressings are placed over the chest tube tracts; in addition, in small infants with thin chest walls, a suture can be placed around the chest tube which is tied down to occlude the wound as the tube is withdrawn. Even a small residual pneumothorax increases the chances for blood and fluid accumulation within the pleural cavity and may lead to postoperative empyema.

HEMOTHORAX AND HEMOMEDIASTINUM

Blood loss and postoperative bleeding are quite variable during and following intrathoracic operations. In cases of lung biopsy, lobectomy, or patent ductus arteriosus ligation, for example, virtually no blood loss is expected. In contrast, massive bleeding and prolonged postoperative drainage may be encountered during and after a re-operation for a complex congenital heart defect. Chest drainage tubes are inserted following an operation within the chest or mediastinum in which even minimal postoperative bleeding is expected. Excessive bleeding requires re-exploration of the chest for control. A table of acceptable rates for postoperative bleeding as a function of the size of the patient has been proposed by Kirklin.[65] Rates of bleeding in excess of these limits require re-exploration. Serious complications may occur as a result of waiting too long in the hope that conservative measures and time will take care of the bleeding. Chest tubes are of only limited effectiveness in draining blood from the pleural cavities and mediastinum. Proper position, suction, and "stripping" are important; but once clots begin to collect within the chest, tube function deteriorates and the likelihood of re-exploration for evacuation of the clot and control of bleeding increases. Accumulation of blood within the chest seriously compromises pulmonary function and cardiac output. Cardiac dysrhythmias and tamponade occur quickly in children and may even require urgent re-opening of the incision in the ICU to prevent death. Prior to re-exploration of the chest, all possible measures should be taken to restore normal blood coagulation, including the administration of fresh frozen plasma, platelets, and protamine. In selected patients, antifibrinolytic agents, fresh whole blood, factor-specific cryoprecipitates, and vitamin K may be indicated. Normal body temperature should be restored as quickly as possible; 5 to 10 cm positive end-expiratory pressure (PEEP) can be tried to reduce postoperative intrathoracic bleeding, and agitation and hypertension should be pharmacologically controlled.[66] In spite of all these potentially useful measures, a very low threshold for re-exploration to control postoperative bleeding and to evaluate a hemothorax or hemomediastinum is the best insurance of a subsequent complication-free recovery.

CHYLOTHORAX

The accumulation of lymph within the pleural cavity is a relatively late complication of intrathoracic operations. The thoracic duct may be injured in either pleural cavity, but it is most often encountered during dissection around the descending thoracic aorta in the left hemithorax. It is particularly at risk during operations for patent ductus arteriosus and coarctations of the aorta. In some cases an unusually large amount of straw-colored or milky-white fluid may be noted in the chest tube drainage before the tube is removed. In such situations the tube should be left in place and the patient kept NPO or at least on a low-fat diet for several more days.

It is more common for a chylothorax to be discovered several days after the chest tube has been removed when the patient has resumed a normal diet. Acute respiratory distress may develop, with respirations becoming increasingly labored and breath sounds diminished over the hemithorax involved. Chest radiograph will reveal an opaque hemithorax or a large accumulation of fluid. A chest tube should be inserted to drain the fluid and fully re-expand the lung. The tube should be left in place for several days, since most leaks in the thoracic duct will seal during this time and no further treatment will be required. Dietary restriction of fat and the use of short-chain triglycerides may facilitate spontaneous closure of the lymph fistula. Exploration and surgical control of the leak may be required if significant drainage continues or if nutritional de-

pletion becomes a problem. The use of total parenteral nutrition during the early management of chylothorax has been useful in prolonging the time before surgical intervention is required and allowing a greater chance for spontaneous sealing of the leak to occur. Even at the time of re-exploration, the surgeon may find it quite difficult to locate and eliminate the source of lymphatic drainage, especially in the small infant.

ATELECTASIS

Postoperative atelectasis is, to a greater or lesser degree, an almost universal occurrence following intrathoracic operations in infants and small children. Surgical manipulation of the small, fragile, and often congested lung, associated with postoperative incisional pain and the child's instinctive reluctance to cooperate with even the most skillfully designed program for pulmonary toilet, often complicate recovery. Children with congenital cardiac defects are frequently weak and debilitated, and increased pulmonary blood flow or pulmonary venous congestion from left ventricular failure futher complicate the problem.

Management of atelectasis in the older child should begin during the preoperative orientation when the child is taught to cooperate with nurses and respiratory therapists during the conduct of chest percussion, deep breathing, coughing, and suctioning. Incentive spirometry is particularly effective in the older child, especially when one of the clown-like or ball-containing "game" devices is used during preoperative training.

When postoperative fever, tachycardia, tachypnea, and diminished breath sounds suggest atelectasis, a chest radiograph usually confirms the presence of areas of uninflated lung. If vigorous chest physical therapy and incentive spirometry fail to eliminate the atelectasis, nasotracheal aspiration is employed. In patients who are still intubated, suction, irrigation, and positive pressure ventilation usually re-expand the atelectatic segments, unless the tube itself is

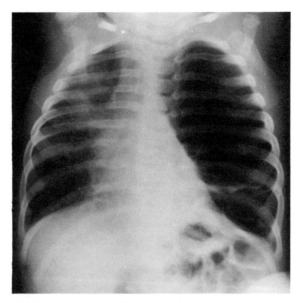

Fig. 16-6 5-month-old male with left upper lobar emphysema. Preoperative chest radiograph showing hyperlucency and decreased vascular markings of left upper lung field, compression atelectasis of left lower lobe, and shift of heart and mediastinal structures toward right.

obstructing one or more bronchi, with the right upper lobe being particularly susceptible to obstruction by an improperly placed endotracheal tube. Re-intubation with endotracheal suctioning and positive pressure ventilation can be used for a few hours in infants with persistent atelectasis. Bronchoscopy may be required to examine each bronchial orifice and directly extract obstructing mucus plugs or blood clots. It is particularly useful following an episode of vomiting and suspected aspiration, and can be done at the bedside in the ICU, even using rigid bronchoscopes.

Children with neuromuscular disorders, scoliosis, small airways, cardiac disease, chronic debilitation, and cystic fibrosis pose particularly troublesome problems and may even require a tracheostomy to manage persistent or recurrent postoperative atelectasis. If atelectasis is not prevented or promptly corrected, pneumonitis and life-threatening sepsis may develop within a few days (Fig. 16-6).

GASTRIC DISTENTION

The use of an uncuffed endotracheal tube with positive pressure ventilatory assistance may lead to the accumulation of a significant quantity of air in the stomach and upper gastrointestinal tract of the infant or child, both during anesthesia and in the postoperative period. This problem is compounded by the swallowing reflex of the infant. Gastric distention may lead to severe bradycardia and respiratory distress acutely, and to subsequent diffuse abdominal distention, pain, ileus, and respiratory insufficiency. Gastric perforation may even occur as a result of gaseous distention of the stomach. These complications are avoided by the presence of a functional nasogastric tube inserted after the induction of anesthesia, and kept in place until after the child is extubated and no longer requires positive pressure ventilation. A sump-type catheter which is irrigated periodically and connected to intermittent suction can be used. Tube position is confirmed in the stomach by auscultation of an injected bolus of air, palpation, aspiration, and x-ray examination.

UPPER AIRWAY OBSTRUCTION

Upper airway obstruction following extubation of the infant or child is far more common than in the adult. The likelihood of such obstruction occurring is increased by a difficult intubation, multiple attempts at intubation, over-hydration, congestive heart failure, and prolonged intubation. If the child has been agitated or overly active during awakening from anesthesia, trauma to the cords and trachea can produce edema which may result in some degree of upper airway obstruction following extubation. The small infant with a large tongue and short neck is particularly at risk, especially those with craniofacial anomalies involving the upper airway or with myxedema.

To minimize the likelihood of post-extubation upper airway obstruction, the intubated child can be heavily sedated and all gases humidified. In those children particularly at risk of obstruction, dexamethasone 0.1 mg/kg should be given 30 minutes prior to extubation, and all equipment necessary for prompt re-intubation should be kept at the bedside until a satisfactory upper airway is assured. When prolonged ventilatory support is required, a tracheostomy should be considered to minimize trauma to the vocal cords and to eliminate the pressure and potential necrosis with subsequent stenosis at the level of the narrow subglottic cricoid ring. With meticulous care, however, infants are now ventilated for many weeks with endotracheal intubation alone.

LOW CARDIAC OUTPUT

Infants and children with cardiothoracic conditions requiring operation are obviously more at risk of having an inadequate cardiac output during the postoperative period than patients with less critical illnesses. The low cardiac output syndrome is characterized by oliguria, obtundation or otherwise abnormal mental status, and progressive respiratory and hepatic deterioration. When it can be determined, the mixed venous oxygen saturation or tension will be low due to the wide arteriovenous oxygen difference, indicative of a large extraction of oxygen.

Five factors determine the adequacy of cardiac output: (1) heart rate, (2) cardiac rhythm, (3) vascular volume, (4) vascular resistance, and (5) myocardial contractility. Proper management of cardiac output in the pediatric thoracic surgical patient requires that bodily demands for cardiac output be kept to a minimum. Fever must be prevented or promptly controlled, and agitation and pain reduced with analgesics and sedatives. The work of breathing is reduced by the use of mechanical ventilatory assistance when necessary. Management of a low cardiac output is discussed in Chapter 18.

ANESTHESIA FOR SOME SPECIFIC
PEDIATRIC THORACIC PROCEDURES
(Tables 16-8 and 16-9)

Bronchoscopy and Bronchography

Therapeutic and diagnostic bronchoscopy in the pediatric patient is not an uncommon procedure and requires skill and cooperation between the endoscopist and anesthesiologist since the airway must be "shared" and each must understand and appreciate the problems of the other (see ch. 9).

The development of the pediatric magnifying bronchoscope* has greatly enhanced the safety and effectiveness of bronchoscopy in infants and children. This system provides sheaths of varying sizes and lengths to be used on even the smallest infants, although

(*Text continues on p. 554*)

---

* Storz Endoscopy Co., Tuttlingen, W. Germany: K. Storz Endoscopy American 658 S. San Vincente Blvd., Los Angeles, CA 90048

Table 16-8
Selected Thoracic Abnormalities and Anesthetic Considerations Requiring Operation in Infants and Children

Condition	Description	Anesthetic and Perioperative Considerations
Achalasia	Motor disturbance of the esophagus in which cardia does not relax during swallowing resulting in esophageal dilation, esophagitis, regurgitation, failure to thrive and often aspiration pneumonitis.	Pre-existing chronic aspiration pneumonitis and poor nutritional status often necessitates postoperative mechanical ventilation and vigorous chest physiotherapy, and sometimes a regimen of total parenteral nutrition.
Agenesis, aplasia, or hypoplasia of lung or lobe(s)	Embryologic defects; symptoms vary from none to severe respiratory insufficiency.	Mediastinum may be markedly shifted toward affected side; trachea may be kinked; therapeutic or diagnostic bronchoscopy often necessary, for severe respiratory infections.
Bronchiectasis	Dilatation of bronchi from inflammatory destruction of bronchial and peribronchial tissues; exudate often accumulates in dependent areas of affected lung.	Bronchoscopy and bronchography is often helpful in defining extent of process and in obtaining cultures directly from affected areas. If medical therapy fails, lobectomy is indicated.
Bronchobiliary fistula	A fistula connecting right middle lobe bronchus and the left hepatic duct.	Bronchoscopy and bronchography for diagnosis and surgical excision of the intrathoracic portion of the fistula. Severe recurrent respiratory infections and atelectasis dictate vigorous pre- and postoperative chest physiotherapy and often repeated therapeutic bronchoscopy.
Chylothorax	Chylous pleural effusion: may be congenital due to birth injury to thoracic duct or due to trauma, especially after palliative cardiovascular procedures involving a left thoracotomy.	Conservative management usually suffices (repeated aspiration and insertion of thoracostomy tube connected to underwater seal). Persistent drainage (longer than 3 or 4 weeks) after appropriate conservative measures may be treated surgically by ligation of the thoracic duct just above the diaphragm. Loss of protein and fats often results in severe nutritional problems, and hyperalimentation is usually required.
Coarctation of the aorta	Narrowing of aorta usually just distal to left subclavian ar-	Symptomatic infants usually have associated cardiovascu-

Table 16-8 (continued)

Condition	Description	Anesthetic and Perioperative Considerations
	tery. Preductal coarctation usually longer segment of narrowing; post-ductal coarctation usually discrete narrow segment.	lar defects, e.g. ventricular septal defects, patent ductus. Beyond infancy, children are usually asymptomatic but often hypertensive. In older children, extensive collateral vessels may result in massive blood loss during thoracotomy. Cross-clamping of the aorta during repair usually results in significant hypertension in vessels proximal to the cross-clamp and requires pretreatment with vasodilators. (See Text.)
Corrosive or caustic burns of the esophagus	Chemical burns of mucosa	Initially, esophagoscopy usually done to determine extent of damage. Burns of epiglottic and laryngeal mucosa may compromise airway and make intubation difficult.
Croup (infectious)	Acute laryngotracheal bronchitis. Non-diphtheritic infections usually caused by viral agents.	Must differentiate from acute epiglottitis (see below). Usually does not progress beyond stridor or slight dyspnea.
Cystic adenomatoid malformation	Malformed bronchi lead to irregular aeration. Air accumulates in the potential cystic structures.	Sudden massive blood loss may result during removal from avulsion of vessels arising from the aorta and entering cystic areas. Preoperative arteriography should define extent and location of blood supply.
Cystic fibrosis	Multisystem disease of exocrine glands especially affecting lungs and pancreas.	Chronic lung disease leading to pulmonary insufficiency in many patients. Pulmonary complications include pneumothorax and massive hemoptysis from erosion of enlarged thin-walled bronchial vessels. Bronchoscopy for therapeutic bronchial lavage or for localization of bleeding site with subsequent resection or embolization of bleeding bronchial vessels may be necessary. For se-

Table 16-8 (continued)

Condition	Description	Anesthetic and Perioperative Considerations
		lected patients with more localized lung disease, pulmonary resection may be done. Respiratory support with tracheal intubation and mechanical ventilation during infectious exacerbations is not uncommon (see text, bronchoscopy).
Cystic hygroma	A cystic tumor arising along the course of the primitive lymphatic sacs.	Most commonly seen in the neck region; they may be very large and impinge on normal airway structures and result in obstruction of the upper airway, making intubation difficult; occasionally may extend into the mediastinum.
Diaphragmatic hernia Foramen of Bochdalek hernia	Postero-lateral (usually left) diaphragmatic defect allowing herniation of abdominal contents into thoracic cavity with compression of ipsilateral lung and shift of mediastinum toward contralateral side.	Often, the most serious of all neonatal surgical problems because of rapidly progressive respiratory failure and early death if not corrected quickly. Resuscitative measures (intubation, ventilation, and treatment of metabolic and respiratory acidosis) must be instituted immediately. (See text.)
Foramen of Morgagni hernia	Retrosternal herniation of portion of bowel. Usually presents later and less dramatically than Bochdalek hernia.	May be asymptomatic; surgical repair indicated when diagnosed due to risk of incarceration; may occur into pericardium resulting in compromise of cardiac output.
Ectopic bronchus (Eparterial bronchus, "pig bronchus")	Origin of right upper lobe bronchus from trachea.	Endotracheal intubation may block right upper lobe bronchus resulting in atelectasis; may be associated with chronic right upper lobe infection and bronchiectasis.
Empyema	Accumulation of pus within the pleural space, often associated with staphylococcal pneumonia.	Large empyemas may compress lung and compromise respiratory function; usually managed with thoracostomy tube placed under local anesthesia; chronic empyema may require decortication of fibrinous covering on parenchymal and pleural surfaces to re-expand affected lung.

Table 16-8 (continued)

Condition	Description	Anesthetic and Perioperative Considerations
Erb-Duchenne palsy	Injury (usually birth trauma) to upper brachial plexus (fifth and sixth cervical nerves) resulting in loss of ability to abduct the arm from shoulder, externally rotate arm, supinate forearm. Muscle function of hand is retained.	This and other forms of brachial plexus injuries may be associated with phrenic nerve injuries with paralysis of the diaphragm on the involved side.
Epiglottitis	Usually bacterial infection (most commonly *H. influenza*) of epiglottis and surrounding structures including larynx.	Severe, life-threatening, rapidly progressive disease which may result in total obstruction of upper airway. Should be managed by nasotracheal intubation under anesthesia *in operating room* with surgeon standing by to do tracheotomy if endotracheal tube cannot be passed. Infectious process rapidly responds to intravenous antibiotics and endotracheal tube can be removed usually in 48 to 72 hours as swelling subsides, as proven by direct laryngoscopy.
Esophageal duplication (enteric cyst)	Spherical or tubular posterior mediastinal structures with muscular walls and lining of any type of gastrointestinal epithelium or ciliated epithelium. Associated anomalies include hemivertebrae of upper thoracic spine and intraabdominal enteric cysts. Usually do not communicate with the lumen of the esophagus but may be connected to the small bowel.	Large cysts may compress the lung. Because they frequently contain acid-secreting gastric mucosa, peptic ulceration may occur and erode into lung, bronchus, or esophagus with resulting hemorrhage.
Esophageal perforation	Usually traumatic caused by instrumentation for pre-existing disease. May occur in newborn, usually on right side, from birth trauma and presents a sudden respiratory collapse accompanied by hydropneumothorax.	Esophagoscopy for pre-existing disease (stricture of esophagus from corrosive burns or tracheo-esophageal fistula) is common procedure in pediatric patients. Anesthesia must be appropriately deep to prevent coughing while esophagoscope is in place. In newborn presenting with hydropneumothorax from esophageal perforation, immediate aspiration is necessary followed by thoracotomy and repair of perforation.

Table 16-8 (continued)

Condition	Description	Anesthetic and Perioperative Considerations
Esophageal stenosis	Rarely, congenital defect associated with tracheo-esophageal fistula without esophageal atresia; or, as isolated congenital stenosis in which esophageal wall contains tissues of respiratory tract origin including ciliated epithelium and cartilage. More often acquired and associated with esophageal reflux.	Excision is required if ectopic tissue is present. Repeated esophageal dilatations either with esophagoscope or by bougienage to alleviate re-stenosis due to scar tissue formation. Esophageal perforation is always a possible complication. Infants are often malnourished and require total parenteral nutrition.
Esophageal stricture	The result of trauma to the esophagus from several causes: tracheo-esophageal fistula repair; corrosive burns of esophagus, congenital esophageal stenosis.	Require repeated dilatations with perforation always a possible complication. Colon interposition (or other visceral esophageal bypass) may be necessary.
Esophagitis	In infants, may be the result of gastroesophageal reflux with or without hiatal hernia; may subside spontaneously by 12–15 months of age if not associated with a large hiatus hernia.	Failure to thrive from recurrent vomiting during early infancy and respiratory infections from repeated aspirations may be quite severe. If symptoms cannot be controlled by propping baby in infant seat to prevent reflux, some form of anti-reflux procedure may be indicated. Anemia may result from chronic blood loss.
Eventration of the diaphragm	Congenital defect of muscular layer of diaphragm allowing usually minor herniation of part of abdominal organs into chest. Usually on right. May be asymptomatic or rarely may present like Bochdalek hernia. Respiratory symptoms depend on extent of herniation of abdominal contents and range from minimal to severe; gastric volvulus may result when there is significant eventration of the left hemidiaphragm.	On chest x-ray there is usually a smooth dome shaped elevation of the diaphragmatic shadow on the affected side with loss of lung volume; small asymptomatic eventration should be corrected whether or not they are symptomatic; if respiratory infection is present, appropriate medical therapy with antibiotics, chest physiotherapy and even therapeutic bronchoscopy is usually indicated prior to correction.
Gastroesophageal reflux (chalasia)	Results from failure of proper valvular function of esophagogastric junction; may or may not be associated with hiatus hernia.	Vomiting, malnutrition, failure to thrive, recurrent respiratory infections, chronic anemia characterize these infants; condition may clear spontaneously by 12-18 months of age with conservative treatment (frequent

Table 16-8 (continued)

Condition	Description	Anesthetic and Perioperative Considerations
		feedings and propping baby in infant seat); hyperalimentation often necessary; indications for anti-reflux procedure include esophagitis, esophageal stricture, significant hiatus hernia, recurrent and unresponsive pulmonary problems resulting from aspiration; ventilatory support after repair is often required due to poor general condition of patient as well as pre-existing pulmonary infection.
Hemothorax and hemopneumothorax	Usually the result of trauma either accidental or surgically induced. Usually there is co-existing pneumothorax.	Must be drained with thoracostomy tube(s) usually employing local anesthesia. Blood loss into chest cavity may be massive; portions of the lung may become trapped by clotted blood which will not drain via thoracostomy tube, and open thoracotomy may be required to remove clot and re-expand lung. Traumatic left sided hemothoraces are more commonly associated with injuries to the great vessels while those on the right are usually due to injury to the pulmonary hilum. Respiratory support may be necessary during recovery.
Hiatal hernia	Herniation of upper part of the stomach into the left hemithorax; sliding type more common than paraesophageal type.	See gastroesophageal reflux and esophagitis above. Treatment is usually directed at associated gastroesophageal reflux. Chronic aspiration and pulmonary pathology may be significant.
Hyaline membrane disease	Idiopathic Respiratory Distress Syndrome primarily seen in premature newborn but may occur in infants of diabetic mothers or those born by Cesarean section and under other stressful conditions at the time of delivery.	Long-term ventilatory support may be required and damage to upper airway may result in subglottic stenosis. Ligation of patent ductus arteriosus may be required. (See text.)
Kartagener's syndrome	Situs inversus totalis, paranasal sinusitis, bronchiectasis	May require excision of bronchiectatic segments of lung.

Table 16-8 (continued)

Condition	Description	Anesthetic and Perioperative Considerations
Lobar emphysema, congenital	Obstructive emphysema usually of one of upper lobes (left upper lobe, most commonly). May be result of defective bronchial cartilage to affected lobe.	May cause severe respiratory symptoms in newborn period requiring immediate surgical intervention or may not become symptomatic for as long as 5 to 6 months. Lobectomy is treatment of choice. Intubation and positive pressure ventilation may further over-inflate the lobe and compromise respiratory exchange in other parts of the lung. During induction of anesthesia spontaneous ventilation should be preserved until chest is opened and emphysematous lobe is brought out of the operative site. *Nitrous oxide should not be used* until after lobectomy is accomplished. After the lobectomy is accomplished the remaining lung tissue should be gently re-expanded *under direct vision* before closure of the thoracotomy is begun.
Lobar emphysema, acquired	Usually the result of localized obstruction from foreign bodies, inflammatory reaction, extrinsic compression of bronchus or bronchiole by lymph nodes or tumor in mediastinum. (Extrinsic bronchial compression usually results in atelectasis but emphysema may rarely result.)	Bronchoscopy is usually required for diagnosis and is therapeutic in the instance of a suspected or known foreign body. (See text—bronchoscopy). Anesthetic considerations similar to those stated above (congenital lobar emphysema).
Lung abscess	In infants and children, usually results from aspiration of infected material when pulmonary defense mechanisms are overwhelmed or when there is serious systemic disease or immunosuppression.	Bronchoscopy may be diagnostic as well as therapeutic. Long term medical therapy with large doses of intravenous antibiotics plus intermittent bronchoscopy to promote drainage usually suffices. Although resection is difficult in children, it may be accomplished using a balloon tipped Fogarty catheter placed in the bronchus during bronchoscopy. (See text—bronchoscopy).

Table 16-8 (continued)

Condition	Description	Anesthetic and Perioperative Considerations
Lung cysts—Bronchogenic	Usually unilobar and thick-walled structures lined with respiratory epithelium; may be located within the lung, mediastinum or pericardial sac adjacent to main bronchi; only occasionally communicating with bronchus.	May not be seen on x-ray but may produce compression of trachea or bronchus. May be difficult to find and to dissect especially if within the mediastinum; injury to phrenic nerve or other mediastinal structures may complicate postoperative course.
True congenital lung cysts	May be unilobar or multilobar with extensive compromise of adjacent lung tissue and other intrathoracic structures.	Communications with bronchial air passages makes infection almost inevitable; appropriate antibiotics and therapeutic bronchoscopy may be indicated prior to excision of cystic lobe but significant compromise of lung function either from compression or infection may make excision urgent. Postoperative ventilator support, especially in the chronically ill and malnourished infant or child, may be necessary.
Mediastinal emphysema (pneumomediastinum)	Air in mediastinum	Often associated with respiratory distress syndrome of prematures and in children with respiratory distress from any cause. Usually associated with pneumothorax which may necessitate drainage via catheter or thoracotomy tube; may be seen after tracheotomy, or esophageal or tracheal perforation. Tension pneumothorax or large pneumopericardium resulting in tamponade requires immediate treatment to remove air. Nitrous oxide should not be used as part of anesthetic management in patients with pneumomediastinum or pneumothorax.
Mediastinal masses, cysts and tumors	Epithelium-lined cystic masses of enteric, neurogenic, bronchogenic or coelomic origin; or solid vascular, or granulomatous tumors, malignant or benign, primary or metastatic	May be asymptomatic even occasionally when quite large; clinical manifestations appear from expanding, space-occupying structure and depend on location; tracheal or bronchial compression may result in respiratory distress making thoracotomy urgent;

Table 16-8 (continued)

Condition	Description	Anesthetic and Perioperative Considerations
		intubation may be difficult if tracheal deviation is present and appropriate measures to cope with difficult intubation should be taken before anesthesia is begun including preparation for bronchoscopy and tracheotomy. Postoperative respiratory support may be necessary.
Mediastinitus	Severe systemic infection of mediastinal structures; may follow pharyngeal, esophageal, or tracheal perforation from any cause, thoracic or cervical operations complicated by wound infection, or rupture of infected mediastinal lymph nodes.	Incision and drainage and massive antibiotic therapy required; may also require intermittent instillation of bacteriocidal solutions (such as Betadyne) via mediastinal drainage tubes. Ventilatory support usually necessary postoperatively.
Myasthenia gravis	Autoimmune disorder in which acetylcholine receptors in muscle are affected resulting in weakness; may be seen in pediatric patient even in neonatal period and should always be suspected in infants of mothers with myasthenia.	In infant of myasthenia gravis mother, may be transient or persistent and may well require ventilatory support in newborn period. Muscle relaxants as adjunctive anesthetic agents are rarely if ever needed in myasthenic patients. Thymectomy may be indicated in patients unresponsive to medical management and postoperative ventilatory support after thymectomy may be necessary.
Pectus deformities —Pectus excavatum	Funnel chest; severity varies from very mild (usually not requiring surgical correction) to severe requiring early surgical intervention. Usually sporadic incidence but familial occurrence not rare; may often be seen in patients with Marfan's syndrome; frequently progressive.	Usually thought to be "asymptomatic" in infancy and childhood, but subtle cardiac and pulmonary abnormalities have been shown to be present in many patients and are related to displacement and compression of the heart and to a decrease in intrathoracic volume. Besides the psychologic, cosmetic, and orthopedic reasons for correction, these patho-physiologic changes may become severe with progression over time. Anesthetic considerations during and after repair include the possibility of pneumothoraces, the produc-

Table 16-8 (continued)

Condition	Description	Anesthetic and Perioperative Considerations
		tion of a "flail chest" if surgical dissection is extensive, and postoperative atelectasis from splinting due to pain.
—Pectus carinatum	Pigeon breast; usually not apparent at birth, but becomes evident at three or four years of age. May be seen in patients with Marfan's syndrome or congenital heart disease.	The more severe forms may cause compression and displacement of the heart and reduction of intrathoracic volume; as may be seen in pectus excavatum deformities. The same perioperative considerations apply (see above).
Pericardial problems —Absence of the pericardium	May be total or partial; left (most common), right or diaphragmatic. May be associated with congenital diaphragmatic hernia or heart disease; arises from defective formation of pleuropericardial membrane or of the septum transversum.	Total absence of the pericardium usually does not require surgical correction; partial defects on the left may result in herniation of ventricles or left artrial appendage with strangulation; right-sided defects may result in obstruction of the superior vena cava. Surgical treatment includes enlargement of defect to prevent strangulation or closure using a portion of the mediastinal pleura. When associated with diaphragmatic hernia or congenital heart disease, clinical findings usually are primarily due to the associated defect.
—Pericardial cysts	Coelomic cyst—rare in childhood	Usually asymptomatic. Surgical removal usually done to establish diagnosis.
—Pericarditis (Acute)	May be primary—e.g. viral, rheumatic, bacterial, postpericardotomy—or a secondary manifestation of systemic disease.	Except for bacterial (purulent) pericarditis, usually self-limited and rarely requires surgical intervention except for removal of fluid if signs of cardiac tamponade are present. Purulent pericarditis is usually secondary to a severe infectious process such as pneumonitis, osteomyelitis, or meningitis—*Staphylococcus aureus* and *H. influenza* most common. Purulent pericarditis requires surgical drainage, vigorous antibiotic therapy and general postoperative support measures with close monitoring.

Table 16-8 (continued)

Condition	Description	Anesthetic and Perioperative Considerations
—Chronic constrictive pericarditis	Rare in childhood; Etiology usually unknown but may follow purulent or viral pericarditis.	Radical pericardectomy via median sternotomy with extensive resection of visceral and parietal pericardium from atria, cavae, and ventricles. Intra- and post-operative monitoring should include arterial and pulmonary artery catheters, and urinary output. Postoperative ventilatory support is usually required.
Pericardial effusion with cardiac tamponade	Unusual in childhood	Cardiac tamponade occurs when blood, fluid, or air within the pericardium interferes with ventricular filling during diastole and reduces stroke volume and cardiac output. Most commonly seen after cardiac surgery and must be considered *first* in differential diagnosis, if a low cardiac output state exists in such patients. Treatment of acute tamponade in postoperative patient is immediate opening of chest incision to relieve compression and to control bleeding; tamponade in other situations (rheumatic, viral or bacterial infections) may be treated initially with needle drainage in emergent situations but almost always requires surgical drainage (see above). Cardiac depressant drugs such as thiopental and the potent inhalational anesthetics should be avoided during anesthesia as in any patient who has a significantly depressed cardiac output.
Pneumomediastinum	Air in mediastinum	(See mediastinal emphysema above)
Pneumopericardium	Air in the pericardium	May be associated with pneumothorax and pneumomediastinum in premature newborns with the respiratory distress syndrome. Sufficient quantities of air, like blood or other fluids, may result in cardiac tamponade and require removal by pericardiocentesis.

Table 16-8 (continued)

Condition	Description	Anesthetic and Perioperative Considerations
Pneumothorax	Air in the pleural space	May occur during anesthesia especially in patients requiring high inflation pressure to expand lungs due to any cause (e.g., infants with idiopathic respiratory distress or congenital diaphragmatic hernia). Treatment of significant pneumothorax (probably greater than 30%) is needle aspiration or thoracostomy tube so that the lung can be expanded. The presence of a pneumothorax precludes the use of nitrous oxide during anesthesia, at least until the chest is opened or a thoracotomy tube is inserted. Tension pneumothorax (see below).
Pneumatocoele	Emphysematous blebs or cysts resulting from rupture of alveoli so that single or multilocular cavities occur; usually the result of *Staph. aureus* pneumonia, but may be congenital (bullous emphysema).	Pneumatocoeles in patients with *Staph. aureus* pneumonia may require thoracostomy drainage to treat respiratory distress or tension pneumothorax. These complications may occur suddenly and without warning.
Phrenic nerve palsy	Traumatic origin	Trauma to either phrenic nerve from birth injury (e.g., breech delivery) or surgical trauma (e.g., Blalock-Taussig or Blalock-Hanlon operation) results in upward displacement and decreased movement of the ipsilateral diaphragm. Lung volume is decreased and ventilatory exchange impaired. Must be differentiated from eventration of diaphragm or diaphragmatic hernia. Spontaneous recovery may occur, but occasionally plication of the diaphragm on the affected side is necessary to improve respiratory function.
Poland's syndrome	A spectrum of defects, usually unilateral, in which there is absence of the pectoralis minor and part of pectoralis major muscles, along with defects of costal cartilages	Paradoxical movement with respirations is seen in larger defects. Usually asymptomatic, but may be surgically corrected to prevent progressive deformity of

Table 16-8 (continued)

Condition	Description	Anesthetic and Perioperative Considerations
	and ribs at the sternal insertions, hypoplasia of subcutaneous tissue, and upward displacement and hypoplasia of the nipple and breast on the affected side. Hand deformities may also be associated.	chest wall; as well as for psychologic and cosmetic reasons. After correction of larger defects, ventilatory support may be required as with more extensive pectus repairs (see above).
Pulmonary artery sling	Anomalous left pulmonary artery arising from right pulmonary artery and coursing toward the left side over the right main stem bronchus and behind the lower trachea between the trachea and esophagus.	One of the most severe types of vascular malformations which compress the trachea and esophagus. Compression of right mainstem bronchus may result in obstructive emphysema and/or atelectasis of right lung. Hypoplasia of distal trachea and right bronchus along with defective tracheal and bronchial cartilages makes ventilatory management difficult. High incidence of associated congenital cardiac defects. (See text—Vascular Rings).
Pulmonary arterio-venous fistula	Fistulous and often aneurysmal connection between pulmonary artery and vein; may be single but often multiple; high incidence in patients with Osler-Weber-Rendu hereditary hemorrhagic telangiectasia.	Signs and symptoms depend on the size and extent of shunt of unsaturated blood into the systemic circulation. Cyanosis and polycythemia may be severe. Brain abscess, hemoptysis, or hemorrhage into the pleural space may occur. Congestive heart failure is rare. Surgery is indicated in most cases unless there are multiple fistulae involving both lungs. Anesthetic considerations are the same as with any patient with a right-to-left shunt. Postoperative ventilatory support may be necessary if the dissection is extensive.
Pulmonary sequestration	Accessory lower lobe almost always located in the left hemithorax. Nonfunctioning pulmonary tissue usually with no connection to airway system or pulmonary arterial tree; blood supply from systemic circulation.	May be asymptomatic or may present as recurrent pneumonia in region of left lower lobe. Surgery indicated because of high incidence of infection in sequestered lobes. Aortography to determine origin of blood supply is helpful in avoiding significant blood loss during surgical removal.

Table 16-8 (continued)

Condition	Description	Anesthetic and Perioperative Considerations
Right middle lobe syndrome	Extrinsic compression and obstruction of right middle lobe bronchus resulting in pneumonitis, atelectasis and eventually bronchiectasis. Compression usually due to mediastinal lymph nodes.	Diagnostic and therapeutic bronchoscopy often required. Persistent or recurrent right middle lobe collapse often makes lobectomy necessary.
Scimitar syndrome	Anomalous venous return from right lung to inferior vena cava with an intact atrial septum.	Correction requires cardiopulmonary bypass; physiology and hemodynamics similar to that found in secundum atrial septal defects. There may be abnormalities of the lung parenchyma, as well as the pulmonary arterial tree on the right.
Sternal clefts	May vary from small V-shaped defects in upper sternum to complete separation of the sternum with the heart outside the pericardium and the chest wall (Ectopia cordis).	With larger clefts, the heart and great vessels are covered only by skin and subcutaneous tissue. Direct closure may compress the heart and lungs. May be associated with diaphragmatic and abdominal wall defects. True ectopia cordis is very rare and carries a grave prognosis, since severe anomalies of the inside of the heart and of the great vessels are invariably present.
Subcutaneous emphysema	Air in the subcutaneous tissues.	Usually due to rupture of alveoli into mediastinal structures with subsequent dissection of air into mediastinum and into subcutaneous tissues of chest, neck, and face. May occur after tracheostomy or be associated with pneumothorax and pneumomediastinum in the respiratory distress syndrome. Treatment directed at underlying cause.
Subglottic stenosis	Narrowing of the cricoid area of the upper airway.	May be congenital, but usually results from trauma due to instrumentation or endotracheal intubation for prolonged periods; usually granulomatous or due to cartilagenous defects. Bronchoscopy often required to determine extent of stenosis and tracheostomy may be re-

Table 16-8 (continued)

Condition	Description	Anesthetic and Perioperative Considerations
		quired. Endoscopic resection of granulomatous lesions may result in relief of obstruction; but, they may recur.
Tension pneumothorax	Air under pressure in pleural space.	When the amount of air in the pleural space is large enough to cause the intrapleural pressure to exceed atmospheric pressure, the collapsed lung, the heart and other mediastinal structures shift to the opposite side compressing the other lung. In addition, venous return is impaired and torsion on the great vessels may markedly impair cardiac function; circulatory collapse may occur. Immediate aspiration followed by insertion of a chest tube is mandatory. This may occur during anesthesia or mechanical ventilation.
Thymus conditions	The thymus normally occupies the anterior-superior mediastinum and may give the impression or cardiac enlargement of mediastinal widening on chest x-rays of young children.	Thymic tissue may extend into the neck, and thymic cysts may occur in these areas, as well as in the mediastinum. Thymic cysts may enlarge rapidly and produce symptoms. Thymic tumors are rare, but may be seen in infancy and childhood.
Tracheal stricture (acquired)		Abnormal mediastinal structures of many varieties may produce significant tracheal (or bronchial) compression and result in severe respiratory distress. Endotracheal intubation or tracheostomy *may not* relieve the obstruction and selective right or left main-stem bronchial intubation or instrumentation with a rigid bronchoscope may be necessary.
Tracheomalacia	Partial or nearly complete collapse of trachea during inspiration.	Common cause of stridor and partial upper airway obstruction in infants and small children. Due to incomplete formation or weakness of tracheal wall; especially cartilagenous rings. Laryngoma-

Table 16-8 (continued)

Condition	Description	Anesthetic and Perioperative Considerations
		lacia produces similar symptoms and is due to weakness or incomplete formation of rigid laryngeal structures. Bronchoscopy and laryngoscopy are often necessary to make the diagnosis and to rule out other causes of upper airway obstructive symptoms, e.g. foreign body, subglottic stenosis, vocal cord paralysis, etc.
Vascular rings	See text.	See text.
Vocal cord paralysis	May result from birth trauma or damage to recurrent laryngeal nerve during surgical procedures involving chest or neck.	Laryngoscopy with patient breathing spontaneously is necessary to diagnose vocal cord paralysis. Common cause of stridor following transcervical approach for division of tracheo-esophageal fistula, or cervical esophagostomy for esophageal atresia. May also follow ligation of a patent ductus, or a Blalock-Taussig shunt.

Table 16-9
Cardiovascular Procedures in Infants and Children not Requiring Cardiopulmonary Bypass

Procedure	Description	Anesthetic and Perioperative Considerations
Blalock-Hanlon atrial septectomy	Surgical excision of atrial septum to increase mixing of systemic and pulmonary venous blood in patients with transposition of the great arteries.	Rashkind balloon septostomy at cardiac catheterization may prove inadequate and surgical intervention needed to provide adequate mixing. Patients are cyanotic and usually manifest the signs and symptoms of congestive heart failure. Surgical septostomy is done through a right thoracotomy and may involve inflow occlusion and cardiac standstill. Resuscitative drugs and the ability to replace blood rapidly are important considerations for the anesthesiologist. Nitrous oxide/narcotic/relaxant anesthetic techniques are usually employed. Postoperative ventilatory support is usually required.

Table 16-9 (continued)

Condition	Description	Anesthetic and Perioperative Considerations
Blalock-Taussig shunt	Anastomosis of the right or left subclavian artery (depending on the presence of a right or left aortic arch) to the pulmonary artery to *increase* inadequate pulmonary blood flow for patients with tetralogy of Fallot physiology (pulmonary stenosis and right-to-left shunt through a ventricular septal defect, atrial septal defect, patent ductus or patent foramen ovale).	Hypoxemia usually severe. Anatomy of intracardiac defects usually precludes total correction although age and size may influence selection of surgical procedure for a given defect. Anastomosis may be surgically difficult due to small size of subclavian artery, and heparinization is necessary to insure patency. This requires the expectation of postoperative bleeding and blood replacement, as well as maintenance of at least partial heparinization to keep shunt from clotting. Postoperative ventilatory support may be necessary but excessive inspiratory pressures must be avoided to minimize the ventilatory effects of intrathoracic blood flow.
Waterston	Anastomosis of the ascending aorta to the right pulmonary artery to *increase* pulmonary blood flow for patients with tetralogy of Fallot physiology (see above).	Same anesthetic considerations as with Blalock-Taussig shunts; Waterston shunts may kink pulmonary artery and result in differential pulmonary blood flow and make total correction of associated defect more difficult. Technically easier to perform than Blalock-Taussig shunt, but more difficult to correct when total correction of defect is anticipated. "Over-shunting" may result which results in congestive heart failure.
Pulmonary artery banding	Employed to *decrease* torrential flow to lungs in large left-to-right shunts in which increased pulmonary blood volume results in congestive heart failure and pulmonary edema. May be employed in conjunction with Blalock-Hanlon atrial septostomy to decrease pulmonary flow while increasing intracardiac mixing in patients with transposition of the great arteries or in patients with associated ventricular septal defects.	Congestive heart failure usually predominates the clinical picture. Preoperative ventilatory support with positive end-expiratory pressure or continuous positive airway pressure is often required prior to surgery as well as in the immediate postoperative period. Nitrous/narcotic/relaxant anesthetic techniques are usually employed for these patients.

Table 16-9 (continued)

Condition	Description	Anesthetic and Perioperative Considerations
Coarctation of the aorta	Symptomatic coarctation of the aorta in infancy is usually associated with other congenital cardiac anomalies including ventricular septal defects, patent ductus, aortic stenosis, and transposition of the great arteries. In childhood but beyond infancy, coarctation of the aorta is usually asymptomatic and is less often associated with other congenital heart defects except for a bicuspid aortic valve with or without stenosis or insufficiency. Systemic arterial hypertension usually accompanies isolated coarctation and may represent the presenting abnormality.	Congestive heart failure from obstructive circulatory disease usually predominates clinically, and preoperative ventilatory support along with medical anticongestive measures are often necessary. After subclavian flap angioplasty or primary repair of infantile coarctation by end-to-end repair, postoperative ventilation is useful in treating residual pulmonary edema. See text for anesthetic and physiologic consideration.
Division of vascular rings	Pathophysiology results from vascular malformations which compress the trachea, bronchi, or esophagus.	(See text).
Ligation and/or division of patent ductus arteriosus	Persistent patent ductus arteriosus occurs as an isolated anomaly, associated with complex congenital heart disease, or with respiratory disorders of the newborn, such as the idiopathic respiratory distress syndrome of the premature or in association with persistent fetal circulation of the stressed newborn.	Asymptomatic persistent patency of the ductus arteriosus requires surgical correction as an elective procedure and should be treated as such by the anesthesiologist. The anesthetic and immediate postoperative considerations are relatively simple and encompass the usual precautions undertaken during any type of elective thoracotomy. Sophisticated monitoring techniques in uncomplicated patent ductus are not usually necessary. An intercostal bupivacaine block from within the thorax prior to closure is often useful in preventing respiratory complications in the immediate postoperative period. Ligation of the ductus arteriosus in the premature newborn with respiratory distress is discussed in the text.

Table 16-9 (continued)

Condition	Description	Anesthetic and Perioperative Considerations
Pacemaker implantation	Implantation of permanent epicardial pacing electrode and abdominal wall power source is required in symptomatic infants with congenital complete heart block and in young patients who develop complete heart block after intracardiac repair of congenital or acquired defects.	Transvenous or temporary epicardial pacing may be warranted prior to induction of anesthesia regardless of the anesthetic technique employed. Since children may require a much higher stimulating threshold than adults, care should be taken at the time of surgery that the diaphragm is not stimulated to contract by the pacing signal. The use of non-depolarizing muscle relaxants may mask diaphragmatic pacing. A carefully controlled constant infusion of succinylcholine can be used at the time of determination of required pacemaker threshold.
Potts' Shunt	Anastomosis of descending aorta to main pulmonary artery to increase pulmonary blood flow in patients with tetralogy of Fallot physiology	Rarely done in recent years because of the higher incidence of "over-shunting" and pulmonary artery hypertension than is seen with Blalock-Taussig shunts.
Central Gortex shunts	Prosthetic material used to connect pulmonary artery to aorta to increase pulmonary blood flow.	Same anesthetic considerations as with Blalock-Taussig shunts. Blood loss through wall of prosthesis may be massive, especially if heparinization is required to prevent thrombosis.
Glenn Shunt	Anastomosis of superior vena cava to main pulmonary artery to increase pulmonary blood flow in patients with tricuspid atresia and decreased pulmonary flow.	Rarely done now due to the relatively high incidence of the superior vena caval obstructive syndrome and late shunt failure requiring some other palliative (Blalock-Taussig shunt) or corrective (Fontan procedure) operation. Same anesthetic considerations as with other aortico-pulmonary shunts.
Aorta-pulmonary artery anastomosis (creation of aortico-pulmonary window)	Done to increase pulmonary blood flow.	Can sometimes be done without cardiopulmonary bypass if anatomy of great vessels allows partial occlusion side-biting clamps to be used during the anastomosis.

ventilation is more difficult with the 3.0 mm instrument due to the resistance of the system itself when the light source and magnifying lens are in place. The larger instruments furnish adequate ventilating capabilities and allow the surgeon to continue the visual examination while the patient is being ventilated via the 15 mm sidearm attached to the anesthesia system. With these larger instruments, small biopsy forceps or grasping forceps can be passed through the instrument channel while ventilation is maintained with the telescope in place. If larger forceps are needed, the telescope must be removed and biopsy or foreign body extraction accomplished without optical magnification via the main channel of the bronchoscope.[67]

Indications for diagnostic bronchoscopy in children include determination of the cause of stridor, such as laryngotracheomalacia, laryngeal webs, post-intubation or post-tracheotomy stenosis; the origin of hemoptysis; the investigation of persistent pneumonia or atelectasis; and in the workup of a suspected tracheo-esophageal fistula (in combination with esophagoscopy).

Therapeutic bronchoscopy in children is usually done to remove aspirated foreign bodies or for the treatment of cystic fibrosis (see below). Removal of foreign bodies may be especially treacherous, depending on the size and nature of the aspirated material, since fragmentation may occur producing glottic, tracheal, or bilateral main-stem bronchus obstruction. In some cases, the endoscopist may be forced to push the foreign material down into the right or left mainstem bronchus to allow ventilation of the unobstructed air passages. If the foreign body is impacted in a bronchus, a Fogarty catheter may be slipped past the object with the balloon deflated, and once beyond the foreign body, the balloon inflated and pulled toward the bronchoscope or even into the bronchoscope.[68] If the foreign body material is vegetal (peanut or bean), *vegetal* or *arachidic* bronchitis will result, particularly if the object has been present for some time. This condition is characterized by cough, a septic fever pattern and dyspnea.[69] Treatment includes removal of the foreign body and appropriate antibiotic coverage, as well as chest physiotherapy and postural drainage.[70]

The anesthetic technique for bronchoscopy is tailored to the condition of the patient and the indication for the procedure. Many patients requiring bronchoscopy, either diagnostic or therapeutic, will arrive in the operating suite with an intravenous infusion in place so that thiopental in appropriate doses may be used for induction. Atropine is usually given prior to bronchoscopy to avoid untoward vagal reflexes during the procedure. Halothane/nitrous oxide/oxygen or halothane/oxygen can be used as an alternative to an intravenous induction if an intravenous catheter has not been placed. If nitrous oxide is used with halothane and oxygen for induction, it should be discontinued several minutes prior to the insertion of the bronchoscope to ensure optimal oxygenation during the procedure. Succinylcholine may be needed to facilitate insertion of the appropriate-sized bronchoscope. Once the bronchoscope has passed the cords, the breathing circuit is attached to the sidearm of the instrument and ventilation assured. Significant leaks and inadequate ventilation may occur until all the openings at the tip of the bronchoscope have passed beyond the vocal cords. In patients with various forms of chronic lung disease in which the upper airways are dilated (e.g., cystic fibrosis), even the largest available bronchoscope may not fill the trachea enough to prevent significant leaks which impair adequate ventilation, particularly in the presence of increased airway resistance. In such cases, the leak can be minimized or eliminated by gently compressing the glottic structures around the bronchoscope with the thumb and index fingers applied to the cricoid cartilage.

Bronchoscopic or laryngoscopic instrumentation of the upper airway always carries with it the possibility of significant laryngeal or subglottic edema, especially in smaller infants and children. Management of this complication includes postoperative humidification of inspired gases, adequate hydration, intermittent positive pressure breathing of racemic epinephrine (0.5 cc racemic epinephrine diluted with 3.5 cc normal saline) every two to three hours, and dexamethasone.[71] Endotracheal intubation may be required if these measures do not suffice.

Bronchography may be necessary to define the extent of certain parenchymal diseases of the lung such as segmental bronchiectasis. Contrast material is introduced with a catheter passed via the bronchoscope or an endotracheal tube, depending on the ease with which the catheter can be placed into the desired area of the bronchial tree. This procedure is usually done in the radiology department in order to utilize fluoroscopy, and the patient may need to be turned into several positions in order to obtain adequate diagnostic films. After the necessary radiographs are obtained, as much of the contrast material as possible is suctioned from the bronchial tree. Anesthesia should be sufficiently deep to prevent coughing when the contrast is introduced, since coughing may spread the material and result in poor quality radiographs.

Anesthesia for bronchography is similar to that for bronchoscopy using either an intravenous induction and halothane/oxygen maintenance or an inhalation induction as described above. If an endotracheal tube is used instead of a bronchoscope to pass the contrast catheter, a curved 15 mm connector with a removable cap "chimney" side-arm is used so that ventilation can be maintained while manipulation of the catheter is underway.

Bronchoscopy and bronchial lavage in patients with cystic fibrosis (and other chronic lung diseases) are done to attempt to open airways obstructed by thick inspissated secretions characteristic of these conditions. Lavage is done using generous amounts of half-normal saline and dilute sodium bicar-bonate as well as diluted acetylcystine (see Ch. 12).

These patients are often quite ill with borderline or overt respiratory failure, superimposed pneumonia, and cor pulmonale. The anesthetic management must take into account all of these factors. The uptake of the inhalation agents is slow due to the lung disease, and the cardiovascular depressant effects of induction doses of barbiturates may preclude their use. Narcotics are also relatively contraindicated in these patients due to their suppression of the cough reflex. Intravenous ketamine (1-2 mg/kg) along with diazepam (0.1-0.2 mg/kg) has been used for induction.[72] Additional doses of each of these drugs may be necessary, but are usually not required if the procedure is not prolonged. Very small incremental doses of thiopental (0.5-1.0 mg/kg) have also been added to this regimen in some patients. Atropine is not contraindicated in patients with cystic fibrosis undergoing bronchoscopy, since its drying properties are minimal if given intravenously prior to the administration of ketamine and succinylcholine. It should be used during bronchoscopy in such patients to avoid undesired vagal responses from succinylcholine and manipulation of the airway.

Esophagoscopy

Indications for upper gastrointestinal tract endoscopy include: management of acquired or congenital esophageal stricture; evaluation of the extent and degree of caustic or acid burns of the esophagus; removal of foreign bodies; determination of the extent of reflux esophagitis in patients with dysfunction of the gastroesophageal sphincter; identification and treatment of esophageal varices; and in conjunction with bronchoscopy for evaluation of a tracheo-esophageal fistula. The flexible fiberoptic esophagogastroscope is sometimes used in children; however, the rigid instruments are usually employed, especially in the removal of foreign bodies and in the management of esophageal strictures, the most common reasons for esophagoscopy in the pediatric patient.[73]

In adult patients, sedation may suffice along with topical anesthesia for upper gastrointestinal endoscopy. However, patient cooperation is necessary; for this reason, general anesthesia is almost always required in the pediatric age group. The exception to this may be for the removal of coins in the esophagus, which can sometimes be accomplished using light sedation and insertion of a Foley catheter into the esophagus through the nose. Under fluoroscopic visualization, the coin is pulled from the esophagus by inflating the balloon tip as it lies beyond the coin.[74]

For many patients undergoing esophagoscopy, a rapid sequence induction using pre-oxygenation, thiopental, succinylcholine, and cricoid pressure is probably the safest method, especially if there is known to be esophageal dilatation above a stricture with the possibility of retained material. A few small infants may require awake intubation (see tracheo-esophageal fistula). Elective esophagoscopy for other conditions can be safely done using an inhalation induction. Maintenance of anesthesia after intubation of the trachea is accomplished with deep levels of inhalational agents, since light levels of anesthesia which allow coughing or movement may result in esophageal or pharyngeal perforation and must be avoided.

In very small infants, the esophagoscope may impinge upon the endotracheal tube and cause obstruction. This complication, as well as the possibility of accidental extubation during the procedure, must be watched for at all times. Stridor may also result after esophagoscopy and should be managed as outlined in the section on bronchoscopy. Sharp foreign bodies may perforate small or major blood vesels, and significant bleeding may require blood replacement.

Congenital Diaphragmatic Hernia

Congenital diaphragmatic hernia is one of the true emergencies that the anesthesiologist encounters in the newborn. It occurs in one of 2200 live births and the signs and symptoms indicating its presence are often manifest very shortly after delivery, with the infant showing severe respiratory distress and cyanosis which does not improve with the administration of oxygen.[75] Other clinical findings indicating the presence of a diaphragmatic hernia include tachypnea, retractions, heart sounds which may be best heard over the right hemithorax, and a scaphoid abdomen. Audible bowel sounds in the chest may be present but their absence does not rule out the condition. A chest radiograph should be taken immediately to confirm the diagnosis, since if the newborn with a symptomatic diaphragmatic hernia is to be saved, early treatment to stabilize the patient and surgery are mandatory (Fig. 16-7, 16-8).

A herniation of the bowel into the chest (most commonly through the foramen of Bochdalek) occurs on the left in 85 percent of cases; 13 percent on the right, and 1 to 2 percent are bilateral.[76] Associated anomalies are often present and include defects of the cardiovascular system (in 23%), the gastrointestinal tract (malrotation in 40%), the genitourinary system, and the central nervous system.[77] In those without other defects, the mortality rate is still 25 percent.[78]

The major result of bowel contents being in the chest is pulmonary hypoplasia which always is present on the side of the hernia; but may also be present on the contralateral side as well, due to a shift of the mediastinal structures away from the hernia. On the affected side, there is an embryological reduction in the number of branches or generations of pulmonary arteries and bronchi due to the compression of the developing lung. The opposite lung is also compressed to varying degrees and its development altered.

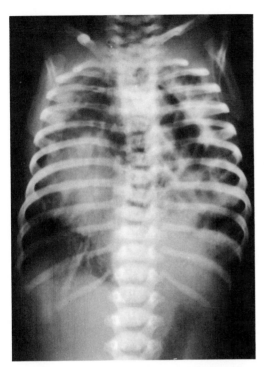

Fig. 16-7 Newborn with congenital diaphragmatic hernia through foramen of Bochdalek. Preoperative chest radiograph showing fluffy gut mostly within the left hemithorax but also some herniation into right side; and absence of most gas shadows from the abdomen, except for a small amount in stomach and descending colon.

Survival probably depends on the degree of hypoplasia of the lung on the unaffected side, as well as the early recognition of the condition and its early appropriate treatment.[79]

Pathophysiologically, the presence of the bowel in the chest results in compression atelectasis of whatever air spaces there are in the lung on the affected side, as well as in the opposite lung due to the mediastinal shift. The atelectasis produces intrapulmonary shunting, hypoxia, and underventilation of the "good lung," leading to hypercarbia. The mediastinal shift may impede venous return to the heart, producing a decrease in cardiac output. This, plus the hypoxemia due to the intrapulmonary shunting, leads to a rapidly developing severe metabolic acidosis. The severe combined metabolic and respiratory acidosis, which is unresponsive to the usual conservative measures, dictates early surgical intervention. Early intubation of the trachea and administration of oxygen is indicated. Mask ventilation using high inspiratory pressures may cause gastric distention and can further compromise already embarrassed pulmonary and cardiovascular systems. After intubation, low levels of positive pressure ventilation should be used, since excessively high pressure may result in alveolar rupture of the "good" lung with subsequent collapse. Tracheal intubation, the administration of oxygen, and correction of the metabolic component of the combined acidosis prior to transport and surgical intervention have been shown to improve markedly the survival of these infants.[80]

Anesthesia for the correction of a diaphragmatic hernia in a newborn is primarily a continuation of resuscitative measures begun preoperatively. Small doses of nondepolarizing muscle relaxants and narcotics are used as needed. Potent inhalational agents are usually not tolerated, due to the infant's decreased myocardial contractility and poor venous return. Nitrous oxide is contraindicated, due to its ability to displace air in the bowel, causing an increase in the size of the mass in the chest. Nitrous oxide also makes it more difficult for the surgeon to replace the bowel in the abdominal cavity which is already too small to accept it. It may be necessary for the surgeon to create a ventral hernia in order for the bowel to be placed into the abdomen.[81]

Patients with congenital diaphragmatic hernias usually arrive in the operating suite with monitoring and intravenous catheters in place. An arterial catheter is mandatory in the pre-, intra-, and postoperative periods for direct measurement of blood pressure and for sampling of arterial blood for blood gases, pH, electrolytes, glucose, and calcium levels. The anesthesiologist must stay in direct visual contact with the operative field to ensure as effective ventilation as possible,

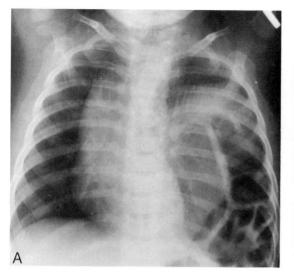

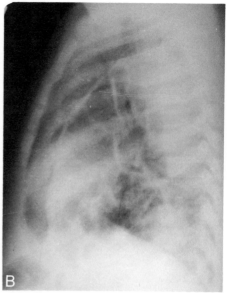

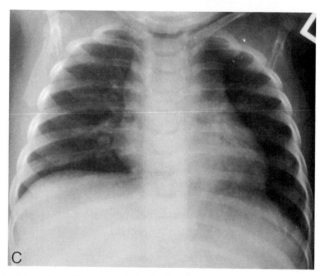

Fig. 16-8 6-month-old male with congenital diaphragmatic hernia through foramen of Bochdalek. Patient was asymptomatic until 6 months of age when he became febrile and a chest radiograph was taken which revealed presence of bowel in left hemithorax. (A and B) Preoperative chest radiograph PA and lateral. (C) Postoperative chest radiograph.

and to make certain that excessive pressure is not applied to the airways. Temperature must be monitored and steps taken to avoid hypothermia, since it will result in worsening of the already severe metabolic acidosis. Adequate amounts of glucose-containing fluids should be given and the glucose level measured frequently to avoid hypo- or hyperglycemia. Blood is usually not required for the repair of a diaphragmatic hernia, but blood loss should be meticulously measured by weighing sponges and careful observation of suction bottles. The volume status of these very sick infants is often borderline, and hypovolemia may need to be treated vigorously with blood or colloid.

After removal of the herniated bowel from the chest, the lung on the affected side cannot be expected to expand to any great degree, and attempts at its expansion by using high ventilatory pressures should be avoided, since rupture of the lung on the opposite side may result. Some surgeons advocate the use of a chest tube connected to underwater seal on *both* sides after repair is accomplished; the one on the unaffected side is placed prophylactically in case a life-threatening collapse should occur. If a chest tube is not placed in the uninvolved side at the time of repair, preparation should be made for its insertion by having the set-up immediately available at the infant's bedside and personnel available for immediate intervention should deterioration take place suddenly in the postoperative period. If a pneumothorax does occur, especially on the contralateral side of the hernia repair, sudden hypoxia may result in cardiac arrest. If this is suspected, time should not be wasted in confirming its presence, but a chest tube should be placed immediately.[82,83]

The postoperative period is difficult more often than not in these patients, and artificial ventilation is required for at least several days. Attempts should be made to keep the PaO_2 between 60 to 80 mmHg and the $PaCO_2$ between 35 to 40 mmHg, if possible. Careful attention should be given to the volume status, as well as the nutritional state of the patient. A gastrostomy is often placed at the time of surgery so that feeding may take place during recovery.

Raphaely and Downes reported, in 1973, that calculation of the $P(A-a)O_2$ while administering 100 percent oxygen via an endotracheal tube shortly after removal of the bowel from the chest cavity is helpful in determining prognosis.[84] If the $P(A-a)O_2$ is less than 400 mmHg, the infant will usually survive, provided there are no other serious defects present. This idea appears valid, since it probably reflects the ability of the lung on

the unaffected side to maintain adequate oxygenation and removal of carbon dioxide.

Several authors have investigated pulmonary dynamics of older patients who had repair of congenital diaphragmatic hernias as infants.[85,86] It appears that there is persistence in the reduction of the number of branches of both bronchi and pulmonary arteries on the affected side, resulting in a decrease in ventilation and perfusion. Pharmacologic manipulation of elevations in pulmonary vascular resistance using vasodilators such as priscoline, chlorpromazine, and acetylcholine has been tried in the postoperative period with some success, but more investigation is needed to warrant any specific conclusions.[87,88] However, Wohl et al found that total lung capacity and vital capacity averaged 99 percent of predicted values.[89] In those that survive without other disturbing defects, lung function may be nearly normal.[90]

Other types of congenital diaphragmatic hernias (foramen of Morgagni or hiatus hernias) usually do not become so dramatically and devastatingly evident in early infancy as do those of the Bochdalek variety. They may be completely asymptomatic for months or years and may present as an incidental finding during investigation of other conditions. The anesthetic approach to these is less fraught with problems for the anesthesiologist.

Esophageal Atresia and Tracheo-esophageal Fistula

Esophageal atresia (EA) with or without a tracheo-esophageal fistula (TEF) is not an uncommon congenital anomaly requiring early surgical intervention. The incidence of these related defects occurs in approximately 1 in 3000 live births.[91]

The presence of polyhydramnios during pregnancy may indicate some form of intestinal obstruction in the fetus; if it is present, the diagnosis of esophaeal atresia can be made at the time of delivery or shortly afterwards by carefully attempting to insert a soft radio-opaque catheter into the stomach either nasally (which may also rule out the presence of choanal atresia) or through the mouth. If atresia is present, the catheter will be seen to coil in the upper blind pouch of the atretic esophagus. If further anatomic definition is needed and contrast medium required, the use of a small amount of dilute barium (2 cc or less) is considered to be the lesser of several evils.[92] The use of oil-based or water-soluble contrast materials may often result in a chemical pneumonitis if an associated TEF exists. Newborn infants do not clear these substances from the lungs and airways, due to an ineffective cough and impaired ciliary function. Any infant showing early signs of gagging and coughing on secretions with feedings, and subsequent respiratory distress and cyanosis, should be suspected of having some form of esophageal defect, and appropriate steps should be taken to make a diagnosis so that early intervention can prevent the development of pneumonia and even death. If an H-type fistula exists (see below), without esophageal atresia, early signs of respiratory distress are not usually present (gagging, coughing, cyanosis, rapid respirations), and the diagnosis may not be suspected until the child is several months old when recurrent pneumonia suggests the presence of this type of defect.

Several anatomic combinations of esophageal atresia and TEF include:

1. Esophageal atresia with the fistula between the distal esophageal segment and the distal trachea (87%).
2. Esophageal atresia without TEF (8%).
3. Tracheo-esophageal fistula without esophageal atresia (H-type) (4%).
4. Esophageal atresia with the fistula between the proximal esophageal segment and the trachea (less than 1%).
5. Esophageal atresia with the fistula between both proximal and distal esophageal segments and the trachea (less than 1%).

There is a very high incidence (perhaps as high as 50%) of associated congenital anomalies in patients with esophageal atresia, with or without a tracheo-esophageal fistula.[93] Calverly and Johnston reported that factors influencing survival in patients with TEFs were associated congenital anomalies, prematurity, and pulmonary complications.[94]

In patients with EA/TEF, cardiovascular defects are present in 15 percent or more and are 25 times more common than in the general population.[93,95] Mortality figures for children with TEF and cardiovascular defects are nearly three times that for infants with TEF and no cardiovascular defects.[93] The more common cardiovascular defects in infants with EA/TEF are ventricular-septal defect, coarctation of the aorta, tetralogy of Fallot and atrial-septal defects.

Anomalies in other parts of the gastrointestinal tract occur in about 20 percent of patients with EA/TEF; the genitourinary system in approximately 10 percent (usually absent kidney); musculoskeletal system in 10 to 30 percent; and craniofacial defects in 5 percent.[95] Further evidence of the importance of associated anomalies with EA/TEF affecting mortality figures has been reported by Barry and Auldist.[96] They conclude that the mortality rate for patients with isolated TEF is 6 percent, but 50 percent for those with TEF and multiple defects. Quan and Smith described the VATER association of defects.[97] VATER is a mnemonic suggesting the association of *V*ertebral anomalies, *A*nal atresia, *T*racheo-*E*sophageal fistula with esophageal atresia, *R*enal anomalies, and *R*adial limb dysplasias.

Low birth weight is not necessarily an indication of prematurity, but most authors reporting series of patients with EA/TEF accept a birth weight of less than 2500 grams as indicating a state of immaturity with its concomitant ramifications for management and survival. Smith reported that the incidence of prematurity or a birth weight of less than 2500 grams is 50 percent in patients with

EA/TEF which is significantly higher than with any other defect.[98] In his series, the premature infant with EA/TEF, unless extremely small (less than 1500 g), posed no particular problem with management because of size or maturity.

Pulmonary complications (atelectasis, pneumonitis, consolidation, and varying degrees of respiratory insufficiency) are related to the age at which the diagnosis is made and surgical intervention undertaken.[94,99] Aspiration of secretions or feedings from the proximal esophageal segment almost always results in atelectasis or pneumonitis of the right upper lobe. Regurgitation of gastric contents via the fistula results in a chemical pneumonitis which is resistant to treatment. The advantages of diagnosis before the infant is fed for the first time are obvious, since the morbidity and mortality observed in infants with this condition is significantly higher if diagnosis and appropriate treatment are delayed.

Pulmonary complications may be avoided or minimized by withholding feedings, inserting a suction system into the upper pouch of the atretic esophagus to remove secretions, and nursing the infant in a 45-degree head-up position. Gastrostomy should be performed as soon as possible to prevent the increased risk of regurgitation of gastic contents, as well as upward displacement of the left hemidiaphragm and a decrease in lung volume associated with gastric distention. Early intubation to protect the lungs and airways may be useful in esophageal atresia without TEF, but is of no use when there is a communication between the trachea and the stomach, since most of the gas will travel into the stomach rather than the lungs.

The intraoperative management of patients with EA/TEF requires great skill and patience from both surgeon and anesthesiologist. Successful outcome depends on recognition that the condition exists, appropriate preoperative therapeutic measures, and meticulous cooperation between surgeon and anesthesiologist since both are required to work in virtually the same small area.

Gastrostomy is usually carried out in the operating suite with local anesthesia using 1 percent lidocaine (2-4 mg/kg). The infant is maintained in the 45-degree head-up position to minimize the possibility of aspiration, and atropine (0.01 mg/kg) is administered intravenously upon arrival in the operating room. The infant should be monitored during the procedure with a precordial stethoscope, blood pressure cuff, and temperature probe. Esophageal stethoscopes and temperature probes are avoided for obvious reasons during gastrostomy, as well as during subsequent procedures for EA/TEF. Appropriate oxygen is given as necessary and careful attention paid to maintenance of body temperature and proper fluid, electrolyte, and glucose administration.

For more definitive repairs of EA/TEF, general anesthesia with endotracheal intubation is required. The monitoring technique is usually dictated by the general condition of the infant: the sicker the infant, the more complex the monitoring regimen. Newborn infants requiring surgery often arrive in the operating room with umbilical arterial (UA) and venous catheters in place which are used for pressure measurements and administration of fluids and blood. Even if a UA catheter is used for direct pressure measurement and blood sampling, a back-up indirect pressure measurement system should be applied in case the UA catheter becomes inoperative during surgery. Heart and breath sounds are monitored with a stethoscope placed against the left hemithorax after the infant is positioned for a right thoracotomy.

Intubation is usually done with the infant awake after pre-oxygenation. The appropriate-sized endotracheal tube (usually 3.0 mm) is passed beyond the vocal cords while breath sounds are monitored on both sides of the chest. After positioning for the right thoracotomy, tube position should be rechecked to ensure ventilation of both lungs. Some leakage through the TEF may occur even with the endotracheal tube tip below the level of the fistula, and this may be quite significant if the TEF is large. Infants are allowed to breathe spontaneously or with gently assisted ventilation until ligation of the fistula is accomplished, after which time controlled ventilation with low pressures can be safely utilized. Intubation of the fistula itself is recognized when the endotracheal tube is within the trachea, but expansion of the lungs is impossible while the stomach becomes distended or the gastrostomy tube leaks air whenever positive pressure is applied. Secretions may be a problem and obstruction of the endotracheal tube can occur. Suctioning of the endotracheal tube should be done carefully and with the knowledge and cooperation of the surgeon. The use of a humidification system in the anesthetic circuit is useful in preventing inspissation of secretions in the endotracheal tube, and has an added advantage in reducing heat loss via the lungs.

After awake intubation and proper securing of the endotracheal tube, anesthesia can be induced and maintained with low concentrations of halothane, enflurane, or isoflurane along with nitrous oxide and oxygen. If significant pneumonia exists, a high inspired oxygen concentration may be necessary to maintain the PaO_2 between 80 to 100 mmHg. If the potent anesthetic agents are not tolerated, a nitrous oxide/narcotic technique can be used, but requires controlled ventilation.

The integrity of the fistula repair can be assured by the surgeon's placing a small amount of saline into the wound, and the anesthesiologist's applying 20 cm H_2O constant positive pressure to the airway and looking for any leak in the tracheal suture line. If, after ligation of the fistula, primary repair of the esophageal atresia is undertaken with anastomosis of the proximal and distal segments, the surgeon may ask the anesthesiologist to pass a small suction catheter into the proximal segment until it can be felt near the end of the atretic esophageal pouch. When the catheter is palpable and placed properly, the anesthesiologist can mark it at the level of the infant's upper alveolar ridge with a su-

ture or umbilical tape with the head in a neutral or slightly flexed position. It is then withdrawn and carefully measured to determine the maximum safe distance that catheters should be inserted for postoperative oropharyngeal suctioning to avoid disruption of the anastomosis. Extension of the neck after repair is avoided for the same reason.

Most infants undergoing repairs for EA/TEF are left intubated for several hours to several days after surgery. Weaning from the ventilator begins as soon as possible after blood gas values and radiologic findings indicate improvement in atelectasis or pneumonia.

Complications after the repair include persistent pneumonia or atelectasis, pneumothorax, leakage or breakdown of the anastomosis, or reopening of the fistula into the trachea. Other tracheal complications (tracheal stenosis or granulomas) are quite rare.[100]

Anesthesia for Repair of Coarctation of the Aorta Beyond Infancy[101]

Coarctation of the aorta is a congenital constriction of the aorta which varies from partial to complete occlusion of the lumen of that vessel. The site of obstruction may be located at any site beyond the aortic valve but most commonly occurs just distal to the origin of the left subclavian artery. Beyond infancy, the most common form of coarctation of the aorta is that located as an isolated segment just distal to the left subclavian artery. This condition produces almost total obliteration of the aortic lumen, and survival depends on the development of collateral arteries which connect the brachiocephalic vessels with the descending aorta. Major collateral pathways include the arteries around the shoulder and those within the muscles of the chest wall, especially the intercostal and internal mammary arterial systems. Extensive anastomoses among these vessels result in the rib-notching evident on the chest radiographs of patients with coarctation, as well as the frequent finding of multiple bruits and thrills over the infrascapular area of the back on physical examination. A bicuspid aortic valve, with or without valve stenosis or insufficiency, is commonly associated with post-ductal coarctation.

Older children with coarctation of the aorta are usually asymptomatic, the diagnosis is usually made when weak or absent femoral or other lower extremity pulses are noted on physical examination along with upper extremity hypertension.

The physical examination is usually remarkable only in that there is a difference in the pulses and measurable blood pressure between the upper and the lower extremities. There may be a precordial murmur transmitted to the suprasternal area, and there may be audible bruits heard in the midportion of the back between the scapulae. Continuous murmurs over the back and upper thorax suggest the presence of adequate collateral vessels around the area of coarctation, although other signs are needed to confirm this important physiologic aspect of the defect.

The chest radiograph in isolated coarctation of the aorta will usually show a normal-sized heart with perhaps a suggestion of left ventricular prominence. The development of adequate collateral vessels around the coarcted segment results in rib-notching. Subtle changes can be observed at the base of the heart, caused by the coarctation itself, as well as pre- and poststenotic dilatation of the aorta: the "3" sign and the "E" sign.

In classical coarctation of the aorta, catheterization data is useful for ruling out associated anomalies, such as aortic stenosis and/or insufficiency, and in defining the adequacy and extent of collateral vessels around the coarctation. Although the pressure gradient across the coarctation is of interest, the range of blood pressure recorded proximal to the coarctation is probably more important to the anesthesiologist in determining an acceptable range of blood pressure during the surgical repair.

Induction of anesthesia can be accomplished either with thiopental or by mask. Supplementation with narcotics is often used to attenuate the hypertensive response to endotracheal intubation. Monitoring of vital signs during induction of anesthesia for young patients with coarctation is accomplished using a precordial stethoscope, blood pressure cuff, and ECG. After the patient is asleep, an arterial catheter is placed in the *right* radial artery, unless there is some indication that the right subclavian artery arises distal to the area of coarctation.

Repair of an isolated post-ductal coarctation is done via a left thoracotomy. In most cases, resection of the narrowed portion of the aorta and direct end-to-end anastomosis is considered the repair of choice. Since cross-clamping of the aorta during the repair is necessary, adequate collateral circulation around the coarctation is imperative if neurological and renal complications are to be avoided. Collaterals should be assessed clinically and angiographically prior to surgery. Before the resection is actually begun, a period of "test" cross-clamping is often carried out. During the "test" cross-clamping, a rise in the systemic arterial pressure of more than 20 to 30 mmHg suggests marginal or inadequate collateral vessels into the descending aorta. If inadequate collateral vessels are suspected, the cross-clamp is removed and intravenous sodium nitroprusside or other vasodilators can be administered.[102–104] The cross-clamp is reapplied when blood pressure is under adequate control. If questionably adequate collaterals are present, the pressure in the descending aorta should be directly monitored to ensure satisfactory perfusion of the spinal cord and the kidneys during the period of aortic interruption. Once the repair has been accomplished, nitroprusside is discontinued and adequate blood should be immediately available, before the cross-clamps are slowly released, distal before proximal. If significant bleeding occurs with release of either cross-clamp, it should be reapplied to control blood loss until surgical hemostasis is accomplished. Blood pressure almost invariably falls with the removal of the cross-clamps, but usually not alarmingly so, if adequate volume replacement has accompanied the infusion of nitroprusside during the cross-clamp period.

Two other aspects of the management of patients with coarctation of the aorta deserve special consideration. (1) *Management of bleeding from collateral vessels.* Blood loss from collateral vessels during opening of the chest and during mobilization of the aorta for the repair may be massive. An adequate supply of blood and blood products for replacement must be available and immediately at hand. It is recommended to have blood hanging in-line with the necessary equipment for rapid infusion before the chest incision is made. Postoperative bleeding may also be significant, even after meticulous hemostatic measures are taken by the surgeon, and measures for rapid blood replacement must be maintained. (2) *"Rebound" hypertension* is not unusual in the immediate postoperative period. If not managed properly, this may result in the "post-coarctation syndrome" with abdominal pain, ileus, mesenteric arteritis, and even bowel infarction. This "syndrome" is more likely to be seen in post-coarctation repair patients who show a delayed onset of *diastolic* hypertension with or without systolic elevation of blood pressure.[105,106] The "post-coarctation" syndrome has not been seen in patients whose diastolic blood pressures have been maintained within the normal range using nitroprusside, propranolol, or reserpine, and in whom decompression of the gastrointestinal tract has been assured by withholding early feedings and by nasogastric tube drainage. The exact etiology of this condition remains unclear, but may be related to the release of norepinephrine and renin.[107] Weaning patients from vasodilator therapy after coarctation repair should be gradual and may require up to five to seven days to accomplish. Propranolol may also be required for several weeks after coarctation repair to maintain an acceptable blood pressure.

Patent Ductus Arteriosus in the Premature Infant

Persistent patency of the ductus arteriosus (PDA) in the infant born prematurely has been well-documented.[108–112] Because of improved techniques for maintaining ventilation in the face of the respiratory distress syndrome, and better understanding of the metabolic and nutritional needs of prematures, the survival of these infants has improved significantly during the last decade.

The vasoconstrictor response of the ductus to an increase in the partial pressure of oxygen in the early neonatal period is proportional to gestational age; the lower the gestational age, the greater the likelihood of patency of the ductus. Forty percent of infants weighing less than 1750 g at birth will have clinical evidence of patency of the ductus; while in those weighing less than 1200 g, the incidence rises to 80 percent.

As with other types of left-to-right shunts, the clinical picture of patency of the ductus depends on the size of the ductus and the relationship of pulmonary resistance to systemic resistance. Because many infants born prematurely have RDS (60%), the severity of this disease determines the amount of left-to-right shunting. The more severe the RDS, the higher the pulmonary resistance is in relation to the systemic resistance, and, therefore, the less the magnitude of the shunt. Indeed, in the most severe forms of RDS, pulmonary resistance is higher than systemic, and right-to-left shunting occurs through the ductus resulting in a lower PaO_2 below the level of the ductus. As RDS improves, pulmonary resistance falls below systemic, the shunt is reversed, and congestive heart failure may ensue and warrant closure either pharmacologically or surgically.[113-115]

Some relationship between the presence of a patent ductus and the development of necrotizing enterocolitis in the premature infant has been suggested because of the vascular effects of a large run-off resulting in a steal phenomenon from the splanchnic circulation, but this has not been clearly defined.[116,117]

Once the decision to close the ductus surgically has been made by the neonatologists, cardiologists, and surgeon, the anesthetic management is usually simply an extension of the preoperative management. These infants will arrrive in the operating room with monitoring and intravenous catheters in place. Some are treated with non-depolarizing muscle relaxants to improve their ventilatory status, and most will be intubated and artificially ventilated using as low an inspired oxygen concentration and peak inspiratory pressure as possible while maintaining adequate oxygenation.[118] Protection from hyperoxia and resulting retrolental fibroplasia must be assured in the infant with a PDA. The PaO_2 should be maintained at 60 to 80 mmHg.[119-124]

Premature infants withstand anesthesia for ligation of a PDA quite well. Nitrous oxide/air/oxygen, a non-depolarizing muscle relaxant, and small doses of narcotics (morphine or fentanyl) are usually used. Continuation of supportive measures is important during the perioperative period and include maintenance of body temperature, provision of proper amounts of fluids, electrolytes, glucose, calcium, and correction of metabolic acidosis using sodium bicarbonate.* Although blood loss is usually minimal,

it should be remembered that the ductus tissue is very friable and mobilization of the structure in order to ligate it may result in tearing and sudden massive blood loss. Therefore, immediate transfusion may be necessary and blood should be readily available in the operating suite. Resuscitation drugs including diluted epinephrine, calcium, and bicarbonate should always be prepared and ready for use.

An important consideration in managing the premature infant with a PDA is the maintenance of adequate levels of hemoglobin. If the hemoglobin level falls, the cardiac output must rise in order to maintain adequate peripheral oxygenation. In the premature infant with a PDA and a significant left-to-right shunt, the myocardium is already compromised and anemia may further compromise it. Even the small amount of blood taken for blood gas analysis may become significant over several days because of the small blood volume of these patients. The hematocrit level should be maintained above 45 percent by transfusion. The administration of stored blood to the anemic premature results in more efficient peripheral oxygen delivery, since fetal hemoglobin is less effective at the tissue level in unloading oxygen than is adult hemoglobin.

Tracheostomy

Fortunately, the need for urgent tracheostomy in infants and children is very rare. Endotracheal intubation is usually possible even in cases of relatively severe acute epiglottitis.[125,126] Tracheostomy can be a difficult and dangerous procedure in the small infant with a short, fat neck, especially when the child is agitated and struggling. Every effort should be made to gain satisfactory control of the airway by endotracheal intubation and/or bronchoscopy, and to perform the tracheostomy under the ideal circumstances of the operating room and general anesthesia with controlled ventilation (see Ch. 13).

---

* An arterial pH of less than 7.30 due to a metabolic component or base deficit of 5 or greater should be corrected using sodium bicarbonate; calculating the dose to be administered using the formula:
mEq $NaHCO_3$ = weight in kg × base deficit correction desired × 0.5
The mEq of $NaHCO_3$ should be diluted with an equal amount of sterile distilled water to lower the very high osmolarity of bicarbonate. Hyperosmolarity has been suggested as a cause of spontaneous intracranial hemorrhage in the premature newborn. Full correction of the total base deficit is not usually recommended. Rather, correction of approximately one-half of the measured deficit is carried out and blood gases remeasured before further correction is attempted.

Tracheostomy is considerably simplified by the presence of a ventilating bronchoscope in the trachea. The rigid instrument can be manipulated by the anesthesiologist to displace the trachea directly anteriorly beneath the skin. Major arteries and veins thus fall to either side, while good ventilation is assured. Supplemental local infiltration anesthesia can be used to allow a "light" level of general anesthesia. The electrocautery is used to dissect and to control bleeding, since even minimal postoperative bleeding can be dangerous and difficult to control.

Tracheostomy tubes of several appropriate sizes should be available in the operating room, and proper adaptors for the ventilation system tested for compatibility. Cuffed tracheostomy tubes are usually not necessary in children, and their use is discouraged since mucosal erosion, necrosis, and subsequent tracheal stenosis are more likely when cuffed tubes are used. The carina is very high in the infant and small child, and it is not unusual to have to shorten the tracheostomy tube in order to assure good ventilation of both lungs. A tracheostomy tube resting on or very near the carina will also be difficult to suction and will provoke paroxysms of coughing.

Postoperatively, a chest radiograph is obtained and the child is observed carefully in the ICU. Many children having tracheostomies will require controlled positive pressure ventilation postoperatively due to the underlying pathology which necessitated the procedure. Even those seemingly healthy children who required tracheostomy for acute upper airway obstruction (epiglottitis) must be observed very carefully. Accidental removal or obstruction of the tube must be detected immediately if life-threatening hypoxemia is to be prevented. Humidified air with the desired FIO_2 should be delivered to the tracheostomy. Removal of a tracheostomy tube that has been in place for several weeks or more should be preceded by a diagnostic bronchoscopy to ensure that the upper airway is patent and that there is no ob-

structing granuloma at the site of the tracheostomy (see appendix).

Vascular Rings

The most common vascular abnormalities requiring operation to relieve airway obstruction include the double aortic arch, a right aortic arch with a left-sided ligamentum arteriosum, and an anomalous origin of the innominate artery (the "innominate arterial compression syndrome"). The first two of the anomalies are true "vascular rings," the trachea and esophagus being squeezed in a circle formed by these continuous vessels.

Vascular rings usually present in early childhood. Symptoms include wheezing, stridor, coughing, noisy breathing, difficulty in feeding, and even frank cardiorespiratory arrest. The diagnosis can usually be established by a chest radiograph with barium swallow, the barium-filled esophagus being indented posteriorly by the vascular structure. Angiography may be used to further delineate the anomaly, although it is probably not necessary in most cases. Bronchoscopy with or without bronchography will clearly demonstrate the flattened and obstructed trachea just above the carina. Simple "air tracheograms" visible on properly performed plain chest radiographs usually demonstrate the abnormality quite satisfactorily.

The tracheal compression caused by the vascular ring can be relieved by division of the ring at an appropriate point, care being required to maintain the proper relationship of vessels needed for circulation to the head and lower body. Operation is usually performed through a left thoracotomy. Anesthetic management must take into consideration the child's airway obstruction, but fortunately ventilation usually improves once an endotracheal tube is in proper position. The trachea is usually compressed just above the carina, so the tube must often be pushed down lower than would ordinarily be the case. Occasionally, direct left mainstem intubation is required with a side-hole in the endotracheal tube facilitating ventilation of the right lung. The surgeon will need to partially collapse the left lung to gain exposure to the vascular structures. Comparison of palpable pulses in the head and arms may assist the surgeon in identifying the proper location for division of the ring.

Correction of the "innominate artery syndrome" requires only that the innominate artery be pulled forward away from the trachea which it is compressing. The artery is usually sutured to the posterior periosteum of the sternum to hold it away from the trachea. The results of operation are excellent in most cases.

Postoperatively, relief of the tracheal obstruction is usually clearly evident and dramatic. Occasionally, however, there will have been substantial tracheomalacia produced by the chronic presence of the offending vessel. Symptoms of airway obstruction may persist for some time, particularly if the child is over-hydrated, suffering from congestive heart failure, or is quite small. A traumatic intubation or the need for prolonged postoperative intubation will increase mucosal edema, producing more symptoms of airway obstruction at an already compromised site in the trachea. Symptoms are more severe when the child is agitated, since the trachea is more likely to collapse during forceful inspiration. Obviously, this is a "vicious circle" which is best interrupted by the judicious use of sedation, fluid restriction, diuretics, steroids, humidified oxygen, and racemic epinephrine.

One form of partial vascular ring, the pulmonary arterial sling, may require the use of cardiopulmonary bypass for correction. In this anomaly, the left pulmonary artery passes to the right of the trachea before crossing back posteriorly to the left lung. This "sling" thus pulls on and compresses the trachea and right mainstem bronchus at the carina. Correction requires division of the left pulmonary artery, removal of the left pulmonary artery from behind the trachea,

and re-anastomosis of the vessel to the main pulmonary artery just distal to the pulmonary valve.

PREVENTION OF BACTERIAL ENDOCARDITIS DURING THORACIC OPERATIONS

Patients with rheumatic or congenital heart disease may require thoracic or other types of surgery which require the administration of antibiotics to prevent infectious endocarditis. While the anesthesiologist may not be completely responsible for ordering the necessary medications, an awareness is necessary of the risks involved if the prophylaxis is omitted, the types of surgical procedures in which antibiotic coverage is needed, and the dosages of the recommended drugs. It must also be remembered that even hemodynamically insignificant defects (e.g., mild mitral regurgitation from old rheumatic fever, a tiny ventricular septal defect, mild aortic or pulmonary valve stenosis, or a bicuspid aortic valve) must be covered with appropriate antibiotics. Infective endocarditis is one of the most serious complications of heart disease and the proper steps in its prevention must be taken.

The Committee on Rheumatic Fever and Bacterial Endocarditis of the Council on Cardiovascular Disease in the Young of the American Heart Association has recommended the following scheme:[127]
Operations requiring antibiotic prophylaxis include the following:

1. Dental procedures that are likely to result in gingival bleeding. Shedding of deciduous teeth is not included.
2. Surgery or instrumentation of the upper or lower respiratory tract including tonsillectomy, adenoidectomy, bronchoscopy, esophagoscopy, or any procedure causing disruption of the respiratory mucosa. Laryngoscopy and endotracheal intubation for anesthesia are excluded

provided trauma to the oral, pharyngeal, or glottic structures does not occur.

3. Genitourinary tract surgery or instrumentation including cystoscopy, urethral catheterization, and prostatic or bladder surgery.

4. Lower gastrointestinal tract or gall bladder surgery or instrumentation.

5. Surgery of the heart and great vessels including a patent ductus arteriosus.

6. Following cardiac surgery. *Exceptions* include patients with uncomplicated atrial septal defects of the secundum variety closed with direct suturing without a prosthetic patch; patients who have had division and ligation of a patent ductus arteriosus more than six months prior to present surgery; patients who have had coronary artery bypass grafts.

7. Surgical procedures involving any infected or contaminated tissues, e.g., incision and drainage of abscesses.

8. Patients who require long-term indwelling vascular catheters, e.g., hyperalimentation.

The patient taking ordinary rheumatic fever prophylaxis cannot be considered to be adequately covered for prevention of endocarditis for the above-mentioned surgical procedures.

The surgical procedure planned dictates the antibiotic regimen to be followed for prevention of endocarditis. Thoracic operations require the administration of appropriate doses of penicillin, both aqueous given intravenously and procaine given intramuscularly, as well as streptomycin or gentamycin given 30 minutes to one hour before surgery and continued postoperatively for three days or longer. Penicillin-sensitive patients may be given erythromycin or vancomycin along with streptomycin. The administration of vancomycin intravenously should be done with caution since rapid injection of this antibiotic has been reported to cause untoward reactions.[128]

REFERENCES

1. Downes JJ, Raphaely RC: Anesthesia and intensive care, p 12. In Ravitch MM, Welch KJ, Benson CD et al. Eds: Pediatric surgery. 3rd ed. Year Book Medical Publishers, Inc., Chicago, 1979

2. Smith CA, Nelson NM: The physiology of the newborn infant. Charles C. Thomas, Springfield, 1976

3. Rudolf AM: The changes in the circulation after birth: their importance on congenital heart disease. Circulation 41:343, 1970

4. Smith CA, Nelson NM: The physiology of the newborn infant. Charles C. Thomas, Springfield, 1976

5. Smith, ibid.

6. Bennett EJ: Fluids for anesthesia and surgery in the newborn and the infant. Charles C. Thomas, Springfield, 1975

7. Williams PR, Oh W: Effect of radiant heaters on insensible water loss in newborn infants. Am J Dis Ch 128:511, 1974

8. Volpe JJ: Neonatal periventricular hemorrhage: past, present, and future. J Peds 92:693, 1978

9. Simmons MA, Adcock EW, Bard H et al: Hypernatremia and intracranial hemorrhage in neonates. NEJM 291:6, 1974

10. Lubchenco LO: The high risk infant. In Major problems in clinical pediatrics, Vol 14. WB Saunders Company, Philadelphia, 1976

11. Avery GB: Neonatalogy, pathophysiology and management of the newborn. JB Lippincott Company, Philadelphia, 1981

12. Aranda JV, Sitar DS, Parsons WD et al: Pharmacokinetic aspects of theophylline in premature infants. NEJM 295:413, 1976

13. Lubchenco LO, Bard H: Incidence of hypoglycemia in newborn infants classified by birth weights and gestational age. Pediatrics 47:831, 1971

14. Bakwin H: Tetany in newborn infants: relation to physiologic hypoparathyroidism. J Peds 14:1, 1939

15. Tsang RC, Chen I, Friedman MA et al: Neonatal parathyroid function: role of gestational age and postnatal age. J Peds 83:728, 1973

16. Schedewie HE, Odell WD, Fisher DA et al: Parathoromone and perinatal calcium homeostasis. Pediatric Research 13:1, 1979

17. Oliver TK, Jr: Temperature regulation and heat production in the newborn. Pediatric Clinics of North America 12:765, 1966

18. Pearlstein PH, Edwards NK, Atherton MD et al: Computer assisted newborn intensive care. Pediatrics 57:494, 1976

19. Roe CF, Santulli TV, Blair CS: Heat loss in infants during general anesthesia and operations. J Ped Surg 3:266, 1966

20. Bland JW, Williams WH: Anesthesia for treatment of congenital heart defects, p 287. In Kaplan JA, Ed: Cardiac anesthesia. Grune and Stratton, New York, 1979

21. Thein RMH, Epstein BS: General surgical procedures in the child with a congenital anomaly, p 88. In Stehling LC, Zauder HL, Eds: Anesthetic implications of congenital anomalies in children. Appleton-Century-Crofts, New York, 1980

22. Noonan JA: Association of congenital heart disease with other defects. Pediatric Clinics of North America 25:797, 1978

23. Greenwood RD, Rosenthal A, Nadas AS: Cardiovascular abnormalities associated with diaphragmatic hernia. Pediatrics 57:92, 1976

24. Barnes LA: Nutrition and nutritional disorders, p 199. In Vaughn VC, McKay RJ, Behrman RE, Eds: Nelson textbook of pediatrics. 11th ed. WB Saunders Company, Philadelphia, 1979

25. Steward DJ: Manual of Pediatric Anesthesia. Churchill Livingstone, New York, 1979, p 21

26. Moffitt EA, McGoon DC, Ritter DG: The diagnosis and correction of congenital cardiac defects. Anesthesiology 33:144, 1970

27. Laver MB, Bland JHL: Anesthetic management of the pediatric patient during open-heart surgery. Int Anesthesiol Clin 13:3, 1975

28. Santoli FM, Pensa PM, Azzolina G: Anesthesia in open-heart surgery for correction of congenital heart diseases in children over one year of age. Int Anesthesiol Clin 14:3, 1976

29. Hansen DD: Anesthesia. In Sade RM, Cosgrove DM, Castaneda AR Eds: Infant and child care in heart surgery. Year Book Medical Publishers, Chicago, 1977

30. Bland JW, Williams WH: Anesthesia for treatment of congenital heart defects, p 291.

In Kaplan JA, Ed: Cardiac anesthesia. Grune and Stratton, New York, 1979

31. Ponce FE: Propranolol palliation of tetralogy of Fallot: Experience with long-term drug treatment in pediatric patients. Pediatrics 52:100, 1973

32. Honey M, Chamberlin DA, Howard J: The effect of beta-sympathetic blockade on arterial oxygen saturation in Fallot's tetralogy. Circulation 30:501, 1964

33. Cummings GR: Propranolol in tetralogy of Fallot. Circulation 41:13, 1970

34. Guntheroth WG, Kawabori I: Tetralogy of Fallot, p 287. In Moss AJ, Alams FH, Emmanouilides GC, Eds: Heart disease in infants, children and adolescents. 2nd ed. Williams & Wilkins, Baltimore, 1977

35. Eger EI, Kraft ID, Keasling HH: A comparison of atropine, or scopolamine, plus pentobarbital, meperidine, or morphine as pediatric preanesthetic medication. Anesthesiology 22:962, 1961

36. Steward DJ: Manual of Pediatric Anesthesia. Churchill Livingstone, New York, 1979, p 22

37. Merin RG: Effects of anesthetics on the heart. Surg Clin North Am 55:759, 1975

38. Schwartz DA, Horwitz LD: Effects of ketamine on left ventricular performance. J Pharmacol Exp Ther 194:410, 1975

39. Traber DL, Wilson RD, Priano LL: The effect of beta-adrenergic blockade on the cardiopulmonary response to ketamine. Anesth Analg 49:604, 1970

40. Gibbs RF: Monitor liability. Anesthesiol News, p. 1, March, 1978

41. Smith RM: The pediatric anesthetist. 1950-1975. Anesthesiology 43:144, 1975

42. Cannard TH, Dripps RD, Helwig J et al: The ECG during anesthesia and surgery. Anesthesiology 21:194, 1960

43. Mazzia VDB, Ellis CH, Siegal H et al: The electrocardiogram as a monitor of cardiac function in the operating room. JAMA 198:103, 1966

44. Nadas AS, Fyler D: Pediatric cardiology. 3rd ed.: WB Saunders, Philadelphia, 1972, p 191

45. Kinsey VE, Arnold HJ, Kalina RD et al: PaO_2 levels and retrolental fibroplasia: A report of the cooperative study. Pediatrics 60:655, 1977

46. Motoyama EK, Cook DR, Oh TH: Respiratory insufficiency and pediatric intensive care, p 632. In Smith RM, Ed.: Anesthesia for infants and children. 4th ed., The CV Mosby Company, St. Louis, 1980

47. James LS, Lanman JT: History of oxygen therapy and retrolental fibroplasia. Pediatrics 57:591, 1976

48. Prince SR, Sullivan RL, Hackel A: Percutaneous catheterization of the internal jugular vein in infants and children. Anesthesiology 44:170, 1976

49. Cote CJ, Jobes DR, Schwartz AJ et al: Two approaches to cannulation of a child's internal jugular vein. Anesthesiology. 50:371, 1979

50. Kaplan JA: Hemodynamic monitoring. In Kaplan JA, Ed: Cardiac anesthesia. Grune & Stratton, New York, 1979

51. Forestner JE: personal communication.

52. Adamsons K, Towell ME: Thermal homeostasis in the fetus and newborn. Anesthesiology 26:531, 1965

53. Stern L, Lees MA, Ledac J: Environmental temperature, oxygen consumption, and catecholamine excretion in newborn infants. Pediatrics 36:367, 1965

54. Buetow KC, Klein SW: Effect of maintenance of "normal" skin temperature on survival of infants of low birth weight. Pediatrics 34:163, 1964

55. Gandy GM, Adamsons K, Cunningham N et al: Thermal environment and acid-base homeostasis in human infants during the first few hours of life. J Clin Invest 43:751, 1964

56. Goudsouzian NG, Morris RH, Ryan JF: The effects of a warming blanket on the maintenance of body temperatures in anesthetized infants and children. Anesthesiology 39:351, 1973

57. Bennett EJ, Patel KP, Grundy EM: Neonatal temperature and surgery. Anesthesiology 46:303, 1977

58. LaFarge CG, Miettinen OS: The estimation of oxygen consumption. Cardiovasc Res 4:23, 1970

59. Sade RM, Cosgrove DM, Castaneda AR: Infant and child care in heart surgery. Year Book Medical Publishers, Chicago, 1977

60. Janssen PJ: Anesthesia for corrective open heart surgery of congenital defects beyond infancy. Int Anesth Clin 14:3:205, 1976

61. Steward DJ: Manual of pediatric anesthesia. Churchill Livingstone, New York, 1979, p 48

62. Rao Cc, Krishna G, Grosfeld JL et al: One lung pediatric anesthesia. Anesth & Analg 60:450, 1981

63. Koka BV, Jeon IS, Andre JM et al: Postintubation croup in children. Anesth Analg 56:501, 1977

64. Burgess GE, Cooper JR, Marino RJ et al: Laryngeal competence after tracheal extubation. Anesthesiology 51:73, 1979

65. Kirklin JW, Karp RB, Bargeron LA: Surgical treatment of ventricular septal defect, p 1044. In Sabiston DC, Spencer FC, Eds: Surgery of the chest. 3rd ed. WB Saunders Company, Philadelphia 1976

66. Ilabaca PA, Ochsner JL, Mills NL: Positive end - expiratory pressure in the management of the patient with a postoperative bleeding heart. Ann Thorac Surg 30:281, 1980

67. Johnson DG: Endoscopy, p 513. In Ravitch MM, Welch KJ, Benson CD et al, Eds: Pediatric Surgery. 3rd ed. Year Book Medical Publishers, Inc., Chicago, 1979

68. Ibid. p. 514.

69. Stern RC: Foreign bodies in the larynx, trachea, and bronchi, p 1198. In Vaughn, McKay, Berhman RE, Eds: Nelson textbook of pediatrics. 11th ed. WB Saunders Co., Philadelphia, 1979

70. Law D, Kosloske AM: Management of tracheobronchial foreign bodies in children: A reevaluation of postural drainage and bronchoscopy. Pediatrics 58:362, 1976

71. Jordan WS, Graves CL, Elwyn RA: New therapy for postintubation laryngeal edema and tracheitis in children. JAMA 212:585, 1970

72. Meyer BW: Pediatric Anesthesia. JB Lippincott Co, Philadelphia, 1981, p 158

73. Johnson DG: Endoscopy, p 518. In Ravitch MM, Welch KJ, Benson CD et al. Eds: Pediatric Surgery. 3rd ed. Year Book Medical Publishers, Inc., Chicago, 1979

74. Campbell JB, Quattromani FL, Foley LC: Catheter technique for removal of foreign bodies. Experience with 100 cases. Ped Radiol 11:174, 1981

75. Thein RMH, Epstein BS: General surgical procedures in the child with a congenital anomaly, p 87. In Stehling LC, Zauder HL, Eds: Anesthetic implications of congenital anomalies in children. Appleton-Century-Crofts, New York, 1980

76. Grosfeld JL, Ballantine TVN: Surgical respiratory distress in infancy and childhood. Curr Probl Ped 6, 7:3, 1976

77. Adelman S, Benson CD: Bochdalek hernias in infants: Factors determining mortality. J Ped Surg 11:569, 1976

78. Greenwood RD, Rosenthal A, Nadas AS: Cardiovascular abnormalities associated with diaphragmatic hernia. Pediatrics 57:92, 1976

79. Holder RM, Ashcraft KW: Congenital diaphragmatic hernia, p 433. In Ravitch MM, Welch KJ, Benson CD, et al, Eds: Pediatric Surgery. 3rd ed. Year Book Medical Publishers, Inc., Chicago, 1979

80. Boles ET, Schiller M, Weinberger M: Improved management of neonates with congenital diaphragmatic hernias. Arch Surg 103:344, 1971

81. Mahour GH, Hays DM: Ventral hernia coverage with silon after correction of congenital diaphragmatic hernia. J Ped Surg 6:75, 1971

82. Thein RMH, Epstein BS: General surgical procedures in the child with a congenital anomaly, p 90. In Stehling LC, Zauder HL, Eds: Anesthetic implication of congenital anomalies in children. Appleton-Century-Crofts, New York, 1980

83. Holder RM, Ashcraft KW: Congenital diaphragmatic hernia, p 439. In Ravitch MM, Welch KJ, Benson CD et al, Eds: Pediatric Surgery. 3rd ed. Year Book Medical Publishers, Inc., Chicago, 1979

84. Raphaely RC, Downes JJ: Congenital diaphragmatic hernia: Prediction of survival. J Ped Surg 8:815, 1973

85. Chatrath RR, El Shafie M, Jones RS: Fate of hypoplastic lungs after repair of congenital diaphragmatic hernia. Arch Dis Child 46:633, 1971

86. Kitagawa M, Hislop A, Boyden EA et al: Lung hypoplasia in congenital diaphragmatic hernia. A quantitative study of airway, artery, and alveolar development. Br J Surg 58:342, 1971

87. Dibbins AW, Wiener ES: Mortality from neonatal diaphragmatic hernia. J Ped Surg 9:653, 1974

88. Dibbins AW: Neonatal diaphragmatic hernia: A physiologic challenge. Am J Surg 131:408, 1976

89. Wohl MEB, Griscom NT, Strieder DJ et al: The lung following repair of congenital diaphragmatic hernia. J Ped 90:405, 1977

90. Thein RMH, Epstein BS: General surgical procedures in the child with a congenital anomaly, p 90. In Stehling LC, Zauder HL, Eds: Anesthetic implications of congenital anomalies in children. Appleton-Century-Crofts, New York, 1980

91. Waterston DJ, Bonhan-Carter RE, Aberdeen E: Congenital tracheoesophageal fistula in association with oseophageal atresia. Lancet 2:55, 1963

92. Ball, TI, personal communication

93. Greenwood RD, Rosenthal A, Nadas AS: Cardiovascular abnormalities associated with diaphragmatic hernia. Pediatrics 57:92, 1976

94. Calverly RK, Johnston AE: The anesthetic management of tracheoesophageal fistula: a review of ten years' experience. Canad anaesth Soc J 19:270, 1972

95. Thein RMH, Epstein BS: General surgical procedures in the child with a congenital anomaly, p 91. In Stehling LC, Zauder HL, Eds: Anesthetic implications of congenital anomalies in children. Appleton-Century-Crofts, New York, 1980

96. Barry JE, Auldist AW: The VATER association: one end of a spectrum of anomalies. Am J Dis Child 128:769, 1974

97. Quan L, Smith DW: The VATER association, vertebral defects, anal atresia, T-E fistula with esophageal atresia, radial and renal dysplasia: A spectrum of associated defects. J Ped 82:104, 1973

98. Smith RM: Anesthesia for infants and children. 4th ed. The CV Mosby Company, St. Louis, 1980

99. Bedard P, Givran DP, Shandling B: Congenital H-type tracheoesophageal fistula. J Ped Surg 9:663, 1974

100. Myers NA, Aberdeen E: Congenital esophageal atresia and tracheoesophageal fistula, p 459. In Tavitch MM, Welch KJ, Benson CD, et al, Eds: Pediatric surgery. 3rd ed. Year Book Medical Publishers, Inc., Chicago, 1979

101. Bland JW: Anesthesia for repair of coarctation of the aorta beyond infancy. In Stehling LC, Ed: A Practical approach to pediatric anesthesia: Recommendation of the experts. Year Book Medical Publishers, 1981. In press

102. Steward DJ: Manual of Pediatric Anesthesia. Churchill Livingstone, New York, 1979

103. Balal FY, Bennett EJ, Salem MR et al: Anaesthesia for coarctation. Anaesth 29:704, 1974

104. Bennett EJ, Dalah FY: Hypotensive anaesthesia for coarctation. Anaesth 29:269, 1974

105. Sealy WC: Indications for surgical treatment of coarctation of the aorta. Surg Gynecol Obstet 97:301, 1953

106. Sealy WC, Harris JS, Young WG et al: Paradoxical hypertension following resection of coarctation of the aorta. Surgery 42:135, 1957

107. Fox S, Pierce WS, Waldhausen JA: Pathogenesis of paradoxical hypertension after coarctation repair. Ann Thorac Surg 29:135, 1980

108. Heymann MA: The ductus arteriosus, p 168. In Moss AJ, Adams FH, Emmanouilides GC, Eds: Heart disease in infants, children and adolescents. Williams & Wilkins, Baltimore, 1977

109. Clarkson PM, Orgill AA: Continuous murmurs in infants of low birth weight. J Peds 84:208, 1974

110. Rudolph AM: Congenital Diseases of the Heart. Year Book Medical Publishers, Chicago, 1974, p 176

111. Neal WA: Patent ductus arteriosus complicating respiratory distress syndrome. J Peds 86:127, 1975

112. Thibeault DW: Patent ductus arteriosus complicating the respiratory distress syndrome in preterm infants. J Peds 86:102, 1975

113. Heymann MA, Rudolph AM, Silverman NH: Closure of the ductus arteriosus in premature infants by inhibition of prostaglandin synthesis. N Engl J Med 295:530, 1976

114. Friedman WF: Pharmacologic closure of patent ductus arteriosus in the premature infant. N Engl J Med 295:526, 1976

115. Nadas AS: Patent ductus revisited (Editorial). N Engl Med 295:563, 1976

116. Davidson M: Neonatal necrotizing enterocolitis, p 992. In Rudolph AM, Ed: Pediatrics. Appleton-Century-Crofts, New York, 1977

117. Hakanson DO, OH W: Necrotizing enterocolitis and hyperviscosity in the newborn infant. J Peds 90:458, 1977

118. Stark AR, Bascom BA, Frantz ID: Muscle relaxation in mechanically ventilated infants. J Peds 94:439, 1979

119. Betts EK, Downes JJ, Schaffer DB et al: Retrolental fibroplasia and oxygen administration during general anesthesia. Anesthesiology 47:518, 1977

120. Kinsey VE, Arnold HJ, Kalina RD et al: PaO_2 levels and retrolental fibroplasia: A report of a cooperative study. Pediatrics 60:655, 1977

121. Phibbs RH: Oxygen therapy: A continuing hazard to the premature infant. Anesthesiology 47:486, 1977

122. Merritt JC, Sprague DH, Merritt WE et al: Retrolental fibroplasia: A multifactorial disease. Anes & Analg 60:109, 1981

123. Adamkin DH, Shott RJ, Cook LN et al: Nonhyperoxic retrolental fibroplasia. Pediatrics 60:828, 1977

124. Kingham JD: Acute retrolental fibroplasia. Arch Ophthal 95:39, 1977

125. Sweeney DB, Allen TH, Steven IM: Acute epiglottitis: Management by intubation. Anaesth Intensive Care 1:526, 1973

126. Oh TH, Motoyama EK: Comparison of nasotracheal intubation and tracheostomy in management of epiglottitis. Anesthesiology 46:214, 1977

127. American Heart Association Committee on Rheumatic Fever and Bacterial Endocarditis: Prevention of endocarditis. Circulation 56:139A, 1977

128. Wilkinson PL, Ham J, Miller RD: Clinical Anesthesia. The CV Mosby Company, St. Louis, 1980, p 165

APPENDIX—RESPIRATORY CARE OF PEDIATRIC PATIENTS

A. *Tracheal airway care* (applies to endotracheal tubes and tracheotomies)
   1. Use sterile tracheal apparatus.
   2. Humidify and warm inspired air.
   3. Instill sterile saline (0.5 ml to 2 ml.) every 1–3 hours to prevent drying of secretions.
   4. Induce coughing or positive pressure to inflate chest with chest physiotherapy.

B. *Suctioning of endotracheal tubes and tracheotomies*
   1. Use sterile equipment (suction catheter, sterile saline, sterile gloved hand).

2. Have second person to ventilate patient with 100 percent oxygen before and after each suctioning and to instill saline for wash.
3. Suction only 10–20 seconds at the time followed by 5–10 positive pressure breaths of 100 percent O_2.
4. After suctioning of endotracheal tube is completed, suction mouth and also nose if necessary.
5. Reconnect patient's endotracheal tube to ventilator or other supportive apparatus.
6. Check ventilator or supportive apparatus (CPAP or PEEP) and observe patient closely.

C. *Removal of endotracheal tubes*
   1. Mildly sedate patient (10–20 mg/kg chloral hydrate) if necessary while patient breathes 100 percent oxygen.
   2. Suction nose and mouth thoroughly. (Remember newborn babies are obligate nose breathers for 3–6 weeks.)
   3. Remove stomach contents by suctioning.
   4. Change to sterile catheter and put on sterile glove for suctioning endotracheal tube *if necessary.*
   5. Ventilate patient with 100 percent oxygen for 2–5 minutes.

6. Remove endotracheal tube at the end of a full inspiration.
7. Place patient in atmosphere with oxygen concentration 20 percent higher than that prior to extubation.
8. Suction mouth and throat q30–60 minutes and p.r.n. for 4–6 hours after extubation depending on the amount of secretions present. Give bag and mask ventilation with 100 percent oxygen after each suctioning and physiotherapy.
9. Preferably feed patient via nasogastric tube (with infants at 45° angle) for at least 8 hours following extubation and supplement with IV fluids.
10. Steroid administration remains controversial but if administered should probably be given intravenously one hour prior to extubation (0.2 mg/kg dexamethasone) as one shot dose.
11. If stridor is present after extubation, racemic epinephrine in 1:8 dilution administered as an aerosol via IPPB may be helpful. Frequency and duration of treatment should not be more often than 5 minutes every 20 minutes for 3 or 4 treatments.

D. *Endotracheal tube sizes*

Endotracheal (Clear) Portex Tubes
Thin Wall—Uncuffed

Internal Diameter (I.D.) (mm)	Age of Patient (approx.)	Length (cm) mid-trachea	
		Oral	Nasal
2.5–3.0	Premature	11	13.5
3.5	Newborn	12	14
4.0	6 months	13	15
4.5	1 year	14	16
5.0	2 years	15	17
5.5	4 years	17	19
6.0	6 years	19	21
6.5	8 years	20	22
7.0	10 years	21	22
7.5	12 years	22	23
8.0	14 years	23	24
8.5	16 years	24	25
9.0	18 years	25	26
9.5	Adult	26	27

Formula: Size of Tube (I.D.) $= \dfrac{\text{Age of Patient} + 4.5}{4}$
(Approx.)

or

Size of Tube (I.D.) $= \dfrac{18 + \text{Age}}{4}$
(mm)

E. *Parameters useful in determining need for respiratory support*

Parameter	Normal	Wean or Extubate
PaO_2 ($FiO_2 = 1.0$)	greater than 600 mmHg	greater than 300 mmHg
PaO_2 ($FiO_2 = 0.21$)	75–100 mmHg	50 mmHg
$PaCO_2$	35–45 mmHg	45–50 mmHg
VC	70 ml/kg	15 ml/kg
Neg insp force	less than -100 mmHg	less than -25 mmHg

F. *Oral vs. nasotracheal intubation*

Oral

 Advantages   *Disadvantages*
 Easier to place   Harder to maintain in place
 Larger size possible   More cord damage possible
 Easier to suction

Nasal

 Advantages   *Disadvantages*
 Better tolerated by patient   Smaller size
 Harder to dislodge in either direction Nasal bleeding
                   More difficult to suction
 Less movement at cord area   Sinus infection
 Better oral hygiene possible
 Oral feedings possible

Some Complications Arising from Nasotracheal Intubation

1. Tracheal stenosis
2. Tracheal and/or vocal cord erosion
3. Pharyngoesophageal perforation
4. Necrosis of nares
5. Granuloma of cords
6. Catheter obstruction
7. Right main stem bronchus intubation

G. *Tracheostomy*

Rare in children because of common use of nasal or tracheal intubation. Should be done electively in controlled conditions in operating room with airway secured with endotracheal tube or bronchoscope.

1. *Indications* (relative)
   1. Inability to maintain adequate airway with endotracheal tube
   2. Profuse secretions requiring almost constant suctioning
   3. Upper airway obstruction not safely managed with endotracheal tube
   4. Ultra-long-term need for ventilatory support
   5. Subglottic stenosis

2. *Complications arising from tracheotomy*
   1. Tracheal stenosis
   2. Tracheal erosion
   3. Mediastinitis
   4. Pneumothorax, pneumopericardium, pneumomediastinum
   5. Hemorrhage or hemothorax
   6. Infection and pneumonia
   7. Surgical error (high tracheotomy, damage to vocal cords)
   8. Erosion into esophagus or into innominate artery
   9. Mechanical obstruction
   10. Accidental decannulation
   11. Difficulties in closing stoma

JAMES R. ZAIDAN, M.D.

17
Pacemakers

The increasing use and complexity of pacemakers make it important for anesthesiologists to understand basic pacemaker physiology, so that the patient may receive better care. The anesthesiologist will be exposed to the pacemaker patient in several situations. First, he might help to analyze the electrode after a pacemaker insertion; second, he might encounter a pacemaker patient who is about to undergo noncardiac surgery; third, he might work with a patient who requires short-term pacing after cardiac surgery; and fourth, he might be required to decide which patient would benefit from temporary pacing in the perioperative period. This chapter will discuss these areas of pacemaker management.

TERMINOLOGY AND NOMENCLATURE

Definitions

As with any new subject, definitions are important.[1] The following definitions will be used throughout the remainder of this chapter.

1. **Pacemaker:** A combination of a pulse generator, lead, and electrode.

2. **Generator:** That part of the pacemaker that contains the stored energy, produces electrical impulses, and detects intrinsic myocardial electrical activity. Many times the generator is mistakenly called the battery.

3. **Electrode:** The electrical conductor which is in physical contact with the atrium or ventricle.

4. **Lead:** The insulated wire which connects the electrode and generator.

5. **Threshold:** The amount of electricity that is just able to stimulate the ventricle to contract.
   a. **Current threshold:** The number of milliamperes required to cause pacing.
   b. **Voltage threshold:** The number of volts required to cause pacing.

6. **Pulse duration:** The number of milliseconds in each pacing impulse. The pulse duration is usually within the range of 0.5 to 1.0 msec.

7. **Bipolar:** A pacemaker circuit in which both the positive and negative electrodes are located in the heart (Fig. 17-1).

8. **Unipolar:** A pacemaker circuit in which the negative (stimulating) electrode is located on the heart and the positive

575

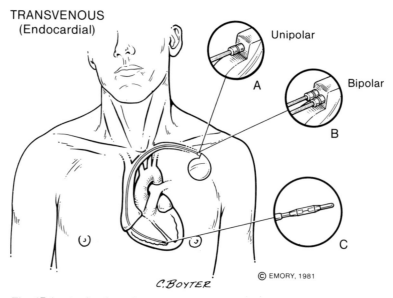

TRANSVENOUS
(Endocardial)

Unipolar

A

Bipolar

B

C

C. BOYTER

© EMORY, 1981

Fig. 17-1 An implanted transvenous pacemaker is shown in this figure. The generator can be positioned at either shoulder with the lead directed through the venous system to the right ventricular apex. *Inset A:* Generator connections for a unipolar system. *Inset B:* Generator connections for a bipolar system. *Inset C:* Electrodes of a bipolar system.

(ground) electrode is located away from the heart. The ground is usually included in the implanted generator. During open heart or thoracic surgery, the ground can be a temporary electrode sewn to subcutaneous tissue (Fig. 17-2).

9. **Endocardial:** The stimulating electrode is in contact with the right ventricular endocardium. Endocardial stimulation can be either unipolar or bipolar. The route of entry is usually through a subclavian or right internal jugular vein. For this reason, an endocardial electrode sometimes is called a *transvenous electrode* (Fig. 17-1).

10. **Epicardial:** The stimulating electrode is applied to the heart through the epicardium. This system, correctly called *myocardial* rather than epicardial, can be arranged in a unipolar or bipolar circuit (Fig. 17-2).

11. **Pulse interval:** This is the number of milliseconds between two consecutive pacing impulses. Divide this number into 60,000 to determine the number of impulses per minute.

12. **Automatic interval:** The automatic interval is basically the same as the pulse interval.

13. **Escape interval:** This interval is the number of milliseconds between a patient's intrinsic R wave and the following paced beat.

14. **Hysteresis:** This is the difference between the intrinsic heart rate when pacing commences and the pacing rate. As an example, if the automatic interval were 833 msec (72 beats per minute), pacing would stop if the patient's heart rate increased to 73 per minute. If the escape interval were 923 msec (65 beats per minute), pacing would not resume until the patient's heart rate decreased to 65. The pacemaker would then begin pacing at a rate of 72. This is an example of seven-beat hysteresis and does not imply abnormal function.

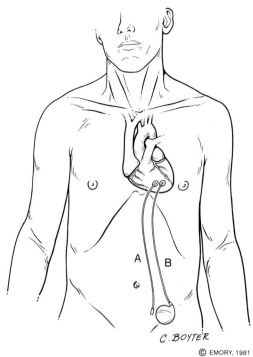

C. BOYTER

© EMORY, 1981

Fig. 17-2 The pacemaker system shown here is epicardial and unipolar. Lead A is a spare for use if the working lead should fail. Lead B is the working lead in that it is connected to the generator. Notice the placement of the generator for an epicardial system compared with that for the transvenous system.

15. **R-wave sensitivity:** This is the number of millivolts required to inhibit a generator. One type of pacemaker can be turned off, or inhibited, by an R-wave amplitude of approximately 2 mV. The R-wave sensitivity on the external generator is adjustable. The R-wave sensitivity is explained more fully under Nomenclature.

Nomenclature

Pacemakers are named according to their location and their mode of action. This system of naming includes three letters.[2] The first letter designates the chamber which receives the current output from the generator;

Table 17-1
Pacemaker Nomenclature

A = Atrium
V = Ventricle
D = Dual (indicates both A and V)
I = Inhibited
T = Triggered
O = Asynchronous or does not apply

the second letter designates the chamber in which sensing of the intrinsic electrical activity occurs; and the third letter indicates the mode of action of the pacemaker. Table 17-1 lists the letters which are used in this system of naming and Table 17-2 gives examples of the five most commonly used pacemakers.

The generator in the asynchronous pacemaker has no electrical circuitry to detect intrinsic R waves. If the patient's heart rate is greater than the pacemaker rate, then competition develops between normal conduction and the pacemaker impulses. This situation exposes the patient with an ischemic ventricle to the possibility of ventricular fibrillation or tachycardia. It is also wasteful of energy. Synchronous pacemakers eliminate both these problems.

The synchronous pacemaker contains a second electrical circuit which detects or senses R waves. These R waves are conducted through the electrode and lead to the generator, in which they turn the pacing circuitry on or off. If the R wave turns on the pacemaker so that it places an impulse in the refractory period of the myocardium, it is called a *ventricular-triggered,* or VVT, pacemaker. A pacemaker that is turned off by an R wave is called a *ventricular-inhibited,* or VVI, pacemaker. It should be understood that the above-mentioned R wave is not that which is seen on the surface ECG but is the voltage change surrounding the electrode as the impulse spreads through the conduction system.

The VVI is the most commonly used permanent pacemaker; however, all the pacemakers in Table 17-2 are available in the implantable form. The VOO, VVI, AOO,

Table 17-2
Five Commonly Used Pacemakers

3 Letter Designation		Explanation
1. VOO	Chamber paced	Ventricle
	Chamber sensed	None
	Mode of action	Asynchronous
2. VVI	Chamber paced	Ventricle
	Chamber sensed	Ventricular R wave
	Mode of action	Inhibited
3. AOO	Chamber paced	Atrium
	Chamber sensed	None
	Mode of action	Asynchronous
4. DVI	Chamber paced	Both the atrium and the ventricle are paced.
(sequential)	Chamber sensed	The R wave in the ventricle is sensed.
	Mode of action	Both the atrial and ventricular pacing circuits are inhibited by the R wave.
5. VAT	Chamber paced	Ventricle
(P-wave synchronous)	Chamber sensed	Atrial P wave
	Mode of action	P wave from the atrium triggers an impulse into the ventricle.

and DVI are the most useful external pacemakers. Many times the VOO is used incorrectly in place of the VVI.

If the patient's heart rate is very slow, the pacemaker can easily override the intrinsic rate. In this situation, a VOO pacemaker is adequate, since competition between the pacemaker and the patient's heart rate is not a problem. A patient with a VOO pacemaker who has third-degree block alternating with sinus rhythm or with atrial fibrillation will develop competition when the ventricular rate increases. This situation is ideal for the VVI pacemaker since it turns off and eliminates competition. This competition between the patient's own impulses and the pacemaker impulses can be dangerous in the ischemic ventricle because of the possibility of initiating ventricular tachycardia or fibrillation.[3, 4] When using the external generator, a VOO can be converted to a VVI simply by turning the R-wave sensitivity dial to about 3 mV. If the sensitivity is set to a lower number, the generator could be turned off by T waves, P waves, and possibly even skeletal muscle potentials. An R-wave sensitivity of 3 mV will permit normal pacing if the patient is shivering but will be inhibited by the patient's intrinsic R waves.

The AOO is most useful in patients with slow sinus rates and slow junctional rhythms with normal atrioventricular conduction. If sequential pacing is necessary, then the DVI is the external generator of choice. These generators are discussed more fully under Cardiovascular Effects of Pacing.

PROCEDURE FOR EVALUATING ELECTRODE PLACEMENT

The importance of evaluating the function of a permanent ventricular electrode immediately after positioning cannot be overemphasized. Only a thorough evaluation of the electrode can assure the patient of trouble-free electrode function and therefore avoid a second operating room experience for electrode replacement. This evaluation is very simple, involving only fluoroscopy and a pacemaker analyzer.

Endocardial Electrode

Fluoroscopy: Fluoroscopy should be used to place the electrode in the apex of the right ventricle on a PA view and pointing anteriorly in the lateral view. Fluoroscopy is not always necessary when placing a temporary transvenous electrode.

Analyzer: The surgeon will attach the negative lead of the cable to the electrode and the positive lead to subcutaneous tissue, then pass the cable to the anesthesiologist. After the cable has been connected to the analyzer (Fig. 17-3), the analyzer is set to a rate 10 percent above the patient's heart rate or to a physiologic rate, a pulse duration of 0.5 msec, and an output of 5 V (Fig. 17-4). The analyzer is turned to "threshold" and the ECG observed for ventricular pacing. The voltage output of the analyzer is slowly decreased until pacing is lost, and the output is then increased until the ventricle is paced once again. The voltage threshold is read on the dial and the current threshold in the digital readout. Approximately 1 V and 2 mA are acceptable thresholds. The resistance is calculated by using Ohm's law:

$$R = 10^3 \ V/mA.$$

An acceptable resistance is less than 750 ohms. Most implantable pacemakers have a voltage output of 5 V and a current output which varies with the resistance according to Ohm's law.

R-wave sensitivity measurement is essential. The pulse is always monitored while evaluating the R-wave sensitivity because the analyzer will stop pacing when the sensing button is depressed. The digital readout will indicate the number of millivolts in the impulse passing the electrode. This impulse is conducted through the electrode and lead to the pacemaker. If this impulse is large enough, it will turn off, or inhibit, the pacing circuitry of the generator. The generator usually will be inhibited by a 2-mV R wave. When the readout has indicated several R waves, the button is released to resume pacing. A patient with no ventricular response obviously does not require evaluation of the R wave. If a patient has a temporary external generator, the R-wave sensitivity will indicate the output of the external generator.

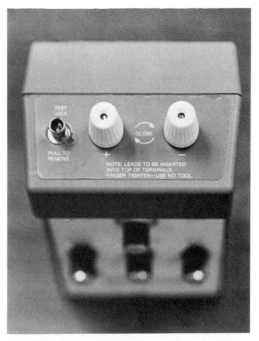

Fig. 17-3 The pacing system analyzer is demonstrated here. The connector labeled "Test Jack" is used to test the generator, and the other two white connectors are used to test the electrode.

Positioning the electrode in an ischemic zone or an infarcted area will result in high current and voltage thresholds, high resistance, and low R-wave sensitivity. If these measurements are in unacceptable ranges, the surgeon should reposition the electrode.

Epicardial Electrode

Fluoroscopy: Fluoroscopy is not necessary since these electrodes are placed by direct vision through a left thoracotomy or a subxiphoid surgical approach.

Analyzer: The same process is used as described for endocardial electrodes.

The analyzer can also be used to test the generator. A separate cable is necessary, the two leads of which are placed by the surgeon on the generator. The anesthesiologist then connects this cable to the analyzer and turns the dial of the analyzer to pulse dura-

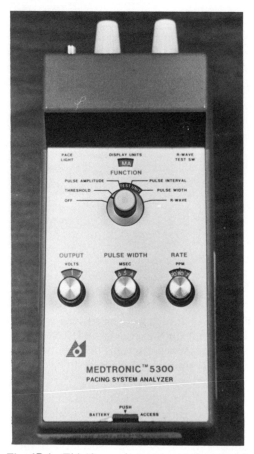

Fig. 17-4 This figure demonstrates the controls of the pacing system analyzer. The pulse width should be adjusted to 0.5 msec and the rate to 10 percent above the patient's heart rate or to a physiologic level in order to test the electrode. When the function switch is turned to "threshold" and the output dial is adjusted to the voltage threshold, the digital readout will indicate current threshold in milliamperes. Resistance can then be determined by using Ohm's law. Turning the function switch to "R-wave" and pressing the "R-wave test SW" will convert the analyzer from a pulse generator to a sensing device. The generator to be implanted is tested simply by turning the function dial to pulse amplitude, pulse interval, and pulse width and observing the digital readout. These numbers for the generator should correspond to the factory specifications.

tion, pulse amplitude, and finally pulse interval. If these three variables correspond to the factory-set specifications, the generator is functioning correctly. The same procedure can be used to evaluate an external generator by simply connecting the analyzer cable to it. The generator is then set to any output and any rate. The analyzer should indicate these settings in the digital readout.

POSITIONING A VENTRICULAR ELECTRODE

Since ventricular pacing can be a life-saving maneuver, the anesthesiologist should be familiar with the technique of inserting a ventricular endocardial electrode. A large-bore needle usually will be included in the package with the electrode (Fig. 17-5, 17-6, 17-7). The right internal jugular and subclavian veins are the most expedient routes to the right ventricle. In an emergency, such as a third-degree block without a ventricular response, one of these veins is cannulated and the electrode is inserted through the cannula while an assistant is connecting the external generator to the pacing leads. The generator is adjusted to an output of 20 mA, an R wave of 3 to 5 mV, and a rate of approximately 70 beats per minute. When ventricular pacing occurs, the advance of the electrode is stopped. This method of inserting a ventricular electrode is recommended only for the most extreme emergency, and, since it is used in the cardiac arrest situation, it is made difficult because of chest compression.

The ECG can be used as a guide to proper electrode placement in less life-threatening situations. Two methods can be used to connect the ventricular electrodes to the ECG. In one method the surface ECG is attached in the usual way and the distal ventricular electrode is connected to the chest lead. The ECG then is set to the chest lead. Another method of obtaining an ECG

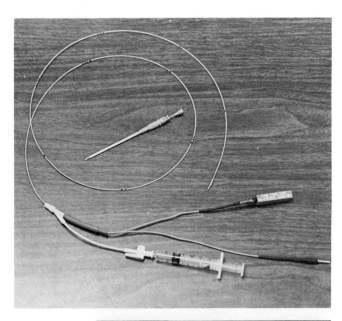

Fig. 17-5 Demonstrated here is a typical transvenous temporary ventricular bipolar electrode. This particular set includes an intravenous cannula, a syringe for balloon inflation, and a connector so that the intracavitary electrogram can be observed during electrode placement.

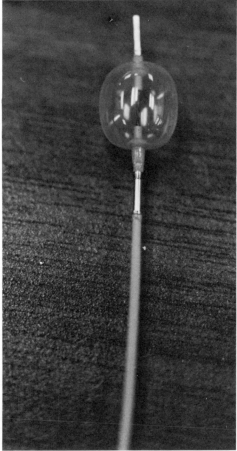

Fig. 17-6 This is the tip of the lead shown in Figure 17-5. Notice that it is bipolar. The balloon should be deflated when an intraventricular electrogram is obtained to prevent knotting in the right ventricle and to simplify insertion to the right ventricular apex.

from the ventricular electrode (Fig. 17-8) is to attach the distal ventricular electrode to the right arm lead and the proximal electrode to the left leg lead. The ECG in this method is set to lead II, and the recorder run at 25 mm/sec. The electrode is advanced through the atrium. The atrial ECG is characterized by very large P waves and very small QRS complexes. As the electrode passes through the tricuspid valve, both the P wave and the QRS complex will become almost isoelectric. Entry into the ventricle will be characterized by very large QRS complexes and, as the electrode approaches the ventricular endocardium, ST elevation. When the electrode is in good position, the external generator is connected to the electrodes and the current output increased until ventricular pacing occurs. If time permits, the electrode position should be analyzed before pacing is initiated.

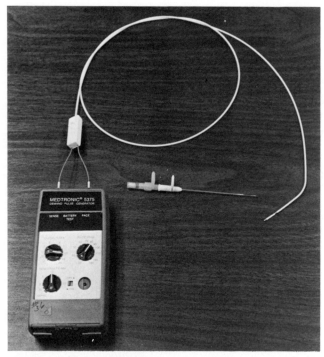

Fig. 17-7 This figure demonstrates a temporary transvenous bipolar electrode system attached to a typical external pacing generator.

INDICATIONS FOR TEMPORARY PACING

Some of the indications for temporary pacing are definite while others are relative and require medical judgment. One definite indication for temporary pacing is third-degree heart block secondary to an acute myocardial infarction (MI). Generally, if a block develops in a patient with an acute anterior MI, it will be a second-degree Mobitz type II which can rapidly deteriorate into a third-degree block. Patients with an anterior MI and block should have a temporary pacemaker. Unfortunately, temporary pacing does not increase the survival rate in this group of patients.[5,6,7] An inferior MI tends to be associated with a second-degree Mobitz I block or Wenckebach phenomenon. Patients with this condition usually do not develop a third-degree block and many times do not require temporary pacing.[5,6,7] Other indications for temporary pacing include very slow

ventricular rates secondary to drug toxicity and a history of multiple episodes of supraventricular tachycardia.

Some controversy surrounds the indications for temporary pacing in the perioperative period. Certainly if a patient with an acute MI and a high-degree block presents for emergency surgery, temporary pacing is indicated. This is true even if the patient has a Mobitz I second-degree block secondary to an inferior MI. Since both enflurane and halothane are known to slow conduction through the atrioventricular (AV) node, third-degree block could develop in these patients during anesthesia.[8,9] Questions arise concerning the patient with bifascicular block. This type of block occurs distal to the AV node. After exiting the AV node, the bundle of His divides into two branches, a left and a right bundle branch. The left bundle branch further divides into an anterior and a posterior fascicle. A block of two of the

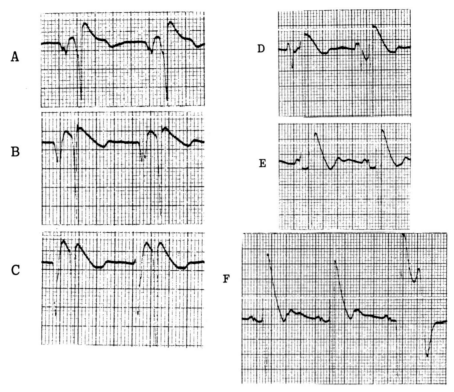

Fig. 17-8 Transvenous electrode progression from the atrium to the right ventricle. The electrodes were connected to the right arm and left leg leads of the ECG. (A) Both electrodes are in the superior vena cava near the right atrium. (B) One electrode has entered the atrium. (C) Both electrodes are in the right atrium. (D) One electrode is in the atrium and one electrode in the ventricle. Notice that the ST segment is beginning to elevate. (E) Both electrodes have just entered the ventricle. (F) The third QRS complex in F demonstrates that the electrodes have just contacted the myocardium. Notice the elevated ST segment.

three main branches of the bundle of His is called a *bifascicular block*. The clinical implication is that since only one fascicle remains to conduct impulses to the ventricle, blockage of this remaining fascicle will cause third-degree heart block. Recent evidence shows that bifascicular block will not deteriorate into a third-degree block during anesthesia.[10]

Another class of patients, who have not been adequately studied, are those with bifascicular block plus a first-degree block. As previously stated, enflurane and halothane are associated with atrial conduction disturbances, and halothane is associated with decreased conduction velocity in the ventricle.

When patients with bifascicular block and first-degree block must undergo major vascular surgery with major fluid and electrolyte shifts, the use of enflurane and halothane is in question. The important point here is that each patient should be eveluted as an individual in relation to the type of surgery, the anesthetic management, and the type of conduction disturbance. It must be remembered that ventricular electrodes are easily positioned if the patient has blood flow through the ventricle, but they are extremely difficult to position during cardiopulmonary resuscitation. Whenever possible, the electrode should be inserted under controlled conditions before surgery. Table 17-3 offers some suggestions concerning the problem of temporary pacing in the patient with bifascicular block.

Patients who require pacemaker implantation and who at the time of induction of anesthesia are not in second- or third-degree block do not need a temporary electrode.

Temporary pacing can also be used to terminate tachyarrhythmias.[11] Type I atrial flutter (regular atrial mechanism with a rate of 250 to 350 beats per minute) is easily converted to sinus rhythm by rapid atrial pacing.

Table 17-3
Bifascicular Block

A. Without First-Degree block
   1. Without symptoms: pacemaker not indicated specifically for anesthesia.
   2. With symptoms: cardiology evaluation suggested for possible permanent implantation. If the consultant states that a permanent pacemaker is not indicated, then it is suggested that the anesthesiologists have a transvenous electrode and external generator immediately available.
B. With First-Degree block
   1. Without symptoms: temporary pacemaker insertions strongly suggested for major vascular or extended surgery associated with large volume shifts and electrolyte changes.
   2. With symptoms: permanent pacemaker implantation is indicated.

Ventricular tachycardia is another tachyarrhythmia that can be converted to a sinus mechanism (Fig. 17-9).

THE DIALS

Many different types of pacemakers are available. Despite this fact, the controls look very much the same. The basic external generator is shown in Fig. 17-10. The connectors are located at the top of the pacemaker. A unipolar circuit, commonly used after cardiac surgery, should have the negative electrode placed on the heart and the positive electrode in subcutaneous tissue. Temporary transvenous leads are bipolar (Fig. 17-6). In the bipolar circuit, it does not matter which electrode is connected to the negative electrode.

All external generators will have the following controls:

1. ON-OFF switch
2. Rate control
3. Current output
4. R-wave sensitivity

The on-off switch has a mechanism to prevent turning off the pacemaker. This mechanism varies with the manufacturer. The rate control generally has a maximum of 180

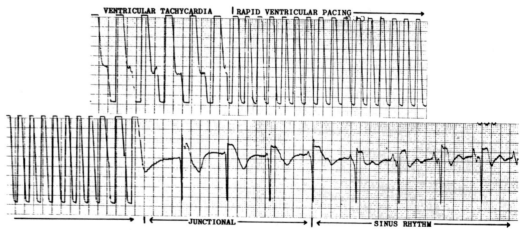

Fig. 17-9 A patient with ventricular tachycardia was converted to sinus rhythm by rapid ventricular pacing.

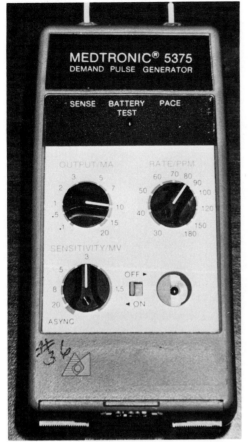

Fig. 17-10 This figure demonstrates a simple external pacing generator. The "sensitivity/MV" dial controls the number of millivolts necessary to turn off the generator. A low number, such as 3 mV, will permit the generator to be inhibited by an R wave of 3 mV or greater. This is a very sensitive setting and would correspond to a VVI pacemaker. Turning the dial to "asynch" makes the generator insensitive to all incoming R waves and corresponds to a VOO pacemaker.

pulses per minute. The rapid atrial pacer, however, has a maximum rate of 800 pulses per minute (Fig. 17-11). The current output is the number of milliamperes in each impulse emitted by the generator. R-wave sensitivity is an important control. It indicates the number of millivolts required to inhibit the external generator. When the dial is set on a very high number, the pacemaker is VOO; however, a low number converts the

generator to a VVI. The rapid atrial pacing generator is asynchronous.

The sequential pacer (Figs. 17-12 and 17-13) sends separate impulses first to the atrium and then to the ventricle. Each external sequential generator will have two sets of connectors, as well as controls that manipulate the atrial and ventricular current outputs and the PR interval. The atrial and ventricular outputs should be set at the threshold plus about 2 to 3 milliamps. The PR or AV interval control adjusts the time interval between the two impulses and is discussed more fully under Cardiovascular Effects of Pacing. A PR interval of 175 msec is a reasonable starting point.

ANESTHETIC MANAGEMENT

Anesthesia for the Patient with a Permanent Pacemaker

One basic idea must be kept in mind concerning the patient with a pacemaker: The pacemaker is not the problem—the underlying disease is the real problem.

PREOPERATIVE PATIENT EVALUATION

The patient's history should be obtained and physical examination performed. These patients have a high incidence of coronary artery disease, peripheral vascular disease, hypertension, and diabetes.[7] Some of the medications that might be encountered are cardiac glycosides, antiarrhythmics, beta blockers, diuretics, antihypertensives, and anticoagulants. Lab work should include hemoglobin, electrolytes, ECG, and a chest radiograph to provide the following information:

Hemoglobin: Is it adequate?
Electrolytes: Is the serum K^+ normal?
ECG: Is the pacemaker impulse present?
Chest radiograph: Is the lead intact?

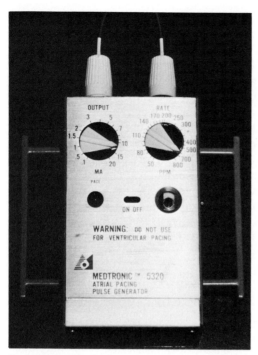

Fig. 17-11 Shown here is a rapid atrial pacer used to terminate atrial tachyarrhythmias. Notice the rate can be increased to 800 pulses per minute.

PREOPERATIVE PACEMAKER EVALUATION

A small FM radio is placed over the generator. If the radio is tuned to a location between stations, each pacemaker impulse will be heard as a loud tick on the radio. The patient's pulse is then palpated. Each tick should correspond to a pulse. Likewise, each paced beat on an ECG should correspond to a pulse. If the pacemaker is a VVI unit and the patient's heart rate is more rapid than the pacemaker rate, then impulses should be absent from the radio and the ECG. If this is the case, then a magnet should be placed over the generator. Impulses should now be heard over the radio. The peripheral pulse, however, will become irregular because competition has developed between the patient's heart rate and the pacemaker's output. A Valsalva maneuver sometimes will slow the heart rate enough to permit activation of

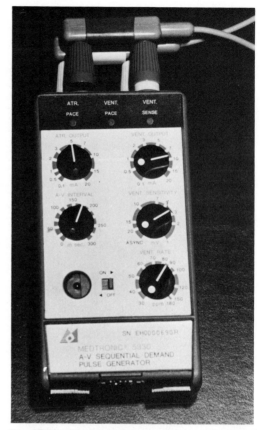

Fig. 17-12 This generator is a DVI or sequential pacemaker. Atrial and ventricular outputs are individually controlled. The "A-V interval" control dial determines the number of milliseconds between the atrial and ventricular pacing impulses and in this example is set to 175 msec. The sensitivity dial is the same as that explained for Figure 17-10.

the VVI pacemaker. Carotid massage, while not definitely contraindicated, should be used only with extreme caution because it might compromise cerebral blood flow.

MONITORING

Patients with a permanent pacemaker do not necessarily require complicated monitoring. Many times, a blood pressure cuff and an ECG are adequate. Decisions concerning central venous pressure and pulmo-

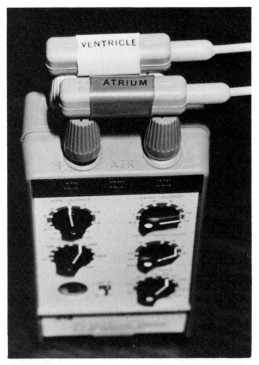

Fig. 17-13 This generator is the same one shown in Figure 17-12 and demonstrates the connections from the patient.

nary artery catheterization should be made in relation to the patient's underlying disease. If the patient has an endocardial electrode, the possibility of electrode dislodgement should be weighed against the information gained from the pulmonary artery catheter. An epicardial (myocardial) electrode will not be dislodged by a pulmonary artery catheter. The presence of a pacemaker should not be the only reason for inserting a pulmonary artery catheter.

Monitoring of intraoperative arterial blood gases and electrolytes is important to ensure adequate oxygenation and ventilation and normal serum potassium.

ANESTHETIC DRUGS

Induction. Thiopental, diazepam, and ketamine have all been used safely in patients with permanent pacemakers.

Muscle Relaxants. The administration of a nondepolarizing muscle relaxant apparently does not result in acute changes in pacing threshold or R-wave sensitivity. The depolarizing relaxants, however, can potentially cause a clinical problem. The VVI can be inhibited by myopotentials, especially in a unipolar circuit.[12] A patient who experiences lightheadedness or dizziness when exercising muscles in the area of the generator raises this possibility. Inhibition of the generator during the period of fasciculation results in cerebral and myocardial ischemia during that period of time. This problem can be eliminated by using nondepolarizing relaxants for intubation or for defasciculation. If inhibition occurs, the magnet must be applied to the generator to convert the VVI to a VOO pacer. The magnet can be removed after the fasciculations are over. The VOO is not inhibited by myopotentials.

Inhalational Agents. Recent information suggests that neither enflurane nor isoflurane alters pacemaker thresholds or R-wave sensitivities.[13,14] The clinical impression is that these drugs are reasonable anesthetics in patients with permanent pacemakers.

Anesthesia for Pacemaker Insertion

ENDOCARDIAL

Local anesthesia with monitoring is adequate for a transvenous electrode insertion. Monitoring should include a blood pressure cuff and an ECG with a recorder. A hand on a peripheral pulse is the best monitor. If the patient has a temporary pacemaker, there must be access to the external generator.

EPICARDIAL

Although epicardial electrodes have been positioned through the subxiphoid approach under local anesthesia, the patients simply are not comfortable. General anesthesia has not resulted in mortality in any patient undergoing epicardial electrode placement at Emory University Hospital. If the patient is not in a third-degree block at the time of induction of anesthesia, then it is not necessary to insert a temporary electrode. A patient who has a third-degree block or extreme sinus bradycardia should have a temporary electrode inserted before the induction of anesthesia. Once again, the monitoring should be adapted to the patient's underlying disease.

DEFIBRILLATING THE PACEMAKER PATIENT

Manufacturers of pacemakers include within the generator circuits which offer protection from large surges of current. An important example of this type of current is defibrillation. More protection is afforded the pacemaker by following the correct defibrillation procedures.[15]

An imaginary line is drawn between the generator and the electrode, and the defibrillator paddles are placed perpendicular to this line. This placement usually results in one paddle in the middle of the back and the other paddle directly over the heart on the anterior chest wall (Fig. 17-14A and B). The paddles should be at least several inches away from the generator. The lowest energy necessary to defibrillate the patient should be used. After defibrillation, the ECG is observed and the carotid pulse palpated to evaluate for effective cardiac output. If pacing does not occur and the patient has no ventricular escape mechanism, basic cardiopulmonary resuscitation must be continued. One of several courses of action is possible at this point. A percutaneous myocardial electrode can be inserted through the subxiphoid route. This is probably the quickest method of inserting an electrode in an extreme emergency. If the percutaneous electrode is una-

vailable, then opening the pacemaker pocket and disconnecting the generator from the lead may be considered. This lead is reconnected to an external generator. The easiest way to do this is to use a cable with sterile alligator clips. One alligator clip is attached to subcutaneous tissue and the other clip to the lead. If the lead is bipolar, either the proximal or distal electrode can be used. The other end of the cable is connected to the external generator and pacing is begun. If pacing still does not occur, then opening the chest and applying the electrodes directly to the heart becomes a possibility. Opening the chest is the last choice.

If the patient has a very slow venticular rate, then there might be time to insert a transvenous electrode as described in another section. In this situation drug therapy is appropriate. Intravenous atropine, 1 to 2 mg, can be tried. Isoproterenol, 2 mg in 250 ml of D_5W infused through microdrop intravenous tubing, should be given at a rate of about 1 to 4 μg/min.

PACEMAKER FAILURE IN THE OPERATING ROOM

A pacemaker that is functioning properly during the preoperative evaluation should continue to work trouble-free throughout the perioperative period. Several situations could occur during anesthesia, however, that would cause improper pacemaker function.

Depolarizing Muscle Relaxants. As discussed above, muscle fasciculations caused by succinylcholine can sometimes inhibit the pacemaker. This inhibition will persist until the fasciculations subside.

Potassium Balance. Potassium is important because it is the ratio of the concentration of K^+ inside the cell to the concentration outside the cell that determines the resting membrane potential (RMP). The

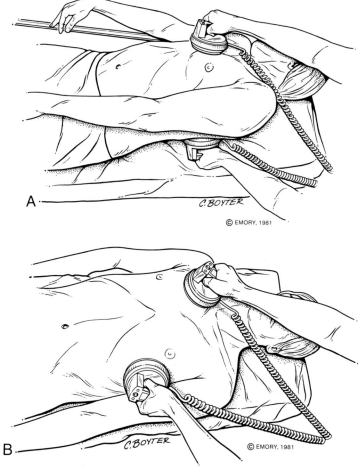

Fig. 17-14 (A) Correct positioning of the defibrillator paddles in a patient with a permanent pacemaker is shown. (B) Placement of the defibrillator paddles as recommended by the American Heart Association is shown here.

RMP is described by the Nernst equation: EMF = $-62 \log [K^+_I]/[K^+_o]$, where EMF is electromotive force or resting membrane potential, $[K^+_I]$ is potassium concentration inside the cell, and $[K^+_o]$ is potassium concentration outside the cell. The ratio $[K^+_I]/[K^+_o]$ is normally about (150 mEq/L)/(5 mEq/L), or 30:1, resulting in an RMP of -90 mV. If this ratio increases, the RMP becomes more negative and therefore more distant from the threshold potential. This is called *hyperpolarization.*

It is more difficult for the pacemaker to depolarize the membrane if that membrane is hyperpolarized. The causes of an acute increase in the $[K^+_I]/[K^+_o]$ ratio are increased $[K^+_I]$ and decreased $[K^+_o]$. This situation occurs clinically in the presence of acute respiratory alkalosis. To illustrate an extreme example, if $[K^+_o]$ suddenly became 1 mEq/L, the ratio would be 150. Calculating the negative logarithm, the RMP becomes -135 mV. A current output that would stimulate the myocardium to contract at an RMP of -90 mV might cause inadequate stimulation if the RMP is -135 mV. A pacemaker

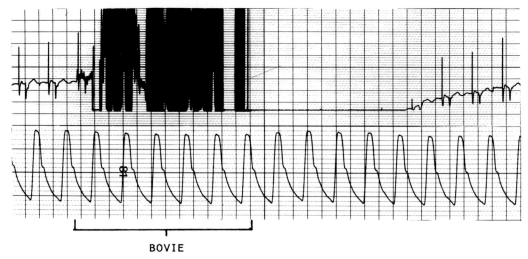

BOVIE

Fig. 17-15 The Medtronic 5330 DVI external generator is not inhibited by the electrocautery. The top trace shows the typical response of the ECG to the cautery, while the bottom trace demonstrates the radial artery pressure tracing. Notice that the heart rate shown by the radial artery pressure tracing does not decrease during use of the cautery. This patient had an intrinsic ventricular rate of 40 beats per minute.

that was previously functioning properly will begin miscapturing. To correct this problem, the PaCO$_2$ should be increased by adjusting the ventilation. Careful monitoring of ventilation with arterial blood gases to ensure maintenance of a normal pH and PaCO$_2$ becomes very important in the patient with a pacemaker.

A sudden increase in $[K^+_o]$ would decrease the ratio, leading to partial membrane depolarization. In this situation, it is easier for the pacemaker to stimulate the myocardium to contract. Clinically this occurs in acute acidosis, either respiratory or metabolic, in acute K^+ replacement, and during myocardial ischemia or infarction with secondary intracellular potassium loss. It is possible for the pacemaker impulse to cause ventricular tachycardia or fibrillation if the membrane is partially depolarized.

Drugs. Therapeutic doses of antiarrhythmics should not alter pacing thresholds, although toxic doses would be expected to cause pacing failure. Mineralocorticoids have been shown to increase the pacing

threshold, while glucocorticoids, ephedrine, and low doses of isoproterenol all decrease it.[16,17]

Electrocautery. The VVI can be inhibited if the surgeon touches the tissue with the electrocautery and then immediately withdraws it. The older VVI pacemakers simply turned off in the presence of an electrocautery. The newer VVI pacemakers, however, convert to VOO if the cautery remains on the tissue for a few seconds. A VOO pacemaker, either external or implanted, will not be inhibited by the electrocautery. The Medtronic 5330 DVI is not inhibited even when set on an R-wave sensitivity of 3 mV (Fig. 17-15).

Self-Inhibition. The atrial impulse from the DVI pacemaker can inhibit the ventricular pacing circuitry (Fig. 17-16). If the patient is in third-degree block and has no ventricular escape mechanism, the atrial impulse will stop all cardiac output. To eliminate this problem, the atrial output should be adjusted to the lowest setting necessary to achieve atrial pacing and the R-wave sensi-

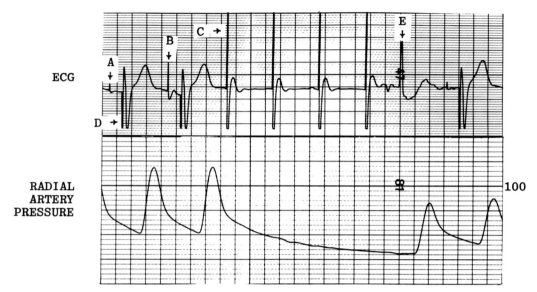

Fig. 17-16 The DVI can inhibit itself. A, B, and C are atrial pacing impulses of increasing current with C having a current of 20 mA. D is a ventricular pacing impulse and E is an escape beat. It is important to see that when the atrial output is high, the ventricular output is inhibited. In this patient the consequences of self-inhibition are obvious by observing the radial artery pressure tracing.

tivity then turned to a slightly higher number. If atrial pacing is lost with the lower atrial output but the higher output inhibits the ventricular pacing circuitry, then the R-wave sensitivity should be adjusted to "asynchronous" (Fig. 17-17). Now, however, this pacemaker will compete with the patient's own R waves, with the possibility of ventricular fibrillation or tachycardia.

VVI Acting as a VOO. This problem could be secondary to a failure in the electrode, lead, or generator and requires a full evaluation. It is possible that the switch that converts the VVI into VOO remained in the VOO position when the magnet was removed.[18] The magnet is placed on the generator and removed once again. Continued VOO pacing will probably require generator replacement. It is probably safe to proceed and change the generator during surgery.

Myocardial Infarction or Ischemia. If pacing is lost very suddenly, the possibility must always be considered that the electrode has been included in an infarcted or ischemic zone. The patient is treated symptomatically, and, if necessary, a new temporary endocardial electrode is inserted.

CARDIOVASCULAR EFFECTS OF PACING

A patient who is experiencing third-degree heart block with a very slow idioventricular rate will derive obvious benefit from ventricular pacing. A simple increase in heart rate will increase the cardiac output. Once the maximum cardiac output is reached, with ventricular pacing at a rate of about 75 to 90, atrial systole and its contribution to cardiac output must be considered.[19] Atrial systole has been found to contribute 10 to 30 percent of the cardiac output and therefore becomes important in patients with minimal cardiac reserve. Since atrial pacing is inappropriate in third-degree block, sequential pacing becomes the obvious choice. In a recent study involving patients with aortic stenosis, aortic insufficiency, and coronary artery disease, it was found that sequential pacing was associated with a higher

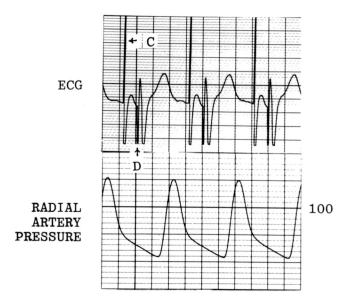

ECG

RADIAL
ARTERY
PRESSURE

100

Fig. 17-17 The situation is the same as described in Figure 17-16. C is a maximal atrial impulse and D is a ventricular impulse. The DVI sensitivity control has been changed to "asynch" so that the atrial output no longer inhibits the ventricular output.

cardiac index than ventricular pacing at the same rate.[20] Sequential pacing at very short PR intervals (e.g., 100 msec) began to look very much like ventricular pacing in terms of cardiac index. It is important to determine the appropriate PR interval for a given heart rate by adjusting the interval to achieve the highest cardiac output. Segel and Samet have made the following recommendations concerning the indications for sequential pacing:[19]

1. In patients with a slow heart rate and congestive heart failure or evidence of significant left ventricular disease, as defined by a very low cardiac output or stroke volume or a systolic ejection fraction of 0.3 or less
2. In patients who have undergone open heart surgery, especially coronary bypass, in the immediate postoperative period
3. In selected patients, for terminating reciprocating reentrant tachycardias.

The presence of an atrial pacing impulse does not guarantee atrial contraction. To ensure that the atrium is actually contracting, the ECG is observed for an atrial depolarization wave after each atrial pacing impulse (Fig. 17-18).

DYSRHYTHMIAS ASSOCIATED WITH PACEMAKERS

As would be expected, patients with pacemakers can have any dysrhythmia. Therefore, premature ventricular contractions and essentially all the atrial dysrhythmias may be seen. A few dysrhythmias are peculiar to the pacemaker and are described below.

Hysteresis. This "dysrhythmia" was described under definitions. The important point is that a pacemaker with hysteresis is functioning normally.

Fusion Beat. A fusion beat occurs when the ventricle is depolarized independently from two entirely different foci (Fig. 17-19).[17] The surface ECG will appear to be a combination of each depolarization. A pacemaker impulse can stimulate the ven-

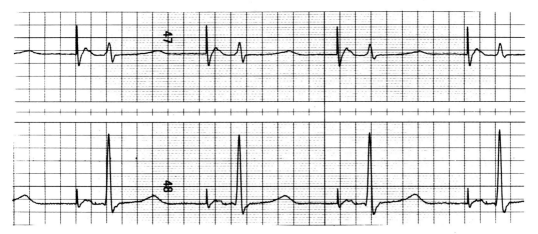

Fig. 17-18 The presence of an atrial pacing spike does not ensure atrial capture unless an atrial depolarization wave is observed on the ECG. Notice the small P wave that follows the atrial pacing spike.

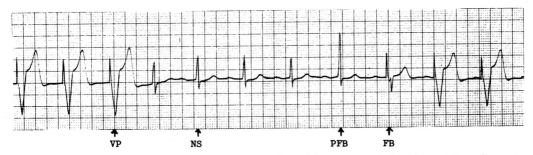

Fig. 17-19 Demonstrated here is normal VVI function with one normal sinus beat (NS) and one fusion beat (FB), one pseudofusion beat (PFB), and ventricular paced beats (VP).

tricle at the same time as the spontaneous depolarization. The surface ECG in this case will look like a combination of the paced beat and the normal beat. Fusion beats occur if the pacemaker rate is very slightly faster than the intrinsic rate. This is not abnormal pacemaker function. Fusion beats should disappear if the intrinsic rate changes.

Pseudofusion Beat. A pseudofusion beat occurs if the pacemaker rate and the intrinsic rate are exactly the same (Fig. 17-19).[17] The ECG will have a nonpaced QRS complex, with a pacing impulse on top of the R wave or in the RS segment. Pseudofusion beats, like fusion beats, are not abnormal and will disappear if the intrinsic rate changes. Ventricular pacing will resume if the intrinsic rate slows, and the pacing im-

pulse will disappear if the intrinsic rate increases. A VVI pacing impulse appearing immediately after the QRS complex is abnormal and implies loss of sensing.

DVI Pacing. It is easy to understand the DVI pacemaker by studying Figure 17-20 and remembering that intrinsic R waves inhibit both the atrial and the ventricular pacing circuits. An RR interval that is shorter than the atrial escape interval will appear as normal sinus rhythm (A). An RR interval that falls between the atrial and ventricular escape intervals will cause atrial pacing (B). Sequential pacing will occur if the RR interval is longer than the ventricular escape interval (C). The DVI pacemaker, then, will be associated with no pacing, atrial pacing, or sequential pacing, depending on the heart rate.

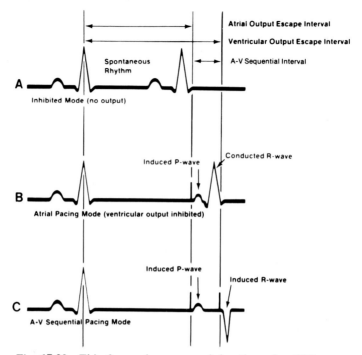

Fig. 17-20 This figure shows normal function of a DVI pacemaker. (With permission of Medtronic, Inc.)

REFERENCES

1. Irnick W, Parsonnet V, Myers G: Compendium of pacemaker terminology, II. Definitions and glossary (Part I). PACE 2 (1): 88-93, 1979

2. Parsonnet V, Furman S, Smyth NPO: Implantable cardiac pacemakers: status report and resource guideline. Circulation 50:A21-A34, 1974

3. Merz W, Jan J, Yoon M: Effects of unipolar cathodal and bipolar stimulation on vulnerability of ischemic ventricles to fibrillation. Am J Cardiol 35:37-41, 1975

4. Preston TA: Anodal stimulation as a cause of pacemaker induced ventricular fibrillation. Am Heart J 86:366-372, 1973

5. Norris RM: Heart block in posterior and anterior myocardial infarction. Br Heart J 31:352-356, 1969

6. Lown B, Kosowsky B: Artificial cardiac pacemakers. N Engl J Med 283:971-977, 1970

7. Furman S: Cardiac pacing and pacemakers. Indications for pacing bradyarrhythmias. Am Heart J 93:523-530, 1977

8. Atlee J, Rusy B: Halothane depression of AV conduction studied by electrograms of the bundle of His in dogs. Anesthesiology 36:112-118, 1972

9. Atlee J, Rusy B: Atrioventricular conduction times and atrioventricular nodal conductivity during enflurane anesthesia in dogs. Anesthesiology 47:498-503, 1977

10. Bellocci F, Santarelli, P, DiGennaro M et al: The risk of cardiac complications in surgical patients with bifascicular block—a clinical and electrophysiologic study in 98 patients. Chest 77:343-348, 1980

11. Waldo AL, Wells JL, Cooper TB et al: Temporary cardiac pacing: applications and techniques in the treatment of cardiac arrhythmias. Prog Cardiovasc Dis 23:451-474, 1981

12. Redd R, McAnulty J, Phillips S et al: Demand pacemaker inhibition by isometric skeletal muscle contractions. Circulation 49 and 50; suppl III, 957, 1974

13. Zaidan JR, Curling PE, Kaplan J.: Effect of enflurane on pacing thresholds. Anesthesiology: 55:A59, 1981

14. Zaidan JR, Curling PE, Kaplan JA: Effect of Enflurane, Isoflurane, and Halothane on Pacing Electrode Function. Presented at the Society of Cardiovascular Anesthesiologists Annual Meeting, May 1982

15. Alyward P, Blood R, Tonkin A: Complications of defibrillation with permanent pacemakers in site. PACE 2:462-464, 1979

16. Nevins M: Drug-pacemaker interactions. J Thorac Cardiovasc Surg 61:610-616, 1971

17. Preston T, Judge R: Alteration of pacemaker threshold by drug and physiologic factors.

Ann NY Acad Sci 167:687-692, 1969

18. Mond H, Sloman J: The malfunctioning pacemaker system. Part II. PACE 4:168-181, 1981

19. Segel N, Samet P: Physiologic aspects of cardiac pacing, pp. 111-148. In Samet P, El-Sherig N, Ed: Cardiac Pacing. Grune & Stratton, New York, 1980

20. Lonergan J, Zaidan J, Waller J, Kaplan J: Hemodynamics of pacing after aortic valve replacement. Anesth Analg 60:263–264, 1981

PART V.

POSTOPERATIVE INTENSIVE CARE

Joel A. Kaplan, M.D.

18
Complications of Thoracic Surgery

Every physician working in the fields of thoracic surgery and anesthesia must realize that even a well-performed surgical procedure can fail due to any one of a multitude of potential complications. These complications can occur intraoperatively or in the postoperative period. The anesthesiologist is most often concerned with complications of the cardiovascular, respiratory, or nervous systems. Table 18-1 is a list of potential complications in patients undergoing non-cardiac thoracic surgery and anesthesia. This chapter will cover a few of these complications in detail; many other complications are covered in the chapters specifically related to them (e.g., tracheostomy and tracheal reconstruction in Ch. 13).

THE LOW OUTPUT SYNDROME

The low cardiac output syndrome consists of hypotension, oliguria, mental obtundation, metabolic acidosis, arterial hypoxemia, and a low mixed venous oxygen tension. This syndrome is commonly seen in the preoperative, intraoperative and postop-

erative periods by anesthesiologists dealing with critically ill cardiovascular patients undergoing thoracic surgery.

Common causes of the low output syndrome are shown in Table 18-2. Cardiogenic shock or acute left ventricular failure is usually due to an acute myocardial infarction. Cardiogenic shock is present when the left ventricular output is insufficient to meet the demands of the body for its normal metabolism and function. This may be seen preoperatively in patients who have had a severe myocardial infarction with mechanical complications, such as a ruptured ventricular septum, or postoperatively in a patient with severe coronary artery disease who suffered an intraoperative myocardial infarction. In addition, right ventricular failure can be seen in patients with acute inferior wall myocardial infarctions, or severe pulmonary disease with cor pulmonale. The right ventricle is then unable to pump the necessary amount of blood needed by the left ventricle to meet the body's demands. Both left and right ventricular failure can also be chronic in nature, as seen with end-stage valvular heart disease. Hypoxemia and myocardial

599

ischemia occurring during thoracic surgery (especially with lung resection) can accentuate the degree of pre-existing cardiac failure to produce the low output syndrome in these patients postoperatively. Supraventric-

Table 18-1
Complications of Thoracic Surgery

I.	*Cardiovascular complications*
	1. Hypotension
	2. Low output syndrome
	3. Dysrhythmias
	4. Postoperative hypertension
	5. Myocardial ischemia and infarction
	6. Pacing problems (Chapter 17)
II.	*Pulmonary complications*
	1. Pulmonary emboli
	2. Bronchopleural Fistula (Chapters 10 and 21)
	3. Empyema and mediastinitis
	4. Pulmonary torsion
	5. Tracheostomy problems (Chapter 13)
	6. Diagnostic procedure complications (Chapter 9)
	7. Chest wall complications
	8. Pleural drainage (Chapter 19)
	9. Pulmonary hemorrhage (Chapter 7)
III.	*Related complications*
	1. Monitoring equipment (Chapter 6)
	2. Neurologic—central and peripheral

ular and ventricular dysrhythmias in the perioperative period can also produce inadequate cardiac output and a severe low output state. The great masquerader in the perioperative period is cardiac tamponade or constriction producing a low output syndrome that is frequently very difficult to diagnose. Other contributing factors to a low cardiac output in the perioperative period include inadequate blood volume, anemia, electrolyte imbalance (especially hypocalcemia and hypokalemia), and metabolic abnormalities such as hypoglycemia or hyperglycemia.

A balance must be maintained between total body tissue oxygen demands and oxygen supply, the latter being primarily determined by the cardiac output. The five factors shown in Table 18-3 determine the cardiac output. Fever, seizures, agitation, and/or excessive respiratory effort increase oxygen demand and hence pose additional demands on the already stressed heart for the delivery of a greater cardiac output. Tissue oxygen delivery is a function of the amount of blood pumped per minute and the amount of oxygen carried in that blood. The latter is, in

Table 18-2
Causes of the Low Output Syndrome

I.	Preoperative	
	A.	Acute myocardial infarction
		1. Cardiogenic shock
		2. Mechanical complications of acute myocardial infarction
	B.	End-stage valvular or coronary artery disease with chronic congestive heart failure
	C.	Poorly controlled congestive heart failure
	D.	Constrictive pericarditis
	E.	Cor Pulmonale
	F.	Trauma
II.	Intraoperative	
	A.	Acute myocardial infarction or ischemia
	B.	Acute dysrhythmias
	C.	Overdoses of depressant drugs
	D.	Hypoxia, acidosis
	E.	Cardiac compression by the thoracic surgeon
	F.	Hemorrhage
	G.	Pneumothorax or hemothorax
III.	Postoperative	
	A.	Acute myocardial infarction
	B.	Myocardial ischemia
	C.	Dysrhythmias
	D.	Cardiac tamponade

Table 18-3

Factors Determining Cardiac Output

I.	Heart rate
II.	Cardiac rhythm
III.	Preload (left and right ventricular filling pressures and volume)
IV.	Afterload
	A. Peripheral vascular resistance for left ventricle
	B. Pulmonary vascular resistance for right ventricle
V.	Myocardial contractility

turn, determined by the hemoglobin concentration, the oxygen saturation, and the position of the hemoglobin-dissociation curve (P_{50}). Since adequate delivery of oxygen to the tissues of the body is the goal of maintaining an adequate cardiac output, it is clear that factors increasing oxygen demand must be minimized, hemoglobin level should be maintained in a normal range, and hypoxemia of pulmonary or cardiac origin avoided.

In the past decade, much information has been obtained about the hemodynamics and biochemical mechanisms of ventricular failure.[1] Sonnenblick and others have looked at structural alterations in the hypertrophied and failing ventricle, which may be of functional importance.[2] Many investigators have studied the abnormal biochemistry in the failing myocardium, including alterations in cardiac muscle metabolism, excitation-contraction coupling, and the contractile process itself. Adenosine triphosphate (ATP) provides the energy for the operation of the contractile machinery and is produced in the mitochondria by oxidative phosphorylation of circulating free-fatty acids and glucose. Some evidence suggests that disturbances of mitochrondrial energy production may contribute to myocardial depression. Other studies have looked at the contractile apparatus itself, consisting of the actin and myosin molecular chains and the modulator proteins, troponin and tropomyosin, which inhibit the actin-myosin reaction. Alterations of the linkage of electrical excitation to mechanical contraction involving calcium and troponin

have been studied. In addition, some believe there may be alterations or abnormalities in the synthesis of some of the myocardial contractile proteins during myocardial ischemia. However, the underlying mechanism by which oxygen deprivation causes depression of the contractile function has yet to be fully clarified. Katz believes that intracellular acidosis, resulting from enhanced anaerobic glycolysis and accelerated lactate formation, may be involved in the abnormal mechanical function of the ischemic heart.[3] He postulates that hydrogen ions compete for calcium binding sites on troponin, thereby maintaining the heart in a state of relaxation. Finally, with depletion of ATP, contracture of the myocardium may develop. This may cause the characteristic disorder of cardiac function in ischemic heart disease; that is, abnormal segmental contraction or dyssynergy. Other investigators have found alterations in cardiac neurotransmitter activity in the failing heart.[1,2] Disturbed local metabolism of the neuron has been shown to lead to decreased norepinephrine stored in the failing heart. In addition to the above factors producing heart failure, concomitant adjustments take place in the peripheral vasculature that serve to support the blood pressure, but often at the expense of further cardiac deterioration. In low output syndromes, the peripheral vasculature usually constricts to increase peripheral resistance and maintain blood pressure; and at the same time, a redistribution of blood flow takes place toward the central life-supporting organs and away from less vital organs such as the kidneys.

Diagnosis of the Low Output Syndrome

CLINICAL SYMPTOMS

It has been customary to divide the symptoms of heart failure into those produced by left-sided failure and those produced by right-sided failure.[4] This clinical description has been useful but is not always physiologically correct, and in the anesthetized patient many of the following symptoms may be difficult to determine. Most types of heart disease primarily affect the left side of the heart. This is true of most patients with coronary artery disease and valvular heart disease. The output from the left atrium may be impeded by mitral stenosis; or the left ventricle may function abnormally as a result of coronary artery disease, primary myocardial disease, aortic or mitral valve disease, or systemic hypertension. Symptoms of left-sided heart failure include dyspnea on exertion, orthopnea and paroxysmal nocturnal dyspnea. Other patients with heart failure complain of cough, insomnia, or even Cheyne-Stokes respiration. In patients with Cheyne-Stokes respiration and heart failure, the pattern of breathing appears to be partially due to a prolonged lung-to-brain circulation time which disturbs the feedback mechanism regulating respiration. "Cardiac asthma," with wheezing due to bronchoconstriction secondary to interstitial pulmonary edema, is common in severe left-sided heart disease. All of these respiratory symptoms of heart failure may progress to the full-blown pattern of acute pulmonary edema. The circumstances surrounding an episode of acute pulmonary edema are varied. It can occur in patients with an acute myocardial infarction, valvular heart disease with volume overload, or in those with a high left atrial filling pressure and low colloid oncotic pressure. The patient is anxious, agitated, pale, and drenched with sweat; while the skin may be cyanotic, cold, or clammy. The respiratory rate is usually rapid and shallow, and the use of accessory muscles of respiration is prominent with large retractions of the intercostal and supraclavicular areas. There may be coughing, expiratory wheezing, and râles and rhonchi filling the chest. The sputum is usually profuse, frothy, watery and blood-tinged. The heart rate is usually rapid and the blood pressure may be elevated. However, in profound left ventricular failure with pulmonary edema, the systolic blood pressure may drop to very low levels.

Other symptoms of congestive heart failure include weight gain and edema formation, oliguria, ascites, and generalized weakness. All of these signs may progress to severe body wasting, called cardiac cachexia, which may occur in the very late stages of chronic, severe, biventricular failure. This multidimensional syndrome results in further myocardial cellular hypoxia. Closely related, and occurring perhaps as a result of oxygen lack, are a voluntary reduction of food intake and a relative or absolute degree of hypermetabolism. A greater reliance on anaerobic glycolysis occurs and prevents the more efficient oxidative utilization of the inadequate supply of nutrients. These patients develop abnormal proteins, and, therefore, abnormal synthesis of the necessary myocardial proteins for ventricular function. These adverse effects of malnutrition should not be forgotten (Chs. 5 and 14), and more attention to the preoperative nutritional status of the patient with chronic congestive heart failure may provide another approach to these patients who are prone to develop a postoperative low output syndrome.

PHYSICAL SIGNS

The physical signs of acute heart failure can be divided into those due to the effects of cardiac failure on other organs, and those present in the heart, arteries, and veins themselves. Physical signs due to the effects of cardiac failure on other organs include pulmonary râles, usually heard at the base of the lungs, and wheezing which is often present during early pulmonary edema. In more severe heart failure, pleural effusions and hydrothorax may be present on both sides, or, more commonly, only on the right side. Peripheral edema and hepatosplenomegaly with ascites appear as late signs of protracted heart failure.

The most classic sign of heart failure is the ventricular gallop sound, or third heart sound. This is the hallmark of either left or right ventricular failure. The sound occurs in early diastole and is associated with a period of rapid ventricular filling in a distended or noncompliant ventricle. A left ventricular gallop sound is best heard at the apex, and a right ventricular gallop sound over the right ventricle. An atrial gallop sound, or fourth heart sound, is not a specific indication of heart failure. It is often associated with a thick-walled ventricle and may be found in patients with hypertension or coronary artery disease who are not in failure. Intraoperatively and postoperatively, these extra heart sounds may be difficult to hear and interpret among the sounds of the ventilators and the chest tubes used for suction and drainage.

Examination of the arterial tracing on an oscilloscope may be useful in diagnosing acute left ventricular failure. *Pulsus alternans* is an early sign of left ventricular failure. This is an alteration in the amplitude of the arterial pulse tracing, despite a regular cardiac rhythm. It has been postulated that sustained pulsus alternans is due to alteration of the contractile state of at least part of the left ventricular myocardium. This may be due to failure of electromechanical coupling in some of the myocardial cells, or to variations in left ventricular filling volume. A premature ventricular contraction transiently accentuates pulsus alternans and makes it more obvious. Observation of the arterial tracing can also lead to the diagnosis of a *dicrotic pulse* in which there appear to be two peaks to the arterial tracing. Left ventricular failure may produce a decreased arterial pressure waveform, with a second accentuated diastolic wave that becomes visible. Reduced stroke volume, a shortened ejection period, or an elevated systemic vascular resistance are the most significant factors producing a dicrotic pulse. Elevation of the systemic vascular resistance appears especially important, since treatment with a vasodilator often returns the arterial tracing to normal. The upstroke of an arterial tracing obtained from the radial artery, or preferably from a more central artery, can also be used to clinically estimate the contractility (dp/dt) of the left ventricle. Good left ventricular contractility produces a sharp upstroke on the arterial tracing; while myocardial depression produces a slow, rounded arterial upstroke representing poor cardiac function.

Abnormalities of the neck veins are also frequently observed during left and right ventricular failure. The neck veins are distended when the patient is in heart failure, with prominent A and V waves and a rapid and deep Y-descent. An abnormal hepatojugular reflux test can also be observed. Observation of the venous pressure tracing on an oscilloscope can also be useful in diagnosing mitral or tricuspid valvular regurgitation (large V waves), a junctional rhythm (cannon waves), or cardiac tamponade.[5]

The diagnosis of cardiac tamponade can often be difficult to make and must be kept in mind, especially in trauma patients, in order not to be overlooked. The patient may be dyspneic, anxious, diaphoretic, ashen-colored or cyanotic, and complaining of chest pain.[6] Beck's triad is frequently present, consisting of (1) neck vein distention which increases with inspiration (Kussmaul's sign), (2) hypotension with a decreased pulse pressure, and (3) distant muffled heart tones. A pericardial friction rub may also be heard. The presence of a *pulsus paradoxus* is an important diagnostic sign of cardiac tamponade.[7] This is an *abnormal* inspiratory fall in the systolic blood pressure. The term is misleading, however, since it is not paradoxical but only an exaggeration of a normal physiologic phenomenon. Normally, the blood pressure during inspiration is 5 mmHg lower than on expiration. This is due to the transmission of intrathoracic pressure and the delay of the increased right-sided blood volume passing through the pulmonary circulation to the left side of the heart. However, any inspiratory decline of the systolic blood pressure by more than 10 mmHg is abnormal, and it is frequently over 20 mmHg in cardiac tamponade. Massumi reported a *paradoxical* pulsus paradoxus, that is the reverse of the usual situation—a rise of the blood pressure on inspiration.[8] This may be seen with left-sided heart failure during positive pressure ventilation, or with isorhythmic ventricular rhythms.

MEASUREMENTS OF THE LOW OUTPUT SYNDROME

In the postoperative period, advanced hemodynamic measurements are used to make the definitive diagnosis of left or right ventricular failure and the low output syndrome. Information is obtained from arterial and venous pressure tracings, as discussed above, and from arterial and venous blood gases. However, the key monitor is the thermodilution pulmonary artery catheter (PAC) which is used to obtain both left and right ventricular filling pressures, pulmonary artery pressures, cardiac output, and the derived parameters of cardiac index, stroke volume, stroke index, left ventricular stroke work index, right ventricular stroke work index, pulmonary vascular resistance, and systemic vascular resistance.[5] From these values, the Frank-Starling curve can be drawn and used in the clinical setting. Insertion of a pulmonary artery catheter is indi-

cated in any thoracic surgical patient in whom the diagnosis of heart failure or the low output syndrome is being entertained. It should be appreciated that the information obtained from the pulmonary artery catheter cannot be accurately obtained by the usual clinical measures. The "old, reliable clinical signs" of cold and blue peripheral extremities, kneecaps, and noses, decreased urine output, and abnormal blood gases do not always correlate with accurately measured cardiac output values. In fact, the cardiac output may be normal, but abnormalities of the peripheral circulation can produce these signs. In other situations, the periphery may look normal while the cardiac output is dangerously low.

The clinically used Starling curve is demonstrated in Figure 18-1. The left ventricular stroke work index (LVSWI) is on the vertical axis and the pulmonary capillary wedge pressure (PCWP) on the horizontal axis. A normally positioned Starling curve is shown, as well as one from a patient with a severely depressed ventricle. On the vertical axis, the LVSWI can be replaced by the stroke volume, cardiac output, or blood pressure. On the horizontal axis, the PCWP

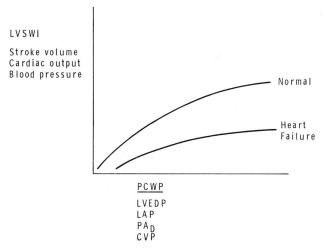

Fig. 18-1 The normal and heart failure Frank-Starling curves. The horizontal axis shows all the measures of preload commonly used, and the vertical axis shows the LVSWI and other values used as measures of cardiac performances.

can be replaced by the left ventricular end-diastolic pressure (LVEDP), left atrial pressure (LAP), pulmonary arterial diastolic pressure, or, occasionally, the central venous pressure (CVP). However, the CVP is by far the least accurate and may, in some cases, be totally misleading. It is important, however, to have both a left-sided measurement of filling pressure, such as the PCWP, and a right-sided measurement, such as the CVP, to be able to determine patients with right ventricular failure or cardiac tamponade.

The true left ventricular preload is the left ventricular end-diastolic *volume*. For clinical purposes, the LVEDP, LAP, or the PCWP are usually substituted. However, it is important to remember that this assumes that there is normal left ventricular *compliance*. In cardiac disease, it is not uncommon to have abnormal left ventricular compliance, where the pressure in the left ventricle as measured by the PCWP may not reflect the true left ventricular preload.[9] In hypertensive cardiac disease, or in patients with hypertrophied, stiff ventricles due to aortic stenosis, the compliance of the left ventricle is frequently decreased. This is a markedly different situation than the heart with chronic volume overload, such as mitral or aortic regurgitation, in which compliance is increased. In addition, it should be remembered that the right ventricle is far more compliant than the left ventricle. In a highly compliant ventricle, large changes in volume are underestimated by changes in ventricular filling pressure. Alternatively, small shifts in volume may be accompanied by large changes in ventricular filling pressures in very stiff ventricles. Thus, in patients with an abnormal ventricular compliance, the PCWP must be carefully interpreted in order to obtain correct information about the left ventricular preload.

Newer diagnostic modalities may occasionally be needed to make the correct diagnosis in patients with a low cardiac output syndrome in the postoperative period. Echocardiography can be used to help rule out the presence of a pericardial effusion and tamponade. Cardiac tamponade can also be diagnosed when a pressure plateau is demonstrated during insertion of a PAC; the right atrial pressure, right ventricular end-diastolic pressure, and pulmonary artery diastolic pressures are all equal.[10] Nuclear cardiology is only beginning to be explored in the intensive care unit. The use of cardiac scanning with radioisotopes and portable scanners is being initiated in some centers to evaluate myocardial contractility on a moment-to-moment basis. A fairly accurate right and left ventricular ejection fraction can be determined with these techniques, as well as the presence of cardiac constriction or valvular abnormalities. Response to therapeutic interventions can also be assessed by the radioisotope scans.

TREATMENT MODALITIES

Rational therapy of postoperative cardiac problems, such as the low output syndrome, depends on a clear understanding by the anesthesiologist or intensivist of the pertinent cardiovascular pathophysiology and pharmacology. Each of the five factors affecting cardiac output shown in Table 18-3 must be considered individually and normalized in order to optimize cardiac function. The pharmacologic and physiologic principles necessary for the use of vasoactive drugs in the setting of thoracic surgery and myocardial dysfunction will be described in detail. Drugs which increase myocardial contractility are called positive inotropic drugs; while drugs which increase systemic vascular resistance (SVR) and blood pressure are usually called vasopressors. However, these terms are frequently used loosely, and interchanged. The peripheral vasodilators decrease systemic vascular resistance, afterload, or left ventricular impedance to ejection.

Bradycardia can be treated pharmacologically or by atrial pacing when atrio-ven-

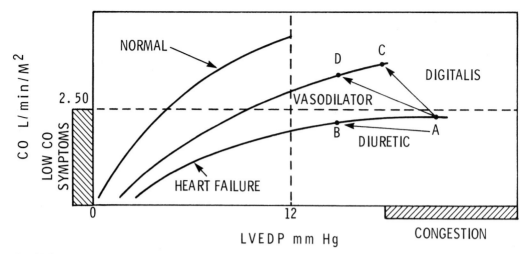

Fig. 18-2 The normal Frank-Starling curve is shown as well as a heart failure curve. Therapeutic interventions are made from point A to point B with the diuretic, point C with digitalis, or point D a vasodilator. Modified from Mason DT: Congestive Heart Failure: Mechanisms, Evaluation, and Treatment. With permission of Yorke Medical Books, Technical Publishing, a division of Dun-Donnelley Publishing Corporation, a Company of Dun & Bradstreet Corporation, 1976.

tricular conduction is intact. In the presence of complete heart block, heart rate can be controlled by atrio-ventricular sequential pacing with an appropriate P-R interval; or if sequential pacing capability is not available, by simple ventricular pacing. Ventricular pacing has the least beneficial effects on cardiac function since the "atrial kick" is lost. Sinus or junctional bradycardias may respond to atropine; while atrio-ventricular dissociation and other slow heart rates may respond to an infusion of isoproterenol.

Tachycardias are often more difficult to control than bradycardias. Treatment of the cause usually results in slowing of the heart rate, however. Ventricular tachycardia is a true emergency and should be immediately treated with lidocaine, in a bolus injection, followed by a constant infusion. If this is ineffective, propranolol, procainamide, or bretylium can be tried, but electrical cardioversion may be needed. The serum potassium level should be checked and restored to normal, if necessary. Supraventricular tachycardias of other than sinus origin may be quite difficult to control. Digitalis is the medication of choice in patients with both heart fail-

ure and dysrhythmias, when digitalis intoxication is not a suspected cause of the dysrhythmia. Propranolol or verapamil may be very useful in the management of some supraventricular tachyarrhythmias, even in patients with heart failure, if the rapid heart rate is contributing to the low cardiac output state by markedly reducing the effective stroke volume (see the section on dysrhythmias).

Therapeutic interventions for intra- or postoperative myocardial dysfunction (acute heart failure) include inotropic drugs, diuretics, and vasodilators, as demonstrated on the Frank-Starling curve in Figure 18-2. The inotropic drugs are represented by digitalis, calcium, and the catecholamines. These drugs move the patient from point A in heart failure toward point C on a higher Starling curve. Signs and symptoms of congestive heart failure are caused by elevated pulmonary and systemic venous pressures and a reduced cardiac output. Inotropic therapy is aimed at treating the elevated ventricular filling pressures and enhancing cardiac output. Conventional therapy in the past has also utilized diuretics to reduce preload (A →

B) in combination with the inotropic drugs. The newest therapeutic intervention is to combine an inotropic drug with a vasodilating drug which reduces left ventricular impedance (A → D).

Inotropic Drugs

A vast array of inotropic drugs can be used to restore the delicate balance of cardiovascular function in a patient with a low cardiac output. Prudent use of these cardiovascular drugs in the critically ill patient depends on a comprehensive knowledge of both their pharmacology and the pathophysiology on which the drug effects are to be superimposed. Used unwisely, these same drugs can further compromise cardiovascular function and survival of the patient.

CARDIAC GLYCOSIDES

Digitalis glycoside preparations are the classic inotropic drugs for the treatment of congestive heart failure.[11] There are a number of digitalis derivatives that share the same pharmacologic actions and differ primarily in terms of potency and pharmacokinetics. These are shown in Table 18-4. The two most likely digitalis preparations to be administered in the postoperative period are digoxin and ouabain. Ouabain is administered only by the intravenous route and has the most rapid onset and shortest duration of action among the cardiac glycosides. Digoxin is slightly slower in onset and somewhat longer-lasting than ouabain, but it has the advantage of being effective after either intravenous or oral administration. The major problem with these drugs is the extremely narrow margin between doses which produce beneficial inotropic effects and those which cause toxicity.

The mechanism of the inotropic action of digitalis has not been fully defined. Digitalis preparations act directly on the myocardial cell membrane and do not depend on the autonomic nervous system to increase contractility. It appears that they increase the availability of ionized calcium to the contractile elements at the time of excitation and coupling. There is a close correlation between the inhibition of sodium-potassium-ATPase by digitalis and its inotropic actions, but the fundamental basis of this relationship is not well understood.

The cardiac effects of digitalis can be described on the Frank-Starling curve. By increasing contractility, digitalis shifts the entire Starling curve upward and to the left, such that for any given filling pressure there is an increased amount of work performed. Another way of looking at myocardial contractility is in terms of the force-velocity relationship; digitalis increases the velocity of shortening of the muscle fiber for any given load (force) imposed upon it. In most cases,

Table 18-4
Digitalis Preparations

Glycoside	Dose		Onset	Peak Effect	½ Life
	Digitalizing	Maintenance			
Digoxin (Lanoxin)	1–1.5 mg	0.125–.50 mg	30 min	1–2 hrs	36 hrs
Ouabain	0.3–.5 mg	—	5–10 min	½–2 hrs	21 hrs
Deslanoside (Cedilanid-D)	0.8 mg	—	10–30 min	1–2 hrs	33 hrs
Digitoxin	1.0 mg	0.1 mg	25–120 min	4–12 hrs	4–6 days

Smith TW: Digitalis glycosides (parts 1 to 4). N Engl J Med 289:945–952, 1010–1015, 1063–1072, 1125–1128, 1973

this effect is expressed as an increased rate of pressure development (dp/dt).

Digoxin produces a dose-related increase in myocardial contractility in both normal and failing hearts.[12] However, the overall hemodynamic effect of digitalis administered to the normal and failing heart is different, since the results from digitalis depend on the conditions existing when it is given, and on the non-cardiac actions and reflex effects induced by the drug. Digitalis acts on the central nervous system and directly on vascular smooth muscle to increase SVR. When it is administered, activation of baroreceptors minimize increases in blood pressure by withdrawing sympathetic tone and increasing vagal activity to the heart. The reduced heart rate offsets increased contractility and prevents any increase in cardiac output in the normal heart. In fact, in the normal heart, a rapidly administered digitalis preparation may lead to a large increase in peripheral resistance and hypertension. In contrast, in the patient with a failing heart, sympathetic nervous system activity is already high. Digitalis improves contractility and cardiac output and, as a result, reflex adjustments lead to a decrease in sympathetic activity and a fall in SVR and venous tone. Pooling of blood in venous capacitance vessels reduces central venous pressure and blood volume. The improved contractility and reduction of both preload and afterload lead to a lower ventricular diastolic volume and wall tension. Hence, the work of the heart is more efficient and oxygen consumption is reduced, while blood pressure is maintained and tissue perfusion improved.

Myocardial ischemia, resulting from coronary insufficiency, may be increased or decreased by digitalis, depending on the functional state of the left ventricle. Changes in oxygen consumption are the net result of opposing effects of digitalis: (1) increased contractility, and (2) decreased wall tension and heart rate. Wall tension is the most important of these factors in determining myocardial oxygen consumption. Mason has shown that in the normal heart digitalis causes an overall increase in myocardial oxygen consumption by increasing the contractile state.[12] However, in the failing heart with a high left ventricular wall tension, digitalis decreases myocardial oxygen consumption by decreasing left ventricular wall tension, in spite of the augmented contractile state of the myocardium. This same principle is true for all the inotropic drugs. If used in the non-failing heart, they will increase myocardial contractility and, therefore, myocardial oxygen consumption. In the failing heart, with an elevated heart rate and wall tension, they may decrease overall myocardial oxygen consumption by decreasing ventricular wall tension while augmenting cardiac function. These drugs can be especially effective if, at the same time that they decrease ventricular wall tension, they do not increase heart rate nor decrease the diastolic blood pressure.

CALCIUM CHLORIDE

Ionized calcium plays an important role in the electrophysiology of excitable membranes and in the contraction of all types of muscle. It is a crucial element of coupling membrane excitation to the contractile process in cardiac muscle. When the membrane depolarizes, ionized calcium is released from the sarcoplasmic reticulum into the cytoplasm where it complexes with troponin. Troponin joined with calcium no longer inhibits the interaction between actin and myosin and the muscle cell contracts. Calcium also plays a role in coupling secretion of neurotransmitters and hormones to excitation of the membranes of nerve endings and endocrine cells.

Ionized calcium exerts a strong influence on cardiac contractility. The intravenous injection of calcium chloride produces a positive inotropic response manifested by increases in stroke volume and in the velocity of ventricular pressure rise (dp/dt). These changes are accompanied by a decrease in left ventricular end-diastolic pressure, and usually an increase in SVR. The hemodynamic effects of intravenous calcium chloride are transient, lasting only about 10 to 15 minutes as a result of the efficient uptake of calcium by bone. On the other hand, acute reductions of ionized calcium, for example, by the administration of citrated blood, are associated with decreased stroke volume and cardiac function.[13]

Bolus doses of 3 to 7 mg/kg of calcium chloride produce a moderate increase in cardiac output and stroke volume for 10 to 15 minutes.[14] Heart rate may slow due to a vagotonic effect of calcium. Additional doses can be given to maintain the effect for longer periods, but other inotropic drugs, such as digitalis or the catecholamines, are usually given instead. The risk of potentiating digitalis-induced dysrhythmias should always be kept in mind when administering calcium to the digitalized patient.[15]

SYMPATHOMIMETICS

Sympathomimetic drugs include many naturally occurring (epinephrine, norepinephrine, dopamine) and synthetic compounds (isoproterenol, dobutamine).[16] There are a number of important differences among these drugs including their chemistry (catecholamine versus non-catecholamine), potency, efficacy, mechanism of action (direct versus indirect), relative potency on different types of adrenergic receptors (alpha versus beta), and on the same type of receptor in different tissues (beta$_1$ versus beta$_2$). Representative examples of the spectrum of sympathomimetic drugs (inotropes and vasopressors) are given in Table 18-5.[5]

Epinephrine (adrenalin) is the prototype drug among the sympathomimetics. Systemic administration of epinephrine is indicated in the therapy of severe cardiac failure and profound hypotension. Its cardiovascu-

Table 18-5
Sympathomimetics

Drug	Dosage		Site of Action		Mechanism of Action
	Intravenous	Infusion	α	β	
Phenylephrine (Neo-Synephrine)	50–100 μg	10 mg/500 ml 20 μg/ml 10–50 μg/min	++++	+	Direct
Norepinephrine (Levarterenol	—	8 mg/500 ml 16 μg/ml 2–16 μg/min	++++	+++	Direct
Epinephrine (Adrenalin)	2–8 μg	4 mg/500 ml 8 μg/ml 2–10 μg/min	+++	+++	Direct
Ephedrine	5–25 mg	—	+	++	Direct & indirect
Dopamine (Intropin)	—	400 mg/500 ml 800 μg/ml 2–15 μg/kg/min	++	+++	Direct
Dobutamine (Dobutrex)	—	250 mg/500 ml 500 μg/ml 2–20 μg/kg/min	+	++++	Direct
Isoproterenol (Isuprel)	1–4 μg	2 mg/500 ml 4 μg/ml 1–5 μg/min		++++	Direct

lar effects result from direct stimulation of both alpha- and beta-adrenergic receptors. Stimulation of cardiac $beta_1$-adrenergic receptors results in an increased heart rate and force of contraction. Very small doses primarily activate $beta_2$-adrenergic receptors in the vasculature and lungs. Moderate-to-large doses stimulate alpha, and $beta_1$-and $beta_2$-receptors, with the effects of alpha receptor stimulation predominating in most vascular beds. The vasculature is constricted in the skin and the kidneys, and dilated in skeletal muscle and splanchnic beds. Intravenous bolus doses of 2 to 8 μg can provide a rapid, though transient, stimulation of cardiac function. A sustained positive inotropic effect can be achieved by continuous infusions of 2 to 10 μg/min in the average 70 kg adult.

There are a number of side effects that can limit the usefulness of epinephrine as an inotropic drug, especially at higher doses. The development of ventricular dysrhythmias may interfere with cardiac output and limit the benefits from its inotropic effect. Supraventricular tachyarrhythmias are less common but more difficult to manage, frequently requiring digitalization to control the heart rate. Large alpha-adrenergic constricting doses of epinephrine, when continued for prolonged periods of time (over 12-24 hours), can significantly impair renal blood flow and renal function and may produce irreversible renal failure. Similarly, vasoconstriction produced when epinephrine is used in large doses can limit blood flow to other tissues and lead to the accumulation of an oxygen deficit and metabolic acidosis. The simultaneous infusion of a vasodilator to produce systemic vasodilatation can be of benefit in improving cardiac output, limiting myocardial oxygen consumption, reducing SVR, and restoring perfusion to the kidneys and other tissues. In fact, in the severely ill patient, the combination of epinephrine and a vasodilator, such as sodium nitroprusside, is one of the most effective therapeutic modalities. This drug combination is administered to obtain the inotropic effect from epi-

nephrine, while reducing the SVR to low normal values with nitroprusside (see below).

Epinephrine is also the principal drug employed in the restoration of cardiac rate and contractility following a cardiac arrest.[17] In this situation, intravenous bolus doses of 0.5 to 1 mg may be used to initiate spontaneous cardiac action or to convert fine ventricular fibrillation to a coarse pattern which is more easily defibrillated. In such circumstances, the alpha-adrenergic activity is extremely important, since the primary objective is to restore blood pressure needed for cerebral and coronary perfusion. Once that is accomplished, the long-term management of the patient should also take the survival and function of other vital organs into account.

Norepinephrine (Levarterenol, Levophed) is the principal chemical transmitter released from peripheral adrenergic nerve endings.[18] Norepinephrine is a less potent stimulant of beta-adrenergic receptors on vascular smooth muscle than is epinephrine. It, therefore, tends to produce arteriolar constriction in all vascular beds and relatively greater increases in SVR than does epinephrine. The peripheral vasoconstriction and hypertension resulting from norepinephrine may lead to baroreceptor activation and reflex slowing of the heart rate. In these situations, norepinephrine may not increase cardiac output, but actually decrease it. However, norepinephrine is a potent cardiac stimulant when its direct actions are not overshadowed by baroreceptor reflex activation. It can be an extremely useful drug in the patient who is markedly vasodilated, possibly due to an anaphylactic reaction or sepsis. It should be administered at low dose to maintain a reasonably normal mean arterial blood pressure and to keep SVR in a low-normal range.

Isoproterenol (Isuprel) is a synthetic and highly specific stimulant of beta-adrenergic receptors, but has no significant effect on alpha-receptors. It is the most potent cardiac stimulant of all the catecholamines.[19] It increases heart rate, automaticity, and contractility, but the net increase in cardiac output may be limited by impairment of cardiac filling, rate and rhythm changes, or decreased venous return to the heart. It dilates all vascular smooth muscle to produce marked reductions in systemic vascular resistance and increased venous capacitance.

Isoproterenol has been shown to be potentially deleterious in patients with coronary artery disease, since it produces tachycardia (increased oxygen demand) and diastolic hypotension (decreased oxygen supply), adversely affecting the myocardial oxygen balance. In addition, some investigators feel that it may cause an intracoronary steal of blood away from ischemic areas of the myocardium.

Isoproterenol is useful in the treatment of complete heart block, valvular heart disease, congenital heart disease, and significant beta-adrenergic receptor blockade. It is administered by intravenous infusion at rates of 1 to 10 µg/min in the average-sized adult. The infusion is usually begun at 1 to 2 µg/min and titrated to effect, or until severe tachyarrhythmias occur.

Dopamine (Intropin) is a chemical transmitter and an intermediate compound in the synthesis of norepinephrine and epinephrine. Specific dopaminergic receptors have been identified in the renal and mesenteric vascular beds and may also exist in the coronary circulation. These receptors are not affected by the usual alpha- and beta-adrenergic receptor blocking drugs, but are selectively blocked by butyrophenones, such as haloperidol, and by phenothiazines, such as chlorpromazine. Dopamine's interaction with these receptors results in vasodilatation of the mesenteric and renal arterioles. In the kidney, dopamine is unique among sympathomimetic drugs in producing a natriuretic effect, possibly as a result of an action on renal tubular cells in addition to its effect of increasing renal blood flow. Dopamine also acts directly on alpha- and beta-adrenergic receptors and can release norepinephrine from nerve terminals.[20]

The major advantage of dopamine, besides its renal effect, is the dose-response relationship apparent in the clinical situation. This is shown in Table 18-6. At low dose, it primarily stimulates dopaminergic receptors with some stimulation of the beta-receptors. In the medium dose range, there is continued stimulation of the dopaminergic receptors with more beta-stimulation and some alpha-stimulation. At high dose, the dopaminergic effect is lost; while there is still beta-stimulation, and a predominance of alpha-stimulation. The dopaminergic effects seen at low and medium doses are major advantages over some of the other drugs, such as epinephrine and norepinephrine, which decrease renal blood flow and urine output. However, at higher doses, dopamine loses these advantages and is essentially the same as norepinephrine.

Dopamine is the most commonly used catecholamine in the postoperative surgical patient, even though it is a less potent car-

Table 18-6
Dopamine

	Dosage (µg/kg/minute)		
	Low	Medium	High
	(2–5)	(5–10)	(>10)
Cardiac output	↑	↑↑	↑↑
Contractility	↑	↑↑	↑↑
Heart rate	↑	↑↑	↑↑
Total peripheral resistance	↓↑	↑	↑↑
Renal blood flow	↑↑	↑	↓
Urine output	↑↑	↑	↓

diotonic drug than either isoproterenol or epinephrine.[21] If large doses are required or it appears to be ineffective, switching to the older, more potent inotropic drugs is indicated.[22] Rapidly increasing the dose of dopamine may lead to detrimental supraventricular tachyarrhythmias. The drug should only be infused through a central line, since infiltration or long-term infusion via a peripheral intravenous catheter can produce a skin-slough in a similar fashion to epinephrine.

Dobutamine (Dobutrex) is the newest catecholamine and is the direct result of specific pharmacologic manipulation of the catecholamine molecule in an effort to design a drug with strong beta-adrenergic activity, immediate onset of action, rapid inactivation, direct action not depending on the release of norepinephrine, minimal peripheral vasoconstriction due to alpha-adrenergic stimulation, little increase in cardiac automaticity, and no adverse redistribution of blood flow away from vital organs. Almost all of these goals have been attained in the development of dobutamine. Two manipulations were made in the basic catecholamine molecule to change it from norepinephrine to dobutamine. First, one hydroxyl group was changed to a hydrogen ion which converted the molecule into dopamine and eliminated some of the alpha-adrenergic stimulation of norepinephrine. This change also produced less chronotropy and less peripheral $beta_2$ stimulation. Next, a dobutyl group was placed on the end of the molecule, instead of an isopropyl group which is present on isoproterenol. This made it a direct-acting drug that had minimal $beta_2$ and alpha peripheral effects with predominant $beta_1$ effects. Thus, a drug was synthesized with almost pure $beta_1$-adrenergic properties, producing large increases in inotropy with less increase in chronotropy than isoproterenol. Its overall effect on SVR is moderate, such that only small increases in arterial blood pressure are observed.

Dobutamine has been used successfully in the therapy of low output syndromes associated with chronic congestive heart failure, myocardial infarction, and surgery.[23-25] Tinker has shown that at a 10 μg/kg/min dose, dobutamine increased mean arterial blood pressure about the same as 10 μg/kg/min of dopamine and somewhat less than 0.02 μg/kg/min of epinephrine.[26] Leier compared dopamine and dobutamine administered for 24 hours to patients with chronic low output syndromes.[27] Dobutamine was administered at 7 μg/kg/min and dopamine at 4 μg/kg/min. At these doses, dobutamine led to greater increases in cardiac index, stroke volume, non-invasive measurements of contractility, and limb blood flow while producing a greater decrease in pulmonary capillary wedge pressure and peripheral resistance. Studies at different doses of either dobutamine or dopamine could yield entirely different results.

NON-CATECHOLAMINE
SYMPATHOMIMETICS

There are a large number of synthetic drugs with sympathomimetic effects based on direct interactions with adrenergic receptors, release of norepinephrine from nerve terminals (indirect action), or a combination of direct and indirect interactions. Generally speaking, these drugs are much less potent than the catecholamines. Some of these drugs, like ephedrine, have significant beta-adrenergic receptor-stimulating properties and can be used in intravenous bolus doses for their cardiotonic effects. Others, such as norepinephrine, have primarily alpha effects and are used as vasopressors for the temporary treatment of hypotension resulting from hypovolemia or vasodilatation.

Diuretics

Furosemide (Lasix) and ethacrynic acid (Edecrin) are potent diuretics that act primarily in the ascending limb of Henle's loop to inhibit sodium reabsorption. Furosemide is usually preferred because it has a broader dose-response range and fewer side effects than ethacrynic acid. Patients vary in their sensitivity to these drugs. Graded responses can be produced by beginning with a small dose and giving progressively larger doses over 10- to 15-minute intervals until the desired response is obtained.

Recent studies have demonstrated that furosemide produces marked systemic venous dilatation prior to the onset of diuresis.[28,29] This rapid increase in venous capacitance and reduction in blood return to the central circulation may explain the almost immediate effects of this drug in the treatment of acute pulmonary edema. Within five minutes of an intravenous dose of furosemide, the average left ventricular filling pressure fell from 20.4 to 14.5 mmHg in one study of 20 patients.[28] The subsequent onset of diuresis further contributes to the reduction in circulating plasma volume and to the delayed resolution of radiologic evidence of pulmonary congestion. In a patient with severe ischemic heart disease and associated heart failure, both the acute and delayed mechanism of reducing left ventricular filling pressure may be beneficial in decreasing myocardial oxygen consumption.

Afterload or Impedance Reduction

The concept of pharmacologically-induced vasodilatation has gained a place in the therapy of inadequate hemodynamic function.[30] Vasodilators are now used for the treatment of refractory heart failure and myocardial ischemia (Table 18-7). There is substantial evidence that hemodynamic performance can be improved when ventricular unloading is achieved.

The mechanism of action of vasodilators in heart failure is fairly clear. Low output states are characterized by increased SVR secondary to increased sympathetic tone in order to support blood pressure in the face of a falling cardiac output. With the increased resistance and increased outflow impedance, left ventricular wall tension remains high during ejection, and stroke volume is decreased. The vasodilators decrease the outflow impedance and thus allow for an increased stroke volume, decreased left ventricular chamber size, and decreased left ventricular work. Indeed, the increase in stroke volume maintains the blood pressure in the face of a decreased SVR.

Studies have shown dramatic improvement in hemodynamics in patients with congestive heart failure using nitroprusside infusions at low doses (10-50 μg/min).[30-32] Cardiac output and renal function improve, SVR and pulmonary capillary wedge pressure decrease, and mean arterial blood pressure remains about the same. In the management of patients with severe low output syndromes and cardiogenic shock, nitroprusside has become a useful adjunct to add to inotropic drugs such as dopamine, dobutamine, or epinephrine. It is particularly indicated if the patient is markedly vasoconstricted and has a high pulmonary capillary wedge pressure.

Vasodilatation can be produced by many drugs with varied sites of action and with different mechanisms of action. All vasodilators do not have similar hemodynamic effects. Drugs that act primarily on the *venous capacitance bed* are represented by sublingual nitroglycerin, which will primarily decrease preload and left ventricular end-

Table 18-7
Indications for Vasodilator Therapy in Low Output Syndromes

1. Chronic intractable heart failure
2. Complicated acute myocardial infarction or ischemia
3. Mitral or aortic regurgitation
4. Postoperative heart failure
5. Intense peripheral vasoconstriction
6. Combined therapy with inotropes when total peripheral resistance is elevated
7. Pulmonary hypertension
8. Cor pulmonale

diastolic pressure. It has minimal effects on afterload and may, in fact, decrease cardiac output, as well as myocardial oxygen demand. Vasodilators with a primary effect on the *arterial bed* include phentolamine, phenoxybenzamine, hydralazine, droperidol, chlorpromazine, and diazoxide. These drugs decrease preload minimally, but markedly decrease afterload and increase cardiac output. The largest group of vasodilators are those which have *mixed actions* on both the arterial and venous vascular beds, including sodium nitroprusside, trimethaphan, intravenous nitroglycerin, prazosin, and combinations of long-acting nitrates with hydralazine. These drugs will decrease both preload and afterload, and when starting with a high left ventricular filling pressure, lead to an increase in cardiac output.

Nitroprusside (Nipride) is a non-selective vasodilator and affects all vascular beds. Therefore, venous capacitance is increased, preload is decreased, and systemic and pulmonary resistances are decreased, resulting in an increased cardiac output and decreased myocardial oxygen consumption. Nitroprusside is most effective in increasing cardiac output when administered in the presence of a markedly elevated left ventricular end-diastolic pressure. The nitroprusside-induced decline in SVR allows the lowered stroke volume to be augmented. However, if the left ventricular end-diastolic pressure is lowered below 12 mmHg, the stroke volume and cardiac output can be decreased by reducing the preload too much and placing the patient back on the ascending limb of the Starling curve. Thus, the most effective therapy is obtained by *afterload reduction* with nitroprusside, while at the same time *augmenting the preload* with a volume infusion to keep the left ventricular end-diastolic pressure in the 12 to 15 mmHg range.[31,32]

Phentolamine (Regitine) is an alpha-adrenergic-receptor blocker chemically related to tolazoline. In addition to alpha-adrenergic blockade, its potent vasodilating properties are also due to direct smooth-muscle relaxation. In addition, it causes cardiac stimulation exceeding that resulting from a reflex response to peripheral vasodilatation. The chronotropic response, which can be marked, may be the result of phentolamine-induced norepinephrine release from nerve endings with blocked re-uptake (alpha$_1$ and alpha$_2$ blockade), and has been associated with the development of dysrhythmias. In patients with severe ventricular dysfunction, phentolamine frequently leads to a decrease in mean arterial pressure and systemic vascular resistance, while stroke volume and heart rate are increased. In comparative studies with nitroprusside, phentolamine was found to have a greater effect on reducing afterload and a lesser effect on reducing preload.[33]

Nitroglycerin's (Tridil) principal action is direct relaxation of smooth muscle in the systemic venous system, thereby increasing the distensibility of the systemic venous capacitance bed. In addition, larger doses of nitroglycerin, when administered intravenously, produce moderate direct systemic arteriolar dilatation.[34] This latter effect can be used to decrease systemic blood pressure and SVR. The predominant venodilatation may decrease cardiac output in some situations. However, the drug may be useful in situations where poor left ventricular function is secondary to acute myocardial ischemia. By reducing left ventricular wall tension and maintaining diastolic coronary perfusion pressure, nitroglycerin may reduce myocardial ischemia, improve left ventricular function, and increase cardiac output.

THERAPY OF CARDIAC TAMPONADE

The treatment of cardiac tamponade is divided into two phases: (1) temporary measures, and (2) definitive treatment. Temporary measures include the following three steps:[5,6]

1. Intravascular blood volume should be expanded in order to increase the central venous pressure above 10 to 15 mmHg. The effective filling pressure of the heart is thereby increased, which opposes the elevated intrapericardial pressure. As the gradient of blood flow among the large veins, atrium, and the right ventricle is restored, stroke volume, pulse pressure, and systolic blood pressure are increased.

2. A positive inotropic drug should be used to augment the action of endogenous catecholamines. In a number of studies using dog models with cardiac tamponade, isoproterenol has been shown to be the most effective inotropic drug during tamponade.[5,6] In one study comparing isoproterenol to norepinephrine, isoproterenol doubled stroke volume, increased heart rate, tripled cardiac output, and dropped SVR by 50 percent while keeping the blood pressure constant. In contrast, norepinephrine increased the resistance and blood pressure by 20 mmHg, but had little effect on heart rate, stroke volume, and cardiac output. Digitalis has been shown not to be very effective in raising the cardiac output during tamponade, due to the large increase in SVR it causes when given intravenously. Studies of the new inotropic drugs, dobutamine and dopamine, have not been performed in patients with cardiac tamponade. However, the pharmacologic effects of these drugs should make them equally effective or more effective than isoproterenol. In studies comparing the effects of isoproterenol to volume infusion, it is apparent that isoproterenol causes an even greater increase in cardiac output than volume augmentation.

3. Metabolic acidosis should be corrected with sodium bicarbonate. It has been shown that catecholamines, especially epinephrine, are significantly less effective in acidotic states and that acidosis by itself further depresses myocardial function.

The definitive treatment of cardiac tamponade is drainage of the fluid. Pericardiocentesis is the treatment of choice for the routine management of a patient with non-traumatic tamponade. Dramatic improvement in blood pressure and cardiac output may occur with removal of as little as 25 ml of fluid. Surgical intervention is the therapy of choice for tamponade due to trauma, especially for penetrating wounds of the heart and great vessels, after surgery, and when fluid reaccumulates or cannot be removed by pericardiocentesis. In many instances, pericardiocentesis serves as a temporizing measure before surgical intervention. Sometimes it is possible to drain the pericardial fluid under local anesthesia prior to the induction of a general anesthetic for exploration of the mediastinum. This is certainly a preferable technique, in order to avoid the risks of anesthetizing a patient with cardiac tamponade.

POSTOPERATIVE DYSRHYTHMIAS

The thoracic surgical patient commonly has minor dysrhythmias during hospitalization, and major life-threatening dysrhythmias also occur during and after pulmonary operations. Patients undergoing pulmonary resection have postoperative supraventricular tachyarrhythmias with a frequency and severity proportional to both their age and the magnitude of the procedure. Optimal management includes anticipation, monitoring, and prompt therapy when appropriate.

Dysrhythmias that are considered significant perioperative problems include supraventricular tachycardias (paroxysmal atrial tachycardia, atrial flutter, atrial fibrillation, and premature atrial contractions); ventricular tachycardia or fibrillation; and conduction disturbances ranging from atrioventricular dissociation to complete heart block. Patients with advanced cardiac disease are most prone to develop cardiac dysrhythmias during or after thoracic surgical procedures. Many factors contribute to the etiology of these dysrhythmias, including underlying cardiac disease, degree of surgical trauma, effects of anesthetic and cardioactive drugs, and metabolic disorders affecting the blood gases and body chemistry.

Bertrand studied 100 patients, using continuous electromagnetic tape recording during surgery, and reported an 84 percent incidence of supraventricular and ventricular dysrhythmias.[35] Dysrhythmias were most common at the time of intubation and extubation of the trachea. Patients with pre-existing cardiac disease had a higher incidence of ventricular dysrhythmias (60% versus 37%) than patients without known heart disease. The dysrhythmias correlated with the severity of the heart disease, the length of the hospital stay, and were responsible for up to 80 percent of surgical mortality.[36]

Hypercarbia, hypocarbia, and hypoxia have all been shown to precipitate the development of dysrhythmias. Edwards showed that hyperventilation to a $PaCO_2$ of 30 or 20 mmHg (pH 7.51 and 7.61) lowered a normal serum potassium level (4.03 mEq/L) to 3.64 and 3.12 mEq/L, respectively.[37] If the serum and total body potassium start at lower levels, it is possible to decrease the serum potassium into the 2 mEq/L range by hyperventilation, and, therefore, precipitate severe cardiac dysrhythmias. Surgical trauma including retraction of the heart, hemorrhage, edema, and hypoxia certainly may contribute to postoperative cardiac dysrhythmias. Cardiac drugs such as digitalis and specific antiarrhythmic drugs may produce dysrhythmias on their own, as well as conduction disturbances.

Postoperative dysrhythmias may result from abnormalities of impulse formation (automaticity), impulse conduction (block, reentry), or both.[38] The cells of the sinoatrial node undergo a rapid spontaneous Phase 4 depolarization and are thus the pacemakers of the normal heart, while ventricular cells normally do not undergo spontaneous Phase 4 depolarization. If, however, the higher pacemaker cells do not fire, the lower cells will undergo slow spontaneous Phase 4 depolarization, taking over as the pacemakers. Factors which selectively decrease the rate of

Phase 4 depolarization of the higher pacemaker sites, while the lower cells are unaffected, favor the movement of the pacemaker to a lower area in the heart. In addition, factors that increase the spontaneous Phase 4 depolarization of a lower pacing site favor the takeover of these lower areas as the cardiac pacemaker. Factors tending to slow pacemaker sites above the atrioventricular (AV) node are vagal influences such as that produced by digitalis or parasympathomimetic drugs. Factors tending to enhance automatic pacemaker activity below the AV node are catecholamines, hypercarbia, hypoxia, and digitalis overdose. Increased automaticity is usually due to an increase in the slope of Phase 4 depolarization, but it may also be caused by an increase in the resting membrane potential or a decrease in the threshold potential.

Abnormal impulse conduction is the second major mechanism of dysrhythmia formation. With a localized abnormality of the conduction system, a reduction in impulse transmission can occur, leading to a form of blocked conduction. In addition, increased impulse transmission may occur when abnormal conduction circuits are formed. These abnormal circuits may be present anatomically (bundle of Kent), develop transiently secondary to various drugs (digitalis), or occur secondary to local tissue abnormalities (ischemia, hypoxia, acidosis) and can lead to the most common form of abnormal conduction called re-entrant excitation.[39] A re-entrant pathway is potentially formed when a difference in the rate of impulse transmission is present in adjacent conductive tissues. In the tissue with abnormal impulse transmission, an antegrade block develops, slowing impulse conduction in a forward direction, but allowing normal retrograde conduction. In the adjacent tissue with normal conduction, the impulse passes the conduction block and proceeds along the normal distal pathways. In addition, the impulse can pass retrograde through the abnormal tissue. This impulse arrives back at the area that conducted normally, finding it re-polarized and capable of rapidly reinitiating impulse formation. Thus, a re-entrant or circus loop is created. For an impulse to complete a re-entrant circuit, it must be unidirectionally blocked, travel slowly over another pathway, and re-excite in retrograde manner the tissue proximal to the block, after its refractory period. This results in a coupled premature contraction. The two key features are slow conduction and unidirectional block in the AV node or Purkinje network. This may be the mechanism of most postoperative supraventricular and ventricular dysrhythmias, since re-entry can occur throughout the conduction system both above and below the AV node.

The mechanism of action of the antiarrhythmic drugs can be integrated with the above discussion. Many of the commonly used antiarrhythmic drugs suppress automaticity in pacemaker cells by decreasing the slope of Phase 4 spontaneous depolarization. For example, propranolol, by reducing beta-adrenergic stimulation, reduces Phase 4 spontaneous depolarization. In addition, re-entrant mechanisms that produce dysrhythmias can be treated by slowing conduction in the abnormal tissue, by converting the unidirectional block to a bidirectional block (propranolol, quinidine), or by reducing or eliminating the unidirectional block by increasing impulse transmission through the AV node (lidocaine).

Treatment of Dysrhythmias

ANTIARRHYTHMIC DRUGS

The mode of action of the antiarrhythmic drugs must be understood in relation to their effects on the various phases of the cardiac action potential, particularly as it relates to the inward and outward membrane currents. In the normal heart, cardiac rhythm is determined by a single dominant pacemaker, a rapid uniform conduction system, and an action potential and refractory period of long duration. Changes in any of these variables will enhance the likelihood of an abnormal cardiac rhythm. Thus, shortening of the action potential, increasing conduction velocity, or decreasing the refractory period may potentiate the development of a dysrhythmia. To better understand the various drugs that are classified as antiarrhythmic agents, it is best to divide them into four electrophysiologic categories.[40,41] All of the drugs have one dominant action on the myocardial cell justifying their classification; however, there is some overlap among groups and continued controversy as to the classification of some of the drugs (Table 18-8).

Class I antiarrhythmic drugs are potent local anesthetics acting on nerve cells as well as myocardial membranes. They are divided into class IA drugs which have the ability to reduce the maximal rate of depolarization in cardiac muscle (block the fast inward sodium channel) and, therefore, increase the threshold of excitability, depress the conduction velocity, produce a marked prolongation in the effective refractory period, and inhibit spontaneous depolarization in automatic cells. These changes occur without any alteration in the action potential duration or resting membrane potential. These drugs include quinidine, procainamide, and disopyramide. Some authors also include propranolol in this class. Lidocaine and diphenylhydantoin differ from the class IA drugs in two ways: (1) they shorten the action potential duration, and (2) they increase conduction velocity and are thus called class IB drugs.

Class II drugs are the beta-adrenergic receptor blocking drugs. Overactivity of the sympathetic nervous system is felt to be significant in the development of certain cardiac dysrhythmias, and this can be inhibited by class II drugs. They work by depressing Phase 4 depolarization with a resultant decrease in cellular automaticity. This group includes propranolol, practolol, metoprolol, oxprenolol, alprenolol, pindolol, and nadolol.

Table 18-8
Anti-Arrhythmic Drugs

Drug	Class	IV Dose	Blood Level Desired	Toxicity
Procainamide (Pronestyl)	I	100 mg q 5 min up to 1000 mg; may infuse at 1–4 mg/min	4–6 µg/ml	Myocardial depression, hypotension, widened QRS; Lupus (chronic)
Quinidine (Quinaglute)	I	200 mg P.O. not IV	4–8 µg/ml	Fever, chills, nausea, diarrhea; Hypotension
Disopyramide (Norpace)	I	150 mg P.O. q 6 HR	2–4 µg/ml	Parasympatholytic symptoms—dry mouth, constipation, nausea, urinary retention, blurred vision; contraindicated in CHF, sick sinus node syndrome, A-V block; may widen QRS
Lidocaine (Xylocaine)	I	1.0–1.5 mg/kg bolus followed by constant infustion 1–4 mg/min	2–5 µg/ml	> 5 µg/ml → CNS excitation, muscle twitching & fasciculations, dizziness, tinnitus, convulsions & respiratory arrest; dosage must be reduced in CHF & liver dysfunction; with A-V block may increase conduction with marked increase in ventricular response
Diphenylhydantoin (Dilantin)	I	100 mg q 5 min. up to 500 mg	8–16 µg/ml	Hypotension & myocardial depression, rapid IV injection → V. fib, asystole, respiratory arrest, death
Propranolol (Inderal)	II	0.5 mg q 2 min up to total dose 5 mg	25–50 ng/ml	Myocardial depression, hypotension, bronchospasm; contra-indicated in CHF, bradycardia and AV block

Drug	Class	Dose	Level	Comments
Bretylium (Bretylol)	III	5 mg/kg diluted in 50–100 ml over 10–20 min; P.O. 600 mg q 6 HR	—	Orthostatic hypotension, myocardial depression, hypotension especially if used subsequent with other anti-fibrillatory agents.
Amiodarone (Cordarone)	III	IV 5–10 mg slowly P.O. 200–800 mg/day	—	Nausea, vomiting, diarrhea; slate grey skin discoloration; thyroid dysfunction; yellowish-brown granular corneal pigments.
Verapamil (Isoptin)	IV	IV 5–10 mg over 15–60 sec (0.145 mg/kg max) Repeat q 30' or infuse 5 μg/kg/min; P.O. 40–80 mg q 8 HR	50–200 ng/ml	Contraindicated in CHF, SA node disease, unstable AV block, hypotension; synergistic depression with beta-adrenergic blockers
Digoxin (Lanoxin)	Glycoside	0.25–0.50 mg → 1.5 mg	2 ng/ml	Bradycardia, CHB; Toxicity potentiated by $K^+ < 3.5$
Ouabain	Glycoside	0.1–0.2 mg → 1.0 mg	—	Bradycardia, CHB; Toxicity potentiated by $K^+ < 3.5$
Edrophonium (Tensilon)	Cholinergic	5–10 mg IV, may use test dose 2 mg esp. in presence digitalis or heart block	—	Sinus bradycardia, AV block, dizziness, abdominal cramps, CARDIAC ARREST.
Phenylephrine (Neosynephrine)	α-adrenergic receptor stimulator	50–100 μg IV	—	Hypertension. ↑ $M\dot{V}O_2$ → ischemia.
Atropine	Parasympatholytic	0.3 to 2 mg	—	Tachycardia, ↑ $M\dot{V}O_2$ → ischemia; fever, dryness.

Class III drugs, such as bretylium and amiodarone, produce prolongation of the action potential and repolarization of both atrial and ventricular muscle. These drugs are not local anesthetics nor beta-blockers. Their lengthening of the effective refractory period reduces the ability for re-entry and constitutes their major antiarrhythmic mechanism.

The class IV drugs are the slow channel calcium inhibitors which block the inward calcium channel at the cell membrane and include verapamil, nifedipine, and diltiazem. These drugs affect Phase 0 repolarization with slowing of the cardiac action potential throughout the conduction system.

Table 18-8 lists the antiarrhythmic drugs, their intravenous/oral doses, therapeutic plasma levels (when known), and toxicities or contraindications. Table 18-9 serves as a rapid reference for the treatment of important cardiac dysrhythmias in the postoperative period. Treatment is divided into the first, second, third, and occasionally a fourth choice for each dysrhythmia.

Four of the new antiarrhythmic drugs are worth expanding upon. Disopyramide (Norpace) is available in oral form to control recurrent premature ventricular contractions and other ventricular dysrhythmias. It appears to be effective in reducing life-threatening dysrhythmias resistant to other treatments, especially those associated with acute myocardial ischemia. This class I drug resembles quinidine, but was thought to have a reduced frequency of side effects; however, more side effects have recently been noted and the drug is not being used to any great extent.

Amiodarone is an experimental antiarrhythmic and antianginal drug without appreciative negative inotropism in the failing myocardium. It produces a decrease in the slope of diastolic depolarization, isolated prolongation of the atrial and ventricular action potentials, and depression of the AV node. This class III drug is useful for chronic prophylaxis of difficult dysrhythmias associated with preexcitation and is effective in both supraventricular and ventricular tachyarrhythmias. The production of corneal pigments, a gray skin discoloration, and thyroid dysfunction must be weighed against its potential benfits. It has also been reported to produce prolonged, severe systemic vasodilatation in patients undergoing cardiac surgery.

Bretylium is capable of markedly reducing the vulnerability to recurrent ventricular tachycardia and fibrillation associated with acute myocardial ischemia. This drug has a biphasic response with an initial release of norepinephrine and an increased conduction velocity, followed by a depletion of norepinephrine stores with a lengthening of the action potential duration and the effective refractory period. It is not useful in the management of supraventricular dysrhythmias, but it can control recurrent resistant ventricular tachycardia or fibrillation, when other drugs have failed.

Verapamil is the most important of the new antiarrhythmic drugs and is a synthetic papaverine derivative which selectively inhibits calcium flux across the cell membrane. By blocking the slow inward current of calcium, Phase 4 diastolic depolarization is prolonged. Its antiarrhythmic effect is produced by slowing atrial depolarization, delaying AV conduction secondary to prolonging the AV refractory period, and impeding the conduction proximal to the bundle of His, without affecting SA nodal or ventricular conduction. Intravenous verapamil is rapidly effective in correcting both atrial and ischemia-induced ventricular dysrhythmias. However, by inhibiting intranodal re-entry or circus-type preexcitation, it is most effective with supraventricular tachycardias. Because of its effect on excitation-contraction coupling, it must be used with caution in patients with significant myocardial dysfunction. It is presently available only in intravenous form, but soon may be available orally. The other calcium channel blockers, such as nifedipine and diltiazem, are much less effective as antiarrhythmic agents.

Table 18-9
Dysrhythmia Treatment Summary

Rhythm	1st Treatment Choice	2nd Treatment Choice	3rd Treatment Choice
Ventricular fibrillation Ventricular tachycardia	Electrical defibrillation 200 watt-sec (3 watt-sec/kg) increase energy as required	Lidocaine (Xylocaine) 1.0–1.5 mg/kg initial bolus Infusion 1–4 mg/min (2 gms/500 cc D$_5$W)	Propranolol (Inderal 0.5 mg q 2 min up to 5 mg 4th-Refractory V. fib. Bretylium 5 mg/kg q s 50–100cc D$_5$W- up to 30 mg/kg total dose
Premature ventricular contractions	Lidocaine (Xylocaine) 1.0–1.5 mg/kg initial bolus; Followed by infusion 1–4 mg/min	Propranolol (Inderal) 0.5 mg q 2 min up to 5 mg	Procainamide (Pronestyl) 100 mg q 5 min up to 1000 mg; may infuse 1–4 mg/min
Atrial fibrillation Atrial flutter	Digitalis 0.25–0.5 mg I.V. (Lanoxin) Ouabain 0.1–0.2 mg I.V. or Verapamil 5–10 mg I.V.	Propranolol (Inderal) 0.5 mg q 2 min to 5 mg	Cardioversion-*External* synchronized- Flutter-50-watt-sec Fibrillation-200 watt-sec *Internal* 5 to 30 watt-sec-synchronized
Paroxysmal atrial tachycardia	Carotid sinus message a) Edrophonium 2 mg → 10 mg can be used to improve response by increasing parasympathetic tone. b) Care must be exercised with carotid vascular disease.	Neosynephrine 50–100 µg/dose ↑ BP and convert via carotid sinus reflex	Propranolol (Inderal) 0.5 mg q 2 min up to 5 mg 4th treatment choice-Verapamil 5–10 mg I.V.
Sinus tachycardia	Usually no treatment required; if ↑HR → Ischemia →→→→	Propranolol (Inderal) 0.5 mg q 2 min up to 5 mg	
Sinus bradycardia	Usually no treatment required; if hypotension or ventricular escape beats present →→→→→→	Atropine 0.3–2.0 mg	Ephedrine 5–10 mg 4th treatment choice-atrial pacing if heart exposed
1° AV block 2° AV block Mobitz I Mobitz II	No treatment required No treatment required More ominous-requires transvenous (Epicardial) pacemaker		
3° AV Block Complete heart block	Atropine 0.3–2.0 mg may be helpful if suprahissian block	Isuprel 1–4 µg/min (1 mg/250 mg D$_5$W)	Transvenous pacemaker (Epicardial)

ELECTRICAL TREATMENT OF
DYSRHYTHMIAS

Since its introduction by Lown in 1962, direct current cardioversion has been widely utilized in the treatment of perioperative cardiac dysrhythmias.[42] It is used to treat ventricular tachycardia and acute or chronic atrial fibrillation or flutter, and is performed by using a synchronized DC shock applied externally to the chest wall. The pulse discharge is synchronized to occur within 20 milliseconds of the peak of the R wave on the ECG, thereby avoiding the period of ventricular vulnerability at the peak of the T wave. The shock depolarizes all the fibers that are excitable at that instant and allows the SA node to reinitiate the normal cardiac rhythm. Synchronization is mandatory to avoid inadvertent ventricular fibrillation which will occur about 2 percent of the time in nonsynchronized cardioversion.[43] All recent cardioverter/defibrillator machines have a synchronizer switch which must be turned on to achieve synchronization.

Atrial flutter is the easiest rhythm to cardiovert, and usually requires about 50 watt/sec externally. For atrial fibrillation or ventricular tachycardia, 200 watt/sec externally is frequently effective, but 300 to 400 watt/sec may be required. Elective external cardioversion is indicated for patients with a recent onset of atrial fibrillation or flutter. However, contraindications to cardioversion include long-term atrial fibrillation, underlying heart block, or digitalis toxicity. Digitalis intoxication is especially dangerous, since cardioversion in its presence can produce serious dysrhythmias or even resistant ventricular fibrillation.

In 1933, Kouwenhoven showed that a dog with a fibrillating heart could be converted to a regular sinus rhythm by an electric countershock. The first human defibrillation was performed by Beck in 1947, with an AC defibrillator. Because of their long discharge time, tendency to produce tissue damage, and the inability to synchronize AC defibrillators, they have been replaced by DC defibrillators.

Considerable controversy exists regarding the proper amount of delivered energy that should be utilized for external DC defibrillation.[44] Adgey et al cite the effectiveness of a 200 watt/sec dose to patients weighing up to 100 kg, with a success rate of 95 percent.[45] If unsuccessful, a second or third dose at the same 200 watt/sec level increases the success rate even further. Various factors exclusive of delivered energy may be important to determine the success of defibrillation: (1) the quality of CPR, (2) the length of delay before the first defibrillation attempt, (3) the underlying disease state, (4) the length of fibrillation, (5) the transthoracic resistance, and (6) the presence of antiarrhythmic drugs. The current American Heart Association guidelines for ventricular defibrillation suggest 3.5 to 6.0 watt/sec/kg should be delivered to patients under 50 kg; while in patients over 50 kg, 400 watt/sec should be utilized initially. However, because of the present trend toward studying delivered energy, many physicians would agree with Adgey that an initial dose of 200 watt/sec of delivered energy or 4 watt/sec/kg should be used and repeated as needed. Only if unsuccessful should the energy be increased to higher levels, since recent studies demonstrated increased myocardial injury when large-dose defibrillation was used.[44]

PULMONARY HYPERTENSION AND COR PULMONALE

Pulmonary hypertension is defined as an elevation of the pulmonary artery pressure above the accepted upper limit of normal. The upper limit of normal is about 25/15 mmHg or a mean pulmonary artery pressure of 13 to 18 mmHg. Under the stress of moderate leg exercise, pulmonary artery pressure does not normally exceed 30/15 mmHg or a mean of 20 mmHg. Pulmonary

Table 18-10

Conditions Producing Pulmonary Artery Hypertension (PAH)

I. PAH produced by elevations of capillary and pulmonary venous pressure
    A. Mitral stenosis, mitral regurgitation
    B. Hypertension, left ventricular failure
    C. Aortic stenosis or insufficiency
II. PAH produced by increases in pulmonary artery blood flow
    A. Congenital lesions: e.g., patient ductus arteriosus, ventricular septal defect
    B. Acquired lesions: post-myocardial infarction ventricular septal defect
III. PAH produced by loss of arterial cross-sectional area
    A. Chronic hypoxia*
        1. Emphysema, chronic bronchitis
        2. High altitude
        3. Chest and airway problems
            a. Pickwickian syndrome
            b. Kyphoscoliosis
    B. Pulmonary Fibrosis
        1. Massive pulmonary fibrosis
           —Silicosis and other pneumoconioses
        2. Interstitial fibrosis
            a. Collagen diseases
            b. Metals
            c. Primary pulmonary disease
                1) Hamman-Rich
                2) Sarcoidosis
            d. Iatrogenic
                1) Radiation
                2) Busulphan therapy
            e. Miscellaneous
                1) Letterer-Siwe
                2) Hand-Schuller-Christian
    C. Pulmonary emboli
        1. Recurrent
            a. Thromboemboli
            b. Parasitic
            c. Fat and tumor emboli
            d. Sickle cell
        2. Solitary emboli
            a. Massive thromboembolism
            b. Amniotic fluid
            c. Air

---

* Conditions producing cor pulmonale
Adapted from: Brooks JL, Kaplan JA: Cardiac diseases, p 268, 312. In Katz, Benumof, and Kadis Eds: Anesthesia in uncommon diseases: pathophysiologic and clinical correlation. Saunders 2nd ed., Phil, 1981

hypertension has been further subdivided into mild, moderate, and severe forms.

Three pathologic conditions can occur which will convert the normally low resistance pulmonary circulation into a high resistance circuit: (1) increases in pulmonary capillary or pulmonary venous pressures, (2) decreases in the cross-sectional area of the vasculature, or (3) increases in pulmonary arterial blood flow. Table 18-10, which lists the causes of pulmonary hypertension, is arranged according to these three pathophysiologic mechanisms.[46]

Increases in pulmonary capillary or pulmonary venous pressure may be caused by conditions such as left ventricular failure, mitral regurgitation, or mitral stenosis. In addition to the passive increase in pulmonary blood volume, active vasoconstriction produced by hypoxia also occurs in the pulmonary vascular bed.[47]

A decrease in pulmonary arterial cross-sectional area results in increased pulmonary vascular resistance, since resistance to flow is inversely proportional to the fourth power of the radius of the vessels. Very small decreases in pulmonary cross-sectional area can thus result in striking increases in pulmonary vascular resistance. Multiple small thrombotic emboli are typical of embolic causes of pulmonary hypertension.

Like systemic arterial hypertension, pulmonary hypertension is characterized by a prolonged asymptomatic period. As pulmonary vascular changes occur, an irreversible decrease in pulmonary cross-sectional area develops, and cardiac output becomes fixed due to the resistance to flow. This results in the symptoms of dyspnea, fatigue, syncope, and chest pain. The diagnostic dilemma presented by pulmonary hypertension is the differentiation of primary pulmonary hypertension from secondary hypertension due to another condition such as left ventricular failure or mitral stenosis. Usually, in the latter circumstances, the symptoms of the primary condition are the most prominent with the pulmonary hypertension being of secondary significance. Right ventricular hypertrophy commonly occurs in response to pulmonary hypertension which may progress to right ventricular dilatation and failure.[48]

Cor Pulmonale

Cor pulmonale is usually defined as right ventricular hypertrophy, dilatation, and failure secondary to pulmonary arterial hypertension due to a decrease in the cross-sectional area of the pulmonary bed. This excludes right ventricular failure, which occurs after increases in pulmonary arterial pressure secondary to increases in pulmonary blood flow, pulmonary capillary or venous pressures. Given this restriction, there

are still numerous causes of cor pulmonale, including pulmonary parenchymal disease, chronic hypoxia, and primary pulmonary arterial disease.[49]

Cor pulmonale is divided into two types: acute and chronic. Acute cor pulmonale is usually secondary to massive pulmonary emboli, resulting in a 60 to 70 percent decrease in the pulmonary cross-sectional area, associated with cyanosis and acute respiratory distress. With acute cor pulmonale there is a rapid increase in right ventricular systolic pressure to 60 to 70 mmHg which slowly returns towards normal, secondary to displacement of the emboli peripherally with increased blood flow past the emboli, lysis of the emboli, and increases in collateral blood flow. These changes often occur within two hours of the onset of symptoms. Massive emboli may be associated with acute right ventricular dilatation and failure, elevated central venous pressure, and cardiogenic shock. Another feature of massive pulmonary emboli is that the pulmonary vasoconstrictive response may be so intense that it persists until after the pulmonary hypertension progresses to acute right ventricular failure, even in the absence of angiograhically demonstrable pulmonary emboli (see the section on pulmonary emboli).

Chronic cor pulmonale presents with a rather different picture. It is associated with right ventricular hypertrophy and a change in the normal crescentic shape of the right ventricle to a more ellipsoidal shape which is consistent with a change from volume-work, which the right ventricle normally performs, to a ventricular geometry more appropriate to the pressure-work required by a high afterload. Curiously, left ventricular dysfunction may occur associated with right ventricular hypertrophy, which cannot be related to any obvious changes in the loading conditions of the left ventricle.[50] Chronic cor pulmonale is usually superimposed on longstanding pulmonary arterial hypertension.

Chronic bronchitis is probably the most common cause of chronic cor pulmonale in adults. Long-standing chronic bronchitis results in an elevation of pulmonary arterial pressure with resulting right ventricular hypertrophy. With any form of respiratory embarrassment, whether it be infection or simply progression of the disease, further increases in pulmonary vascular resistance increase pulmonary arterial pressure, and right ventricular failure supervenes. With the onset of respiratory problems in a patient with chronic bronchitis, a number of changes occur which can make pulmonary hypertension more severe and precipitate right ventricular failure. A respiratory infection produces further abnormalities of the blood gas values with a decline in PaO_2 and elevation in $PaCO_2$. The patient with chronic bronchitis normally has an increase in airway resistance made worse during acute respiratory infections due to secretions and edema, further reducing the caliber of the small airways. These patients also have a loss of structural support from degenerative changes in the airways, and from a loss of the stinting effect of the pulmonary parenchyma. For these reasons, the patient's small airways tend to collapse during exhalation, and there is a rise in airway pressure due to this "dynamic compression" phenomenon. Therefore, with the onset of respiratory embarrassment in the chronic bronchitic, there are increases in pulmonary artery pressure, airway resistance, afterload, and the work requirement of the right ventricle which may result in right ventricular failure.

TREATMENT

The primary focus of therapy is the underlying lung disease, since the right ventricular pressure-workload must be reduced. If right ventricular failure has not appeared, the goal must be to prevent its onset. When it appears it should be treated, but the response will not be good unless right ventricular work is reduced by control of the pulmonary hypertension.

Relief of hypoxemia is of prime impor-

tance in reducing pulmonary hypertension. This can be done either by treating the underlying disease, or by the administration of oxygen. Hopefully, the oxygen will relieve some of the hypoxic pulmonary vasoconstriction and allow for better blood gas exchange. In patients with chronic obstructive pulmonary disease, other supportive therapy with bronchodilators, antibiotics, physical therapy, and the administration of sodium bicarbonate may be useful. When cor pulmonale supervenes, direct cardiac therapy with digitalis, diuretics, and other inotropes and vasodilators may be required. In addition, fluid overload should be corrected and phlebotomy utilized to reduce the hematocrit to allow for better pulmonary blood flow properties.

Digitalis has been used for many years in the treatment of cor pulmonale, but there is still debate concerning its effectiveness and potential dangers.[51] The improvement in cardiac output and the reduction of right ventricular filling pressures are not great when digitalis is administered in the presence of cor pulmonale. Clearly, the beneficial effects of digitalis are not as obvious as they are when used to treat left ventricular failure. Furthermore, patients with pulmonary disease taking digitalis exhibit a high incidence of dysrhythmias compatible with digitalis intoxication, especially during episodes of acute respiratory failure; and they occur in the face of serum digitalis levels that are not usually associated with toxicity. Thus, there appears to be an increased sensitivity to the drug during acute respiratory failure superimposed on cor pulmonale. This high incidence of dysrhythmias limits the usefulness of digitalis in these patients with chronic lung disease

Circulatory supportive measures in the setting of right ventricular failure do not differ theoretically from measures employed in managing left ventricular failure (Table 18-11). Therapy is directed at ventricular preload, inotropic state of the ventricle, and ventricular afterload. Right ventricular pre-

Table 18-11
Abbreviated Pulmonary Vascular Pharmacopaeia

Drug	PA Pressure	PCWP	Pulmonary Blood Flow	SAP	HR	PVR
alpha & beta agonists						
1. Norepinephrine 0.1–0.2 µg/kg/min	↑	↑ to ↑↑	—**	↑↑	↓	NC* to ↑
2. Methoxamine 5–10 mg	↑	↑	—	↑↑	↓↓	—
3. Phenylephrine 50–100 µg	↑↑	—	↓	↑↑	↓↓	↑↑
4. Epinephrine .05–.20 µg/kg/min	↑	NC or ↓	↑	↑↑	↑	↑
5. Dopamine 2–10 µg/kg/min	NC	NC or ↓	↑	NC or ↑	↑	NC
6. Dobutamine 5–15 µg/kg/min	—	↓	↑↑	NC or ↑	↑	↓
7. Isoproterenol 0.015–0.15 µg/kg/min	SL†↓	↓	↑↑	↓	↑↑	↓
beta-antagonist						
Propranolol .5–2 mg	—	NC to ↑	NC to ↓	NC to ↓	↓	NC to ↑
alpha-antagonist						
Phentolamine 1–3 µg/kg/min	↓	↓	↑	↓	↑	↓
Smooth muscle dilators						
1. Aminophylline 500 mg	↓	↓	—	—	↑	↓
2. Sodium nitroprusside .5–3 µg/kg/min	↓	↓	↑↑	NC to ↓	↑	↓
3. Nitroglycerin .5–5 µg/kg/min	↓↓	↓↓	NC to ↑	↓	↑	↓

* NC = No change
** — = Data unavailable
† SL = Slight
Adapted from: Brooks JL, Kaplan JA: Cardiac diseases, p 268, 312. In Katz, Benumof, and Kadis Eds: Anesthesia in uncommon diseases: pathophysiologic and clinical correlation. Saunders 2nd ed., Phil, 1981

load can be assessed by measurement of central venous pressure, preferably as part of full hemodynamic monitoring with a pulmonary artery catheter. Preload can be augmented with judicious use of fluid infusions, or decreased with a vasodilator, such as nitroglycerin, which primarily affects the venous capacitance bed in low doses. The right ventricular contractile state can be estimated by the cardiac output, in addition to observing the right ventricular response to volume infusion. Inotropic support, in addition to the use of digitalis, is often required in the setting of right ventricular failure with chronic cor pulmonale. The inotropic drug selected should be based on its effects on the pulmonary circulation, as well as its systemic hemodynamic effects. For example, in the setting of right ventricular failure, norepinephrine can dramatically increase pulmonary artery pressure and pulmonary vascular resistance, and, therefore, it is relatively contraindicated. On the other hand, dobutamine tends to reduce pulmonary artery pressure and pulmonary vascular resistance, and, therefore, it would be one of the inotropic drugs of choice in right ventricular failure.[52]

Just as in left ventricular failure where the reduction of left ventricular afterload can produce an increase in stroke volume and cardiac output, reduction of right ventricular afterload can produce similar effects during right ventricular failure. Vasodilators found to be effective in some cases in reducing the afterload of the right ventricle include phentolamine, sodium nitroprusside, and nitroglycerin. Aminophylline may be especially useful in the setting of pulmonary hypertension, right ventricular failure, and bronchospasm, since the drug is a direct pulmonary artery dilator, as well as a bronchodilator, and tends to reduce pulmonary artery pressure. Though it may occasionally produce some mild tachycardia and has an arrhythmogenic potential, it is a potentially useful drug in patients with cor pulmonale.[53]

Positive pressure ventilation may produce a fall in right ventricular preload and an increase in pulmonary artery pressure by reducing the cross-sectional area of the pulmonary vasculature during the positive phase of ventilation. The use of PEEP may be detrimental to the patient in right ventricular failure secondary to pulmonary hypertension, since it produces a fall in venous return and right ventricular preload, and an increase in pulmonary vascular resistance and pulmonary artery pressure. The functional residual capacity is already increased in these patients, and the use of PEEP has little to offer in terms of improving ventilation-perfusion matching.

PULMONARY EMBOLISM

Pulmonary embolism is the most common form of acute pulmonary disease in the adult population, and is one of the most common causes of death in both medical and surgical patients. Pulmonary emboli are found in approximately 10 percent of all autopsies. In a general surgical population and in patients dying of congestive heart failure, data indicate an incidence of 30 to 50 percent.[54]

In over 90 percent of cases, the site of formation of the thrombus that eventually finds its way to the lungs is in the calves of the legs. The volume of involved material depends on the extent of venous propagation and the point at which the thrombus breaks loose from the leg. A clot extending from the calf to the iliac vein has a volume of approximately 100 ml. Another area that is a frequent site of clot formation is the pelvis. Emboli also originate in the right atrium in patients with chronic congestive heart failure and atrial fibrillation; however, the volume of clot is much less than that released from the legs or pelvis.

Virchow first described three factors in the genesis of thromboemboli: stasis, damage to the innermost wall of the vessel, and hypercoagulability of the blood. Additional factors adding to the risk of venous thrombosis and pulmonary emboli are: advanced age, prolonged bed rest, obstruction of venous blood flow, heart failure, varicose veins, shock, trauma, major surgery, polycythemia, dehydration, carcinoma, smoking, and the use of oral contraceptive therapy.[55] Chronic congestive heart failure is by far the most important condition predisposing to pulmonary thromboemboli. The most clear-cut example of a hypercoagulable state is the deficiency of antithrombin III.[56] Other abnormalities of the clotting system that may predispose to pulmonary emboli include thrombocytosis, sickle-cell anemia, or the presence of cold agglutinins or macroglobulins.

When a thrombus embolizes, it usually breaks up and follows the distribution of blood flow in the lungs, thus going mainly to the lower lobes on both sides. The pulmonary artery pressure rises as a result of the emboli and vasoactive materials are released which futher augment the pulmonary hypertension. The emboli may produce pulmonary infarctions if the bronchial collateral circulation is not sufficient to maintain the viability of the parenchymal tissue. Acute cor pulmonale may occur if the emboli are sufficiently massive to occlude more than 50 percent of the pulmonary circulation.

McIntyre documented the hemodynamic response to pulmonary emboli in 20 patients free of prior cardiopulmonary disease.[57] Arterial hypoxemia occurred in 95 percent of the patients, and the mean pulmonary artery pressure was increased in 70 percent of the patients. Good correlation was found between the mean pulmonary artery pressure and the angiographic estimation of the pulmonary artery obstruction. Surprisingly, the mean pulmonary artery pressure was found not to exceed 40 mmHg, even with massive obstruction in some patients.

Vasoactive substances released from platelets contribute markedly to the pulmonary pressor response and hypoxemia found following pulmonary microemboli.[58] In dogs embolized with glass beads, it was found that treatment with heparin or sulfinpyrazone, which blocked platelet function, reduced the pulmonary hypertension and hypoxemia by more than 50 percent. Platelet-inhibiting drugs might therefore be useful in the therapy of pulmonary microembolism.

The rate of resolution of acute pulmonary emboli in man has been studied extensively by Dalen et al.[59] In 15 patients with documented pulmonary emboli treated with heparin, sequential studies showed only minimal angiographic and hemodynamic signs of resolution after 7 days. By 10 to 21 days, pressures in the right side of the heart had decreased to near normal levels and there was angiographic evidence of resolution. In some patients, angiographic and hemodynamic abnormalities persisted for weeks after the emboli.

Approximately 10 percent of patients with pulmonary emboli die almost immediately. The natural history of patients who survive the first hour after emboli is dependent on whether the diagnosis is made and therapy is initiated. Dalen found that the diagnosis was not made in approximately 70 percent of patients who survived the first hour, and 30 percent of these individuals succumbed to recurrent emboli.[60] The fate of the patients in whom pulmonary emboli are diagnosed is quite good. The overall hospital mortality of patients treated for acute pulmonary emboli is 8 percent and is dependent on the presence of associated pulmonary disease.[61] Even patients with massive pulmonary emboli do well with therapy directed at preventing further embolization. Recurrence of pulmonary emboli is rare in patients who are adequately treated and in whom appropriate prophylaxis is undertaken against further episodes of emboli.

Diagnosis

The diagnosis of a pulmonary embolus is rarely easy or straightforward in the postoperative period. The embolus must be large before any symptoms appear, and even then they may not be sufficiently characteristic to allow for the proper diagnosis. Pulmonary infarction may be easily confused with other respiratory problems, such as atelectasis or pneumonia, and acute cor pulmonale may at first appear to be an accentuation of preexisting heart disease or an acute myocardial infarction. Many times pulmonary emboli masquerade as an asthmatic attack in a patient with chronic bronchitis, with the primary symptom being wheezing.[62]

Pulmonary emboli are especially difficult to diagnose in patients with a history of chronic congestive heart failure. Clues to the proper diagnosis include: (1) thrombophlebitis of the legs, (2) unexplained dyspnea or tachypnea, (3) blood-streaked sputum, (4) pleuritic chest pain, (5) unexplained fever or tachycardia, and (6) unexplained deterioration in cardiopulmonary status.

Special radiographic techniques have

greatly enhanced diagnostic capability in patients with pulmonary emboli. Pulmonary angiography and lung scanning should be regarded as complementary tests in making this diagnosis. Angiography is currently the most accurate method of establishing the specific diagnosis. Lung scans using ^{131}I tagged human serum albumin are also useful in making the diagnosis of pulmonary emboli. The scans are most consistent with pulmonary emboli when they show abnormalities in the presence of a normal chest radiograph. When there are chest radiographic abnormalities, the scan must be carefully interpreted in relation to these prior abnormalities. A normal lung scan can exclude pulmonary emboli as the cause of respiratory symptoms.

Treatment

When there is a strong suspicion that pulmonary emboli have occurred, treatment should be instituted immediately because of the likelihood of further episodes and the increasing mortality with repeated emboli. Treatment should not be deferred until the diagnosis is confirmed by x-ray examination, ECG, blood gases, lung scan, or pulmonary angiogram. The patient should receive 7,500 to 10,000 units of heparin intravenously, oxygen should be administered, and morphine used for pain or agitation. Hypotension and shock may require intravenous infusions of inotropic drugs, such as isoproterenol or norepinephrine, with the rate of infusion being determined by the blood pressure.[63,64]

The exact regimen of maintenance heparin therapy is still controversial. However, at the present time, the continuous intravenous infusion method with doses ranging from 1,000 to 1,500 U/hr by an infusion pump is most often used. Although the subcutaneous route seems more convenient, the variability and unpredictability of absorption from the injection sites over a period of time makes it less reliable. Warfarin therapy is usually begun on the fifth or sixth day if the patient is stable, with a total changeover from heparin taking place on approximately the eighth to twelfth day.

The role of fibrinolytic therapy for pulmonary emboli is still not clear.[65] The two drugs that have been most extensively studied are streptokinase and urokinase. In a trial of urokinase therapy by the National Heart and Lung Institute, two groups of patients were compared with either heparin therapy or urokinase therapy. The hospital mortality was the same for both groups and there were more hemorrhagic complications in the urokinase group.[66]

Emergency pulmonary embolectomy (Trendelenberg operation) was introduced in the early 1900s for the treatment of massive pulmonary emboli. The introduction of cardiopulmonary bypass has made the performance of this operation technically feasible, but the surgical mortality is still above 50 percent.[67] The primary indication for emergency embolectomy is the presence of right ventricular failure and shock, resistant to vasopressors, in a patient with bilateral central pulmonary emboli documented by pulmonary angiography. In this situation, the embolectomy may be lifesaving.

NEUROLOGIC INJURIES

Both central and peripheral neurologic injuries can occur during intrathoracic procedures. Such injuries often result in serious and disabling loss of function and are very distressing to the patient.[68] Peripheral nerves can be injured either in the chest or in other parts of the body by pressure or stretching. It has been recognized for years that the majority of these postoperative neuropathies are due to malpositioning of the patient on the operating table with subsequent stretching or compression of the nerves.[69,70] Stretching or direct compression of a nerve results in ischemia, and if ischemia is maintained for sufficient time, necrosis of the nerve occurs. In addition, stretching of a nerve can produce rupture of capillary vessels and a consequent hematoma in the nerve bundle itself. If the hematoma is large, the nerve fibers become completely necrotic due to the pressure, with ultimate scarring of the nerve trunks.

The nerve injury may be apparent immediately after surgery, or may not become obvious until several days later. The patients often complain of a variety of unpleasant sensations including hyperaesthesia, paraesthesia, coldness, pain, or anesthesia in the area supplied by the affected nerves.[71] If early recovery does not occur, there is eventual muscle wasting, contractures, stiffening of joints, atrophy, and ulcers, all developing in the area of the nerve injury. Recovery may be complete within a few days to months, or permanent weakness and sensory loss may remain. The longer the period spent in an abnormal position, the worse the ultimate prognosis.

The brachial plexus is especially vulnerable to trauma during thoracic surgery and anesthesia. The muscle tone of the patient is reduced or completely abolished by muscle relaxants and anesthetic drugs, and, therefore, the extremities are susceptible to nonphysiologic positioning. The brachial plexus has a long superficial course in the axilla between two points of fixation, the vertebra above and the axillary fascia below. In addition, the plexus lies in close proximity to a number of freely movable bony structures. Stretching is the chief cause of damage to the brachial plexus, with compression having only a secondary role. Stretching of the plexus is produced by any factor which increases the distance between the two points of fixation including abduction, external rotation, dorsal extention of the arm on an armboard, or suspension of the arm from an ether screen.

Certain congenital abnormalities render the brachial plexus more vulnerable to injury. These include hypertrophy of the scalenous medius muscles, a cervical rib, an ab-

normal slope of the shoulder, or a higher or lower than normal derivation of the brachial plexus.

Branches of the brachial plexus may also be injured lower in the arm. For example, the radial nerve may be compressed by an ether screen against the humerus, if it is allowed to sag off the operating table. Clinically, this will often produce a wrist-drop postoperatively. The ulnar nerve can be injured by compressing it between the upper condyle of the humerus and the edge of the operating table if incorrectly tucked along the side.[72] Severe injuries of the ulnar nerve can lead to a "claw hand."

A properly positioned patient in the thoracotomy position is shown in Figure 18-3. Note the position of the legs as well as that of the arms. Nerve injuries of the lower extremities involving the peroneal nerves, saphenous nerves, and sciatic nerves can occur with incorrect positioning.

Intrathoracic nerves can be directly injured during the surgical procedure by being transected, crushed, stretched, stripped of their blood supply, or cauterized. The intercostal nerves are the ones most frequently injured during intrathoracic surgical procedures. A rib fracture occurring at the time of the thoracotomy can compress the intercostal nerve with development of an intercostal neuritis, manifest by radicular pain in the postoperative period. When excessive stretching and tension are placed on the intercostal nerve roots while the chest is being opened, postoperative intercostal neuralgia may be quite severe. In addition, the chest tubes can produce a neuroma or neuritis by compression of the intercostal nerves.

The recurrent laryngeal nerve can become involved in lymph node tissue and injured at the time of a node biopsy, especially when done through a mediastinoscope. This nerve can also be injured during tracheostomy, substernal thyroidectomy, and radical pulmonary dissections, as well as during repair of certain congenital cardiac defects such as patent ductus arteriosus.

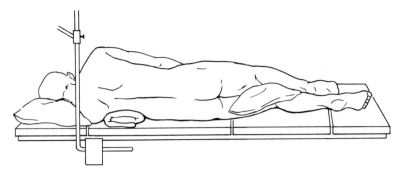

Fig. 18-3 A patient is shown correctly positioned for a thoracotomy procedure. Note the axillary role and padding between the legs which are properly flexed. The upper arm will be carefully positioned on the ether screen in order to avoid stretching the brachial plexus. (This picture is courtesy of Dr. George Silvay.)

The phrenic nerve can be injured during pericardiectomy, radical pulmonary hilar dissections, implantation of pacemakers, division of the diaphragm during esophageal surgery, and during dissection of mediastinal tumors. The vagus nerves may also be injured during esophageal dissection and radical pulmonary dissections.

Cranial nerve injuries also may occur in the thoracotomy position, and these injuries may have serious consequences for the patient. The optic nerve can be injured by pressure against the eyeball, especially in conjunction with hypotension, which can lead to thrombosis of the central retinal artery with potential blindness upon awakening from anesthesia. Deliberate hypotension in the lateral thoracotomy position can lead to this injury if any pressure is put on the down eye. Other cranial nerve injuries have occurred during thoracotomy from pressure being applied to the supraorbital nerve, facial nerve, and trigeminal nerve. Recently, Jaffe and McLeskey reported a case of a transient postoperative Horner's syndrome resulting from prolonged, exaggerated intraoperative lateral flexion of the hand and neck.[73]

Prevention is the treatment of choice for all of these intraoperative nerve injuries. If a nerve palsy does occur, analgesics may be necessary for the first few days to control pain, and the skin may have to be protected from injury and ulceration. All joint mobility should be maintained by frequent physical therapy, and contractures prevented by appropriate splinting. Certain injuries, such as those to the intercostal nerves, can be treated with nerve blocks. By the judicious use of repeated temporary intercostal nerve blocks, both early and late postoperative intercostal pain can be significantly reduced. Injuries to the recurrent laryngeal nerve or phrenic nerve usually show return of function within 6 weeks to 9 months. If vocal cord function does not return after recurrent laryngeal nerve injury, the involved vocal cord may have to be injected with steroids, often leading to return of function. In rare cases, surgical procedures including the injection of Teflon may have to be performed on the involved cord to improve its function. If phrenic nerve paralysis persists, and produces marked respiratory embarrassment due to paralysis of the diaphragm, it is possible to implant a phrenic nerve stimulator to correct respiratory insufficiency.[68]

In summary, numerous complications may occur in the postoperative period to patients undergoing major thoracic diagnostic and therapeutic procedures. These can range from the most severe cardiovascular or respiratory complications to relatively minor but distressing neurologic complications. All of

these can be diagnosed accurately by the as-
tute physician using his clinical skills and
advanced hemodynamic monitoring. Increased understanding of the pathophysiology and pharmacologic interventions allows
for an improved prognosis for some of these
complications

REFERENCES

1. Mason DT: Congestive heart failure: mechanisms, evaluation and treatment. York Medical Books, New York, 1976
2. Sonnenblick EH: Correlation of myocardial
   ultrastructure and function. Circulation
   38:29-44, 1968
3. Katz AM, Hecht HH: The early pump failure
   of the ischemic heart. Am J Med 47:497-502,
   1969
4. Hurst JW, Logue RB: The heart. 5th ed.
   McGraw Hill, New York, 1982
5. Kaplan JA: Cardiac anesthesia. Grune &
   Stratton, New York, 1979
6. Kaplan JA, Bland JW, Dunbar RW: The
   peroperative management of pericardial tamponade. South Med J 69:417-419, 1976
7. Guntheroth WG, Morgan BG, Mullin S: Effect of respiration on venous return and
   stroke volume in cardiac tamponade: mechanism of pulsus paradoxus. Circ Res 20:381-
   390, 1967
8. Massumi RA, Mason DT, Vera Z et al: Reverse pulsus paradoxus. N Engl J Med
   289:1272-1275, 1973
9. Thomas SJ: Valvular heart disease. In Philbin, DM, Ed: Anesthetic management of the
   patient with cardiovascular disease. Little
   Brown & Co., Boston, 1979
10. Weeks KR, Chatterjee K, Block S et al: Bed-
    side hemodynamic monitoring: its value in
    the diagnosis of tamponade complicating car-
    diac surgery. J Thoracic Cardiovas Surg
    71:250-252, 1976
11. Smith TW: Digitalis glycosides (parts 1 to 4).
    N Engl J Med 289:945-952, 1010-1015, 1063-
    1072, 1125-1128, 1973
12. Mason DT: The cardiovascular effects of digi-
    talis in normal man. Clin Pharmacol Ther
    7:1-16, 1966
13. Denlinger JK, Narwold ML, Gibbs PS et al:
    Hypocalcaemia during rapid blood transfu-

sion in anaesthetized man. Br J Anaesth
48:995-1000, 1976
14. Denlinger JK, Kaplan JA, Lecky JH et al:
    Cardiovascular responses to calcium admin-
    istered intravenously to man during halo-
    thane anesthesia. Anesthesiology 42:390-397,
    1975
15. Nola FT, Pope S, Harrison DC: Assessment
    of the synergistic relationshp between serum
    calcium and digitalis. Am Heart J 79:499-507,
    1970
16. Kones RJ: The catecholamines: reappraisal of
    their use for acute myocardial infarction and
    the low cardiac output syndromes. Crit Care
    Med 1:203-220, 1973
17. Standards for cardiopulmonary resuscitation
    (CPR) and emergency cardiac care (ECC).
    JAMA (Suppl.) 227:833-868, 1974
18. Meuller H, Ayers SM, Gregory JJ et al: He-
    modynamics, coronary blood flow, and myo-
    cardial metabolism in coronary shock: re-
    sponse to l-norepinephrine and isoproterenol.
    J Clin Invest 49:1885-1902,1970
19. Beregovich J, Reicher-Reiss H, Kunstadt D et
    al: Hemodynamic effects of isoproterenol in
    cardiac surgery. J Thorac Cardiovasc Surg
    62:957-964, 1971
20. Goldberg LI: Dopamine: clinical uses of an
    endogenous catecholamine. N Engl J Med
    291:707-710, 1974
21. Holloway EL, Stinson EB, Derby GC et al:
    Action of drugs in patients early after cardiac
    surgery. I. Comparison of isoproterenol and
    dopamine. Am J Cardiol 35:656-659, 1975
22. Goldberg LI: Cardiovascular and renal ac-
    tions of dopamine: potential clinical applica-
    tions. Pharmacol Rev 24:1-29, 1972
23. Loeb HS, Bredakis J, Gunnar RM: Superior-
    ity of dobutamine over dopamine for aug-
    mentation of cardiac output in patients with
    chronic low output cardiac faiure. Circulation
    55:375-381, 1977
24. Gillespie TA, Ambos HD, Sobel BE et al: Ef-
    fects of dobutamine in patients with acute
    myocardial infarction. Am J Cardiol 39:588-
    594, 1977
25. Sakamoto T, Yamada T: Hemodynamic ef-
    fects of dobutamine in patients following
    open heart surgery. Circulation 55:525-533,
    1977
26. Tinker JH, Tarhan S, White RD et al: Dobu-
    tamine for inotropic support during emer-

gence from cardiopulmonary bypass. Anesthesiology 44:281-286, 1976

27. Leier CV, Webel J, Bush CA: The cardiovascular effects of the continuous infusion of dobutamine in patients with severe cardiac failure. Circulation 56:468-472, 1977

28. Dikshit K, Vydan JK, Forrester JS et al: Renal and extrarenal hemodynamic effects of furosemide in congestive heart failure after acute myocardial infarction. N Engl J Med 288:1087-1090 1973

29. Austin SM, Schreiner BF, Kramer DH et al: The acute hemodynamic effects of ethacrynic acid and furosemide in patients with chronic postcapillary pulmonary hypertension. Circulation 53:364-362, 1976

30. Guiha NH, Cohn JN, Franciosa JA et al: Treatment of refractory heart failure with infusion of nitroprusside. N Engl J Med 291:587-592, 1974

31. Miller RR, Vismara LA, Williams DO et al: Pharmacological mechanisms for left ventricular unloading in clinical congestive heart failure: differential effects of nitroprusside, phentolamine, and nitroglycerin on cardiac function and peripheral circulation. Circ Res 39:127-133, 1976

32. Chatterjee K, Parmley WW: The role of vasodilator therapy in heart failure. Prog Cardiovasc Dis 19:301-325, 1977

33. Williams DO, Hilliard GK, Cantor SA et al: Comparative mechanisms of ventricular unloading by systemic vasodilator agents in therapy of cardiac failure: nitroprusside versus phentolamine. Am J Cardiol 35:177-178, 1975

34. Mason DT, Zelis R, Amsterdam EA: Actions of the nitrates on the peripheral circulation and myocardial oxygen consumption: significance in the relief of angina pectoris. Chest 59:296-305, 1971

35. Bertrand CA, Steiner NV, Jameson AG et al: Disturbances of cardiac rhythm during anesthesia and surgery. JAMA 216:1615-1617, 1971

36. Angelini L, Feldman MI, Lufschonowski R et al: Cardiac arrhythmias during and after heart surgery: diagnosis and management. Prog Cardiovasc Dis 16:469-495, 1974

37. Edwards R, Winnie AL, Ramamurthy S: Acute hypocapnic hypokalemia: an iatrogenic anesthetic complication. Anesth Analg (Cleve) 56:786-792, 1977

38. Cranefield PF, Wit AL, Hoffman BF: Genesis of cardiac arrhythmias. Circulation 47:190-204, 1973

39. Moe GK, Mendez C: Physiologic basis of premature beats and sustained tachycardia. N Engl J Med 288:250-253, 1973

40. Carson IW, Lyons SM, Shanks RG: Antiarrhythmic drugs. Br J Anaesth 51:659-670, 1979

41. Singh BN, Collett JT, Chew CY: New prospectives in the pharmacologic therapy of cardiac arrhythmia. Prog Cardiovasc Dis 22:243-301, 1980

42. Glassman E: Direct current cardioversion. Am Heart J 82:128-130, 1971

43. Resnekov L: Present status of electroversion in the management of cardiac dysrhythmias. Circulation 47:1356-1363, 1973

44. Tacker WA, Ewy GA: Emergency defibrillation dose: recommendations and rationale. Circulation 60:223-225, 1979

45. Adgey AA: Ventricular defibrillation: appropriate energy levels. Circulation 60:219-223, 1979

46. Brooks JL, Kaplan JA: Cardiac diseases, p 268, 312. In Katz, Benumof, and Kadis Eds: Anesthesia in uncommon diseases: pathophysiologic and clinical correlation. Saunders 2nd ed., Phil, 1981

47. Harris P, Heath D: Causes of pulmonary arterial hypertension, p 226-242. In The human pulmonary circulation, Churchill Livingstone, 1977

48. Stein PD, Babbah HN, Maryilli M: Performance of the failing and non-failing right ventricle of patients with pulmonary hypertension, Am J Cardiol 44:1050-1055, 1979

49. Ross JE: Chronic cor pulmonale, p 1243-1249. In Hurst JW, Ed: The heart. 5th ed. McGraw-Hill, 1982

50. Baum SL, Schwartz A et al: Left ventricular function in chronic obstructive lung disease. N Engl J Med 285:361-365, 1971

51. Green LH, Smith TW: The use of digitalis in patients with pulmonary disease. Annals of Int Med 87:459-465, 1977

52. Harris P, Heath D: Pharmacology of the pulmonary circulation, p 182-210. In The human pulmonary circulation. Churchill Livingstone, 1977

53. Webb-Johnson DC, Andrews JL: Bronchodilatory therapy (Parts I & II), N Engl J Med 297:476-482, 758-764, 1978

54. Dexter L, Alpert JS, Dalen JE: Pulmonary embolism, infarction, and acute cor pulmonale, p 1227-1242. In Hurst JW, Ed: The heart. McGraw-Hill, N.Y., 1982

55. Price DJ: Pulmonary embolism. Anaesthesia 31:925-932, 1976

56. Rosenberg RD: Actions and interactions of antithrombic and heparine. N Engl J Med 292:146-151, 1975

57. McIntyre KM, Sasahara SA: The hemodynamic response to pulmonary embolism in patients without prior cardiopulmonary disease. Am J Cardiol 28:288, 293, 1971

58. Mlczoch J, Lucher S, Weir EK et al: Platelet mediated pulmonary hypertension and hypoxia during pulmonary microembolism. Chest 74:648, 653, 1978

59. Dalen JE, Bauas JA, Brooks HL et al: Resolution rate of acute pulmonary embolism in man. N Engl J Med 280:1194-1199, 1969

60. Dalen JE, Alpert JS: Natural history of pulmonary embolism. Progress in Cardiovascular Diseases 17:259-270, 1975

61. Alpert JS, Smith K, Carlson J et al: Mortality in patients treated for pulmonary embolism. JAMA 236:1477-1480, 1976

62. Olazabal F, Roman-Irigarry LA, Oms JD et al: Pulmonary emboli masquerading as asthma. N Engl J Med 278:999-1001, 1968

63. Rosenberg JC, Hussain K, Lenaghan R: Iso-

proterenol in norepinephrine therapy for pulmonary embolism shock. J Thor Cardio Surg 62:144-150, 1971

64. Sasahara SS: Therapy for pulmonary embolism. JAMA 229:1795-1798, 1974

65. Dalen JE: The case against fibrinolytic therapy. J Cardiovas Med 5:799-807, 1980

66. Jenton E, Hersh J: Observations on anticoagulant and thrombolytic therapy in pulmonary embolism. Prog Cadiovasc Dis 17:335-343, 1975

67. Sautter KD, Myers WO, Ray JF et al: Pulmonary embolectomy: review and current status. Prog Cardiovasc Dis 17:371-389, 1975

68. Hatcher CR, Miller JI: Operative injuries to nerves during intrathoracic procedures, p 363-365. In Cordell RA, Ellison RG, Eds: Complications of intrathoracic surgery. Little, Brown, Boston, 1979

69. Clausen EG: Postoperative paralysis of the brachial plexus. Surgery 12:933-942, 1942

70. Ewing MR: Postoperative paralysis in the upper extremity. Lancet I: 99-103, 1950

71. Britt BA, Gordon KA: Peripheral nerve injuries associated with anesthesia. Canad Anaest Soc J 11:514, 536, 1964

72. Miller RG, Camp PE: Postoperative ulnar neuropathy. JAMA 242:1636-1639, 1979

73. Jaffe TB, McLeskey CH: Position-induced Horner's syndrome. Anesthesiology 56:49–50, 1982

John B. Downs, M.D.

19
Postoperative Respiratory Care

Patients who require thoracotomy often have preexisting pulmonary disease, which, when combined with the operative procedure itself, is likely to result in significant pulmonary dysfunction, the leading cause of postoperative morbidity. This likely explains the vigor with which clinicians have developed, initiated, and sustained numerous respiratory care treatment regimens, often in spite of sparse evidence supporting their efficacy. This chapter will review several clinical considerations of post-thoracotomy respiratory care.

It is important to quantitate the degree of preoperative pulmonary insufficiency. Only with such information can attempts be made to restore and maintain the preoperative level of pulmonary function in the postoperative period. To achieve this goal, it is imperative that staff and equipment be utilized in an efficient manner. Patient-initiated, self-administered respiratory care techniques that create the least amount of patient discomfort should be employed. Tasks that utilize expensive ancillary equipment, that are time-consuming, or that cause patient discomfort are not necessarily beneficial.

Respiratory therapy often is directed at prevention and treatment of atelectasis, the most common postoperative complication. Arterial hypoxemia, a reduction in arterial oxygen tension, is secondary to pulmonary venous admixture and is present to some degree in all patients who undergo thoracotomy. Successful prevention and treatment of arterial hypoxemia may be approached from several radically different directions, aspects of which will be discussed. Post-thoracotomy pleural drainage frequently is poorly understood by paramedical personnel, house officers, and, occasionally, staff surgeons. Such misunderstanding may cause life-threatening complications. A myriad of drugs aimed at altering postoperative respiratory function may be administered both topically and systemically with varying degrees of success. The rationale for use of several of these drugs will be discussed. Finally, the decision whether or not to reintubate the trachea remains subjective and emotional. All these considerations are important to the successful care of patients who undergo operative procedures involving the thorax. A physiologic approach to the prophylaxis and treatment of such patients is likely to result in the most efficient utilization of equipment and personnel. In addition, such an approach is likely to result in patient cooperation and therapeutic benefits.

PREVENTION AND TREATMENT OF POSTOPERATIVE PULMONARY COMPLICATIONS WITH EMPHASIS ON ATELECTASIS

Individuals who have significant preoperative pulmonary dysfunction have an increased incidence of postoperative pulmonary insufficiency. Therefore, an accurate preoperative history and physical examination are necessary to identify such patients. When indicated, laboratory data should be obtained to provide supporting information. When patients with significant pulmonary dysfunction are identified preoperatively, an effective prophylactic regimen should be instituted. Such practice may decrease postoperative morbidity and mortality.[1]

Atelectasis, the most significant cause of postoperative morbidity, has been reported to occur in up to 84 percent of patients undergoing cardiopulmonary bypass for operative procedures on the heart and in 100 percent of patients undergoing thoracotomy for pulmonary resection. There is some disagreement concerning the frequency with which the left and right lungs are affected, but there is general agreement that atelectasis occurs more frequently in the basal lobes than in the middle and apical lung regions. Although some authors have attempted to correlate intraoperative fluid administration with the incidence of atelectasis, it is most commonly believed that restriction of normal respiratory effort secondary to pain, intrathoracic blood and fluid accumulation, and decreased lung compliance lead to rapid, shallow, and constant tidal volumes. Such a respiratory pattern may cause small airway closure and obstruction with inspissated mucus, both of which result in resorption of alveolar air and terminal airway collapse.

Diagnosis of atelectasis may be confirmed by chest roentgenograms, clinical findings, and arterial blood analysis for oxygen tension. However, there is a low positive correlation among these three methods. The reported incidence of atelectasis, therefore, may vary considerably, depending upon the criteria utilized for diagnosis. Patients who undergo thoracotomy have a significant reduction in arterial oxygen tension. Clinical signs of atelectasis, such as increased respiratory rate, decreased tidal volume, increased body temperature, and increased heart rate, may be absent. Even though clinical, roentgenographic, and laboratory evidence of atelectasis may not agree, removal of airway obstruction will lead to resolution of all symptoms of atelectasis in many cases. In contrast, symptomatic treatment, such as administration of antibiotics, which may prevent the increase in body temperature, will not improve the roentgenographic picture and will not relieve arterial hypoxemia. Similarly, administration of oxygen may improve the arterial oxygen tension but may promote the loss of lung volume and cause deterioration of the roentgenographic picture. A chest roentgenogram obtained during deep inspiration may show resolution of atelectasis, but a return to normal shallow tidal breathing will rapidly cause recollapse, arterial hypoxemia, and clinical signs of atelectasis. Only when therapy is directed at the underlying problem will complete resolution be obtained. Successful prophylaxis and treatment of postoperative respiratory problems require an understanding of the disease process and treatment regimens. Therefore, consideration will be given to the physiology of respiration, airway collapse, and airway reexpansion.

Atelectasis, or loss of expiratory lung volume, can be resolved only if there is an increase in the resting lung volume, that is, an increase in functional residual capacity (FRC). Inflation of the lung is dependent upon only two variables: (1) lung compliance (C_L); and (2) the distending pressure across the lung or the transpulmonary pressure (P_L), which is the difference between airway and intrapleural pressures (Fig. 19-1). Any change in lung volume must equal the product of C_L and ΔP_L. Therefore, an increase in FRC can occur only if there is an increase in

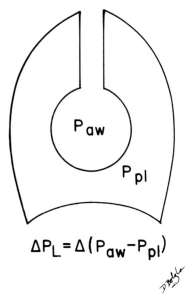

$$\Delta P_L = \Delta (P_{aw} - P_{pl})$$

Fig. 19-1 Lung volume is directly proportional to the difference between airway pressure (Paw) and intrapleural pressure (Ppl), which is defined as the transpulmonary pressure (PL).

P_L, an increase in C_L, or both. In evaluating any therapeutic maneuver, the clinician should question the ability of the maneuver to increase either of these two variables. Similarly, potentially undesirable side effects may be predicted following analysis of the effects of a maneuver on P_L and C_L.

It is extremely important that the reader avoid the common error of equating transpulmonary pressure with airway pressure. For example, increasing airway pressure to 50 cm H_2O with a mechanical ventilator will increase lung volume; whereas an increase in airway pressure to 50 cm H_2O during a cough or use of a blow bottle system will cause a marked decrease in lung volume. By considering the change in intrapleural pressure, the effect of each maneuver on lung volume is easily explained. Mechanical ventilation will raise airway pressure and, to a lesser extent, intrapleural pressure; therefore, it will also increase transpulmonary pressure. Forced expiratory maneuvers, such as coughing and use of blow bottles, cause intrapleural pressure to increase to a greater

extent than airway pressure, so that transpulmonary pressure and lung volume must decrease. The effects of respiratory equipment and maneuvers on lung compliance and on airway, intrapleural, and transpulmonary pressures must be considered in order to assess their physiologic effects. The following sections examine some of the maneuvers and devices suggested for the prevention and treatment of postoperative atelectasis.

Prolonged Postoperative Endotracheal Intubation and "Prophylactic" Mechanical Ventilation

The advent of extracorporeal blood oxygenators during the late 1950s and early 1960s to sustain life for complex operative procedures on the heart led to the widespread belief that postoperative mechanical ventilatory support for 1 to 2 days was a safe and desirable procedure to reduce metabolic demands in the early postoperative period. Such beliefs, although widely held, were not based on the findings of well-controlled prospective investigations. Recent information suggests that the practice is fraught with complications. An endotracheal tube renders the glottis incompetent, making an effective cough nearly impossible. Even a sterile suctioning procedure induces a degree of mucosal trauma, which may set the stage for pulmonary infection. Reflex airway closure may occur, causing widespread loss of lung volume and atelectasis. Also, sedation, which may be required to aid the patient's tolerance of the endotracheal tube and mechanical ventilator, will cause respiratory depression.

Current practice in many institutions dictates that the patient's trachea be extubated as soon as possible following all types of operations in order to reduce the need for narcotics and sedation, to reduce the risk of tracheal contamination and trauma, and to allow better humidification of inspired gases by the patient's natural airway. Occasionally, a postoperative patient may have a significant reduction in body temperature. In this instance, inspired gas may be heated to 40° C and humidified to 100 percent, allowing the lungs to act as a heat sink to effectively increase body temperature. This remains a valid indication for prolonged postoperative endotracheal intubation.

Pain Relief

For years surgeons have recognized the need for adequate postoperative pain control in order to ensure adequate respiratory effort. Many have suggested that vigorous chest physiotherapy, deep breathing exercises, and coughing be encouraged only after administration of systemic analgesic agents. More than 30 years ago, Burford recommended that intercostal nerve blocks be utilized to control pain in patients with thoracic trauma in order to prevent compromise of respiratory function.[2] Subsequent investigators have documented a marked decrease in respiratory function secondary to post-thoracotomy pain which may last up to 2 weeks. Administration of narcotic analgesic drugs may improve pulmonary function slightly, but 50 mg of meperidine has been found to be relatively ineffective in allowing patients to increase their coughing pressure. Therefore, many clinicians have suggested that intercostal nerve blocks be performed prior to, during, or following thoracotomy. Some authors have documented a marked decrease in requirement for systemic pain medication in the immediate postoperative period and others have claimed a decrease in required length of hospital stay. Although there is little doubt that pain may be decreased following intercostal nerve blockade, some authors have expressed a fear that bilateral intercostal nerve blockade may decrease cough effectiveness.

Injection of local anesthetic agents into the epidural space appears to be an efficient and effective means of decreasing postoperative pain and improving pulmonary function. Many studies have documented a marked increase in FRC and vital capacity when epidural analgesia is utilized in the postoperative period. Recently, injection of 2 to 10 mg of preservative-free morphine sulfate into the epidural space has produced marked decreases in thoracotomy pain. Vital capacity and expiratory flow rates are significantly increased, so that cough effectiveness is improved following epidural morphine injection. Since patients have a decreased level of pain but are without significant systemic depressing effects of morphine, they are more mobile and should have improvement in pulmonary function secondary to early ambulation. The technique appears to be safe, with only a few reports of respiratory depression following epidural morphine injection. Each injection produces significant pain relief for 16 to 24 hours; therefore, the technique is more efficient for producing postoperative pain relief than other methods. The technique must be considered experimental at this time, but it is likely that it will be available generally in the near future, since effective pain relief without respiratory depression is the ideal goal.

Positioning

It has been realized by pulmonary physiologists that changes in body position alter the distribution of gas within the lungs during inspiration. For example, dependent lung regions receive the majority of gas flow during inspiration; similarly, gravity directs the preponderance of pulmonary blood flow to dependent lung regions. Therefore, ventilation and perfusion are relatively well matched in spontaneously breathing individuals. Knowledge of these effects may be utilized to explain various clinical observations and to promote resolution of some pathologic respiratory conditions. For example, the patient with atelectasis of the right lung will have a significant decrease in arterial blood oxygen tension. In the right lateral decubitus position, it would be anticipated that the arterial oxygen tension would be even lower, secondary to increased blood flow to areas of lung that are poorly ventilated. Placing the individual in the left lateral decubitus position might be expected to produce an increase in arterial oxygen tension. In addition, drainage of the collapsed right lung would be promoted. On the other hand, were the patient to be placed in a right lateral decubitus position, increased ventilation would be directed towards the collapsed right lung, promoting reexpansion. Depending upon the immediate goal, different positions might be encouraged. Piehl and Brown found that altering the position of five patients with severe respiratory distress, requiring high levels of positive end-expiratory pressure (PEEP), caused a significant increase in arterial oxygen tension.[3]

In a recent editorial, Al-Jurf questioned the efficacy of the time-honored cough.[4] He suggested that the cough is important only in promoting a precough deep breath and that frequent turning of the patient to alter regional ventilation, in combination with deep breathing to cause lung expansion, would be sufficient postoperative therapy in the majority of patients. As mentioned previously, assumption of the upright position by patients will allow the diaphragm to descend and lung volume to increase. Ultimately, matching of ventilation and perfusion will be improved.

Chest Physiotherapy

Physical therapy, or physiotherapy, is one of the oldest and best-accepted forms of therapy aimed at prevention and treatment of various pathologic respiratory conditions. Techniques include postural drainage, breathing exercises, vibration, deep breathing, coughing, and percussion. Most clinicians feel that chest physiotherapy is beneficial in spite of data insufficient to support the clinical impression.

Postural drainage depends greatly upon gravity for its beneficial effects. Although postural drainage often is ordered as routine postoperative treatment following thoracic operative procedures, there is little rationale for its use in patients who do not have difficulty with increased secretions or who have an effective cough mechanism. However, postural drainage is effective in aiding in the clearance of secretions of patients with severe chronic obstructive lung disease or in patients who have an ineffective cough following their operation. In patients who incur atelectasis secondary to retained secretions, postural drainage should be directed towards the affected segments (Fig. 19-2A through L). Often, postural drainage is combined with percussion, also known as *tapotement*. Recently, there have been conflicting reports regarding the efficacy of percussion in speeding the central movement of peripheral secretions.

The postoperative patient also may need assistance with coughing in the postoperative period. Pressure may be applied to specific chest regions in order to increase the expiratory flow of gas and thus assist the cough mechanism in moving secretions from the periphery. Application of hand pressure to the thoracic cage during exhalation is claimed to be particularly effective for removing peripherally-retained secretions in intubated patients who are receiving mechanical ventilatory support. Some clinicians feel that a vibratory movement may be added in order to free tenacious secretions. However, there is no critical evidence that vibration is of benefit.

As early as 1928, Sante realized that atelectasis may be more effectively treated by allowing the patient to lie on the affected side, thus increasing ventilation to the atelectatic lung.[5] It was Sante's feeling that this maneuver, combined with an effective cough, usually would be more effective than bronchoscopy for resolving atelectasis. Soon

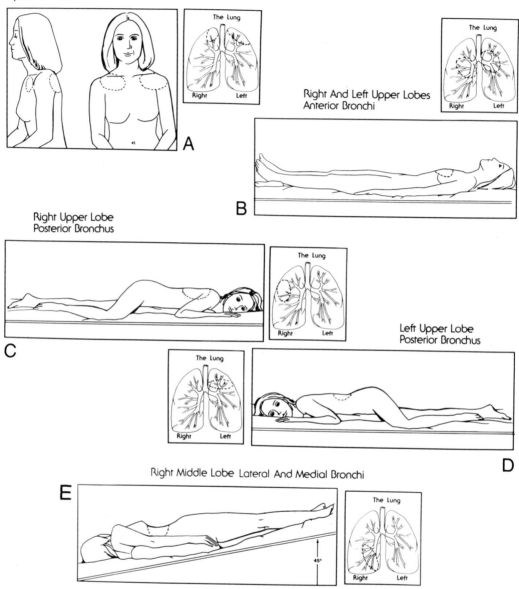

Fig. 19-2 Position requirements for postural drainage of various lung regions (drawings by Mark Friedman). (A) The patient sits upright and leans slightly backward with percussion anteriorly, then slightly forward with percussion posteriorly. (B) The patient lies on his back. (C) The patient lies on the left side with the right side of the body turned forward to an angle of about 45°. The bed is flat. A pillow is placed in the left armpit and under the left chest for support. (D) The patient lies on the right side with the left side of the body turned forward to an angle of about 45°. The bed is flat. The pillow is placed in the right armpit and under the right chest for support. (E) The patient under the shoulder to the right hip elevating the right side of the body slightly. The foot of the bed is elevated to approximate a 45° angle.

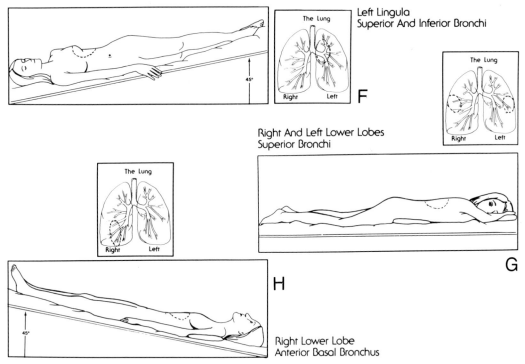

Fig. 19-2 (*continued*)   (F) The patient lies on his or her back. A pillow is placed under the left shoulder to the left hip elevating the left side of the body slightly. The foot of the bed is elevated to approximate a 45° angle. (G) The patient lies facing downward with a pillow under the abdomen in order to flex the trunk. The bed is flat. (H) The patient lies on his or her back turned slightly onto the left side. The foot of the bed is elevated to approximate a 45° angle.

thereafter Winifred Linton, the superintendent physiotherapist at Brompton Hospital, developed the previously discussed physiotherapeutic techniques for patients with chest diseases (Fig. 19-2A through L). Recently, some critical reviews have questioned the efficacy of chest physiotherapy in preventing or resolving atelectasis. However, Marini et al found that chest physiotherapy was as effective as fiberoptic bronchoscopy for this purpose.[6] Although there is likely to be no improvement in oxygenation following chest physiotherapy, there has been documented improvement in lung-thorax compliance, indicating expansion of previously nonventilated lung regions. Stein and Cassara found that application of chest physiotherapy to a group of "poor risk" patients during the pre- and postoperative period significantly re-

duced morbidity and mortality due to pulmonary complications.[1] Chest physiotherapy has been shown to be ineffective in patients who have pneumonia, but, this finding was not unexpected, since pneumonia usually does not cause retention of sputum and atelectasis.[7]

Literature reviewing the physiologic effects of chest physiotherapy is sparse. However, there is a general consensus that chest physiotherapy is beneficial in selected patients, especially those who have difficulty in clearing copious secretions. In other patients, chest physiotherapy appears to offer no benefit when compared with other, less time-consuming maneuvers, such as blow bottles and incentive spirometry. In view of the expense involved in supplying a chest physiotherapist to patients who require postoper-

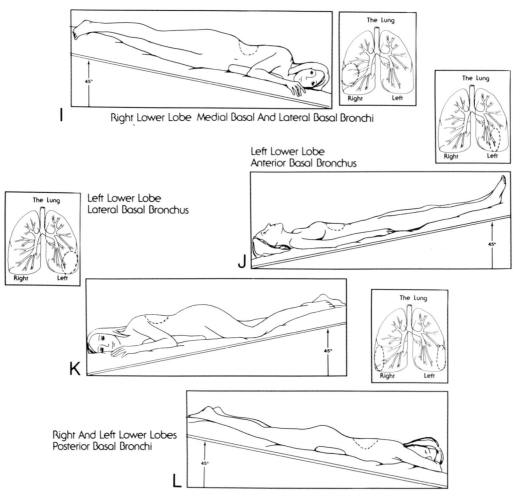

I — Right Lower Lobe Medial Basal And Lateral Basal Bronchi

Left Lower Lobe Anterior Basal Bronchus

Left Lower Lobe Lateral Basal Bronchus

J

K

Right And Left Lower Lobes Posterior Basal Bronchi

L

Fig. 19-2 (*continued*)   (1) The patient lies on the left side and hugs pillow. The foot of the bed is elevated to approximate a 45° angle (J) The patient lies on his or her back with the body turned slightly onto the right side. The foot of the bed is elevated to approximate a 45° angle. (K) The patient lies on the right side and hugs pillow. The foot of the bed is elevated to approximate a 45° angle. (L) The patient lies on his or her abdomen with pillow under hips. The foot of the bed is elevated to approximate a 45° angle or higher.

ative therapy, chest physiotherapy should be administered only to selected patients.

Transtracheal Catheterization

In 1960, Radigan and King suggested the percutaneous placement of a small polyethylene tube for instillation of irritant materials into the trachea.[8] They found that atelectasis then could be eliminated in their postoperative patients and suggested that all patients who undergo thoracotomy should have a transtracheal catheter inserted. Subsequent investigators have suggested injecting pancreatic dornase or mucolytic agents through a transtracheal catheter. However, few studies have documented the effectiveness of the technique. Injection of irritant materials through a transtracheal catheter will stimulate vigorous coughing for 24 to 48 hours. However, following that period of time, patients seem to grow tolerant of the injections and they become less effective.

With time, evidence of significant complications began to appear in the literature. Subcutaneous emphysema, pneumomediastinum, hemoptysis, paratracheal abscess, fatal dysrhythmia, hematoma, air emboli, bleeding, and aspiration pneumonitis all have been reported. In view of the significant complications that may occur and the lack of documented efficacy, transtracheal catheterization cannot be recommended as a routine postoperative procedure.

Tracheobronchial Suction

Occasionally, patients may be unable to clear secretions from their airways and may require endotracheal suction with a small-bore plastic catheter. This maneuver is performed to ensure adequate removal of secretions from large airways and to maintain airway patency. Several considerations are important for proper tracheobronchial suctioning. The procedure should be performed in a sterile manner in order to prevent contamination of the patient's airway, which may lead to antibiotic-resistant bacterial pneumonia in susceptible patients. After the procedure has been carefully explained to the patient, his head should be placed in a "sniffing" position and preoxygenation performed with any of the devices to be discussed later. A sterile glove is placed on the right hand, which is used to grasp a sterile, appropriately sized suction catheter. A light coating of sterile lubricant is placed on the distal third of the catheter, which is slowly advanced through the nose during inspiration. During exhalation, the vocal cords are more closely approximated, making advancement into the trachea less likely. Increasing loudness of breath sounds may be detected through the suction catheter as the tip approaches the larynx. If the catheter slips into the esophagus or coils in the oropharynx, breath sounds will diminish or disappear, which indicates that the catheter should be retracted slightly and readvanced.

Grasping the patient's tongue may prevent him from swallowing the catheter. Once the catheter is in place, humidity will be seen to precipitate within the tube during exhalation and will clear during subsequent inspiration. Vigorous coughing may be stimulated by advancing the catheter into the oropharynx. Therefore, gagging and coughing cannot be used as definitive signs of proper placement of the suction catheter. Once proper position of the suction catheter is verified, oxygen tubing should be connected to the proximal end of the catheter and oxygen should be administered to the patient at a rate of 2 to 5 L/min in order to continue preoxygenation.

Following 2 to 5 minutes of preoxygenation, intermittent suction should be applied to the catheter, which may be alternately advanced and withdrawn 1 to 2 inches. If this is not productive of sputum, consideration should be given to injection of 5 ml of sterile normal saline into the suction catheter in order to stimulate coughing and central movement of secretions. Suction should be applied to the catheter intermittently; it should not be applied continuously for more than 10 seconds, as to do so might cause a decrease in lung volume and severe arterial hypoxemia. It has been suggested that the clinician exhale and hold his breath while applying suction to the patient's trachea. The sensation of dyspnea will indicate when the procedure should be terminated.

A similar procedure is employed for endotracheal suctioning through an endotracheal tube. When an endotracheal tube is in place, preoxygenation of the patient may proceed more rapidly. If the patient is breathing spontaneously, the inspired oxygen should be increased to 80 to 100 percent for 2 to 5 minutes. A sterile suction catheter then should be advanced through the endotracheal tube and suction applied intermittently. Lavage with 5 ml of sterile normal saline may be performed during the period of preoxygenation. In patients who are receiving mechanical ventilatory support, the rate of the mechanical ventilator should be adjusted to 10 to 12 breaths per minute and the fractional concentration of inspired oxygen increased to 0.8 to 1.0. Following 2 to 5 minutes of preoxygenation and ventilation, suctioning may proceed. Some clinicians have advocated that manual compression of a 5-L anesthesia bag with a continuous flow of oxygen be used to provide positive pressure breaths with a high inspired oxygen concentration. Such systems are readily contaminated and have no documented beneficial effects that cannot be duplicated by the patient's mechanical ventilator. Also, some patients may not require large-tidal-volume mechanical ventilation with high inspired oxygen concentrations for preoxygenation. For example, patients with severe chronic obstructive lung disease may require only a moderate increase in inspired oxygen concentration and ventilator rate prior to the suctioning procedure.

Haight described the use of nasotracheal suctioning in the management of postoperative atelectasis in 1938.[9] Since that time, the procedure has been extremely popular among clinicians in order to stimulate deep breathing and coughing. Some investigators have suggested that it be performed routinely at least once in order to use the technique as an ongoing threat to the less cooperative patient. Thus, the procedure has been suggested as punitive as well as therapeutic. Many investigators have suggested different maneuvers in order to ensure entry by the catheter into the left main-stem bronchus. Recent investigations have suggested that turning the head to the opposite side or using the contralateral nostril will not increase the success rate of left main-stem catheterization. It is likely that the best way to ensure a left main-stem bronchus cannulation is to use a catheter with a curved tip with the patient in a left lateral decubitus position. A fiberoptic bronchoscope may be utilized to ensure that the left lung is suctioned if it is important to aspirate secretions from the left main-stem bronchus.

Sackner suggested that endotracheal suction may produce significant mucosal trauma, which subsequently may act as a nidus for infection.[10] He claimed that catheter design is one of the major offending problems in producing mucosal damage. In a later article, Jung and Gottlieb suggested that mucosal damage did not occur secondary to catheter design fault; rather, it was secondary to repetition, vigor, and amount of applied suction.[11] Regardless of the immediate etiology, it is evident that endotracheal suction may cause significant mucosal damage, may cause contamination of the patient's airway, and therefore may cause morbidity. Vigorous suctioning also has been shown to cause a significant reduction in lung volume, especially in infants, severe arterial hypoxemia secondary to deoxygenation of the lung, and severe cardiac dysrhythmias in a high percentage of patients when preoxygenation is not employed. Many of these complications may not be readily reversible. For example, the loss of lung volume following suctioning in infants may take 30 minutes to 1 hour to resolve. Because of the potential risks of nasotracheal suction and the largely undocumented potential benefits, some authors feel that the technique never should be applied. It is this author's feeling that nasotracheal suction may be indicated on occasion but that other methods are more likely to produce beneficial results with less risk of complications.

Bronchoscopy

Some authors have suggested that bronchoscopy be performed immediately after thoracotomy in any patient with roentgenographic evidence of atelectasis. This will ensure the absence of any occluding foreign body and will allow removal of any obstruction. The hypoxemic individual is likely to suffer progressive arterial hypoxemia during the procedure; therefore, the clinician should be prepared to ventilate the patient with a high inspired oxygen concentration. Frequently, anesthesia personnel are requested to stand by for the procedure to provide such assistance. It should be kept in mind that bronchoscopy is effective at removing only secretions found in the large airways. Peripheral secretions are not obtainable with a bronchoscope. Furthermore, bronchoscopy is almost always unpleasant for the patient, is time-consuming for the clinician, and therefore, cannot be repeated frequently.

Some authors have suggested that fiberoptic bronchoscopy is less traumatic for the patient and less likely to cause a decrease in arterial oxygen tension than nasotracheal suction; and it also allows aspiration of secretions from distal lung regions. However, ventilation during fiberoptic bronchoscopy is more difficult than during rigid bronchoscopy. Although there is some debate concerning the ability of fiberoptic bronchoscopy to cause resolution of atelectasis, there are sufficient reports which document the efficacy of this technique, indicating that fiberoptic bronchoscopy must be considered to be beneficial for a large percentage of patients with atelectasis.

Following aspiration of secretions through a rigid bronchoscope, positive airway pressure may be applied in order to promote reinflation of a collapsed lung. In 1974, Bowen et al described the use of a rigid bronchoscope with a balloon cuff at its distal end and manual compression of an anesthesia bag for generation of positive pressure.[12] Thus, increased airway pressures could be applied to specific areas of lung to encourage reexpansion. Several years later Millen and his colleagues described the use of a balloon-tipped fiberoptic bronchoscope to accomplish the same result.[13] Thus, although there is some disagreement, it is clear that bronchoscopy will provide a controlled means of aspirating secretions from the airway and will permit application of positive pressure to specific regions of the lung to promote lung inflation. When conservative respiratory therapy techniques fail, fiberoptic or rigid bronchoscopy should be utilized.

Sustained Inflation

During thoracotomy, sustained hyperinflation of the lung is manually accomplished by vigorous compression of the anesthesia reservoir bag. All surgeons and anesthesiologists have observed recruitment of collapsed lung units, which may occur during a 5- to 10-second period of sustained lung inflation. Surprisingly, this treatment has not been routinely applied in the postoperative period. It is likely that the difficulty of placing an endotracheal tube in the awake, tachypneic, agitated, and uncooperative postoperative patient with atelectasis is responsible for the lack of popularity of this technique.

Commonly, pediatric patients who have undergone thoracotomy and who have recurrent right upper lobe atelectasis may benefit from periodic endotracheal intubation for application of positive airway pressure, immediately followed by tracheal extubation. Unfortunately, the psychologic and physiologic trauma to the patient and the time required by the clinician are factors that are likely to prevent routine application of this treatment modality.

Rebreathing

In the past, some clinicians have recommended that patients be instructed to rebreathe exhaled gas from a reservoir. By so doing, in effect the patient will have an increase in physiologic dead space and will require an increase in minute ventilation in order to maintain a normal arterial carbon dioxide tension. Thus, deep and rapid breathing may be promoted. Although early investigations suggested a beneficial effect of such therapy, it is now realized that significant arterial hypoxemia may occur during rebreathing. Most patients who are able to cooperate for rebreathing treatments should be able to take and sustain a deep breath, a maneuver which should produce the same beneficial effect. Therefore, rebreathing of exhaled gas can no longer be recommended.

Blow Bottles

Decades ago clinicians felt that forced exhalation against a resistance would create an increase in airway pressure and cause inflation of the lung. Thus, water-filled bottles with submerged tubing were designed and patients were instructed to blow vigorously into a water-filled bottle in order to displace fluid into a second bottle. Once accomplished, the task was to be repeated several times. Several investigators found the use of blow bottles to be associated with an increase in FRC. Since blow bottles are cheaper than many other forms of respiratory therapy, they have been advocated and widely applied, especially in thoracic surgical services. Recently, Bartlett et al suggested that blow bottles are useful only because of the deep inspiration preceding the forced exhalation and are less efficient than incentive spirometry.[14] Nunn et al found that vigorous forced exhalation caused a significant decrease in arterial oxygen tension, and this effect was even more significant when oxygen was added to the inspired air.[15] Physiologically, a forced exhalation will decrease expiratory transpulmonary pressure and lung volume, which suggests that blow bottles should be avoided in postoperative patients. Not only is the maneuver fatiguing, but it may have a detrimental effect on pulmonary blood flow, cardiac output, FRC, and arterial oxygen tension. If there is any benefit from blow bottles, it likely is secondary to the deep breath that must precede the forced expiratory maneuver.

Intermittent Positive Pressure Breathing (IPPB)

For more than three decades, intermittent positive pressure breathing has been used for the prevention and treatment of postoperative atelectasis. Surprisingly, few if any studies have established the benefits of this form of therapy, and the results of numerous studies have been negative. Advocates of IPPB state that such investigations failed to provide proper administration techniques, equipment, etc.; opponents claim that IPPB is used primarily because of the financial rewards attendant on its application. As stated by Gold, "... the overwhelming evidence against IPPB therapy in the surgical patient calls for its abandonment and the substitution of other (less harmful and expensive) approaches...."[16] Since chest physiotherapy, incentive spirometry, blow bottles, and standard conservative respiratory therapy are less expensive in terms of equipment and personnel than IPPB, most authors agree with Gold and have recommended discontinuation of IPPB.

There is general agreement that for IPPB to be effective, adequate volumes must be delivered to the patient's lungs. Recent investigations reporting beneficial effects of IPPB have utilized higher peak inflation pressures, sustained inspiratory airway pressures, and greater inspired volumes than earlier investigations. Currently, it is recommended that if IPPB is used, it should be volume-limited rather than pressure-limited, as is common in practice. Thus, IPPB should be administered to a preset tidal volume rather than to a preset airway pressure.

In addition, several investigations have indicated that IPPB may produce harmful side effects. Iverson et al found that patients who received IPPB therapy had an increased incidence of pulmonary complications (30 percent) compared with a similar group of patients who received incentive spirometry or blow bottle therapy (16 and 9 percent, respectively).[17] Browner and Powers found that postoperative patients receiving IPPB experienced a significant subsequent fall in FRC; Lareau, Wright, and Shim each observed a significant fall in PaO_2 following IPPB.[18-21] The observations of Paul et al may explain the decrease in FRC and PaO_2 observed following IPPB.[22] Patients who underwent major thoracic operative procedures each had a pleural catheter inserted in the right hemithorax. Postoperatively, each patient had expiratory transpulmonary pressure measured during and following 15 minutes of IPPB. Each patient was observed to hyperventilate during treatment and to hypoventilate following treatment. During hypoventilation following IPPB, the expiratory transpulmonary pressure decreased in each patient. Presumably, hypoventilation was accompanied by absorption of oxygen from small airways, resulting in a decrease in FRC and a significant fall in PaO_2.

Since even properly administered IPPB with large tidal volumes may result in hyperventilation and associated ill effects, it may be contraindicated for the majority of postoperative patients. A conservative recommendation would be to apply IPPB only to patients who cannot generate an inspiratory transpulmonary pressure of sufficient magnitude to significantly increase lung volume, who require assistance in the clearance of secretions, and who require delivery of topical medications. Certainly IPPB should not be applied routinely to postoperative patients.

Incentive Spirometry

In 1966, Ward et al suggested that a prolonged deep breath is the most efficient way for postoperative patients to prevent and reduce atelectasis.[23] These authors equated this maneuver with a sigh or yawn. Subsequently, Bartlett and his colleagues described a device to encourage such activity.[24] Their incentive spirometer has become the most widely utilized postoperative respiratory care device in the United States. Several other investigators have performed prospective comparisons of incentive spirometers with IPPB, blow bottles, chest physiotherapy, and other maneuvers and have found that incentive spirometry is associated with a lower complication rate and less atelectasis than other treatment regimens. Several investigators have found that patients who have a de-

creased FRC and arterial hypoxemia, presumably secondary to ventilation-perfusion mismatching, will experience a significant increase in PaO_2 following several deep breath maneuvers. Similarly, some investigators have found a reduction in atelectasis as diagnosed by chest roentgenogram following incentive spirometry. Bartlett performed a prospective investigation in patients who had undergone thoracotomy and provided the first sound physiologic basis for incentive spirometry.[24] He was able to show that the deep-breath maneuver created an increase in *inspiratory* transpulmonary pressure, indicating an increase in lung volume. Similar measurements during IPPB failed to reveal a significant increase in transpulmonary pressure, which indicated lack of a deep breath during IPPB. Based on these results, incentive spirometry has become more popular than IPPB for the prevention and treatment of postoperative atelectasis. It is important to note that Bartlett failed to report *expiratory* transpulmonary pressures during either IPPB or incentive spirometry. Therefore it was not possible to determine whether or not an increase in FRC was likely to have occurred in his patients. It has rather been assumed that a large inhaled volume will cause expansion of an atelectatic lung and that the expanded areas will remain open. Although this is a reasonable assumption, it represents the same presumptive thinking that led to the popularity of IPPB during the last two decades and it may not be correct. Future studies should be directed toward resolution of this question.

Since the introduction of the incentive spirometer, several different types of devices have been developed. Originally, the incentive spirometer required the patient to inhale deeply and sustain the inhalation for several seconds. A breath counter was incorporated into the design of the spirometer so that the clinician could ensure patient cooperation.

Recently devices have been introduced which do not require that a preset inhaled volume be taken and do not ensure that the deep breath will be sustained. Many devices

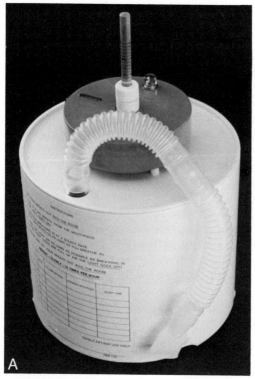
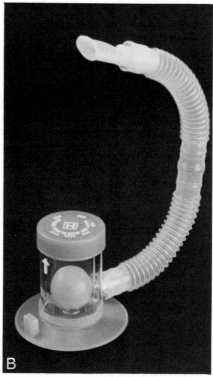

Fig. 19-3 (A) A volumetric incentive spirometer with volume indicator and counter. (B) A flow rate–sensitive incentive spirometer.

encourage a rapid inspiratory flow rate rather than a large inhaled volume. These devices technically are simpler and less expensive than volume-directed devices (Fig. 19-3A and B). Lederer et al compared three currently-used devices and found no significant difference in their effects.[25] It is difficult to determine from available evidence whether or not measurement of the inhaled volume is necessary or desirable. However, it is likely that devices designed to ensure a large inspired volume are preferable.

Several investigations have failed to find a beneficial effect of incentive spirometry. It is likely that uncooperative patients or patients who are experiencing significant postoperative pain will not cooperate to perform a deep-breath maneuver. In such instances, it is foolish to expect that a bedside device will prevent atelectasis. Similarly, if patients are not given adequate instruction or if they

misuse the device, it is unlikely that the device will be effective. Although some patients may be self-motivated sufficiently to not require supervision at all times, many will require immediate bedside attention. In such instances, incentive spirometry will be no more economical than IPPB or other respiratory care devices and maneuvers.

Continuous Positive Airway Pressure (CPAP)

As stated earlier, the goal in the treatment of atelectasis is to increase the FRC of the lung and to prevent small airway collapse. Such an increase in lung volume can occur only if there is an increase in lung compliance or an increase in expiratory transpulmonary pressure. It is unlikely that any respiratory therapy maneuver will directly increase lung compliance. Therefore, an increase in FRC is most likely to occur following an increase in expiratory transpulmonary pressure. Clinically it is possible to increase transpulmonary pressure in two ways. Whenever airway pressure remains constant, a decline in intrapleural pressure will cause an increase in transpulmonary pressure and an increase in lung volume. A decrease in expiratory intrapleural pressure may be created by relieving abdominal distension, by reducing tension in abdominal and thoracic musculature, and by having patients assume a more upright position, causing abdominal contents to provide traction on the diaphragm.

Surgeons have known for decades that assumption of the upright position often causes improvement in postoperative pulmonary function. For that reason, early postoperative ambulation is a goal of most surgeons. Unfortunately, patients who undergo thoracotomy may not tolerate immediate ambulation postoperatively. In such patients, other means of preventing pulmonary complications must be provided. Application of positive pressure to the airway will cause intrapleural pressure to increase, but to a lesser extent than the increase in airway pressure. Therefore, transpulmonary pressure will increase as will lung volume. This, of course, is the rationale for IPPB. During IPPB the lung will sustain an increase in volume only during the inspiratory phase of the respiratory cycle. If an individual is assumed to inhale for 1 second and to do so 12 times per minute, he will spend 80 percent of the respiratory cycle in exhalation, during which there is no significant increase in airway pressure. Therefore, if there is an increase in FRC, it must be secondary to a residual effect of positive pressure applied during inspiration. Since the goal is to increase *expiratory* lung volume, a more logical approach would be to apply positive pressure to the airway during the expiratory phase of respiration. As a result, expiratory transpulmonary pressure will be increased, as will FRC.

Application of positive end-expiratory pressure (PEEP) to the ventilatory pattern of patients with the adult respiratory distress syndrome (ARDS) who require mechanical ventilatory support has been commonly employed for many years. Continuous application of positive pressure to the airway of spontaneously breathing patients throughout the respiratory cycle (CPAP) was practiced in the 1930s and 1940s for the treatment of congestive heart failure and "traumatic wet lung" and recently has been utilized in infants with idiopathic respiratory distress syndrome, as well as in some adults with the ARDS.[2] However, CPAP has not been commonly employed to prevent atelectasis in postoperative patients. Physiologically, this would seem a most reasonable approach to the prevention of atelectasis. Using methodology similar to that described by Bartlett, Paul and Downs measured transpulmonary pressure of patients who underwent aortocoronary bypass grafting.[22,26] Expiratory transpulmonary pressure was measured before, during, and every 5 minutes after treatment with an incentive spirometer, IPPB, or CPAP applied with a face mask. They found that IPPB and CPAP both increased expiratory transpulmonary pressure during treatment. Because of pain, patients refused to inhale deeply during incentive spirometry and expiratory transpulmonary pressure was not increased, even during treatment. Following IPPB, there was a significant decrease in expiratory transpulmonary pressure. Presumably, this was secondary to a period of hypoventilation following treatment. Following CPAP there was a significant decrease in expiratory transpulmonary pressure, but it remained above baseline levels for the ensuing 30 minutes. Not surprisingly, there was no significant alteration in expiratory transpulmonary pressure following incentive spirometry. In a similar group of patients, Downs and Mitchell determined that 6 cm H_2O CPAP was required to maintain FRC at preoperative levels.[27] Fowler et al reported data from four patients who had atelectasis unresponsive to chest physiotherapy, tracheobronchial suction, and fiberoptic bronchoscopy, and in whom 5 to 15 cm H_2O PEEP was effective in causing resolution of atelectasis in all patients in 24 hours or less.[28] Other similar cases have been reported.

Early reports expressed fear that continuous application of positive pressure to the airway might force distal migration of secretions and worsen atelectasis secondary to small airway obstruction. However, recent evidence suggests that collateral channels to ventilation may be recruited during application of CPAP, causing inflation of previously unventilated lung regions.[29] If so, positive pressure distal to small airway obstruction may cause central migration of offending secretions and improvement in pulmonary function.

CPAP applied by face mask was originally decribed by Barach in the mid-1930s. Subsequently, CPAP was applied clinically during the next two decades. However, this form of treatment fell into disuse as a result of facial trauma induced by hard-rubber, ill-fitting face masks, fear of gastric distension, vomiting, aspiration, and poor understanding of the dangers of endotracheal intubation. Greenbaum et al utilized a transparent, cushioned mask to treat 14 patients with significant arterial hypoxemia with up to 14 cm H_2O CPAP.[30] For eight patients endotracheal intubation was avoided. Subsequent to this report in 1976, many patients have been treated with CPAP without significant complications, and endotracheal intubation has been avoided. Recently, Andersen et al applied an average of 15 cm H_2O CPAP and chest physiotherapy with postural drainage to a group of postsurgical patients with atelectasis.[31] CPAP was applied once an hour for 25 to 35 respirations with the highest tolerable airway pressure, and within 12 hours most patients had improved dramatically. In contrast, a control group who received chest physiotherapy, postural drainage, and endotracheal suction had insignificant resolution of atelectasis. These authors concluded that

CPAP applied with a face mask could be used to treat atelectasis. There is uniform agreement that when CPAP is applied with a mask, the clinician must ensure that gastric distension, regurgitation, and aspiration do not occur. In addition, proper equipment must be utilized, including a soft, self-sealing face mask which will not induce facial trauma.

Presently, CPAP applied continuously, or periodically, appears to be the most physiologically sound approach to the prevention and treatment of postoperative atelectasis. The technique requires little patient cooperation and will not induce fatigue, as will many other respiratory therapy techniques. In fact, CPAP may be applied to the sleeping patient, unlike any other noninvasive form of respiratory therapy. Further prospective evaluation of this technique will be required, but preliminary investigations indicate greater efficacy for face-mask CPAP than for other forms of treatment.

PREVENTION AND TREATMENT OF POSTOPERATIVE HYPOXEMIA

It is not the purpose of this section to discuss in detail the physiology of postoperative oxygenation. However, some basic principles must be covered in order to arrive at a rational treatment plan for the postoperative patient. Too frequently a low arterial oxygen tension is presumed to be secondary only to right-to-left intrapulmonary shunting of blood. Although this is a frequent cause of deficient arterial oxygenation, it is by no means the only major factor. Frequently, patients who require thoracotomy have preexisting pulmonary disease, with areas of lung with low but finite ventilation/perfusion ratios. Most patients with severe chronic obstructive lung disease have a low arterial oxygen tension for this reason, and not because of significant fibrotic lung disease, which may produce low arterial oxygenation by causing a diffusion block to oxygen transfer from the alveolar space to the pulmonary capillary blood. However, all three mechanisms may explain the presence of inadequately oxygenated blood in the arterial circulation of some patients. That is, venous blood may pass through the lung without becoming fully oxygenated, which is the so-called venous admixture. Whether inadequate oxygenation of arterial blood occurs because of a diffusion defect, low but finite ventilation/perfusion ratio, or absolute right-to-left intrapulmonary shunting of blood, other variables may also have a significant influence on the ultimate arterial oxygen tension. For example, either an increase in oxygen consumption secondary to a marked increase in metabolic rate or a decrease in cardiac output may cause returning venous blood to have a decreased oxygen content. When venous oxygen saturation is low, arterial blood will have a much lower oxygen tension than might be explained on a basis of venous admixture alone. Similarly, a low hemoglobin concentration will result in a decrease in mixed-venous oxygen saturation and amplification of arterial hypoxemia.

Such factors must be considered in evaluating the patient with arterial hypoxemia; otherwise, inappropriate therapy may be instituted. For example, a patient with a low cardiac output secondary to intravascular hypovolemia may be hypoxemic in the absence of elevated levels of intrapulmonary shunting of blood. Application of PEEP and/or vigorous diuresis in an attempt to improve arterial oxygenation could impede thoracic venous inflow of blood, resulting in further depression of cardiac output and thereby further deterioration of systemic oxygenation. Because the arterial oxygen tension is so greatly dependent on the arterial-venous oxygen content difference, it is imperative that mixed-venous oxygen content and saturation be evaluated in patients with significant arterial hypoxemia in the postoperative period. In the absence of any clinical evidence to indicate deficient cardiac output or increased metabolic rate, a decrease in ar-

terial oxygen tension may be considered to be secondary to venous admixture. However, if there is any doubt, a pulmonary artery catheter should be inserted and a mixed-venous blood sample obtained for analysis. Assumption of a fixed arterial-venous oxygen content difference in calculating right-to-left intrapulmonary shunting of blood is likely to lead to significant error in a large portion of postoperative thoracic surgical patients and therefore is not recommended.[32] This is especially the case in patients who have undergone cardiopulmonary bypass procedures, in whom a low cardiac output, decreased hemoglobin concentration, and increased oxygen consumption are likely to occur.

Evaluation of arterial oxygenation is complicated further by the effect of the inspired oxygen concentration on venous admixture and calculated right-to-left intrapulmonary shunting of blood (Fig. 19-4). For example, individuals with low but finite ventilation/perfusion ratios will have significant arterial hypoxemia when breathing room air. It is not unusual for individuals with severe chronic obstructive lung disease to have arterial oxygen tensions between 40 and 50 mmHg. However, when the inspired oxygen concentration is elevated slightly, there is a dramatic increase in arterial oxygen tension. When right-to-left intrapulmonary shunting of blood is calculated before and after administration of oxygen, a dramatic decrease in the calculated shunt fraction secondary to a masking effect of oxygen on low but finite ventilation/perfusion ratios is observed. The same effect will occur when a diffusion defect contributes to arterial hypoxemia.

It has long been felt that oxygen has little or no effect on absolute right-to-left intrapulmonary shunting of blood. However, recent investigations have disclosed a significant increase in right-to-left intrapulmonary shunting of blood when high inspired oxygen concentrations are administered.[33] Although several mechanisms have been postulated in an attempt to explain this

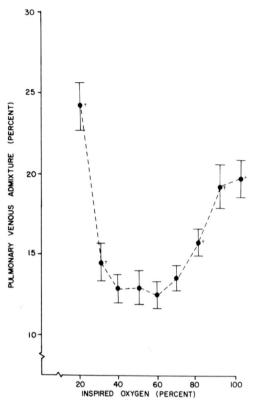

Fig. 19-4 Calculated pulmonary venous admixture depends greatly upon the fractional concentration of inspired oxygen (FIO$_2$). When FIO$_2$ is low, venous admixture may be elevated as a result of ventilation-to-perfusion mismatching, diffusion impairment, and right-to-left intrapulmonary shunting of blood. When the FIO$_2$ is increased, venous admixture is greater, owing to increased intrapulmonary shunting of blood. († = significantly greater than at FIO$_2$ = 0.5.)

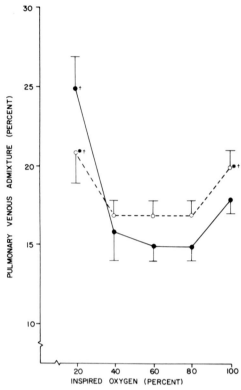

Fig. 19-5 Pretreatment with steroids may decrease venous admixture when inspired oxygen is low. However, an elevated FIO$_2$ may cause increased right-to-left intrapulmonary shunting of blood following administration of steroids. (Steroids = o - - - o; placebo = ●——●.) (Reproduced from Douglas ME, Downs JB, Shook D: Response of pulmonary venous admixture: a means of comparing therapies? Chest 77:764–770, 1980.)

observation, it is likely that high inspired oxygen concentrations will lead to rapid resorption of gas from terminal airways in areas of lung with low but finite ventilation/perfusion ratios. This phenomenon has been termed *absorption atelectasis* and was described by Lansing and Jamieson in 1963.[34] Subsequent investigators have observed significant atelectasis when 100 percent oxygen is inspired. It is likely that the presence of nitrogen in the inspired gas will prevent this effect, but application of positive pressure to the airway, even to 25 cm H$_2$O, is

unlikely to prevent it. Therefore, the prevalent opinion that high inspired oxygen concentrations may be safely utilized for up to 24 hours because they may not cause oxygen toxicity should be considered inaccurate. Oxygen should be viewed as any other drug and should be applied only when clinically indicated and in an amount required to produce the clinically desired effect.

The above described response of venous admixture to alteration in inspired oxygen concentration may be altered by different therapeutic regimens. For example, Douglas et al found that patients who had undergone

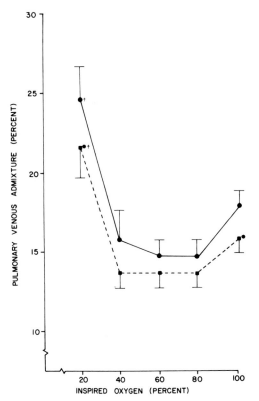

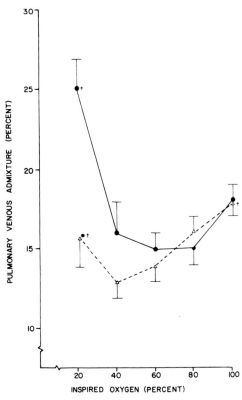

Fig. 19-6 Application of continuous airway pressure (CPAP) will reduce pulmonary venous admixture at all inspired oxygen concentrations following cardiopulmonary bypass. (CPAP = ●----●; No CPAP = ●——●.) (Reproduced from Douglas ME, Downs JB, Shook D: Response of pulmonary venous admixture: a means of comparing therapies? Chest 77:764–770, 1980.)

Fig. 19-7 Following cardiopulmonary bypass, steroids and CPAP appear to have different modes of action and may have addictive effects. Therefore, pulmonary venous admixture is markedly decreased when the patient is breathing room air and remains unchanged at high inspired oxygen concentrations. (CPAP and steroids = △----△; Control = ●——●.) (Reproduced from Douglas ME, Downs JB, Shook D: Response of pulmonary venous admixture: a means of comparing therapies? Chest 77:764–770, 1980.)

cardiopulmonary bypass and who breathed room air had a significant decrease in right-to-left intrapulmonary shunting of blood if steroids were administered intravenously prior to the bypass (Fig. 19-5).[35] However, when these patients breathed pure oxygen, the degree of right-to-left intrapulmonary shunting of blood was increased compared with that in patients who had received placebo. It is possible that steroids cause an increase in perfusion to poorly ventilated lung regions, which thus explains the increase in calculated shunt fraction when patients breathed pure oxygen. Steroids may decrease small airway resistance, thus improving the

ventilation/perfusion ratio in other lung regions. Such an effect would cause an increase in arterial oxygen tension when patients breathe room air. Douglas also found that application of CPAP significantly decreased calculated shunt fraction regardless of the inspired oxygen concentration (Fig. 19-6).[35] Thus, when patients received steroids and CPAP, arterial oxygen tension was increased from 52 ±2 mmHg to 62 ±3 mmHg (mean ± SEM, p < .05). The significant increase in arterial oxygen tension appears to be due to an additive effect of steroids and CPAP on areas of lung with low but finite ventilation/perfusion ratios (Fig. 19-7).

Patients who undergo thoracotomy often require oxygen administration in the immediate postoperative period, usually to maintain the arterial oxygen tension greater than 60 to 80 mmHg. Numerous devices have been described for the administration of oxygen to these patients, including face shields, face masks, rebreathing masks, venturi masks, oxygen tents, and nasal prongs. Available information suggests that no currently available device will give an accurate concentration of inspired oxygen at all times. Therefore, the device used to administer oxygen to the postoperative patient should be chosen with consideration of the desired objectives. If the clinician is concerned with limiting the inspired oxygen concentration in order to prevent depression of the patient's hypoxic drive to breathe, then a venturi mask would be the most logical choice. If the objective is merely to increase the inspired oxygen concentration in order to ensure that the patient does not become hypoxemic, then a device should be utilized that will remain in place and will increase the inspired oxygen concentration at most times, especially when the patient is active, eating, or ambulating. In these instances face masks and face shields are less likely to remain in proper position than nasal prongs. It has been determined that oxygen administration at 3 L/min through nasal prongs will provide the patient with an inspired oxygen concentration of 0.25 to 0.30. When a higher inspired oxygen concentration is desired, a face mask is utilized to deliver high flows of oxygen-enriched gas to the patient's face. Special care then must be taken to ensure that the device remains in place at all times. Usually, when 30 percent oxygen is inadequate to create satisfactory arterial oxygen tension, other means, such as CPAP, are utilized.

A marked decrease in arterial oxygen tension may be secondary to a significant increase in right-to-left intrapulmonary shunting of blood due to small airway closure. If so, therapy should more appropriately be directed at increasing lung volume than at increasing the inspired oxygen concentration. Oxygenation of pulmonary capillary blood occurs predominantly during the expiratory phase of respiration. Therefore it is the expiratory lung volume, the FRC, that is responsible for the efficiency of arterial oxygenation. As discussed previously, an increase in FRC can occur most efficiently when expiratory transpulmonary pressure is increased. Therefore it is not surprising that CPAP has been found to be efficacious for increasing arterial oxygen tension in many patients with small airway closure. Although many clinicians have suggested that PEEP and CPAP be applied only if the patients otherwise require "toxic" levels of inspired oxygen, CPAP is applied early in a patient's treatment regimen, even when a face mask is used. Often the increase in lung volume that occurs with low levels of CPAP may increase lung compliance and cause a dramatic increase in FRC. This frequently is indicated clinically by a sharp fall in the patient's respiratory rate, which is evidence that the work of breathing has been significantly reduced. Furthermore, arterial oxygen tension is often increased. When increasing inspired oxygen concentration and application of CPAP by face mask are inadequate to provide the desired arterial oxygen tension, consideration must be given to endotracheal intubation and mechanical ventilation.

PLEURAL DRAINAGE

Drainage of the pleural cavity was described first by Hewett in 1876 for the treatment of empyema.[36] In 1911, Kenyon described the use of an underwater seal system, a rather simple means of maintaining a closed pleural space.[37] As time progressed, thoracostomy tubes have become routine after thoracotomy for many operative procedures and often are placed as a means of treating pneumothorax, hemothorax, empyema, and pleural effusion. Because of the frequency with which pleural drainage is applied and because of the serious nature of complications, it is essential that all personnel dealing with pleural drainage systems be familiar with the mechanics and physiology involved. Although simple in concept, the underwater seal system for maintaining negative pressure within the pleural space frequently is misunderstood. The different systems for accomplishing pleural drainage are too numerous to discuss individually. The configuration of bottles, application of suction, and daily management of pleural drainage systems are based more on local custom than on precise physiologic principles. Therefore, only the basic principles will be discussed in any detail.

Thoracostomy Tubes

Thoracostomy tubes frequently are placed to treat various pathologic conditions, but occasionally placement of thoracostomy tubes is recommended for prophylactic reasons. Insertion of a thoracostomy tube should not be considered a benign procedure and should be accomplished only by, or under the supervision of, an individual with considerable experience and judgment. Misplacement of the tube, especially when using the trochar technique, may cause laceration of the lung, liver, spleen, diaphragm, stomach, colon, and kidney. If the tube is too large or too stiff or is placed too superficially, the pleural space may not be sufficiently separated from the atmosphere, and recurrent pneumothorax may result. Often, subcutaneous emphysema results from thoracostomy tube insertion, and infection of the ribs has been reported. Intercostal artery and vein laceration may occur, resulting in significant bleeding. Almost universally, significant pain at the insertion site limits respiratory excursion. If possible, chest roentgenograms should be obtained in order to confirm the presence of significant pneumothorax or effusion, and thoracostomy tubes should be inserted only when necessary.

Drainage System

In an attempt to improve pleural drainage, various modifications of the basic underwater seal system, consisting of one-, two-, and three-bottle systems (Figs. 19-8 and 19-9), have been suggested. Recently, disposable plastic systems have been devised which circumvent many of the problems inherent in locally assembled systems, such as breakage and restrictive flow. However, inadequate suction may cause significant problems even with the disposable systems. If the flow rate of the suction system cannot exceed the rate of leakage of air into the pleural space, a tension pneumothorax will occur. In this instance, the patient would be safer with a simple underwater seal system than with applied wall suction. Complications such as these have been discussed in detail by Emerson and McIntyre and by Van Way.[38,39] In general, it is best to have negative pressure generated by a variable-control turbine pump rather than by a diaphragm regulator, which may have limited flow capability.

Munnell and Thomas polled 442 members of the Southern Thoracic Surgical Association and 48 nonmember thoracic surgeons to determine which drainage systems they employed; 53 percent used a system with a single bottle and 36 percent utilized a two-bottle system.[40] A dry trap first bottle may

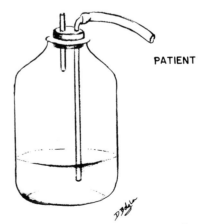

Fig. 19-8 Standard underwater seal pleural drainage system.

PATIENT

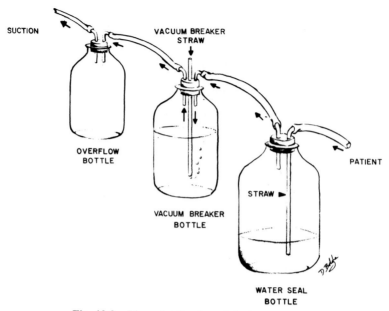

SUCTION

VACUUM BREAKER
STRAW

OVERFLOW
BOTTLE

VACUUM BREAKER
BOTTLE

PATIENT

STRAW ▶

WATER SEAL
BOTTLE

Fig. 19-9 Three-bottle pleural drainage system.

allow reverse air flow, especially when the suction gradient is low. Therefore many practitioners use an underwater seal bottle first and a dry trap bottle second to protect the suction source from frothing and spill-over. The three-bottle system employs a dry trap, a low-negative-pressure water limiter bottle, and a water seal, usually in that order (Fig. 19-9). The most commonly applied disposable systems utilize this principle. Since there is a low-negative-pressure limiter, usually set at 15 cm H_2O, there is no point in applying flow in excess of that necessary to create bubbling throughout the respiratory cycle. Any further negative pressure or flow applied to the system will result only in further entrainment of atmospheric air.

Management

Management of the pleural drainage system is fraught with confusion and often inappropriate action. For example, Heimlich stated that the chest drainage tube must be clamped during transport, even though he

recognized that air and blood could accumulate in the chest, causing lung collapse.[41] Munnell and Thomas found that 35 percent of respondents clamped the thoracostomy tube during transport of the patient.[40] It should be apparent that if the underwater seal bottle is held above the patient, fluid may be siphoned from the underwater seal bottle into the patient's chest. Hence, the bottle must be kept below the level of the patient's chest at all times. Only during the brief period of time when it is necessary to elevate the chest-tube drainage bottle above chest level should the tube be clamped. Therefore the classical instruction given to nurses and other paramedical personnel to clamp chest tubes whenever the system is broken or the patient is moved should be condemned.

Suction applied to the thoracostomy drainage system is *never* lifesaving. On the contrary, limited flow by the suction system may prevent adequate drainage of air from the pleural space. Whenever there is doubt regarding the adequacy of drainage, the suction system should be disconnected and a simple underwater seal system instituted.

Such a system will prevent significant buildup of pressure within the pleural space and will allow drainage of fluid as long as the tubing is patent. In order to ensure patency of the tubing, "milking" the chest tube (pushing air and fluid back into the chest) and "stripping" the tube (a distal movement to create vacuum within the tubing to suck fluid and/or air from the chest) have been recommended to be performed at regular intervals. In individuals who have significant drainage and/or bleeding, these maneuvers may be required every 5 minutes. If the temperature of the tubes approaches body temperature, it is likely that bleeding is active and there is an increased risk of clotting of the thoracostomy tube.

The thoracostomy drainage system should not be broken for routine procedures. For example, the bottle should not be emptied for intake and output measurements. Such procedures are likely to result in contamination of the system and may cause recurrent pneumothorax. Once the thoracostomy tube is placed, a dry sterile dressing should be left in place for 24 to 48 hours. When removing the tube, the clinician should ensure that pleural pressure is above atmospheric to prevent air entrainment and pneumothorax. Therefore the patient should be instructed to take a deep breath and to perform a Valsalva maneuver during removal of the tube. A sterile occlusive dressing should be placed over the thoracostomy insertion site and should remain in place for at least 24 hours to ensure closure of the tube tract.

Thoracostomy tube drainage may be lifesaving. However, complications and errors in treatment may cause significant morbidity and mortality. Therefore, all physicians, nurses, and other personnel dealing with patients in whom thoracostomy tube drainage is necessary should have a good understanding of the mechanics and physiology involved. Several texts are available which describe the physiology of thoracostomy drainage in detail, and the reader is urged to consult these for further information.[42]

DRUG THERAPY

Perhaps surprisingly, drug therapy plays little role in the routine respiratory care of the postoperative patient requiring thoracic surgery. For years, respiratory stimulants were administered to patients in an effort to reverse the respiratory depressant effects of anesthesia. However, such stimulants are not without untoward side effects and may cause significant increases in cardiac output, apprehension, and shortness of breath. Careful administration of general anesthesia should ensure an insignificant depression of respiratory drive in the postoperative period. There is no evidence that administration of respiratory stimulants will decrease the incidence of postoperative pulmonary complications, and postoperative respiratory depression can be treated in more appropriate ways. Therefore, administration of respiratory stimulants is rarely, if ever, necessary.

Some patients who undergo thoracotomy may have reactive airway disease with significant postoperative bronchospasm. Most patients will have had pulmonary testing prior to their operation to document the existence of bronchospastic disease and its reversibility with topical bronchodilators. Occasionally, patients may be operated upon without acquisition of such preoperative data and may require administration of bronchodilators in the postoperative period. If so, racemic epinephrine, isoproterenol, isoetharine, metaproterenol, terbutaline, and salbutamol may be administered topically to promote bronchodilatation. Racemic epinephrine also may decrease mucosal edema secondary to airway trauma and has often been used in the postoperative period. The pharmacologic action of these drugs is beyond the scope of this discussion (see Ch. 5). However, all can be administered easily with a hand-held nebulizer, although in patients who are unable to inhale sufficiently, intermittent positive pressure breathing may be a more efficient means of delivery. Table 19-1 shows the drugs and inhaled doses.

Parenteral bronchodilators such as the methylxanthines and catecholamines may also be administered to patients in the postoperative period. Increased levels of cyclic adenosine monophosphate (AMP) may cause relaxation of bronchial smooth muscles. Therefore drugs such as the methylxanthines, which inhibit phosphodiesterase, the enzyme responsible for breakdown of cyclic AMP, may be useful. Additionally, drugs such as the catecholamines may stimulate adenylate cyclase, which will increase production of cyclic AMP. Such drugs will have an additive effect and may be used in combination.

Administration of bronchodilators should not be routine practice. Only when objective evidence of increased airway resistance, such as wheezing and prolonged exhalation, is present should bronchodilators be administered. Commonly, bronchodilators stimulate the myocardium and may cause dysrhythmias. Furthermore, most such drugs reverse hypoxic pulmonary vasoconstriction and may cause rapid and significant right-to-left intrapulmonary shunting of blood and arterial hypoxemia. Therefore, most patients who require administration of bronchodilators should also receive supplemental oxygen.

In patients with known bronchospastic disease, consideration should be given to administration of steroids prior to, during, and following operation. There is some evidence that topical steroids such as beclomethasone may be effective in preventing bronchospasm in the postoperative period. Similarly, cromolyn sodium may be useful when administered prophylactically to patients who have known bronchospastic disease. It should be emphasized that cromolyn sodium is not a bronchodilator and has no role in the treatment of active bronchospasm.

For several years some clinicians have recommended administration of mucolytic agents to the respiratory tract. However, most series which have examined the effectiveness of topically administered mucolytics have found that they have no significant influence on the incidence of postoperative atelectasis. There is no question that administration of mucolytic agents will cause an increase in the production of sputum of some patients. However, it is not clear that mucolytic-enhanced sputum production is therapeutic. For example, most mucolytics are sufficiently irritating to the respiratory tract that increased production of sputum may occur in reaction to the irritant. In patients who have difficulty in clearing secretions, administration of a mucolytic agent may cause deterioration in pulmonary function. Furthermore, if an individual has difficulty in raising secretions, further liquefaction of the secretions may cause them to run distally into peripheral airways rather than causing them to be cleared more easily. Since these agents are irritating, expensive, and potentially dangerous, they should not be used without very specific indications. Certainly, they cannot be recommended as a routine prophylactic measure.

Topical application of antibiotics to the respiratory tract has been recommended by various authors. Amphotericin-B, bacitracin, polymyxin, neomycin, and mycostatin are antibiotic agents that have been recommended for topical administration, since their systemic toxicity would be too great if administered parenterally. In addition, carbenicillin, gentamycin, and kanamycin also have been recommended for topical use. Initially, topical administration was accomplished by nebulization. However, evidence has accumulated to indicate that nebulization of potent antibiotics leads to rapid creation of resistant bacteria in the environment. Furthermore, these antibiotics are just as effective when instilled directly into the trachea. Subsequently, several investigators have found no beneficial effect of either prophylactic or therapeutic administration of

Table 19-1
Respiratory Inhalant Products

Trade Name (Manufacturer)	Active Constituents	Usual Dosage
Sympathomimetics:		
Micronefrin (Bird Corp.) Vaponefrin (Fisons)	Racemic epinephrine, 2.25%	0.25–0.5 ml* 4–6 times daily
Medihaler-Epi (Riker)	Epinephrine, 0.7%	1–2 metered inhalations (0.16–0.32 mg) 4–6 times daily
Alupent (Boehringer Ingelheim) Metaprel (Dorsey)	Metaproterenol sulfate as a micronized powder in an inert propellant	2–3 metered inhalations (1.30–1.95 mg) not to exceed 12 inhalations daily
Alupent (Boehringer Ingelheim) Metaprel (Dorsey)	Metaproterenol sulfate, 0.5%	0.2 to 0.3 ml* 4–6 times daily
Aerolone (Lilly)	Isoproterenol HCl, 0.25%	0.25 to 1.0 ml* 4–6 times daily
Ventolin (Glaxo)	Microcrystalline suspension of albuterol in propellants	2 metered inhalations (90 μg) 4–6 times daily
Isuprel (Breon)	Isoproterenol HCl, 0.5% or 1%	0.25–0.5 ml* of 0.5% soln. 4–6 times daily
Norisodrine Aerotrol (Abbott)	Isoproterenol HCl, 0.25%	1–2 metered inhalations (120–240 μg) 4–6 times daily
Isuprel Mistometer (Breon)	Isoproterenol HCl, 0.25%	1–2 metered inhalations (125–250 μg) 4–6 times daily
Medihaler-Iso (Riker)	Isoproterenol HCl, 2 mg/ml	1–2 metered inhalations (75–150 μg) 4–6 times daily
Norisodrine Sulfate Aerohalor (Abbott)	10% Aerohalor cartridges (powder)	2–4 Aerohalor inhalations (0.090–0.180 μg) 4–6 times daily
Norisodrine Sulfate Aerohalor (Abbott)	20% Aerohalor cartridges (powder)	2–4 Aerohalor inhalations (0.180–0.360 μg) 4–6 times daily
Bronkosol (Breon)	Isoetharine Hcl, 1%	0.25–0.5 ml* 4–6 times daily
Bronkometer (Breon)	Isoetharine mesylate, 0.61%	1–2 metered inhalations (340–680 μg) 4–6 times daily
Corticosteroids:		
Vanceril (Schering)	Beclomethasone dipropionate	1–2 metered inhalations (42–84 μg) 3–4 times daily
Beclovent (Glaxo)	Beclomethasone dipropionate	1–2 metered inhalations (42–84 μg) 3–4 times daily
Mucolytics:		
Mycomyst (Mead Johnson)	Acetylcysteine, 10% or 20%	2–4 ml† of 10% solution 4–6 times daily
Cromolyn sodium:		
Intal spinhaler (Fisons)	Cromolyn sodium as a micronized powder	One capsule (20 mg) via Spinhaler 4 times daily

* Dilute with 2 to 5 ml diluent and give over 10 to 15 minutes by IPPB or compressor.
† By IPPB or compressor. Simultaneous bronchodilator administration will decrease possible increased airway resistance caused by acetylcysteine.

antibiotics topically. Finally, topical administration of drugs such as polymyxin may lead to significant bronchospasm in susceptible individuals. Therefore, in the absence of information demonstrating a beneficial effect of topically administered antibiotic agents, their use should be restricted to occasional cases, in which other modes of therapy have failed.

REINTUBATION OF THE TRACHEA

Following operation, if a patient's respiratory status deteriorates significantly, consideration must be given to reintubation of the trachea. Pediatric thoracic surgeons have utilized the technique of reintubation for many years in the treatment of atelectasis, especially of the right upper lobe. In such infants the endotracheal tube usually is placed without anesthesia or muscle relaxation and a small amount of saline solution is instilled through the tube; this is followed by vigorous manual ventilation and suction. Following repetition of this sequence 3 or 4 times, extubation is accomplished and the infant allowed to breath spontaneously. This treatment has not gained favor in adult respiratory care, probably because of the difficulty involved with intubating awake adults. It may be necessary to produce a brief period of anesthesia and muscle relaxation in patients who require reintubation. Usually this can be accomplished with a short-acting intravenous barbiturate anesthetic agent and a short-acting muscle relaxant.

Some patients ventilate inadequately in the postoperative period and may have significant elevation of arterial carbon dioxide tension. Fortunately, hypoventilation resulting in hypercarbic acidosis is an infrequent postoperative problem. The individual with postoperative carbon dioxide retention may be somnolent with shallow tidal breathing and a decreased respiratory rate. In such cases, respiratory depression is usually the result of parenteral administration of respiratory depressant drugs, such as narcotics or barbiturates, or is secondary to the insidious onset of hypercarbia causing decreased respiratory drive. The latter problem usually exists only in patients who have a hypoxic drive for respiration and who receive an excessive concentration of oxygen in the postoperative period. Analysis of arterial blood for carbon dioxide tension and pH is the most accurate means of diagnosing this problem. However, clinical observation of the patient is the only efficient means of knowing when to analyze arterial blood samples. Routine orders for blood sampling often will not be adequate for detecting or preventing this problem. A high degree of suspicion based on preoperative assessment is essential.

Numerous authors have detailed clinical tests to be utilized in determining when an individual requires reintubation and institution of mechanical ventilatory support. However, Browne and Pontoppidan found that only two clinical measurements correlated significantly with a patient's ability to maintain adequate spontaneous respiration, namely, vital capacity and the negative pressure created by an inspiratory effort against a closed airway.[43] The peak negative pressure generated against a closed airway is a direct reflection of the patient's muscular ability to generate negative intrapleural pressure and therefore of his neuromuscular ability to breathe spontaneously. In contrast, the vital capacity maneuver requires adequate lung compliance in addition to muscular stength. For example, a patient may have normal respiratory muscle strength to breathe, but the lung may be so stiff that adequate spontaneous respiration cannot occur. Therefore, the combination of a peak negative pressure measurement and vital capacity measurement likely will tell the clinician if a patient has deficient respiratory muscle strength and/or decreased lung compliance. If an individual is able to generate a vital capacity of 15ml/kg and a peak negative pressure of -20 cm H_2O or greater, he should be able to support spontaneous ventilation. The clinician should be careful to note that these maneuvers are independent of respiratory drive. An individual may have sufficient strength and compliance to support spontaneous ventilation, but if respiratory drive is inadequate, respiratory failure and acidosis will ensue.

Failure of the patient to support adequate spontaneous respiration, resulting in respiratory acidosis, is much less frequent than the problem of inadequate postoperative oxygenation. Patients with arterial hypoxemia may require intubation, but ventilation is infrequently required to treat postoperative arterial hypoxemia (Fig. 19-10). If CPAP cannot be adequately delivered by mask, the patient may require tracheal intubation for consistent delivery of higher levels of CPAP. When necessary, this should be done early and prior to the administration of an excessive inspired oxygen concentration.

Once a decision is made to reintubate the patient, mechanical ventilator settings should be appropriate to treat and prevent further respiratory acidosis. In addition, some care should be taken to ensure that respiratory alkalosis does not occur. Prior investigations have revealed that an alveolar ventilation of approximately 4L/min will provide a normal arterial carbon dioxide tension in the majority of postoperative patients. During mechanical ventilatory therapy, physiologic dead space is elevated and the dead space/tidal volume ratio approaches 0.50. Therefore, a minute ventilation of approximately 8L/min is required for most postoperative adult patients.[44]

A ventilator rate of up to 10 breaths per minute and a tidal volume of 8 to 12 ml/kg may be necessary to prevent respiratory acidosis and a further decrease in FRC. Intermittent mandatory ventilation is used to maintain a normal arterial blood pH. Care should be taken to ensure that adequate humidity is supplied to the patient at all times. Even short exposure to cool, unhumidified

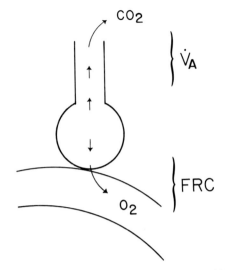

Fig. 19-10 Maintenance of functional residual capacity (FRC) is necessary to ensure optimum oxygenation of arterial blood, thus preventing right-to-left intrapulmonary shunting. Bulk flow of gas into and from the alveolar spaces is unnecessary to maintain this function. In contrast, efficient carbon dioxide excretion from alveolar spaces depends upon bulk flow of gas from the lung. Therefore, alveolar ventilation ($\dot{V}_A$) may be manipulated to ensure maintenance of proper arterial carbon dioxide tension, and a continuous positive pressure may be applied to the airway to maintain approximate FRC and arterial oxygenation.

gas may cause significant tracheal mucosal damage and inspissation of secretions, with further compromise of respiratory function.

Once the patient is reintubated, care should be taken to maintain the sterility of the patient's airway. Therefore, the connection between the endotracheal tube and the breathing circuit should be broken only for necessary maneuvers. For example, suctioning of the tracheobronchial tree should occur only when auscultation of the patient's chest reveals the need for such treatment. Routine suctioning should be avoided. The patient's position should be changed frequently in order to prevent atelectasis and retention of secretions in dependent airways. The endotracheal tube should be equipped with a high-residual-volume, low-pressure cuff, and cuff pressure should be documented to be less than 20 mm Hg. Inflation of the cuff should occur with no more air than is required to just prevent an air leak. Intubation of the trachea is fraught with complications and should not be considered a benign form of therapy. Finally, once the patient is intubated, thought should be given to weaning the patient from oxygen, mechanical ventilation, and CPAP, and to extubating him as soon as possible.

REFERENCES

1. Stein M, Cassara EL: Preoperative pulmonary evaluation and therapy for surgery patients. JAMA 211:787-790, 1970
2. Burford TH, Burbank B: Traumatic wet lung. J Thorac Surg 14:415-424, 1945
3. Piehl MA, Brown RS: Use of extreme position changes in acute respiratory failure. Crit Care Med 4:13-14, 1976
4. Al-Jurf AS: Editorial—Turn, cough and deep breaths. Surg Gynecol Obstet 149:887-888, 1979
5. Sante L: Massive (atelectatic) collapse of the lung. Ann Surg 88:161-177, 1928
6. Marini JJ, Pierson DJ, Hudson LD: Acute lobar atelectasis: a prospective comparison of fiberoptic bronchoscopy and respiratory therapy. Am Rev Respir Dis 119:971-978, 1979
7. Graham WGB, Bradley DA, Kleczek R et al: Efficacy of chest physiotherapy and intermittent positive-pressure breathing in the resolution of pneumonia. N Engl J Med 299:624-627, 1978
8. Radigan LR, King RD: A technique for the prevention of postoperative atelectasis. Surgery 47:184-187, 1960
9. Haight C: Intratracheal suction in the management of postoperative pulmonary complications. Ann Surg 107:218-228, 1938
10. Sackner MA, Landa JF, Robinson MJ et al: Pathogenesis and prevention of tracheobronchial damage with suction procedures. Chest 64:284-290, 1973
11. Jung RC, Gottlieb LS: Comparison of tracheobronchial suction catheters in humans. Chest 69:179-181, 1976
12. Bowen TE, Fishback ME, Green DC: Treat-
ment of refractory atelectasis. Ann Thorac Surg 18:584-589, 1974
13. Millen JE, Vandree J, Glauser FL: Fiberoptic bronchoscopic balloon occlusion and reexpansion of refractory unilateral atelectasis. Crit Care Med 6:50-55, 1978
14. Bartlett RH, Gazzaniga AB, Geraghty TR: Respiratory maneuvers to prevent postoperative pulmonary complications—a critical review. JAMA 224:1017-1021, 1973
15. Nunn JF, Coleman AJ, Sachithanandan T et al: Hypoxaemia and atelectasis produced by forced expiration. Br J Anaesth 37:3-12, 1965
16. Gold MI: Is intermittent positive pressure breathing therapy (IPPB RX) necessary in the surgical patient? Ann Surg 184:122-123, 1976
17. Iverson LIG, Ecker RR, Fox HE et al: A comparative study of IPPB, the incentive spirometer, and blow bottles: the prevention of atelectasis following cardiac surgery. Ann Thorac Surg 25:197-200, 1978
18. Browner B, Powers SR Jr: Effect of IPPB on functional residual capacity and blood gases in postoperative patients. Surg Forum 26:96-98, 1975
19. Lareau S: The effect of positive pressure breathing on the arterial oxygen tension in patients with chronic obstructive pulmonary disease receiving oxygen therapy. Heart Lung 5:449-452, 1976
20. Wright FG Jr, Foley MF, Downs JB et al: Hypoxemia and hypocarbia following intermittent positive-pressure breathing. Anesth Analg (Cleve) 55:555-559, 1976
21. Shim C, Bajwa S, Williams MH Jr: The effect of inhalation therapy on ventilatory function and expectoration. Chest 73:798-801, 1978
22. Paul WL, Downs JB: Postoperative atelectasis. Arch Surg 116:861-863, 1981
23. Ward RJ, Danziger F, Bonica JJ et al: An evaluation of postoperative respiratory maneuvers. Surg Gynecol Obstet 123:51-54, 1966
24. Bartlett RH, Krop P, Hanson EL et al: Physiology of yawning and its application to postoperative care. Surg Forum 21:222-224, 1970
25. Lederer DH, Van de Water JM, Indech RB: Which deep breathing device should the postoperative patient use? Chest 77:610-613, 1980
26. Bartlett RH, Brennan ML, Gazzaniga AB et al: Studies on the pathogenesis and prevention of postoperative pulmonary complications. Surg Gynecol Obstet 137:925-933, 1973

27. Downs JB, Mitchell LA: Pulmonary effects of ventilatory pattern following cardiopulmonary bypass. Crit Care Med 4:295-300,1976

28. Fowler AA III, Scoggins WG, O'Donohue WJ Jr: Positive end-expiratory pressure in the management of lobar atelectasis. Chest 74:497-500, 1978

29. Stone DR, Downs JB: Collateral ventilation and PEEP in normal and edematous lungs of dogs. Anesthesiology 53:S186, 1980

30. Greenbaum DM, Millen JE, Eross B et al: Continuous positive airway pressure without tracheal intubation in spontaneously breathing patients. Chest 69:615-620, 1976

31. Andersen JB, Olesen KP, Eikard B et al: Periodic continuous positive airway pressure, CPAP, by mask in the treatment of atelectasis—a sequential analysis. Eur J Respir Dis 61:20-25, 1980

32. Mitchell LA, Downs JB, Dannemiller FJ: Extrapulmonary influences on A-aDO$_2^{1.0}$ following cardiopulmonary bypass. Anesthesiology 43:583-586, 1975

33. Douglas ME, Downs JB, Dannemiller FJ et al: Change in pulmonary venous admixture with varying inspired oxygen. Anesth Analg (Cleve) 55:688-695, 1976

34. Lansing AM, Jamieson WG: Mechanisms of fever in pulmonary atelectasis. Arch Surg 87:184-190 1963

35. Douglas ME, Downs JB, Shook D: Response of pulmonary venous admixture. A means of comparing therapies? Chest 77:764-770, 1980

36. Hewett C: Drainage for empyema. Br Med J 1:317, 1876

37. Kenyon JA: A preliminary report on a method of treatment of empyema in young children. Med Rec 80:816, 1911

38. Enerson DM, McIntyre J: A comparative study of the physiology and physics of pleural drainage sytems. J Thorac Cardiovasc Surg 52:40-46, 1966

39. Van Way CW III: Persisting pneumothorax as a complication of chest suction. Chest 77:815-816, 1980

40. Munnell ER, Thomas EK: Current concepts in thoracic drainage systems. Ann Thorac Surg 19:261-268, 1975

41. Heimlich HJ: Valve drainage of the pleural cavity. Dis Chest 53:282-287, 1968

42. von Hippel A: Chest Tubes and Chest Bottles. Charles G Thomas, Springfield, Ill., 1970

43. Browne AGR, Pontoppidan H: Abstacts of Scientific Papers, Annual Meeting of The American Society of Anesthesiologists, 69-72, 1972

44. Downs JB, Marston AW: A new transport ventilator: an evaluation. Crit Care Med 5:112-114, 1977

T. James Gallagher, M.D.

20
Etiology and Treatment of Respiratory Failure

ETIOLOGY OF ACUTE RESPIRATORY FAILURE

Terminology

Acute respiratory failure (ARF) serves as a catch-all phrase for many different changes occurring in the lung. The pathophysiology, precipitating event, presentation, and treatment of ARF differ tremendously depending on whether the lungs were otherwise healthy or already had some preexisting underlying disease. However, considerable insight and understanding of ARF have been acquired and effective treatments, resulting in dramatically decreased morbidity and mortality, have been developed during the last decade.

The terminology of this disease has varied greatly over the years. *Shock lung* was a very early term, which was based on the assumption that hemorrhagic or hypovolemic shock was a major causative factor. It is now known that shock by itself, while responsible for some ultrastructural changes of the pulmonary architecture, does not directly contribute to the development of respiratory

failure.[1,2] More likely, the injuries commonly associated with hypovolemia, such as multisystem trauma, are the true culprits.

Pump lung was another early term, indicating the close association of postoperative respiratory failure with cardiopulmonary bypass. With continued equipment improvement, this problem has become rare; in fact, nowadays most post-cardiopulmonary bypass patients are extubated the night of or the morning following surgery.[3]

The term *congestive atelectasis* often appeared in the literature.[4] At one time, many felt the atelectasis which developed during ARF was a major contributor to or precursor of the phenomenon. However, as will be described, atelectasis develops late in the course of the entire process and plays an insignificant role in the early alterations of blood gas exchange. At autopsy the lung maintains its shape and form surprisingly well, and very little collapse can be detected.[5] Although it may develop in response to other pathologic events, atelectasis is not a major precipitator of adult respiratory distress syndrome.

The *wet lung syndrome* was first de-

665

scribed during World War II.[6] This surprisingly accurate clinical description later gave way to such terms as *Da Nang lung*. During the Vietnamese conflict, ARF often developed after resuscitation with large amounts of balanced electrolyte-containing solutions. Some felt that the ensuing hemodilution and reduction of colloid oncotic pressure caused the fluid accumulation in the pulmonary interstitial space. This debate centering on the appropriate resuscitation fluid still rages and will be discussed in detail later.

Today, the most frequently used descriptive terms include *acute respiratory insufficiency* (ARI), *adult respiratory distress syndrome* (ARDS), and ARF. Within limits, these are quite interchangeable, but the term *acute respiratory failure* will still be primarily used.

Clinical Characteristics and Diagnosis

The earliest, most subtle changes of ARF are first detected by blood gas analysis. Depending upon the precipitating event, it may be as long as 48 hours before these abnormalities actually begin to manifest themselves (Table 20-1). The arterial oxygen pressure (PaO_2) will be less than expected for the inspired oxygen concentration (FIO_2); moreover, it does not respond to an increase in the administered oxygen percentage. For example, in most patients a PaO_2 of 65 mmHg on 40 percent inspired oxygen is less than normally expected. The patient with ARF may then have the PaO_2 rise to only 80 mmHg despite an increase in the inspired oxygen concentration to 80 or 90 percent.

Table 20-1
Early Signs of Acute Respiratory Failure

Hypoxemia
Hypocarbia
Tachypnea
Decreased compliance
Increased venous admixture

Normally, the PaO_2 should be over 600 mmHg when the FIO_2 reaches 0.9.

The second characteristic of ARF includes failure to improve oxygenation despite the addition of mechanical ventilation. Contrary to what might be expected, positive pressure ventilation by itself does not markedly improve the poor oxygenation characteristic of respiratory failure.

In contrast to the neonate who develops hyaline membrane disease, maintenance of $PaCO_2$ is usually not a problem in the adult with acute respiratory failure.[7,8] Only in the late stages of the disease process does CO_2 retention become significant. Spontaneous respiratory rates of 40 to 50 per minute contribute to hypocarbia and a resultant respiratory alkalosis early in the disease. Arterial PCO_2 commonly averages 30 to 35 mmHg. Close inspection may reveal nasal flaring as well as involvement of the accessory muscles of respiration.[9]

Radiographic changes contribute little to the diagnosis of ARF. In the very early stages severe blood gas derangements may occur, yet the chest radiograph may still be interpreted as entirely normal. Only later, usually as a preterminal event, are interstitial or alveolar infiltrative changes routinely present. Actually, at any stage of ARF very little correlation exists among the patient's clinical course, blood gas exchange, and radiologic presentation (see Ch. 3).

Pulmonary mechanics also deteriorate during ARF. Lung volumes, including functional residual capacity (FRC), routinely decrease. At the same time pulmonary compliance worsens and the lungs become stiffer. This means it will take an increasingly greater transpulmonary pressure gradient to deliver the same tidal volume.[7] Since transpulmonary pressure is the difference between airway and intrapleural pressure, during mechanical positive pressure ventilation the respirator will need to develop higher inflation pressures during inspiration in order to deliver the same tidal volume.

Later on some minimal atelectasis may

occur, but it is usually not evident on chest radiography. Most often the major pathophysiologic change involves a ventilation-perfusion mismatch. Perfusion remains largely unaltered while significant hypoventilation develops in many lung units. Characteristically, venous admixture or intrapulmonary shunt increases. Severe defects in oxygenation may accompany an almost completely normal chest film. Therefore, failure to document radiographic deterioration does not rule out the syndrome. In the very late stages of the disease, the familiar bilateral, fluffy infiltrates indicative of interstitial and alveolar fluid accumulation appear. At this so-called preterminal stage, CO_2 retention is more likely than hypocapnia. By this time, significant changes in compliance have already developed.

A variety of heterogenous events may eventually result in or cause the syndrome of acute respiratory failure. Regardless of the precipitating event, the pulmonary response appears to be both nonspecific and predictable. The clinical features and the pathophysiologic changes of acute respiratory failure are quite reproducible.

The clinical scenario just described always produces a very high mortality rate, and an autopsy reveals several significant findings. The lungs usually weigh about 3 to 4 times normal. When they are excised and cut in cross-section, pink-tinged fluid flows out of both the alveolar and interstitial spaces. It is extremely difficult to specifically identify either space, let alone normal areas. The lung takes on a very beefy red appearance, a so-called hepatization. Light microscopy reveals alveolar infiltration by red and white blood cells, including granulocytes, eosinophils, and other debris. Hyaline membranes may be seen both in the terminal airways and in the interstitial space. Significant interstitial edema can be demonstrated.[10] In fact, the untrained eye may fail to recognize the specimen as pulmonary tissue.

A more detailed inspection by electron microscopy indicates further derangement.[11] Normally, the alveolar epithelium and capillary endothelium are in very close juxtaposition, separated only by a very thin basement membrane. With ARF, significant swelling of the interstitial space separates the two surfaces. Edema of the alveolar walls can also be easily recognized and, when the walls are engorged, they may actually bulge into the terminal airways. Perivascular cupping also develops in response to the edema.

Pathophysiology

Characterization of the pathologic changes in ARF is begun by a study of lung volumes. Figure 20-1 depicts a typical, normal spirogram tracing.[12] The tracing demonstrates normal tidal volume changes and a vital capacity maneuver—maximal inhalation followed by maximal exhalation. Despite this maximal effort some gas known as the *residual volume,* always remains in the lung. No matter how much a person exhales, that volume remains and it can be considered for this discussion as relatively constant. The difference between the lung volume at end-tidal ventilation and residual volume is the *expiratory reserve volume.* Together, the expiratory reserve volume and the residual volume make up the FRC. However, since residual volume is more or less constant, changes ascribed to FRC principally relate to changes in the expiratory reserve volume.

Closing volume (Fig. 20-2) represents the lung volume required to prevent small airway or alveolar collapse. Closing volume is not actually a volume that is routinely measured but in fact can be better appreciated as a concept.[13] It includes the lung volume necessary to balance any extra-alveolar forces tending to cause alveolar collapse. In normal circumstances, closing volume about equals the residual volume. This means that a vital capacity maneuver will not lead to airway collapse.

Several disease processes contribute to or require an increase in closing volume.

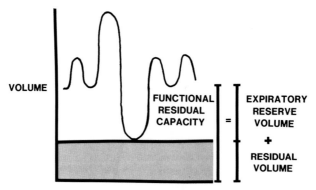

Fig. 20-1 A normal spirogram tracing. The small upward excursions represent normal tidal volume excursions followed by a vital capacity maneuver. The shaded area at the bottom represents the residual volume, which remains constant. The expiratory reserve volume and the functional residual capacity are also illustrated.

Obstructive pulmonary disease, the aging process, chronic smoking, ventilation-perfusion mismatch, and interstitial water accumulation all cause an increase in closing volume. Not only interstitial water but also increased interstitial pressure secondary to the water requires an increased closing volume. As might be expected, inactivation or loss of surfactant contributes to the same types of changes in closing volume.

During respiratory failure, alterations can affect both FRC or, more precisely, expiratory reserve volume and closing volume. Most causes of decreased FRC are familiar

(Table 20-2). Massive obesity, as well as the supine and lithotomy positions, contributes to a reduced FRC. Obesity can prevent adequate chest wall expansion; the supine and lithotomy positions both move the diaphragm cephalad, contributing to a loss of lung volume. Intra-abdominal manipulations, including surgical packing, peritonitis, and pancreatitis, as well as aspiration or near drowning, can severely decrease FRC.

Therefore, the reduction of FRC for the reasons listed in Table 20-2 and an increase in lung closing volume will combine to produce small airway collapse, a major reason

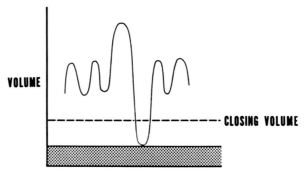

Fig. 20-2 A normal spirogram tracing. Closing volume, illustrated here, is greater than residual volume. If this patient were to exhale to residual volume, airway collapse might begin to occur.

Table 20-2
Origins of Decreased FRC

Obesity
Smoking
Supine position
Lithotomy position
Upper abdominal surgery
Thoracic surgery
Peritonitis
Aspiration syndrome
Lung contusion

for blood gas derangement in ARF (Table 20-3). A change in one parameter alone could cause the same problem, but that would require significantly greater volume shifts. When both volumes are altered, the degree of change in each does not have to be as significant to cause severe pulmonary dysfunction.

The loss of FRC or residual volume means that pulmonary gas volumes are diminished at the end of tidal ventilation. If at the same time closing volume has been elevated, airway collapse will occur when the changes are great enough that at end exhalation resting lung volume remains less than the closing volume (Fig. 20-3).

To recapitulate, in respiratory failure lung volume changes occur. Expiratory reserve volume decreases while closing volume moves in the opposite direction. Airway collapse takes place when both changes are

Table 20-3
Predisposing Factors for Acute Respiratory Failure

1. Multiple-system trauma
2. Pancreatitis
3. Peritonitis
4. Abdominal sepsis
5. Prolonged intra-abdominal or thoracic surgery
6. Pneumonia
7. Near drowning
8. Aspiration of gastric contents
9. Inhalation of noxious agents
10. Fat embolism
11. Flail chest
12. Pulmonary embolism

large enough to produce a resting lung volume that is less than closing volume. The resultant airway collapse produces hypoxemia, as documented by blood gas analysis.

Fluid Flux Across The Lung

In order to better appreciate the lung volume changes in acute respiratory failure, a detailed, in depth understanding of the anatomic derangements commonly present in ARF is needed. In reality, the alveolus is surrounded by the blood in much the same way a ball might sit in a bucket of water. The perivascular interstitial space separates the alveolar and capillary epithelial and endothelial linings and blood gas exchange takes place across these membranes. The interstitial space behaves more as a potential than as a real space. The larger arterioles and venules, as well as the lymphatics, reside in the central or peribronchiolar interstitial compartment.

The lymphatics drain any excess or accumulated fluid back into the central circulation.[14] The lymph flows to the thoracic duct, which in turn empties into the azygos system. Lymph flow removal operates under the control of several different mechanisms. Elevated interstitial or capillary pressures accelerate flow, while the intrinsic motion of the lung during spontaneous respiration also encourages lymphatic drainage. The lymphatic vessels also have their own peristaltic motion, which contributes to maintaining the parenchyma in essentially a dry state.

The alveolar capillary interface actively participates in many of the derangements occurring during acute respiratory failure.[15] A series of endothelial cells line the capillary wall. These elongated cells are not tightly bound to each other but are actually separated by junctions on the order of 40 angstroms (Å) in diameter. Albumin molecules normally measure about 80 to 100 Å, which permits the cleft to act as a filtering mechanism to inhibit most albumin movement

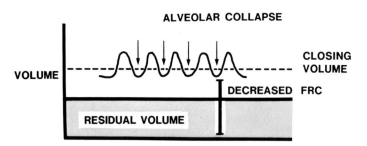

Fig. 20-3 While expiratory reserve volume has decreased, closing volume has increased. At the end of normal tidal ventilation, the closing volume exceeds gas volume left in the lungs. Therefore airway collapse and hypoxemia begin to develop.

across the membrane.[16] The epithelial cells lining the alveoli form a very tight boundary and render that stucture watertight to any fluid from the interstitial space.

Water can move across the capillary membrane by active transport, by vesicle movement, or directly through the interendothelial clefts. In ARF the major fluid shifts principally take place by fluid fluxes through the aforementioned endothelial junctions. The remaining mechanisms do not play a major role. Because of the pore size only water and small protein molecules can pass, while under normal circumstances most of the albumin remains in the vascular compartment.

The perivascular interstitial space is more a potential than a real space and most often fluid does not accumulate in it but instead moves to the central or peribronchiolar space and eventually finds its way into the lymphatic circulation. Mucopolysaccharides reside primarily in central interstitial areas and their osmotic properties help draw any fluid to that area. The lymphatics then clear water and any protein, including albumin, which might accumulate.[17]

Several opposing factors influence the fluid flux across the alveolar capillary-endothelial junctional clefts.[18] The pulmonary capillary hydrostatic or microvascular pressure tends to move fluid in the direction of the interstitial space. Capillary pressure

should not be confused with pulmonary capillary wedge pressure (PCWP), since capillary pressure cannot be measured clinically and must be estimated. Several different formulas have been proposed and most authorities accept an estimate of about 40 to 50 percent of the difference between pulmonary capillary wedge and pulmonary venous pressure. Additionally, the pressure changes with position. When the lung is upright, apical microvascular pressures are close to zero while capillary pressures at the bases are usually much higher than alveolar pressures. The low-pressure pulmonary circulation distribution changes in response to gravity and therefore can vary markedly from one area of the lung to the next, depending on position.[19]

The interstitial space itself usually contains a small amount of fluid and albumin or other small protein molecules. An oncotic pressure develops, primarily dependent on the albumin concentration. That oncotic pressure exerts its influence to draw fluid from the capillary to the interstitial space. Methods to sample interstitial-fluid oncotic pressure are not readily available to the clinician. Therefore, this factor cannot be accurately determined during any particular illness. Obviously, a large movement of non–protein-containing fluid into the interstitial space would reduce tissue oncotic pressure.

Two other forces act to oppose fluid egress from the capillary bed. Most protein remains in the plasma, where it exerts a large oncotic effect tending to prevent water from moving out of the capillary compartment. Several devices are now available which permit clinical determinations of oncotic pressure. Normal values range up to 20 to 25 mmHg.[20]

Any fluid tending to accumulate in the interstitial portions of the lung will obviously develop its own hydrostatic pressure. While interstitial pressure normally has a slightly negative value, very small accumulations of fluid will rapidly convert that pressure to positive.[21] The pressure elevation then acts to oppose further fluid shifts. Like oncotic pressure, interstitial hydrostatic pressure remains extremely difficult to determine. Various techniques, including use of micropipets or implanted capsules, all markedly alter this delicate space and make any pressure determinations unreliable, especially during changing conditions. The best estimates and extrapolations from chronic animal implantations indicate that human hydrostatic pressure usually remains subatmospheric, at about −7 cm H$_2$O. The negative pressure in part results from lung expansion and deflation during spontaneous ventilation.[22]

Fluid flux across the capillary also depends on the filtration coefficient (K$_{F,C}$ in the Starling equation), which varies with capillary surface area. Not all the pulmonary vessels are open at once; the degree of patency reflects pulmonary blood flow. Thus, the greater the flow, the larger the area of perfusion and the larger K$_{F,C}$ and the greater the fluid movement or flux across the alveolar-capillary membrane.[23]

The filtration coefficient varies in response to permeability changes if such changes do indeed exist. Permeability will be discussed later, but the mechanism appears to involve an alteration of the endothelial pore size or diameter and most likely represents a reversible phenomenon. This evidence comes from laboratory animals which were infused with so-called permeability substances and eventually returned to normal without other than supportive care.[24] Since flow correlates with the fourth power of the radius, even small changes in radius have quite pronounced effects on fluid fluxes. If the radius were to double, flow would increase by a factor of 16. Therefore, any fluid changes are much more pronounced when permeability has been altered.

The reflection coefficient (θ_c) reflects solute movement across a membrane.[22] A solute that cannot cross has a value of 1; if the solute can freely cross, then θ_c approaches a value of zero. The value of θ_c changes in each vascular bed in any species and probably equals about 0.9 in human lung. This means that normally very little protein moves across the alveolar-capillary membrane.

These effects are described by the Starling equation (sometimes referred to as "Starling forces"):

$$J_U W = K_{F,C} (P_c - P_t) - \theta_c (\pi C - \pi T)$$

where $J_U W$ = net volume movement
  $K_{F,C}$ = filtration coefficient
  Pc = capillary hydrostatic pressure
  Pt = tissue hydrostatic pressure
  θ_c = reflection coefficient
  πc = capillary oncotic pressure
  πt = tissue oncotic pressure

The Starling equation *describes the forces present;* it of course does not itself influence or cause net fluid flow. It mathematically expresses the interrelationship of the various forces present.

Lung Water and Disease States

Under normal circumstances, the balance of all the forces produces a slow but continuous fluid movement into the perivascular interstitial space at a rate of about 10 to

20 ml/hour. This slow influx permits easy removal by the lymphatics. Acute respiratory failure develops when other events alter this delicate balance.

Several different events can influence microvascular pressure.[25] A simple example is an obstructive phenomenon such as a pulmonary embolus. Vascular occlusion precedes cessation of flow, and capillary pressure soon increases. If none of the other Starling forces were to change, then the equilibrium would be unbalanced and fluid movement across the capillary membrane would accelerate.

Left ventricular failure also can increase microvascular pressure. Forward flow diminishes and the eventual backup in the pulmonary vascular bed elevates microcapillary pressures. These changes do not occur immediately, since, as previously described, the pulmonary bed is never fully patent. Therefore, before any pressure increase secondary to congestive heart failure might develop, vascular bed recruitment must be maximized. Increases in flow or cardiac output do not usually elevate capillary pressure because of the recruitment phenomenon. Not until flow exceeds 250 percent of baseline values does pressure increase[26] (see Ch. 7).

Intense vasoconstriction from the release of vasoactive amines or secondary to hypoxic pulmonary vasoconstriction can also locally affect microvascular pressure.[27,28] These localized changes explain some of the infiltrates which develop after pulmonary embolus and which previously were ascribed to pulmonary infarction. In fact, these infiltrates represent fluid accumulation caused by the high pressures.

Serum oncotic pressure relates to serum albumin levels. If oncotic pressure alone decreases while all the other Starling factors remain unchanged, then fluid flux into the interstitium increases. Massive hemodilution secondary to infused balanced electrolyte solutions will reduce serum oncotic pressure. Hypoalbuminemia also develops during chronic illness when albumin production diminishes and fails to replace the eventual loss of circulating molecules. The stress of illness and surgery, combined with inattention to the suddenly increased nutritional needs, quickly worsens the problem. Unfortunately, exogenously administered albumin has little or no effect on restoring serum levels to normal since most of the protein moves out of the circulating volume and into various storage depots.[29,30]

Some reports have indicated that an increased fluid flux and eventual water accumulation in the interstitium will occur whenever the serum oncotic pressure or the serum oncotic–pulmonary capillary wedge pressure (COP-PCWP) gradients were reduced.[31] However, despite total elimination of the gradient, several clinical trials have failed to show any derangement in pulmonary function as judged by PaO_2, venous admixture, or intrapulmonary shunt (Qsp/Qt).[32]

Until recently, interstitial or extravascular lung water accumulation could not be clinically measured. However, with the advent of a microprocessor to measure extravascular lung water by the thermal dye technique, these data should be forthcoming. Early reports have demonstrated a very poor correlation between extravascular lung water and blood gas exchange.[33,34]

The thermal dye method utilizes fluid at 0 °C to equilibrate rapidly with all lung water during one circuit through the pulmonary bed. Since transit time and concentration are known, total lung water can be calculated. The indocyanine green combines with albumin and therefore permits measurement of vascular water. Subtracting vascular from total lung water gives extravascular or interstitial water.

It really is not feasible to predict lung water changes based on information from a single parameter (Fig. 20-4). A change of one Starling factor while all others remain fixed would obviously lead to a major imbalance. The rate and direction of any fluid shift will

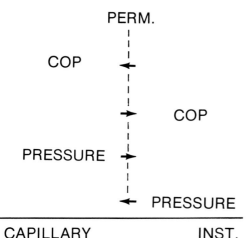

Fig. 20-4 The Starling forces balanced across the capillary membrane. Change of one factor will not influence a fluid shift unless all others remain unchanged.

be dependent on its degree and on the particular factor affected. However, alteration of only one force rarely happens. A decreased colloid oncotic pressure tends to produce more water movement into the lung parenchyma. However, as water begins to move in that direction and accumulate, other changes simultaneously occur. The increased water in the interstitium elevates tissue hydrostatic pressure, which then opposes further fluid egress from the vascular compartment. Simultaneously, the water dilutes the albumin already present, decreasing the tissue oncotic effect; this further opposes fluid accumulation and movement across the capillary membrane. Finally, loss of intravascular water lowers pulmonary blood volume and microvascular pressure. The reduced vascular pressure also opposes further interstitial water accumulation. It remains virtually impossible to change one aspect of the Starling equation without effect on all or most of the others.

Since accurate measurement of any parameter except serum oncotic pressure is not possible, predictions of lung water accumulation are difficult. As previously shown,

when one factor changes, its eventual influence on all the others cannot yet be accurately determined. All the numbers may change, but when placed back into the equation they may balance, so that no net increase in fluid actually takes place. It is not difficult to see that predictions of pulmonary function or extravascular lung water based only on serum oncotic pressure could be quite inaccurate.

A third major factor influencing lung water changes is pulmonary capillary permeability. Most investigators believe that significant alterations of capillary integrity can occur at the previously-described endothelial junctions. Any increase in size dramatically affects fluid movement, including albumin leakage.[5] Alterations of pulmonary capillary permeability occur primarily during sepsis.[34] Either direct bacterial action or secondary endotoxin release can initiate the events. The bacteria or toxin apparently interact with the capillary endothelium. Damage to the vessel wall causes platelets to accumulate and adhere to the injured surface. Serotonin released from the platelets can locally alter the capillary integrity as well as elevate microvascular pressure.

Histamine can be released by stimulated pulmonary mast cells. Histamine also has the ability to alter permeability, and its effects can be reversed by administration of antihistamines. Other factors influencing permeability include the toxic substances inhaled after combustion and other chemical agents too numerous to list here.[24,35] These substances affect both capillary and alveolar integrity.

Some authorities have questioned the existence of permeability alterations.[22] If permeability changes are a real phenomenon, then compared with the effects of pressure elevations, fluid flux should increase dramatically. Since flow relates directly to the radius, any increase will measurably affect the fluid flux rate. If they are not different from pressure-related changes, then the fluid flux rate should be about equal, given the same circumstances.

Fluid flux across the lung cannot be directly measured, but pulmonary lymph flow rate acts as an excellent indirect indicator of both quantity and quality of the fluid movement. The greater the protein in lymph, the more likely are permeability changes.

In laboratory studies in sheep, lymph flow rate and lymph protein concentration were measured at the same pulmonary microvascular pressure.[36,37] The lymphatics draining the lung were cannulated to collect all lymph flow. One group of sheep received a supposed permeability-altering substance (live *Pseudomonas* vaccine) while the other did not. Microvascular pressures were kept identical in both groups. Marked differences in flow rate and albumin concentration at the same pressure occurred in the *Pseudomonas* group compared with the control group, and these differences were ascribed to permeability changes.[38] However, some of the data have been questioned, and it is still unclear to some authorities whether or not permeability is a real factor.

Treatment of so-called permeability alteration remains mostly nonspecific. As previously mentioned, antihistamines may be of benefit in the treatment of histamine-induced changes. Prostaglandin E$_1$ appears to have a non-hemodynamic influence on the changes occurring after pulmonary emboli.[39] However, no other modalities for specifically interfering with capillary membrane alterations are available. Although steroids have been advocated to restore capillary integrity to normal, there is very little evidence to substantiate such claims.[40] In fact, there are such contradictory data regarding the efficacy of steroid usage in respiratory failure that the reader is urged to make his own determination.

Interstitial fibrosis and hyaline membranes develop in relation to the amount of protein flux. Fibrosis first begins about 6 days after the onset of interstitial water accumulation.[5] The pathologic alterations are

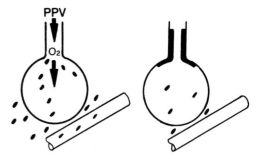

Fig. 20-5 Hyaline membrane formation. Protein in the alveolus is dried. Hyaline membranes form at the terminal air space and alter ventilation.

primarily in the interstitial space and consist of increased collagen deposition. The more severe forms of fibrosis occur in those cases categorized as having altered permeability. Once it occurs, pulmonary interstitial fibrosis is irreversible. It probably is responsible for the radiographic changes and altered pulmonary function in some patients after recovery from acute respiratory failure. Fibrosis can also account for chronic, fixed alterations of compliance.

Hyaline membrane formation does not result from alteration of type I alveolar histocytes, but instead appears to correlate with the appearance of increased permeability.[5] The greater the protein leakage, the more likely hyaline membrane formation. The chemical makeup of hyaline membranes consists of albumin, globulin, and fibrin. The first step most likely includes leakage of protein-laden edema fluid into the alveoli. This may explain the reduced incidence following cardiogenic pulmonary edema. If mechanical ventilation with high inflation pressure commences, drying, denaturation, coagulation, and inspissation of the secretions will accelerate deposition of hyaline membranes in the terminal airways.

Hyaline membrane lining of the terminal airways narrows the lumen (Fig. 20-5). This may contribute to a decrease in pulmonary compliance and prolongation of the ventilatory time constant of the involved units.

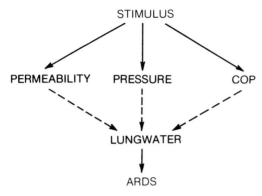

STIMULUS

PERMEABILITY   PRESSURE   COP

LUNGWATER

ARDS

Fig. 20-6 The factors leading to acute respiratory failure. Either alone or in combination, capillary permeability, microvascular pressure, and/or serum colloid oncotic pressure is altered. When lung safety mechanisms fail, lung water increases.

Not every imbalance of the Starling forces leads to interstitial fluid accumulation or acute respiratory failure (Fig. 20-6). In fact, only the few extremes ever require therapy. The lung functions with at least three protective or safety-valve mechanisms, the pulmonary lymphatics being the first line of defense. Conflicting evidence at this time makes evaluation of lymphatic efficiency difficult since it varies in different species.[41] However, in man, flow can increase at least 5 to 7 times over basal rates to aid in the removal of any excess fluid accumulation. As might be expected, protein and excess water are removed equally effectively.

Once the lymphatic mechanism exhausts itself, the interstitial space bears the major burden for ensuring continued normal gas exchange (Fig. 20-7). The pulmonary interstitial space functions as a two-compartment model consisting of the perivascular and peribronchiolar compartments. The peribronchiolar area, as previously mentioned, contains the lymphatics as well as the larger venules and arterioles.

The explanation of water accumulation in the lung can be extrapolated from various animal and laboratory data, including work on the isolated intact hind limb of the dog.[21] The analogy is based on intact parietal and visceral pleurae. When alterations of the Starling forces occur, fluid first leaks into the perivascular areas, but the volume of this potential space is apparently quite limited. At rest, alveolar expansion helps maintain a slightly negative pressure. The perivascular areas connect to the peribronchiolar space via high-resistance pathways. Slightly increased perivascular volume increases the negative pressure to about 0 cm H_2O, and the connecting channels to the peribronchiolar compartment begin to open.

Once fluid begins to move into the peribronchiolar areas, little further increase in interstitial pressure is detected (Fig. 20-8). The lung acts as a reservoir to soak up the increased fluid, increasing its capacity by a factor of 8, while blood gas exchange remains essentially unaffected.[41] However, pressure-sensitive receptors in the interstitium detect the slight changes, and hyperventilation ensues. Careful measurement may determine a decrease in pulmonary compliance, and larger transpulmonary pressure gradients (the difference between intrapleural and airway pressure) are required to deliver the same tidal volume.

Once the interstitial absorptive capacity

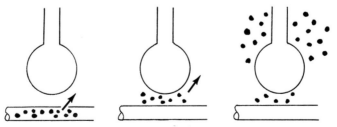

Fig. 20-7 When water moves into the lung, it first collects in the perivascular space and then moves to the peribronchiolar areas.

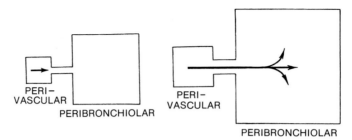

Fig. 20-8 Small amounts of fluid in the perivascular space overcome the high-resistance pathways and fluid moves into the peribronchiolar areas.

exhausts itself, the interstitial pressure begins to increase. At this stage, gas exchange deteriorates and becomes clinically detectable. The increased pressure does not change alveolar geometry but first impinges on the terminal airways. These untethered units are not really attached to any other nearby structure and are easily influenced by any increase of interstitial pressure. The elevated pressure constricts the airways and relative hypoventilation ensues, while simultaneously perfusion continues unimpaired (Fig. 20-9).[5]

A significant ventilation-perfusion imbalance occurs at this point.[42] The narrowed terminal airways cause an increase of the time constant required to ventilate or move oxygen molecules into the alveoli. Since any oxygen already present in the alveolus rapidly moves into the capillary blood, that unit may at least momentarily be devoid of oxygen while perfusion continues unchanged and blood departs that alveolar-capillary unit not completely saturated. In the pulmonary venous system, this blood combines with blood having normal amounts of oxygen coming from unaffected areas. The net effect is a dilution of the overall oxygen content. Clinically, arterial PO_2 decreases and venous admixture or intrapulmonary shunt increases.

If interstitial pressure continues to increase, the terminal airway may occlude and alveolar collapse follows. However, it should be stressed again that atelectasis does not re-flect the primary pathologic changes occurring in ARF. The process is a continuum which begins with ventilation-perfusion alterations. Even at autopsy, true segmental atelectasis represents a rare finding. Obviously, compliance and resistance further deteriorate as interstitial pressure continues to increase.

The third pulmonary safety-valve mechanism involves the alveoli themselves. Eventually, with continued increases in interstitial pressure secondary to fluid inflow, water and protein eventually make their way into the alveoli. Although the alveolar walls themselves become edematous, the epithelial lining remains intact. Water most likely makes its way through the terminal airways and not the alveolar wall. Alveolar fluid accumulation appears to be an all-or-none phenomenon, with the entire lung filling almost at once.[43] The various interconnecting chan-

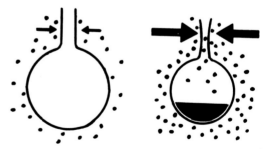

Fig. 20-9 The effects of pulmonary interstitial water. High interstitial pressures begin to narrow terminal airways and alter ventilation. Eventually fluid accumulates in the alveoli.

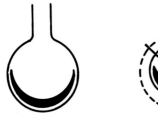

ALVEOLAR EDEMA: ↓ ALVEOLAR SIZE

Fig. 20-10 Fluid in the alveoli interferes with surfactant. Surface tension increases, causing a decrease in alveolar volume and FRC.

nels, such as the pores of Kohn, provide an easy access route for this process.[44] At this stage, pulmonary water increases by over 1,-500 ml, and the easily recognizable clinical signs of pulmonary edema, rales and frothy sputum, are detectable.

The accumulated water inactivates the alveolar surfactant as well as the type I cells responsible for its production (Fig. 20-10). Since surfactant normally reduces surface tension, its inactivation causes a decreased alveolar volume. The water already present prevents complete collapse. However, lung volume, including FRC, measurably decreases and blood gas function further deteriorates. The water also obviously interferes with gas exchange.

Causes of Acute Respiratory Failure

Clinical situations associated with a high incidence of ARF (Table 20-3) include major, multiple-system trauma, especially when associated with direct chest injuries.[45–47] Obviously, the resultant chest contusion can cause major disruption of the pulmonary gas exchange system. The response to generalized trauma is not often predictable. Most times, unlike direct penetrating injuries, blunt trauma invariably affects more than one organ system. The exact mechanism of pulmonary involvement remains unclear but may include a number of factors such as interference with normal

clotting mechanisms and release of free fatty acids from both long bone fractures and soft tissue injuries. Both responses may work alone or synergistically. Coagulation deficits may result in multiple peripheral thrombi in the pulmonary vascular bed. The pulmonary circulatory bed primarily acts as an efficient filtering system. At any one time, a large percentage of the vascular channels have little or no flow. Obliteration secondary to clots or thrombi in the patent vessels does not initially result in hypertension but instead in recruitment of previously non-patent pathways. In fact, 70 percent of the pulmonary vascular bed must be occluded before any increase in pulmonary artery pressure occurs.

Once microvascular pressure does increase, pulmonary interstitial water accumulation is much more likely to occur. In fact, some authorities feel that the most important effect of Starling forces on water movement involves alteration of pulmonary microvascular pressure.[48,49] All other alterations appear to be of secondary importance. The release of free fatty acids after soft tissue injuries leads to the same type of alterations in the pulmonary circulatory bed as might be expected in the fat embolism syndrome.

Acute peritonitis from any cause, including perforation of large or small bowel, or pancreatitis with or without abscess formation can cause a very severe form of ARF.[50–53] Again, the precise factors have not been well elucidated. Release of endotoxins, live bacteria, and/or viruses may interfere with capillary integrity, cause permeability alterations, and eventually increase lung water.

Additional changes take place during acute peritoneal inflammation. The small and large intestine develop marked distention from both the secondary ileus and bowel gas retention, as well as bowel wall edema. The abdominal inflammation and bowel distention produce significant diaphragmatic elevation, with a decrease in FRC and pulmonary compliance.

Many authors still feel that endotoxin release operates as a primary cause of ARF, although this has never been well documented. The endotoxin not only alters capillary permeability but also leads to intense vasoconstriction and marked pulmonary hypertension.[54]

Respiratory failure may develop after major surgery, especially upper abdominal or intrathoracic procedures. Risk factors identified include smoking, morbid obesity, abnormal pulmonary function testing, and length of operation. These predictors are useful for problems involving alveolar hypoventilation and CO_2 retention but are not nearly as useful for predicting hypoxic difficulties.[55]

Oxygenation can deteriorate because of patient refusal or inability to make maximal sustained inspiratory efforts. Failure to cough and take deep breaths leads to progressive partial, and eventually complete, atelectasis.[56] Since perfusion remains unchanged, PO_2 decreases. Although adequate documentation is lacking, protracted surgical manipulation, especially of the small bowel, may possibly lead to progressive hypoxemia. Since no other causes have been described, some have felt this response resulted from release of endogenous substances which affect the integrity of the alveolar capillary membrane.

Respiratory failure can also appear during an acute pneumonic process.[57] The familiar lobar pneumonia of bacterial origin is relatively easy to distinguish and has little bearing on the variety of ARF described here. However, the interstitial form of either viral or bacterial origin presents an entirely different picture. The invasion of bacteria or viruses may affect the alveolar capillary membrane, and the gradient for fluid movement may shift in the direction of the interstitial compartment. If lymphatic involvement develops, ability to rapidly remove any accumulating water may be severely compromised. The interstitial inflammation can affect fluid flux rates, which may increase in

proportion to the relative effectiveness of the various safety-valve mechanisms. That, plus the inflammatory process itself, contributes to ultrastructural derangements and the eventual increased interstitial pressure. The clinical picture appears similar to other causes of respiratory failure—hypoxemia and tachypnea develop while lung mechanics deteriorate. The usual mechanical disruptions include altered compliance and loss of lung volume.

The changes brought about by lobar pneumonia not only are different but do not respond to the same treatment modalities as the more common forms of respiratory failure. In these circumstances, the alveoli fill with proteinaceous debris and the ventilation-perfusion alterations occur because of alveolar rather than interstitial derangements. Until that clears, the patient is unlikely to respond to the usual treatment modalities so effective in ARF. In fact, increased airway pressures during unilateral lung disease may actually cause deterioration of pulmonary function. The pressure will be directed to the noninvolved, more compliant lung and not really affect the diseased portion. The high airway pressures may interfere with the pulmonary circulation. Being a low-pressure system, the pulmonary circulation is responsive to both gravitational and alveolar pressure. Flow can therefore be directed away from the non-involved healthy lung to the poorly ventilated, involved side, producing the very worst matching of ventilation to perfusion. Most gas is delivered to the non-involved healthy lung, while perfusion redirects itself to the diseased portion. A radiographically-significant lobar pneumonia may have minimal influence on gas exchange. Both alveolar ventilation and perfusion may alter to such a degree that significant ventilation-perfusion changes do not take place.

Alterations of the alveolar side of the alveolar-capillary membrane interface also contribute to the development of ARF. Aspiration of fresh- and salt-water, as well as of gastric contents, represent common problems.[58] Salt-water drowning very closely mimics fulminant pulmonary edema, since the fluid-filled alveoli cannot enter into gas exchange. Fortunately, in time, the salt-water is absorbed and the alveoli generally do not suffer any long-term ill effects. The major clinical challenge is to provide adequate support until resolution begins. The water absorbed may cause some increase in intravascular volume; however, this is usually not of clinical importance. Likewise, hemolysis or electrolyte disturbances are not major factors in salt-water drowning. The immediate and most important life-saving function involves early restoration of blood gas exchange using mechanical ventilation and positive end-expiratory pressure (PEEP). After near drowning, attempts to remove water are not very successful since aspirated volumes are usually not large and alveolar absorption begins almost immediately.

Fresh-water drowning represents a more difficult clinical problem. Not only are the alveoli filled with fluid, but the fresh-water inactivates the surfactant lining the alveoli. The surfactant produced by the type II alveoli cells lines the alveolar surface and reduces surface tension, preventing cell collapse. The type II cells are also inactivated or destroyed by the fresh-water. Since those cells must regenerate, the period of dysfunction is markedly lengthened. All these factors serve to make fresh-water drowning a more difficult clinical problem to treat than salt-water drowning. When compared with salt-water drowning, the unstable alveoli after fresh-water aspiration are more likely to require both mechanical ventilatory support and PEEP/CPAP for an increased interval.[59] As in salt-water drowning, electrolyte and hemolytic disturbances are actually of secondary importance. If they are severe enough to present a problem, the patient has usually already had an early, overwhelming hypoxic insult.

Aspiration of gastric contents can lead to several different sequelae.[60,61] Large particulate matter can become lodged in and obstruct the airway at any level. The gastric fluid can fill the alveoli in a manner similar to that in drowning and interfere with oxygenation and CO_2 elimination. Aspiration of fluid with a pH less than 2.5, as well as a large volume, has been associated with both high morbidity and high mortality. The acid causes severe damage to the alveolar capillary membrane, with loss of integrity and eventual interstitial fluid accumulation. Since Mendelson's description of acid aspiration, ingestion of antacids has become a popular prophylactic measure against acid aspiration, especially in the preanesthetic period.[62] However, alkali aspiration can have clinical effects as severe as those after acid aspiration.[63]

Aspiration may occur after active vomiting or silent regurgitation. Reports have demonstrated appearance of gastric contents in the lung despite protection of the airway with a cuffed endotracheal tube. During induction of anesthesia, cricoid pressure and the head-up position have been recommended to prevent aspiration. However, these are not 100 percent effective and the clinician must always be on the alert. As in the case of drowning, removal of the aspirate does not affect outcome unless large particulate material obstructs the airway.

ARDS may also develop after the inhalation of various substances, including the products of combustion. Toxic substances are often released, owing to burning of synthetic materials in closed spaces. The major pathological disruptions occur either to the alveolar-capillary membrane or to the alveoli themselves. Identification or listing of all such toxic products is not possible, but the severity of the problems usually relates to both the particular substance and the inspired concentration. The inflammation of the alveolar walls and destruction of the surfactant in general are not dissimilar to the changes after aspiration. However, certain substances can have very specific actions, such as interference with particular aspects of cellular function.

Some pulmonary changes may develop as a direct result of the hypoxia due to carbon monoxide inhalation.[64] This may account for some of the capillary membrane changes which disrupt the normal pathways of fluid movement in and out of the lung. Most likely, the immediate deaths in these instances are due to the hypoxia rather than to any specific effect of the various substances. However, carbon monoxide has other direct effects besides hypoxia. Poisoning of the cytochrome oxidase system rapidly destroys most cellular respiration.

Fat embolism syndrome can also contribute to or act as a precursor of acute respiratory failure.[65] Patients most at risk include those with long bone fractures or major soft tissue injuries. It can also occur in conjunction with major orthopedic surgery of the femur, hip, or pelvis. In all these circumstances, large fat globules are released from the marrow into the venous circulation and make their way to the pulmonary circulatory bed.

The fat itself is not the major problem; rather, the free fatty acids which are released are the actual culprits.[66] After arrival in the pulmonary artery, they may begin to alter and interfere with the normal capillary wall architecture. Platelets are then attracted to the injured area of the capillary, where they agglutinate and release serotonin. Not only do the fatty acids directly increase pulmonary vascular permeability, but the serotonin also alters capillary integrity and, in addition, promotes an intense pulmonary vasoconstriction. The resulting alteration of the previously balanced Starling forces means that conditions now favor water movement across the capillary bed into the pulmonary interstitium. If the pulmonary safety-valve mechanisms are overwhelmed, interstitial water accumulates and the fine reticular pattern characteristic of interstitial edema will become evident on the chest radiographs. Diagnosis of the fat embolism syndrome

is difficult.[67] The reputed characteristic findings do not appear with any regularity. Hypoxia, in association with the previously mentioned events, predominates as the most consistent finding. The chest radiograph may have the ground-glass appearance due to interstitial water. The mental confusion, often present, develops as a result of either the hypoxia or the petechial hemorrhages present in the cerebral cortex. The free fatty acids interfere with the normal clotting mechanisms, and petechiae can also develop in the eye grounds and nail beds. However, these changes are not always present and the diagnosis may require correlation of a history of long bone fractures with unexplained hypoxia. Even fat globules in the urine are not all that common a finding.

Special therapeutic maneuvers, including administration of heparin and intravenous alcohol, appear to have no specific benefits. Both supposedly help clear the fat, one by decreasing and the other by increasing serum lipase activity. Neither has been very successful in ameliorating the course of the disease. The traditional methods of treatment for ARF work as well in this circumstance as in any of the others.[68] Perhaps the most helpful ancillary measure includes immobilization of the involved extremity to prevent further release of fat particles.

Flail chest represents another specialized form of acute respiratory failure. Direct blunt trauma to the thorax usually causes the injury.[69] A flail chest has at least two consecutive ribs fractured in at least two places. Each rib section between the two fracture sites essentially floats free. During normal spontaneous breathing, as the diaphragm moves down and the chest wall out, intrathoracic pressure, which at rest is between -3 and -5 cm H_2O, becomes even more negative. This difference between intrathoracic and ambient or airway pressure permits gas to move freely into the lungs. With a flail chest, however, each time intrathoracic pressure becomes more negative, the free segment moves inward instead of out with the rest of the chest wall. This is the often decribed paradoxical motion. Since the chest wall moves inward, pulmonary expansion may be altered or decreased in the area underlying the injury site.

Not all cases of flail chest result in hypoxia.[70] Oxygenation deteriorates not because of the flail but because of the underlying pulmonary contusion resulting from the same impact originally causing the flail. The contusion is an area of edema and hemorrhage. If, as is usually the case, the edema interferes more with ventilation than with perfusion, a ventilation-perfusion mismatch may develop and hypoxemia follow. The rapid shallow respirations and chest wall splinting occur in response to the decreased oxygenation and interstitial fluid accumulation as well as to the pain.

This respiratory pattern accentuates the flail. Early observers interpreted this finding as evidence that the altered oxygenation resulted directly from the flail. The use of PEEP and/or continuous positive airway pressure (CPAP) with intermittent mandatory ventilation (IMV) has helped delineate the problem.[71] As end-expiratory pressure increases independently of any ventilator rate changes, the tachypnea subsides owing to the improved oxygenation. Once the spontaneous rate decreases, the flail becomes much less pronounced. Decreasing PEEP/CPAP and recurrence of hypoxemia cause a resumption of the hyperventilation, and the paradoxical motion resumes anew.

It is clear that any therapy must concentrate first and most importantly on the lung contusion and not on the flail. Measures to internally or externally stabilize the chest wall are not required. These methods have previously included wire fixation, towel clips, and controlled mechanical ventilation. Prolonged, controlled mechanical ventilation and patient paralysis neither improve nor alter the course of the disease. Spontaneous respiration will not interfere with the healing process of the fractured ribs, provided the hypoxia secondary to the contusion is ade-quately corrected with expiratory positive pressure. This appreciation of the important pathologic changes can measurably shorten the time of ventilatory support. The normalization of blood gas exchange responds to appropriate PEEP or CPAP therapy and can usually be discontinued within 5 to 7 days. Mechanical support can then be easily weaned. Even after withdrawal of all ancillary support, some flailing may still be clinically detectable but will have no effect on blood gas exchange provided hypoxemia is no longer present. When cases of flail chest are described as not requiring mechanical ventilation, no doubt any underlying parenchymal damage is only minimal and hypoxemia does not constitute a major problem.

Pulmonary embolism may also lead to the development of ARDS; however, the major changes are vascular in origin and are not directly germane to the present discussion.

With an understanding of the basic pathophysiologic changes occurring in ARF, the rationale behind the various treatment modalities can more readily be understood. In summary, respiratory failure develops secondary to disruption of the Starling forces. When the lung safety-valve mechanisms are overwhelmed, water accumulation produces alterations in normal ventilation-perfusion relationships. Lung volumes decrease, and in the final stages the alveoli are overwhelmed by the sudden inflow of water and protein.

TREATMENT OF RESPIRATORY FAILURE

Effective treatment of ARF presumes the correct diagnosis has been made. All other causes of reduced PaO_2 or increased intrapulmonary shunt must have been evaluated and, if present, appropriately treated. These include copious pulmonary secretions, altered FiO_2, pneumothorax, atelectasis, right mainstem intubation, severe bronchospasm, pneumonia, increased oxygen consumption, decreased cardiac output, and other similar events.[72,73]

Oxygen Therapy

Once the basic pathophysiologic derangements present in ARF are understood, the clinician can plan a specific treatment regimen. The initial therapeutic response to the hypoxia includes supplemental oxygen therapy. This will usually correct or prevent severe hypoxemia and buy time until events can be sorted out and the patient begun on the most efficacious therapy. However, prolonged high inspired oxygen concentrations might eventually prove detrimental. Sufficient data exist which demonstrate an actual increase in intrapulmonary shunt when breathing oxygen at close to 100 percent concentrations.[74,75]

A major alteration in acute respiratory failure is ventilation-perfusion mismatching secondary to narrowing of the terminal airways. In essence the time constants are extended, which means it requires a finitely longer time to deliver the same gas volume in the alveoli. At an FIO_2 of 0.5 or less, nitrogen comprises a large component of the alveolar gas mixture. Nitrogen acts as an inert gas, and at ambient pressure blood and tissues are already saturated with nitrogen molecules. Although nitrogen continually moves between the alveoli and the blood and between blood and tissue, no net accumulation occurs in any of the compartments. Hence the label *inert gas*. During ARF, elevated interstitial pressures increase the likelihood of airway and eventually alveolar collapse. Sufficient lung volume will prevent or oppose those effects; when adequate nitrogen is in the mixture, there are no real problems.[76] Although oxygen rapidly exits from the alveoli via capillary perfusion, enough of the inert nitrogen remains behind to act as a splint and maintain alveolar patency by preventing collapse due to the elevated interstitial pressures.

When the ARF patient breathes 100 percent oxygen, blood perfusing the alveoli rapidly extracts all the oxygen present. The increased time constants mean a prolongation of the time the alveoli contain little if any gas. The alveoli, now devoid of any gas, cannot continue to oppose the elevated interstitial pressure and begin to collapse, and the calculated intrapulmonary shunt increases. Unfortunately, these changes are not prevented by the application of PEEP or CPAP.

When this mechanism is operative, the increase in intrapulmonary shunt is accompanied by a reduction in lung volume, specifically FRC. Therefore, a therapeutic maneuver originally designed to increase oxygenation may actually contribute to a further deterioration of pulmonary function.

High inspired oxygen concentrations can also blunt the protective mechanism of hypoxic pulmonary vasoconstriction (HPV).[27] Normally, a low alveolar oxygen pressure (PAO_2) represents alveolar hypoventilation secondary to ventilation-perfusion mismatch or alveolar collapse. Capillary perfusion continues basically unaltered despite the ventilation changes resulting from events such as terminal airway narrowing. A major ventilation-perfusion mismatch is prevented by the protective HPV response. The vasoconstriction diverts blood from altered areas of ventilation to noninvolved areas. The reduced flow to the hypoventilated areas helps preserve V/Q relationships and maintain oxygenation, thus preventing deterioration of the shunt fraction. A high FIO_2 blunts this response; localized tissue hypoxia remains minimal and perfusion continues or increases to the involved areas.[77] Intrapulmonary shunt may actually increase. Since the amount of pulmonary vascular smooth muscle is minimal, a large intrapulmonary blood volume, indicated by high capillary wedge pressures, can also ablate the entire HPV mechanism.[78,79]

High inspired oxygen concentrations may also lead to pulmonary oxygen toxicity.[80] Most available evidence indicates that lung changes begin after breathing 100 percent oxygen for as little as 6 hours. The pathophysiology resembles ARF. In fact, the two conditions are often indistinguishable, particularly if extremely high O_2 concentrations are delivered for any length of time during respiratory failure. The derangements develop in response to the accumulation of superoxide, hydrogen peroxide, and other toxic radicals. Alveolar infiltration, interstitial edema, and hyaline membrane formation are all demonstrable. The changes at atmospheric pressure are related to both the exposure time and concentration of inspired oxygen. Most authorities agree that at an FIO_2 of less than 0.5, the risk of O_2 toxicity is quite minimal. At an FIO_2 above 0.6, changes may appear after 48 hours; whereas substantial chest pain may begin as early as 6 hours after breathing 100 percent oxygen. The earliest detectable findings include a reduction of vital capacity.

A high inspired oxygen concentration can be excluded as a helpful adjunctive maneuver in ARF. Not only does it have its own peculiar problems, as previously described, but oxygenation does not markedly improve despite the increase in delivered concentration.

Oxygen can improve the hypoxia secondary to V/Q mismatch.[81] The effective therapeutic ranges appear to include an FIO_2 between 0.21 and 0.35. The increased oxygen concentration has the effect of converting hypoventilated units to more-normally ventilated areas apparently by minimizing the amount of time the alveoli are devoid of oxygen. Alveoli always have some gas present so that perfusion to totally unoxygenated units does not develop. If ventilation is absent altogether, as eventually happens in most units, an increased FIO_2 cannot significantly alter the ventilation-perfusion relationships and thereby improve oxygenation.

Adjuvant Therapy

Is there any role for steroid therapy in the treatment of ARF? Recent evidence has demonstrated that complement activation, particularly C5-A, may play a direct role.[40] Conditions associated with ARF such as sepsis, pancreatitis, and multiple system trauma can all activate the complement system.

The specific complement factor, C5-A, interacts with leukocytes to cause plugging of the pulmonary vascular bed. Steroids may have a role in decreasing the effects of C5-A. The key may be early dosage since the white cell plugging occurs only very transiently, being dissipated in less than 1 hour.

Both diuretic therapy and albumin infusions have been extensively used as treatment modalities during ARF.[82-84] Proponents have argued that since the diuretics increase free water clearance and decrease intravascular volume, the eventual reduction of intravascular pressure and concomitant elevation of colloid oncotic pressure will influence the Starling forces so that the direction of any fluid shift will be from the pulmonary interstitial to the intravascular space.[85] Unfortunately, these methods have been uniformly unsuccessful in reversing the clinical syndrome and have not improved the mortality rate. The events originally responsible for the imbalance in the Starling forces are apparently still active; neither diuretics nor albumin, even in high doses, has enhanced oxygenation; presumably, therefore, they cannot change the gradient for fluid movement.

Much has been written about the relationship of acute respiratory failure and pulmonary hypertension.[86,87] When present, pulmonary hypertension does represent a severe form of respiratory dysfunction. However, not all severe cases of ARF necessarily involve pulmonary hypertension.[88] Therefore, the cause-effect relationship of pulmonary hypertension remains unclear.

Pulmonary hypertension has several detrimental aspects. The elevated pressures contribute to changes in the Starling forces favorable to fluid movement into the interstitium. Additionally, elevated pulmonary artery pressure may severely affect right ventricular afterload and ultimately cardiac output.

Specific therapy aimed at the reduction of pulmonary hypertension has had mixed or unpredictable results. The most popular agent, sodium nitroprusside, has been found to increase intrapulmonary shunt. However, when shunt does change, it appears to relate to reductions in cardiac output rather than to direct alterations of pulmonary artery pressure.[89,90]

If cardiac output increases with nitroprusside, as hoped for, intrapulmonary shunt does not necessarily change. Nitroprusside, as well as all other vasodilators, does not have specific effects on the pulmonary circulation. Unfortunately, while used in attempting to lower pulmonary artery pressure, it also profoundly affects the systemic circulation.

Respiratory alkalosis theoretically acts as a pulmonary vasodilator and reduces pulmonary artery pressure.[19] However, the mechanical rate needed to achieve significant alkalosis may itself have detrimental effects.

As previously indicated, clinical data have demonstrated that interstitial lung water accumulation, while often responsible for acute respiratory failure, does not correlate with the degree of hypoxemia.[91-93] Therefore, even if some decrease in lung water occurs after diuretic and albumin therapy, it is probably not of sufficient magnitude to influence gas exchange.[94]

Ventilator Therapy

The initial response after lung water begins to accumulate includes tachypnea and hyperventilation. However, because of the interstitial derangements, including altered compliance, spontaneous breathing cannot increase ventilation to most of the affected lung units. The patient cannot generate a large enough transpulmonary pressure gradient to overcome the extra-alveolar forces or pressures which were originally responsible

for the total or partial terminal airway collapse. As terminal airway narrowing worsens, the units become essentially devoid of all gas, and alveolar collapse ensues. Even combined diaphragmatic and chest wall movement cannot develop a pressure gradient large enough to expand the collapsed units. The patient continues to hyperventilate but to no avail. The newly collapsed units remain nonventilated while perfusion continues and the intrapulmonary shunting and ventilation-perfusion mismatch continue.[95] While oxygenation does not improve, the linear carbon dioxide dissociation curve permits easy removal of that gas via the remaining ventilated units and accompanying increase in minute ventilation. In fact, CO_2 elimination proceeds without difficulty until actual alveolar infiltration develops.

The next logical step in the development of an effective treatment regimen for ARF includes the addition of the mechanical ventilator. Since the primary problem was one of breathing or respiration, then employment of such a device seems logical. However, the mechanical ventilator by itself does not enhance oxygenation.

Consideration of the lung as a two-unit model can improve understanding of the problem. The positive pressure ventilation will significantly increase airway pressure. If the pressure generated is sufficient to open the collapsed units, then gas will move into those areas during the mechanical inspiratory phase. Since perfusion continues unchanged throughout the entire process, some improvement in blood gas exchange would be expected. However, oxygenation does not significantly increase. This is due to the fact that when the mechanical ventilator cycles into the exhalation phase, airway pressure rapidly reverts to the baseline or ambient level. Any distending force on the affected alveolar units is removed and the terminal airways or alveoli recollapse. Perfusion continues and once again marked alterations of ventilation-perfusion relationships persist.

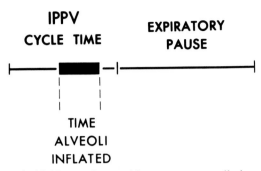

**IPPV
CYCLE TIME**   **EXPIRATORY
PAUSE**

TIME
ALVEOLI
INFLATED

Fig. 20-11 During positive pressure ventilation the airway pressure sufficient to keep alveoli expanded accounts for only a small portion of the inspiratory phase of ventilation.

Examination of the entire inspiratory-expiratory cycle illustrates why positive pressure ventilation does not alleviate the problem (Fig. 20-11). Gas exchange can only improve when alveoli are both ventilated and perfused. Mechanical ventilation reexpands the collapsed alveoli only during mechanical inspiration and even then not during the entire time of inspiration. In fact, evaluation of the entire inspiratory-expiratory cycle indicates that alveolar reexpansion occupies only a small portion of the entire ventilatory cycle. Under those circumstances no real improvement in gas exchange can be expected.

To provide better understanding of these events, an explanation of some aspects of pulmonary physiology is in order. The reasoning can apply to the lung as a whole or to an individual alveolus. During conditions of increased interstitial pressure, the lung requires elevated airway pressures to maintain full expansion. As airway pressure diminishes, so does lung volume. Eventually a pressure is reached below which complete collapse occurs. This point represents the critical closing pressure (CCP). Efforts to reexpand the involved portion require airway pressure application in excess of the closing pressure. The critical opening pressure refers to that point when the alveoli begin to re-expand.[96] That pressure usually exceeds the CCP. Once it is reached, expansion proceeds

quite easily without much further pressure increase.

With the patient attached to a mechanical ventilator, the following scenario takes place. During mechanical inspiration, the respirator develops an airway pressure greater than the terminal airway units' critical opening pressures. With alveolar recruitment, blood gas exchange begins. However, during exhalation, the airway pressure drops below opening pressure; no further blood gas exchange takes place in the affected units. However, if airway pressure is not permitted to reach CCP, then collapse will not recur and blood gas exchange will be markedly enhanced. Positive end-expiratory pressure prevents airway pressure from falling below CCP, and oxygenation continues improved.[97] PEEP and mechanical ventilation appear to work in tandem. The ventilator generates significantly high airway pressures to overcome the interstitial pressure effects and re-expands the collapsed alveoli while PEEP prevents their recollapse. The overall effect includes sustained improvement in gas exchange as well as restoration of resting lung volume.[98] Neither PEEP nor mechanical ventilation alone can successfully reverse the changes described. Rather, both must function in tandem, one to recruit and the other to sustain the acquired changes.

PEEP versus CPAP

Confusion still exists regarding the difference between PEEP and CPAP. Comparison of spontaneous breathing patterns demonstrates the differences (Fig. 20-12). Both have an elevated baseline or resting airway pressure. During CPAP the spontaneous effort reduces airway pressure. However, at no time does the inspiratory airway pressure reach atmospheric or become subambient. The amount of reduction in pressure depends on the patient's breathing effort and the type of spontaneous breathing system.

PEEP implies that during spontaneous

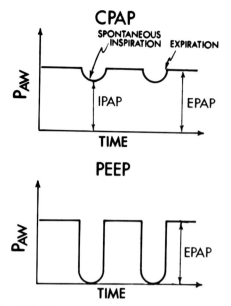

Fig. 20-12 PEEP and CPAP spontaneous breathing patterns. With CPAP, despite negative deflections airway pressure remains positive during the entire cycle. PEEP maintains positive airway pressure only during the exhalation phase. Inspiratory positive airway pressure (IPAP) refers to the lowest positive airway pressure. It is determined by the inspiratory effort. Expiratory airway pressure (EPAP) represents the baseline pressure.

breathing airway pressure does reach ambient or subambient levels. Positive pressure develops only at end-expiration, hence the designation *positive end-expiratory pressure*.

Attachment to a mechanical ventilator does not alter the terminology. If during mechanical ventilation the baseline pressure is elevated and the patient does not breathe spontaneously, then CPAP is in effect. This has previously been designated *continuous positive pressure breathing* (CPPB). When mechanical ventilation and spontaneous breathing coexist, as with intermittent mandatory ventilation (IMV), then either CPAP or PEEP may be operative. If the spontaneous effort reduces airway pressure to ambient or subambient levels, then intermittent mandatory ventilation with PEEP is the appropriate terminology. On the other hand, if airway pressure does not reach ambient levels,

then the system is IMV with CPAP. Depending on the patient's respiratory effort, the mode may actually change from breath to breath.

During spontaneous breathing, the greater the reduction in airway pressure, the greater the enhancement of venous return.[99, 100] However, the greater the airway pressure change, the greater the work of breathing.[101] Clinically, an attempt is made to reach a middle ground, maximizing venous return but not at the cost of a markedly increased work of breathing.

When utilizing PEEP or CPAP, the clinician must initially select an appropriate endpoint. Various plans have been proposed.[102, 103] Many have advocated PEEP/CPAP levels which restore PaO_2 to a level consistent with adequate oxygen saturation while the patient breathes less than toxic concentrations of oxygen. At a normal pH, a PaO_2 of 70 mmHg or higher indicates a hemoglobin saturation of 90 percent or more. Pulmonary oxygen toxicity has not been reported with an FiO_2 of 0.5 or less.

The usual clinical response to developing hypoxia almost always includes an increase in supplemental oxygen. Once all the other causes of a reduced PaO_2 have been ruled out and ARF appropriately diagnosed, PEEP/CPAP therapy is begun; initial levels of 3 to 5 cm H_2O are incrementally increased.[104] As PaO_2 improves, the FiO_2 can be concurrently reduced. Once the endpoint (an arterial saturation of 90 percent on an FiO_2 of less than 0.5) is reached, therapy is considered complete. Any further reduction in PaO_2 will require an appropriate increase in PEEP/CPAP. At times the disease process will further deteriorate, requiring another upward adjustment of the end-expiratory pressure.

As will be discussed, high levels of PEEP/CPAP may interfere with cardiac function. Therefore, some clinicians advocate arbitrary upper limits for CPAP/PEEP, arguing that high levels may seriously impair cardiac function. The usual limits prescribed are 15 to 18 cm H_2O. However, at least one clinical study has demonstrated that a substantial number of patients with apparently severe forms of ARF did not respond to PEEP/CPAP levels up to 15 cm H_2O. Not until PEEP was increased, in some cases far in excess of 15 cm H_2O, did any real improvement in oxygenation occur.[105] If those patients had been arbitrarily maintained at the recommended lower levels, they would not have experienced any improvement in oxygenation. The choice should be predicated on physiologic parameters rather than on arbitrary selection of an end point. The parameters may vary with the clinician, but the eventual PEEP/CPAP levels will more nearly relate to the underlying disease process.

Another proposed endpoint has been pulmonary compliance.[106] Compliance is calculated as the volume delivered divided by the airway pressure differential required to deliver that volume. Either dynamic or static compliance can be chosen. Static compliance includes changes in both lung and chest wall. Clamping the expiratory limb of the circuit after delivery of the breath while performing an inflation hold helps determine static compliance. Dynamic compliance utilizes the peak inflation pressure developed during mechanical inspiration, including airway resistance.

Several studies have attempted to demonstrate a correlation between compliance and oxygen delivery, which includes cardiac output and arterial oxygen content. When compliance is maximized, oxygen delivery also appears maximal. However, further increases in PEEP/CPAP, while demonstrating a reduction in both compliance and oxygen delivery, result in marked improvement in other parameters of oxygenation, namely PaO_2 and intrapulmonary shunt. Oxygen delivery decreases in response to a reduction in cardiac output. It is now known that appropriate cardiovascular interventions will maintain cadiac output, which further emphasizes the lack of correlation between

compliance and other factors. In fact, other studies have also failed to show any consistent relationship between oxygenation and compliance.

Optimal PEEP/CPAP

Gallagher et al popularized the concept of optimal PEEP/CPAP.[107] Intrapulmonary shunt or venous admixture reduction to 15 percent identified the optimal therapeutic goal. For critically ill patients, it is recommended to calculate shunt rather than to follow PaO_2 since many patients have multisystem failure. Either increased oxygen consumption, decreased cardiac output, or a combination of both can cause a reduction in mixed venous or pulmonary artery oxygen content. With any degree of pulmonary dysfunction, only a fixed amount of oxygen is delivered to the blood. Therefore, the amount of oxygen in blood returning to the lungs will determine the PaO_2.[73]

Intrapulmonary shunt or venous admixture, on the other hand, changes only in relation to pulmonary changes. Shunt indicates the portion of cardiac output not oxygenated during flow through the lungs. Cardiac output has less influence on shunt fraction, and therefore intrapulmonary shunt more directly reflects only pulmonary changes.

Certain errors may develop when calculating intrapulmonary shunt.[95] Occasionally, authors have advocated calculating shunt by the modified shunt equation. Since this method assumes a constant oxygen consumption, it should not be used in critically ill patients who often have a continually changing rate of oxygen consumption. The shunt equation assumes 100 percent saturation in the pulmonary capillary bed; therefore, the inspired oxygen concentration must exceed 30 percent to guarantee total saturation.

Venous admixture or intrapulmonary shunt accounts for all disruptions of blood gas exchange in the lung. These include true anatomic shunting, such as lack of perfusion after a pulmonary embolus. True anatomic shunt may develop during high-altitude pulmonary edema when profound arteriolar constriction directs blood away from ventilated areas. Shunting may also develop when ventilation is completely impaired while some perfusion continues. Atelectasis exemplifies these types of change. Most times, the major pathophysiologic events in ARF relate not to true shunting but rather to ventilation-perfusion mismatch in areas where ventilation is less than normal in comparison with the degree of alveolar perfusion.

Major alterations in cardiac output can directly influence the shunt fraction. Since shunt varies with ventilation-perfusion relationships, any large change in pulmonary blood flow might conceivably alter the shunt calculation. In fact, various vasoactive agents, including dopamine and nitroprusside, have been implicated in these changes.[108] Most of the changes happen with alteration of cardiac output. The patency of the pulmonary vascular system depends more on flow than on pressure. As cardiac output varies, flow and hence ventilation-perfusion relationships also change. If cardiac output does not markedly change, shunt remains the same.

The goal of a reduction of intrapulmonary shunt to 15 percent developed because it corresponds to most authorities' definitions of respiratory failure.[109] An alveolar-arterial oxygen gradient [$P(A-a)O_2$] of 300 to 350 mmHg ($FIO_2 = 1.0$) equals about a 15 percent shunt when cardiac output is undisturbed. Since most have advocated initiating therapy at an $P(A-a)O_2$ of 350 mmHg, it does not seem unreasonable to initiate treatment which could restore pulmonary function to that level. The results indicate that the goal can be easily achieved without any untoward risk to the patient. The incidence of pulmonary barotrauma and cardiac depression is similar to that with other ventilatory modes, and the vast majority of patients require less than 25 cm H_2O of PEEP or CPAP. The

mortality rates strictly from respiratory failure equal or are less than those with other methods. To date there is no definitive evidence indicating the best method to treat respiratory failure, since mortality rates do not appear to differ. However, more subtle differences may relate to such things as duration of therapy, complications from the therapy, and length of hospital stay. Until questions of this type are settled, a clear-cut answer as to the preferred treatment regimen does not exist.

When all patients are treated to the same endpoint, for example shunt reduction to 15 percent, there are means of comparing the severity of the illness. Since the criteria remain the same, those requiring greater levels of raised-airway-pressure therapy to attain the same therapeutic endpoint must have a more significant pulmonary injury. In addition, other interventions, including adjustment of the rate and duration of IMV, can also be applied on the basis of objective criteria and thus utilized to compare ARF in different patient populations.

Once PEEP/CPAP has attained a therapeutic endpoint, how long should the modality remain in effect at that particular level? There is no known correct answer. Clinicians usually select some arbitrary minimal time. In general, the longer it takes to reach a preselected level or the higher that level, the longer one should wait before attempting to reduce PEEP/CPAP. When levels of over 20 cm H_2O are in effect, each 24-hour period may see the original level reduced by only one-third to one-half. Weaning from PEEP/CPAP should proceed in the same organized, incremental manner as titration to optimal levels, provided shunt remains within the same acceptable range. Blood gas exchange continues to act as a more sensitive indicator than any other method, including radiography or pulmonary mechanics.

Face-mask CPAP can be utilized for mild forms of ARF.[110] Essentially, the method provides continuous distending pressure to the airway while avoiding the ne-

Table 20-4
Indications for CPAP Mask

Mild ARF
Spontaneous respiration
Normocarbia
Awake-cooperative

cessity of intubation. A continuous flow of gas at a specified FIO_2 through a system similar to a ventilator circuit constitutes all that is necessary. However, the ventilator itself is not actually required. The patient must have adequate spontaneous respiration ($PaCO_2 <$ 45 mmHg) and be alert and cooperative (Table 20-4).

Detrimental effects of the CPAP mask include patient discomfort and gastric distention. Air does accumulate in the stomach and a nasogastric tube should always be placed during face-mask CPAP therapy.

When levels above 10 cm H_2O are required, intubation and mechanical ventilation at low rates may be more efficacious. The ventilator delivers the higher pressures necessary to reach critical opening pressures, while CPAP will maintain the levels which prevent airway closure. If CPAP alone is used, high levels will be required to open the airway units, while actually lower pressure levels could be maintained with an occasional higher pressure during the inspiratory phase of mechanical ventilation.

Complications of PEEP/CPAP

Major problems identified with PEEP/CPAP therapy include interference with cardiac output.[111,112] Several factors appear to operate at different points in the cardiopulmonary circulation. With the initiation of positive airway pressure therapy, any degree of hypovolemia frequently causes a reduced cardiac output. In reality, the patient may act normovolemic, but the raised airway pressure imparts some reduction of venous return to the right heart. The elevated airway pressures are transmitted across the

pulmonary parenchyma to the intrathoracic space. The normally negative intrathoracic pressure may become positive and interfere with superior and inferior vena cava blood return. Dye studies during positive pressure mechanical inspiration have demonstrated actual narrowing of both structures during their intrathoracic course.[113] Stroke volume decreases and cardiac output falls. The arterial blood pressure trace on the oscilloscope may indicate the onset of the problem. Soon after the mechanical breath, the amplitude of the arterial trace markedly diminishes, eventually returning to baseline levels before the next breath. Further evidence of the problem often includes a low central venous or pulmonary capillary wedge pressure (PCWP). Spontaneous breathing reduces intrathoracic pressure and can enhance venous return and restore cardiac output.

During positive pressure breathing the high airway pressures can also influence pulmonary artery pressure.[114-116] As before, each positive pressure breath elevates all intrathoracic pressures, including pulmonary artery pressure. Pulmonary vascular resistance increases, and right ventricular afterload also subsequently rises. Radionuclide scanning can demonstrate heretofore unsuspected changes. Normally, the right ventricle, a thin-walled chamber, operates at low pressures and generates only about one-tenth the work of the left ventricle. In response to an increased pulmonary vascular pressure and resistance, right ventricular dilatation ensues and the intraventricular septum begins to bulge into the left ventricle.[117,118] At this point, right and left ventricular end-diastolic pressures must equilibrate.[119] The left ventricle, being a much thicker muscle, cannot dilate nearly so easily and is also constrained by the rigid pericardium. The septum bulges into the left ventricular outflow tract, interfering with stroke volume. Appropriate therapy should include positive inotropic support, primarily to support right ventricular function. Spontaneous ventilation in lieu of positive pressure mechanical breaths will also limit those pressure effects by reducing the number of intrusions each hour on the pulmonary artery.[120-122]

Distention by PEEP/CPAP of terminal airway units can eventually influence the pulmonary vascular bed. As lung volume increases, and especially with overdistention, several changes occur in the pulmonary capillary bed. Again, positive pressure breathing further complicates the problem. Each mechanical breath can trap blood in the pulmonary circulation, leading to decreased left ventricular preload and eventually decreased stroke volume. Overdistention of the airway may impinge upon capillary diameter and flow. Pulmonary vascular resistance increases, and right ventricular function can deteriorate.

One laboratory study has demonstrated the probable release of endogenous cardiac depressants.[112] After one animal was placed on mechanical ventilation with PEEP, cardiac output decreased. Blood from that first animal was then cross-circulated to a second animal not mechanically ventilated, and the cardiac output of the second animal also decreased. The evidence points to release of some endogenous substance, perhaps secondary to lung expansion.

Data also suggest possible altered ventricular compliance. Again in animals, cardiac output fell after the introduction of PEEP/CPAP and mechanical ventilation. Despite return of transmural PCWP (wedge pressure minus intrathoracic pressure) to original values, stroke volume remained less than before the institution of mechanical ventilation.[116] This suggests altered ventricular contractility or compliance. The authors postulate that pulmonary parenchymal overdistention could cause the lung to come in close contact with the left ventricle, perhaps changing compliance and interfering with ventricular function (Fig. 20-13).

Another clinical problem associated with PEEP/CPAP therapy involves accurate PCWP measurements. By convention, pressures are recorded at end-expiration and the

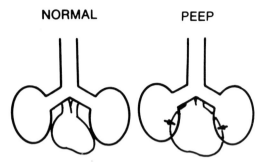

NORMAL   **PEEP**

Fig. 20-13 One effect of PEEP on ventricular function. Overdistention of the lung may compress and interfere with left ventricular function and/or compliance.

catheter tip zeroed to the right atrium. As previously stated, alveolar overdistention interferes with and constricts the pulmonary circulation. Therefore, any measurement of pulmonary vascular pressure can reflect both intra- and extravascular forces. Reports have appeared indicating that the position of the catheter tip itself influences the pressures recorded. If the tip lodges in the so-called zone I, where alveolar pressure is normally higher than vascular pressure and where there is little actual blood flow, PCWP readings can be meaningless. In zone II alveolar pressure is less than pulmonary arterial but greater than venous pressure. Alveolar pressure changes still exert an influence on recorded wedge pressure. The same interrelationships are operative, but less so in the dependent zone III areas, where vascular pressures are usually greater than alveolar pressure. High airway pressures can obviously impact here and, at times, change these relationships. Fortunately, clinical studies have demonstrated that most times the catheter tip is in either zone II or zone III.[123] Also, in the supine position most, if not all, of zone I is eliminated. Therefore, provided the catheter is properly zeroed, the tip location does not constitute a major problem.

The problem still remains of how to measure PCWP during mechanical ventilatory support. In order to remove all effects of PEEP and give true vascular pressures, some clinicians have advocated disconnecting the patient from the ventilator. However, sudden removal of PEEP can trigger a large influx of blood into the pulmonary vascular bed. This effect can be imagined as similar to the opening of a dam in the intrathoracic superior and inferior vena cava. In the space of one or two heart beats a massive inflow of blood dramatically increases the pulmonary vascular volume.

It should be apparent to the reader that any interpretation of wedge pressure during mechanical ventilation and expiratory positive pressure risks error. At times, little correlation exists between left ventricular end-diastolic volume and wedge pressure, especially with pre-existing myocardial disease. Clinical evaluation in light of all data will be required to determine the meaning of a wedge pressure of 20 mmHg recorded during 15 cm H_2O of raised airway pressure therapy. The values change and do not always accurately reflect the true hemodynamic relationships during PEEP/CPAP.

Various mathematical formulas have been proposed to predict the effect of the various PEEP/CPAP levels on wedge pressure. However, since the data for these calculations come from small series of patients, they usually cannot be accurately applied to any individual case.

A different approach involves subtracting intrathoracic from measured wedge pressure in order to calculate transmural or true intravascular capillary wedge pressure. An esophageal balloon catheter can estimate intrathoracic pressure. However, real doubt exists about the validity of the measurement obtained in the supine position because of the influence of the mediastinal structures. Direct catheterization of the intrathoracic space to measure intrapleural pressure, while feasible, does increase patient morbidity and cannot be advocated as standard therapy.[124] In addition, the location of the catheter may preclude measurement of overall intrathoracic pressure.

Recent data have called into question the entire validity of the PCWP during mechanical ventilatory support.[125] Normally, it is assumed that wedge pressure eventually reflects left ventricular end-diastolic pressure (LVEDP). Studies on animals treated with mechanical ventilation and CPAP demonstrate even a marked discrepancy between transmural wedge pressure and LVEDP. In all instances transmural wedge was significantly higher than transmural LVEDP. It appears that in the absence of spontaneous breathing, airway pressure neither is equally transmitted nor equally impinges upon all the intrathoracic pressures. Left heart filling pressures are not nearly as high as would be indicated by wedge pressure. This study may explain some of the difficulty encountered when assessing cardiac function during raised airway pressure therapy. The reported low cardiac outputs may actually indicate inadequate left ventricular filling pressures and volume. Whether blood has remained trapped in the lungs is not clear.

A further complication of raised airway pressure therapy includes the changes in renal function.[126,127] Clinically these most often manifest themselves as a decrease in urine flow.[128] Further laboratory determinations may indicate an elevated vasopressin level as well as changes in urinary sodium excretion.[129] Glomerular filtration rate also falls during positive pressure therapy.

The clinical alterations are clear but the responsible mechanisms are not. Also, spontaneous breathing may mitigate some of the responses. Very few attempts have been made to investigate the apparent differences in renal function when continuous positive pressure therapy is replaced by a method permitting spontaneous breathing.

When animals have no spontaneous respiratory efforts, positive airway pressure decreases carotid sinus and aortic arch baroreceptor activity, and all the above-mentioned changes in renal function take place. When animals breathe spontaneously, changes in sodium excretion and vasopressin are not as large as in the group without spontaneous breathing. These differences may be explained by a greater transmural inferior vena cava pressure in the spontaneous group. It is probably safe to conclude that more than one mechanism operates to produce these observed variations in renal physiology.

Intermittent Mandatory Ventilation

While raised airway pressures can be applied in connection with any form of mechanical ventilation, there may be particular reasons to primarily employ IMV.[130] The technique is explained in detail in chapter 21. Suffice it to say here that IMV promotes spontaneous breathing while simultaneously limiting the number of positive pressure breaths. Spontaneous breathing has several theoretical and proven benefits.

Mechanical positive pressure breathing, in addition to recruitment and re-expansion of collapsed airway units, primarily determines alveolar ventilation. Clinically, the $PaCO_2$ indicates the adequacy or level of the ventilatory process. As stated previously, CO_2 elimination during ARF does not ordinarily present a problem. However, in pre-terminal situations in which alveolar infiltration is present with fluffy infiltrative changes on the radiograph, hypercapnia may be more prone to develop. Earlier, $PaCO_2$ is usually low, 30 to 32 mmHg, with its straight-line dissociation curve facilitating its elimination.

In view of this concept, an understanding of gas exchange suggests that controlled positive pressure breathing is not the ideal therapeutic approach. The philosophy of IMV relates to delivering mechanical ventilation only at a rate necessary to supplement the patient's own spontaneous activities. It limits the mechanical impact on the system.

Arbitrary criteria of the appropriateness of the spontaneous ventilatory efforts includes a $PaCO_2$ of 35 to 45 mmHg, a pH of greater than 7.35, and a spontaneous rate of fewer than 30 breaths per minute. A pH of 7.35 provides a more reasonable basis of

evaluation in normally hypercapnic patients. Attempts to lower their $PaCO_2$ to the previously-indicated range might result in apnea. Some patients also compensate for metabolic alkalosis by retaining CO_2, and again pH becomes a more useful clinical tool.[131] A spontaneous breathing rate above 30 per minute indicates an unnecessarily high level of work to maintain $PaCO_2$. While $PaCO_2$ and pH may be normal, these levels are at the cost of a marked increase in the work of breathing. Somewhere at rates above 40 breaths per minute exhalation changes from a passive to an active maneuver, markedly increasing the physiologic cost.

Studies on healthy subjects indicate that during spontaneous ventilation gas distribution is primarily to the dependent lung portions.[132] In the upright position these are the basilar units, while in the supine position they are the posterior aspects. Several factors are responsible for this distribution pattern.

Both the weight of lung parenchyma and the pulmonary blood volume act to compress the lung segments or alveoli. In the upright position the basilar alveoli are more compressed than those in the apex. However, compared with the apical units, the volumes of the basilar alveoli are such that they are on a much more favorable portion of the pressure-volume curve. Smaller changes in transpulmonary pressure gradients result in larger volume changes than in their less dependent counterparts, which are already at maximal volume and in which large pressure changes are required to effect any volume increase (See Ch. 7).

Similarly, position also influences pulmonary blood flow. The pulmonary circulation, being a low-pressure system, remains quite gravity-dependent. The majority of the right ventricular outflow goes to dependent lung portions. In comparison, ventilation to those same areas does not match the amount of blood flow; an average ventilation-perfusion ratio approaches about 0.6 to 0.7.[12] However, both the volume of blood flow and ventilation to the dependent lung portions exceed that to any other lung area. Therefore, the dependent units, basilar in the upright and posterior in the supine position, are those most involved in blood gas exchange.

Studies in healthy volunteers have demonstrated that in a supine, spontaneously breathing subject, more diaphragmatic motion occurs in the posterior or dependent position.[133] The radius of curvature of the diaphragm promotes more excursion in that plane, which enhances the ventilation already directed to those areas. During paralysis and controlled mechanical ventilation, diaphragmatic motion involves the anterior or non-dependent portion. The passive diaphragmatic motion responds secondarily to increases in intrathoracic pressure. Simultaneously, the abdominal contents push upward on the diaphragm and provide resistance to any movement of the posterior-dependent portion. Therefore, controlled ventilation results in poor matching of ventilation to perfusion, since ventilation flows to the anterior or non-dependent lung units while blood remains in the basilar segments.[134] In fact, the redistribution of blood flow contributes to an increase in calculated physiologic dead space, and units are greatly overdistended in proportion to the amount of circulation. Normally, with controlled, positive-pressure breathing, tidal volumes of 10 to 15 ml/kg are delivered. These represent at least twice the volumes used during spontaneous efforts, and such large volumes contribute to a spillover effect. Once the non-dependent areas are filled, gas moves into the dependent units, which are better situated to participate in gas exchange. Without this hyperventilation during mechanical breathing, $PaCO_2$ would increase and atelectasis would soon develop.

IMV, since it promotes spontaneous breathing activity, exemplifies a theoretically sounder method of ventilation. It provides the best matching of ventilation to perfusion and should therefore maximize oxygenation while optimizing ventilation-perfusion relationships.

Since IMV allows for spontaneous breathing and also limits the number of positive-pressure breaths, interference with cardiac function remains minimal. In fact, almost a linear relationship exists between cardiac output and the mechanical ventilator rate. Spontaneous breathing reduces intrathoracic pressure, enhancing venous return, and also reduces overall mean airway pressure (Fig. 20-12).[135] Both effects minimize cardiovascular deterioration. Limiting the number of ventilator breaths also contributes to a lowered mean airway pressure, since the reduced number of positive-pressure inflations limits the number of transient increases in pulmonary artery pressure (Figs. 20-14 and 20-15). Therefore, interference with right ventricular afterload is minimized.

Newer evidence indicates that pulmonary barotrauma, including pneumothorax, pneumomediastinum, and pneumoperitoneum, correlates with both the frequency and the absolute peak inflation pressure of the positive-pressure breath; limiting the ventilator frequency should have a favorable influence. In fact, the incidence of barotrauma with IMV and high PEEP levels is equal to that obtained when controlled mechanical ventilation and low-level PEEP are employed.

Since the patient can breathe spontaneously on IMV, the need to control respiratory effort by paralysis, sedation, or hypocapnia does not arise. The patient does not "fight" the ventilator. Respiratory alkalosis, with its attendant problems of cardiac dysrhythmias and increased oxygen consumption, does not develop. Since the patient no longer requires paralysis, accidental disconnection from the ventilator does not pose quite the same hazard it would if controlled ventilation were employed.

IMV was originally proposed as a weaning technique (Table 20-5). However, in that aspect it is not superior to any other technique. Patients will be weaned from mechanical support when ready, regardless of

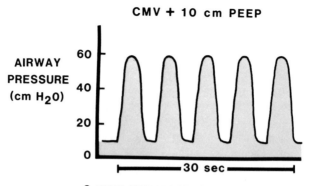

Fig. 20-14 Controlled mechanical ventilation and 10 cm H_2O PEEP/CPAP. Area under curve represents mean airway pressure of 30 cm H_2O.

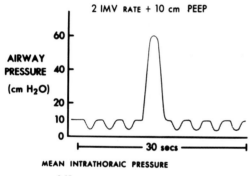

Fig. 20-15 Intermittent mandatory ventilation and 10 cm H_2O PEEP. Negative deflections of the baseline represent spontaneous breathing. The number of mechanical breaths per minute is also decreased. The result is a much lower mean airway pressure than in Figure 20-14. Cardiac output has less impairment.

the method. However, weaning with IMV requires fewer direct nursing interventions.

On controlled ventilation the practice involves transferring a patient receiving 100 percent machine support of respiration to a continuous flow system. Weaning usually is based on some objective criteria, which might include a negative inspiratory force of more than -25 cm H_2O, a vital capacity of at least 1.0 to 1.5 L, and/or a dead space to tidal volume ratio (V_D/V_T) less than 0.6. The actual choices will vary with the physician. The patient must abruptly supply 100 percent of his ventilatory requirements. The patient remains off the ventilator for a very short period the first time and, if all goes well, he is then taken off the machine for progressively longer periods. Ventilatory support alternates continually between 100 and 0 percent. Obviously this method requires close, continual nursing supervision.

With IMV, on the other hand, weaning proceeds in a smooth, stepwise fashion from total mechanical ventilatory support to complete self-support over a time course determined by the patient's physiologic response. Those parameters measured include the aforementioned pH, $PaCO_2$, and spontaneous breathing rate. Other values, such as V_D/V_T, are not required.

As a general rule, patients who develop acute respiratory failure and who are treated early on can be weaned in the first 24 hours to a ventilator rate of 2 to 3 breaths per minute. As long as the patient meets the criteria, the rate can be incrementally reduced by 1 to 2 breaths per minute each change. The pa-

Table 20-5
IMV Weaning Criteria

pH > 7.35
$PaCO_2$ 35–45 mmHg
Spontaneous rate < 30 per minute

tient usually begins at an IMV rate of 8 per minute. With a 12 ml/kg tidal volume, faster rates are normally not required. Periodic hyperinflation or sighs are not used because low-level PEEP/CPAP (less than 5 cm H_2O) ensures that the lung always remains at least at FRC. Discontinuation of all mechanical ventilatory support requires a functional return to normal of all systems. Adequate oxygenation implies an FiO_2 below 0.5 and at least a 90 percent hemoglobin saturation with less than 5 to 6 cm H_2O PEEP/CPAP. Also, on totally-spontaneous breathing the respiratory rate remains less than 30 per minute, while pH exceeds 7.35, and $PaCO_2$ remains at the original baseline levels. Obviously, the patient must be able to maintain his own airway, and all other criteria for extubation must be satisfied. At this juncture, extubation can be safely carried out.

REFERENCES

1. Proctor HJ, Moss GS, Homer LD et al: Changes in lung compliance associated with hemorrhagic shock and resuscitation. Ann Surg 169:82-92, 1969

2. Moss GS, Das Gupta TK, Newson B et al: The effect of saline resuscitation on pulmonary sodium and water distribution. Surg Gynecol Obstet 136:934-940, 1973

3. Klineberg PL, Geer RT, Hirsh RA et al: Early extubation after coronary artery bypass graft surgery. Crit Care Med 5:272-274, 1977

4. Jenkins MT, Jones RF, Wilson B et al: Congestive atelectasis: A complication of intravenous infusion of fluids. Ann Surg 175:657-664, 1950

5. Teplitz C: The core pathobiology and integrated medical science of adult acute respiratory insufficiency. Surg Clin North Am 56:1091-1133, 1976

6. Brewer LA, Burbank B, Sampson PC et al: The "wet lung" in war casualties. Ann Surg 123:343-362, 1946

7. Pontoppidan H, Geffin B, Lowenstein E: Acute respiratory failure in the adult. N Engl J Med 287:626-698, 743-752, 799-806, 1972

8. Farrell P, Avery Me: Hyaline membrane disease. Am Rev Respir Dis 111:654-688, 1975

9. Ashbaugh DG, Bigelow DB, Petty TL et al: Acute respiratory distress in adults. Lancet 2:319-323, 1967

10. Hopewell PC, Murray JF: The adult respiratory distress syndrome. In Shibel EM, Moser KM, Eds: Respiratory Emergencies. C. V. Mosby Co., St. Louis, 1980

11. Schneeberger-Keeley EE, Karnovsky MJ: The ultrastructural basis of alveolar capillary membrane permeability to peroxidase used as a tracer. J Cell Biol 37:781-793, 1968

12. West JB: Respiratory Physiology. Williams & Wilkins Co., Baltimore, 1974

13. Craig DB, Wabba WM, Don HF et al: "Closing volume" and its relationship to gas exchange in seated and supine position. J Appl Physiol 31:717-721, 1971

14. Hall JG, Morris B, Wooley G: Intrinsic rhythmic propulsion of lymph in unanesthetized sheep. J Physiol 180:336-349, 1965.

15. Jones JG, Grossman RF, Berry M et al: Alveolar membrane permeability. Am Rev Respir Dis 120:399-410, 1979

16. Teplitz C: The ultrastructural basis for pulmonary pathophysiology following trauma—pathogenesis of pulmonary edema. J Trauma 8:700-703, 1968

17. Szidon JP, Pietra GG, Fishman AP: The alveolar-capillary membrane and pulmonary edema. N Engl J Med 286:1200-1204, 1972

18. Staub NC: The forces regulating fluid filtration in the lung. Microvasc Res 14:45-55, 1978

19. Borgofsky EH: Mechanisms underlying vasomotor regulation of regional pulmonary blood flow in normal and disease states. Am J Med 57:378-394, 1974

20. Weil MH, Morissette M, Michaels S et al: Routine plasma colloid osmotic pressure measurements. Crit Care Med 2:229-234, 1974

21. Guyton AC: Interstitial fluid pressure. II

Pressure-volume curves of interstitial space. Circ Res 26:452-460, 1965

22. Gabel JC: Relationship of pressure and permeability in the pulmonary vasculature. Ann Refresher Course, Am Soc Anesthesiology, San Francisco, 1976

23. Fishman AP, Hecht HH: The pulmonary circulation and interstitial space. Univ Chicago Press, Chicago, 1969

24. Pietra GG, Szidon JP, Leventhal MM et al: Histamine and interstitial pulmonary edema in the dog. Circ Res 24:325-337, 1971

25. Demling RH: Correlation of changes in body weight and pulmonary vascular pressures with lung water accumulation during fluid overload. Crit Care Med 7:153-156, 1979

26. Muller WH: Observations on the pathogenesis and management of pulmonary hypertension. Am J Surg 135:302-311, 1976

27. Fishman AP: Hypoxia on the pulmonary circulation: How and where it works. Circ Res 38:221-237, 1976

28. Scanlon TS, Benumof JL, Wahrenbrock EA et al: Hypoxic pulmonary vasoconstriction and the ratio of hypoxic lung to perfused normoxic lung. Anesthesiology 49:117-181, 1978

29. Rothschild MA, Oratz M. Schreiber SS: Extravascular albumin. N Engl J Med 301:497-498, 1979

30. Rowe MI, Arango A: The choice of intravenous fluid in shock resuscitation. Pediatr Clin North Am 22:269-274, 1975

31. Guyton AC: A concept of negative interstitial pressure based on pressures in implanted capsules. Circ Res 16:452-460, 1963

32. Virgilio RW, Smith DE, Zarins CK: Balanced electrolyte solutions: experimental and clinical studies. Crit Care Med 7:98-106, 1979

33. Hopewell PC: Failure of positive end expiratory pressure to decrease lung water content in alloxan-induced pulmonary edema. Am Rev Respir Dis 120:813-819, 1979

34. Hill SL, Elings VB, Lewis FR: Changes in lung water and capillary permeability following sepsis and fluid overload. J Surg Res 28:140-150, 1980

35. Fein A, Leff A, Hopewell PC: Pathophysiology and management of the complications resulting from fire and inhaled products of combustion. Review of the literature. Crit Care Med 8:911-998, 1980

36. Vreim CE, Snashall PD, Demling RH et al: Lung lymph and free interstitial protein composition in sheep with edema. Am J Physiol 230:1650-1653, 1976

37. Bowers RE, Brigham KL, Owen PJ: Salicylate pulmonary edema: The mechanism in sheep and review of the clinical literature. Am Rev Respir Dis 115:261-268, 1977

38. Brigham KL, Woolverton WC, Blake LH et al: Increased sheep lung vascular permeability caused by Pseudomonas bacteremia. J Clin Invest 54:792-804, 1974

39. Weir EK, Grover RF: The role of endogenous prostaglandins in the pulmonary circulation. Anesthesiology 48:201-212, 1978

40. Jacob HS: Damaging role of activated complement in myocardial infarction and shock lung: Ramifications for rational therapy. Crit Care State Art 1:1-18, 1980

41. Taylor AE, Granger DN, Brace RA: Analysis of lymphatic protein flux data. I. Estimation of the reflection coefficient and surface area product for total protein. Microvasc Res 13:297-313, 1977

42. West JB: Ventilation-perfusion relationships. Am Rev Respir Dis 116:919-943, 1977

43. Parker JC, Guyton AC, Taylor AE: Pulmonary interstitial and capillary pressures estimated from intra-alveolar fluid pressures. J Appl Physiol 44:267-276, 1978

44. Macklem PT: Collateral ventilation. N Engl J Med 298:49-50, 1978

45. Gallagher TJ, Civetta JM, Kirby RR et al: Post traumatic pulmonary insufficiency: a treatable disease. South Med J 70:1308-1310, 1977

46. Walker L, Eiseman B: The changing pattern of post-traumatic respiratory distress syndrome. Ann Surg 181:693-697, 1975

47. Demling RH, Selinger SL, Bland RL et al: Effect of hemorrhagic shock on pulmonary microvascular fluid filtration and protein permeability in sheep. Surgery 77:512-519, 1975

48. Staub NC: Pulmonary edema. Physiol Rev 54:678-811, 1974

49. Robin ED, Cross CE, Zelis R et al: Pulmonary edema. N Engl J Med 288:239-246, 292-304, 1973

50. Anderson RR, Holliday RL, Driedger AA et al: Documentation of pulmonary capillary

permeability in adult respiratory distress syndrome accompanying human sepsis. Am Rev Respir Dis 119:869-876, 1979

51. Craddock PR, Fehr J, Brigham KL et al: Complement and leukocyte-mediated pulmonary dysfunction in hemodialysis. N Engl J Med 296:769-774, 1977

52. Bachofen M, Weibel ER: Alterations of gas exchange apparatus in adult respiratory insufficiency associated with sepsis. Am Rev Respir Dis 116:589-615, 1977

53. Clowes GHA, Hirsch MFE, Williams L et al: Septic lung and shock lung in man. Ann Surg 181:681-692, 1975

54. Sibbald W, Peters S, Lindsay RM: Serotonin and pulmonary hypertension in human septic ARDS. Crit Care Med 8:490-494, 1980

55. Tisi GM: Preoperative evaluation of pulmonary function. Validity indications and benefits. In Murray J, Ed: Lung Disease. Am Lung Assoc., New York, 1980

56. Bartlett RH, Brennan MI, Gazzaniga AB et al: Studies on the pathogenesis and prevention of postoperative pulmonary complications. Surg Gynecol Obstet 137:925-933, 1973

57. Powner DJ, Eross B, Grenvik A: Differential lung ventilation with PEEP in the treatment of unilateral pneumonia. Crit Care Med 5:170-172, 1977

58. Modell JH: The Pathophysiology and Treatment of Drowning and Near Drowning. Charles C Thomas, Springfield, Ill, 1971

59. Modell JH, Graves SA, Ketover A; Clinical course of 91 consecutive near drowning victims. Chest 70:231, 1971

60. Stewardson RH, Nyhus IM: Pulmonary aspiration: an update. Arch Surg 112:1192-1197, 1977

61. Marx GF: Aspiration pneumonitis. JAMA 201:129-130, 1967

62. Mendelson CL: The aspiration of stomach contents into the lungs during obstetric anesthesia. Am J Obstet Gynecol 52:191-205, 1946

63. Gibbs CP, Schwartz DJ, Wynne JW et al: Antacid pulmonary aspiration in the dog. Anesthesiology 51:380-388, 1979

64. Goldbaum LR, Rami Rez RG, Absalom KB: What is the mechanism of carbon monoxide toxicity? Aviat Space Environ Med 46:1289-1291, 1975

65. Gossling HR, Ellison LH, Degraff AC: Fat embolism: the role of respiratory failure and its treatment. J Bone Joint Surg 56:1327-1337, 1974

66. Nixon JR, Brock-Utne JG: Free fatty acid and arterial oxygen changes following major injury: a correlation between hypoxemia and increased free fatty acid levels. J Trauma 18:23-26, 1978

67. Murray DG, Racz GB: Fat embolism syndrome: A rationale for treatment. J Bone Joint Surg 56:1338-1349, 1974

68. Kusajima K, Webb WR, Parker FB et al: Pulmonary response of unilateral positive end expiratory pressure (PEEP) on experimental fat embolism. Ann Surg 181:676-680, 1975

69. Jensen NK: Recovery of pulmonary function after crushing injuries of the chest. Dis Chest 22:319-346, 1952

70. Trinkle JK, Richardson JD, Franz JL et al: Management of flail chest without mechanical ventilation. Ann Thorac Surg 19:355-363, 1975

71. Cullen P, Modell JH, Kirby RR et al: Treatment of flail chest: use of intermittent mandatory ventilation and positive end expiratory pressure. Arch Surg 110:1099-1103, 1975

72. Cheney FW, Colley PS: The effect of cardiac output on arterial blood oxygenation. Anesthesiology 52:496-503, 1980

73. Prys-Roberts C, Kelman GR, Greenbaum R: The influence of circulatory factors on arterial oxygenation during anesthesia in man. Anaesthesia 22:257-275, 1967

74. Turaids T, Nobrega FT, Gallagher TJ: Absorptional atelectasis breathing oxygen at simulated altitude: prevention using inert gas. Aerospace Med 38:189-192, 1967

75. Oliven A, Abinader E, Bursztein S: Influence of varying inspired oxygen tensions on the pulmonary venous admixture (shunt) of mechanically ventilated patients. Crit Care Med 8:99-101, 1980

76. Dubois AB, Turaids T, Mammen RE et al: Pulmonary atelectasis in subjects breathing oxygen at sea level or at simulated altitude. J Appl Physiol 21:828-836, 1966

77. Suter, PM, Fairley HB, Schlobohm RM: Shunt, lung volume and perfusion during short periods of ventilation with oxygen. Anesthesiology 43:617-627, 1975.

78. Benumof JL, Rogers SN, Moyce PR et al:

Hypoxic pulmonary vascular pressures with lung water accumulation during fluid overload. Crit Care Med 7:153-156, 1979

79. Benumof JL, Wahrenbrock EA: Blunted hypoxic pulmonary vasoconstriction by increased lung vascular pressures. J Appl Physiol 38:846-850, 1975

80. Winter PM, Smith G: The toxicity of oxygen. Anesthesiology 37:210-241, 1972

81. Douglas ME, Downs JB, Dannemiller FJ et al: Change in pulmonary venous admixture with varying inspired oxygen. Anesth Analg (Cleve) 55:688-695, 1976

82. Bone RC: Treatment of adult respiratory distress syndrome with diuretics, dialysis, and positive end expiratory pressure. Crit Care Med 6:136-139, 1978

83. Richardson JD, Franz JL, Grover FL et al: Pulmonary contusion and hemorrhage—crystalloid versus colloid replacement. J Surg Res 16:330-336, 1974

84. Granger DN, Gabel JC, Drake RE et al: Physiologic basis for the clinical usage of albumin solutions. Surg Gynecol Obstet 146:97-104, 1978

85. Puri VK, Weil MH, Michaels S et al: Pulmonary edema associated with a reduction in plasma oncotic pressure. Surg Gynecol Obstet 151:344-348, 1980

86. Zapol W, Snider MT: Pulmonary hypertension in severe acute respiratory failure. N Engl J Med 296:476-480, 1977

87. Sibbald WJ, Patterson NAM, Holliday RL et al: Pulmonary hypertension in sepsis. Crit Care Med 73:583-591, 1975

88. Gallagher TJ, Civetta JM: Normal pulmonary vascular resistance during acute respiratory insufficiency. Crit Care Med 9:647-650, 1981

89. Colley PS, Cheney FW, Hlastala MP: Ventilation-perfusion and gas exchange effects of sodium nitroprusside in dogs with normal edematous lung. Anesthesiology 50:489-495, 1979

90. Gallagher TJ, Etling T: Failure to alter intrapulmonary shunt with sodium nitroprusside. Abstr Sci Papers, Soc Crit Care Med 90, 1978

91. Hill SL, Elings VB, Lewis FR: Changes in lung water and capillary permeability following sepsis and fluid overload. J Surg Res 28:140-150, 1980

92. Hechtman HB, Weisel RD, Vito L et al: The independence of pulmonary shunting and pulmonary edema. Surgery 74:300-306, 1973

93. Demling RH, Staub NC, Edmunds LH Jr: Effect of end expiratory airway pressure on accumulation of extravascular lung water. J Appl Physiol 38:907-912, 1975

94. Tranbaugh RF, Lewis FR, Christensen JM et al: Lung water changes after thermal injury: the effects of crystalloid resuscitation and sepsis. Ann Surg 192:479-490, 1980

95. Cane RD, Shapiro BA, Harrison RA et al: Minimizing errors in intrapulmonary shunt calculations. Crit Care Med 8:294-297, 1980

96. Ashbaugh DG, Petty TL: Positive end-expiratory pressure: physiology, indications and contraindications. J Thorac Cardiovasc Surg 65:165-170, 1973

97. Powers SR: The use of PEEP for respiratory support. Surg Clin North Am 54:1125-1136, 1974

98. Dueck R, Wagner PD, West JB: Effects of positive end expiratory pressure on gas exchange in dogs with normal and edematous lungs. Anesthesiology 47:359-366, 1977

99. Downs JB, Douglas ME, Sanfelippo et al: Ventilatory pattern, intrapleural pressure and cardiac output. Anesth Analg (Cleve) 56:88-96, 1977

100. Sturgeon CL, Douglas ME, Downs JB et al: PEEP and CPAP: cardiopulmonary effects of high positive and expiratory pressure. Anesthesiology 43:533-539, 1975

101. Gherini S, Peters RM, Virgilio RW: Mechanical work on the lungs and work of breathing with positive end-expiratory pressure and continuous positive airway pressure. Chest 76:251-256, 1979

102. Demers RR, Irwin RS, Braman SS: Criteria for optimum PEEP. Respir Care 22:596-601, 1977

103. Powers SR, Mannal R, Neclerio M et al: Physiologic consequences of positive end expiratory pressure (PEEP) ventilation. Ann Surg 178:265-271, 1973

104. Downs JB, Klein EF Jr, Modell JH: The effect of incremental PEEP on PaO_2 in patients with respiratory failure. Anesth Analg (Cleve) 52:210-215, 1973

105. Kirby RR, Downs JB, Civetta JM et al: High level positive end expiratory pressure (PEEP) in acute respiratory insufficiency. Chest 67:156-163, 1975

106. Suter PM, Fairley HB, Isenberg MD: Optimum end expiratory airway pressure in patients in acute pulmonary failure. N Engl J Med 292:284-289, 1975

107. Gallagher TJ, Civetta JM, Kirby RR: Terminology update: optimal PEEP. Crit Care Med 6:323-326, 1978

108. Berk JL, Hagen JF, Tong RK et al: The use of dopamine to correct the cardiac output resulting from positive end expiratory pressure. A two-edged sword. Crit Care Med 5:269-271, 1977

109. Gallagher TJ, Civetta JM: Goal-directed therapy of acute respiratory failure. Anesth Analg (Cleve) 59:831-834, 1980

110. Smith RA, Kirby RR, Gooding JM et al: Continuous positive airway pressure (CPAP) by face mask. Crit Care Med 8:483-485, 1980

111. Quist J, Pontoppidan H, Wilson RS et al: Hemodynamic responses to mechanical ventilation with PEEP: The effect of hypervolemia. Anesthesiology 42:45-55, 1975

112. Patten M, Liebman PR, Hechtman HB: Humorally mediated decreases in cardiac output associated with positive end expiratory pressure. Microvasc Res 13:137-139, 1977

113. Natori H, Tamaki S, Kira S: Ultrasonographic evaluation of ventilatory effect on inferior vena caval configuration. Am Rev Respir Dis 120:421-427, 1979

114. Howell JBL, Permutt S, Proctor DF et al: Effect of inflation of the lung on different parts of pulmonary vascular bed. J Appl Physiol 16:71-76, 1961

115. Hobelmann CF, Smith DE, Virgilio RW et al: Hemodynamic alterations with positive end expiratory pressure: the contribution of the pulmonary circulation. J Trauma 15:951-958, 1975

116. Robotham JL, Lixfeld W, Holland L et al: The effects of positive end expiratory pressure on right and left ventricular performance. Am Rev Respir Dis 121:677-683, 1980

117. Manny J, Patten MT, Liebman PR et al: The association of lung distention, PEEP and biventricular failure. Ann Surg 187:151-157, 1978

118. Cassidy SS, Gaffney FA, Johnson RL: A perspective on PEEP. N Engl J Med 304:421-422, 1981

119. Laver MB, Strauss HB, Pohost GM: Right and left ventricular geometry: adjustments during acute respiratory failure. Crit Care Med 7:509-519, 1979

120. Kirby RR, Perry JC, Calderwood HW et al: Cardiorespiratory effects of high positive end expiratory pressure. Anesth Analg (Cleve) 56:88-96, 1977

121. Jardin F, Farcot JC, Boisante L et al: Influence of positive end-expiratory pressure on left ventricular performance. N Engl J Med 304:387-392, 1981

122. Banner MJ, Gallagher TJ, Bluth LI: A new, microprocessor device for mean airway pressure measurement. Crit Care Med 9:51-53, 1981

123. Kronberg GM, Quan SF, Schlobohm RM et al: Anatomic location of tips of pulmonary artery catheters in supine patients. Anesthesiology 51:467-469, 1979

124. Downs JB: A technique for direct measurement of intrapleural pressure. Crit Care Med 4:207-210, 1976

125. Downs JB, Douglas ME: Assessment of cardiac filling pressure during continuous positive-pressure ventilation. Crit Care Med 8:285-290, 1980

126. Fewell JE, Bond GC: Role of sinoaortic receptors in initiating the renal response to continuous positive-pressure ventilation in the dog. Anesthesiology 52:408-413, 1978

127. Laver MB: Dr. Starling and the ventilator kidney. Anesthesiology 50:383-386, 1979

128. Marquez JM, Douglas ME, Downs JB et al: Renal function and cardiovascular responses during positive airway pressure. Anesthesiology 50:393-398, 1979

129. Ueda H, Neclerio M, Leather RP et al: Effects of positive end expiratory pressure ventilation on renal function. Surg Forum 23:209-211, 1972

130. Downs JB, Klein EF Jr, Desautels D et al: Intermittent mandatory ventilation: a new approach to weaning patients from mechanical ventilators. Chest 64:331-335, 1973

131. Gallagher TJ: Metabolic alkalosis complicating weaning from mechanical ventilation. South Med J 72:766-787, 1979

132. Milic-Emili J, Henderson AM, Dolovich MB et al: Regional distribution of inspired gas in the lung. J Appl Physiol 21:749-759, 1966

133. Froese AB, Bryan AC: Effects of anesthesia and paralysis on diaphragmatic mechanism in man. Anesthesiology 44:247-255, 1974

134. Weinstein ME, Rich CL, Peters RM et al: Hemodynamic and respiratory response to varying gradients between end expiratory pressure in patients breathing continuous positive airway pressure. J Trauma 18:231-235, 1978

135. Douglas ME, Downs JB: Cardiopulmonary effects of intermittent mandatory ventilation. Int Anesth Clin 18:97-121, 1980

James R. Hall, M.D.

21
Techniques of Ventilation and Oxygenation

Support of breathing will be divided into two categories—support of oxygenation and support of ventilation. Since the underlying physiologies of oxygenation and ventilation are different although interrelated, *support* of oxygenation and ventilation must be considered separately when therapy for either or both must be undertaken in a patient.

Support of ventilation is based upon mechanical ventilatory provision of part or all of the *alveolar* ventilation, since this is the means by which carbon dioxide is eliminated, thereby determining alveolar carbon dioxide tension:

$$P_{A}CO_2 \propto (\dot{V}CO_2 / \dot{V}_A).$$

Support of oxygenation is achieved by providing supplemental oxygen (increasing the fraction of oxygen inspired, FIO_2) or improving ventilation-perfusion relationships by increasing resting lung volume. The use of supplemental oxygen can improve the state of oxygenation by increasing the driving pressure for oxygen to enter the blood, i.e., increasing alveolar oxygen tension:

$$P_{A}O_2 = (P_{BAR} - P_{H_2O}) \times FIO_2 - (k) \times P_{A}CO_2$$

where $k = (FIO_2 + (1 - FIO_2)/R) \simeq 1.2$. Note that the lowering of $P_{A}CO_2$ by mechanical ventilation has very little *direct* effect on $P_{A}O_2$, especially as FIO_2 increases above 0.21. The mechanisms by which alteration in resting lung volume and functional residual capacity (FRC) may improve oxygenation are elucidated in Chapter 19. Techniques for this form of therapy are discussed in this chapter.

FEATURES COMMON TO OXYGENATION AND VENTILATION

Although many technical aspects of the support of oxygenation and of ventilation differ, including the breathing circuits, there are three features common to both: (1) provision of fresh gas, including gas flow rate and inspired oxygen concentration; (2) provision of water vapor to the airways; and (3) provision of drugs via the airways. Since these three features are applicable to systems used for support of oxygenation or ventilation, they will be covered in this introductory section.

701

Provision of Fresh Gases into Circuits

A flow of fresh gases can be provided into breathing circuits by using either flow-meters or demand valves. Selection of the flow-metering device depends upon applications of the circuit and economy. For circuits in which continuous or intermittent gas flow rates are high, the use of demand valves may provide savings in oxygen and air costs. Some ventilators have demand valves incorporated into their circuits to provide gas flow for mechanical breaths or for the patient's spontaneous breaths. Appropriateness of their use is discussed later in the chapter.

The provision of different concentrations of inspired oxygen (F_IO_2) can be attained in three ways: (1) relative flow metering, (2) air-oxygen blending, or (3) air entrainment devices.

Relative Flow Metering. This technique utilizes one flowmeter for oxygen and one for air. Their outputs are mixed in a proximal part of the breathing circuit, and adjustment of their relative flow rates provides the desired concentration of oxygen. There are two distinct disadvantages to this system: (1) analysis of the gas mixture and adjustment of flow rates are performed by skilled personnel—an expensive endeavor; and (2) changes in total circuit flow require adjustment of both flowmeters and repeat analyses of the oxygen concentration of the gas mixture—time-consuming and expensive. For these reasons, relative flow metering is not the method of choice for providing accurate fractional inspired oxygen concentrations.

Air-Oxygen Blenders. These are commercially available devices which permit delivery of known concentrations of oxygen by adjustment of a single control. The flow rate of the resulting gas mixture then can be adjusted by using a single flowmeter. Although the inspired oxygen concentration

from this device or any device should be measured periodically (e.g., during each 8-hour shift), adjustments in gas flow from the blender can be made without repeat oxygen analysis, thus effecting considerable savings in personnel time and costs. Air-oxygen blenders, even though they represent an initial capital investment, are the means of choice for oxygen delivery into circuits which need high and/or temporally varying flow rates.

Air Entrainment Devices. These devices, which operate on the Venturi principle (Fig. 21-1), are used to provide different oxygen concentrations. The concentrations of oxygen may be provided at several preset levels or over a wide range, depending upon the type of entrainment mechanism in the device. The type of entrainment mechanism also may limit the measurement accuracy of the oxygen concentration delivered. Air entrainment devices are suitable for providing different concentrations of inspired oxygen to simple oxygen delivery devices (e.g., face masks and face shields) but are not suitable for use with ventilator breathing circuits or non-rebreathing circuits used with distending airway pressure therapy.

Provision of Water Vapor

The provision of adequate humidification is important for two reasons: (1) prevention of excessive water loss via the airways with subsequent inspissation of secretions; and (2) prevention of excess heat loss via the airways (heat of vaporization of water requires 540 Cal/g). Inspired gases reach the patient's body temperature and reach 100 percent relative humidity at that temperature within the conducting airways (this point is the isothermal saturation boundary, or ISB).[1] Since many patients undergoing various forms of breathing support will have had their natural air conditioning system bypassed with use of an artificial airway, it is

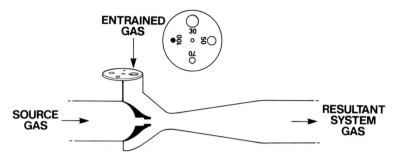

Fig. 21-1 Venturi principle. The source gas, which generally is oxygen, provides the driving flow for a venturi device. The entrained gas generally is room air, which has an oxygen concentration of 21 percent. The resultant system gas is a mixture of the source gas and the entrained gas, and its flow rate is the sum of the source gas and entrained gas rates. Many devices operating upon the venturi principle permit selection of the resultant FIO_2 by adjustment of a variable orifice, which limits inflow of the entrained gas.

important that adequate humidification and heat be provided with the inspired gases in order that the ISB remain as proximal as possible in the airways.

Water vapor is provided by humidifiers. Particulate water is provided by nebulizers, but this is not the primary form desired for routine provision of water via the airways (see below). The amount of water contained in an air sample compared with the capacity of that sample for water vapor is the relative humidity of the sample. To minimize heat and water loss during support of breathing, it is ideal to *deliver* the gases at a temperature very near the patient's body temperature and 100 percent relative humidity.

Water vapor content, as delivered by humidifiers, is a function of three factors: (1) temperature of the system, (2) surface area for water-gas contact within the system, and (3) duration of time for that contact. Although commercially available humidifier systems for use with breathing circuits vary these three factors in many different ways, they basically can be grouped into four categories: (1) pass-over humidifiers, (2) bubble and jet humidifiers, (3) aerosol-generating humidifiers, and (4) wick humidifiers. The principle for each type of humidifier is illustrated in Figures 21-2 through 21-5. Each of the four types may or may not be heated.

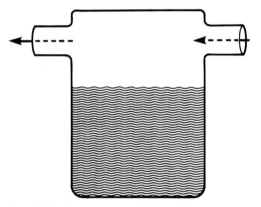

Fig. 21-2 Pass-over humidifier. Water content will vary depending upon duration of gas-water contact, temperature of the system, and surface area for contact, which is fixed by the manufacturing design but may vary in some systems depending upon water level. Heating the system is an option employed by several manufacturers.

Since heating can improve humidification (Fig. 21-6), this is a desirable feature on all systems used for long-term breathing support in adults and on all systems used with neonates and small children.

The efficiency of available systems varies widely, and some systems cannot maintain adequate heat production and/or produce sufficient relative humidity to provide satisfactory performance for long-term patient care. Wick humidifiers with a heater incorporated into the system are the most efficient type available.[2]

Less efficient systems, even those without heaters, may be used when the patient's natural air conditioning system has not been bypassed. This includes use with face masks, nasal cannulae, face shields, etc.

The position of the humidifier in the breathing circuit has an important effect both in minimizing heat and water vapor losses before the inspired gases reach the patient and in decreasing and controlling rain-out of water in the circuit tubing. To minimize heat and water losses, the distance between the humidifier and the patient should be as short as safety and patient care practices permit. Heat also can be maintained by heating the inspiratory limb of the circuit with a heating element, although this may produce additional costs and safety problems. Rain-out of

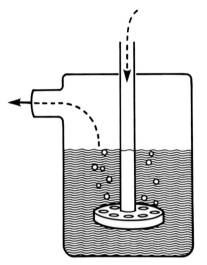

Fig. 21-3 Bubble humidifier. Water content of the respiratory gases is determined by the air-water interface, duration of contact, and temperature of the system—all of which may be variable. Increased surface area for air-water contact increases this system's efficiency above that of the pass-over humidifier.

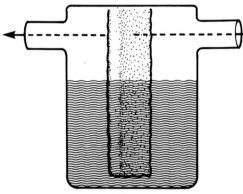

Fig. 21-4 Wick humidifier. Respiratory gases pass through a water-saturated wick, which provides a large surface area for evaporation. The system may be heated to improve efficiency further.

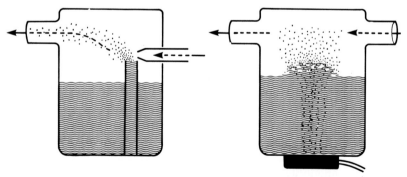

Fig. 21-5 Aerosol-generating humidifiers. Each of these aerosol generators functions as a humidifier in that the particulate water serves as a source of evaporation for water in the respiratory gas atmosphere; each also provides particulate water into the respiratory tract. (Left) Aerosol is generated by the breakup of water emanating from the capillary tube. (Right) Particulate water is generated by an ultrasonic transducer, which is below and physically separated from the water within the system.

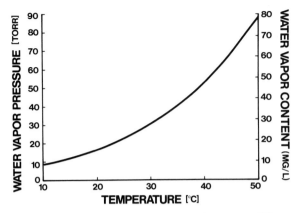

Fig. 21-6 Water vapor pressure and content. Water vapor pressure is a function of system temperature. Water vapor content is shown for saturated conditions (100 percent relative humidity).

water in the breathing circuit may pose a problem, especially with the very efficient systems or with systems in which there is also an aerosol generator. For this reason it is best to maintain the proximal end of the inspiratory limb, including the humidifier, more dependent than the distal end's connection to the patient. Water traps will provide means of collecting condensate in the inspiratory limb. Water traps should always be placed in breathing circuits when moderate to high levels of distending airway pressure are used so that the circuit is never opened to ambient pressure for the removal of condensate.

Provision of Medication via the Airways

Drugs may be administered via the airways by utilizing *nebulizers* inserted into the breathing circuit. Deposition of drugs, like that of water which is nebulized, will depend upon particle size as well as particle density and physical characteristics of breathing and gas mixing.[3,4] Deposition of solute-containing particles also will depend upon their hygroscopicity. Particles larger than 1 micron will be deposited primarily in the nasopharyngeal airways, and particles larger than 50 micron may rain out into the breathing

circuit. Particles between 0.3 and 1 micron will be deposited in the small airways. For many of the bronchoactive and vasoactive drugs that are nebulized in the nonintubated patient, action will not be limited by "loss" in the upper airways since there is uptake from mucosa and respiratory tract epithelium. Loss in the breathing circuit, though, is not acceptable.

The location of the nebulizer is important to optimize delivery of as much of the prescribed drug dose as possible. The ideal location for the nebulizer is between the breathing circuit and the patient's airway. This is important especially with breathing circuits in which there are high gas flows. If the nebulizer is inserted in the inspiratory limb and continuous nebulization is used, a significant portion of the drug may then be lost out of the expiratory limb. Use of an in-line nebulizer between the breathing circuit and the patient will prevent this (Fig. 21-7). The gas driving this nebulizer may be air or oxygen, as dictated by patient needs. Care must be taken in utilizing certain types of nebulizers to make sure the chamber containing the drug remains in a dependent position throughout the period of nebulization.

Orders for administration of drugs via the airways should include the name of the drug, amount to be administered, and total

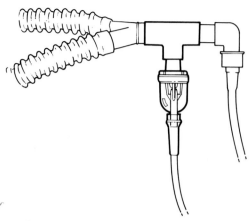

Fig. 21-7 Medication via the airways. An aerosol generator, which can be driven with either air or oxygen, is applied by utilizing a T-connector between the breathing circuit and the connection to the patient's airway. Note the dependent position required for this aerosol generator.

volume to be administered or duration or administration. Drugs should never be ordered or administered by volume or concentration alone.

SUPPORT OF OXYGENATION

Support of oxygenation can be undertaken by two different means. The simpler of the two is the provision of supplemental oxygen via any one of several devices. The second, more complex method is an alteration in resting lung volume, i.e., functional residual capacity (FRC), by application of distending airway pressure. Each approach may produce an increase in arterial oxygen tension, but only the distending airway pressure therapy is directed at the underlying pathophysiology of an oxygenation disability.

Provision of Supplemental Oxygen

OXYGEN DELIVERY DEVICES

Increasing the inspired oxygen concentration can be achieved with any one of several commercially available devices. This ap-

proach to improving arterial oxygen tension and content, though, does have limits. The constraints placed upon this technique include the necessity for gas flows high enough to meet inspiratory needs, an adequate reservoir to meet inspiratory needs, and maintenance of the device consistently on the patient. This last constraint is one which must be met in each and every patient for whom it is desired to have a guaranteed minimum inspired oxygen concentration greater than that of room air. Patients will remove masks and face shields because of discomfort, for suctioning, for eating, to be out of bed, etc. Therefore, a device which can be applied easily and will remain continuously in place is desirable. This describes the nasal cannula and *not* any of the mask devices in routine use. Fourteen devices used routinely for the provision of supplemental oxygen are considered separately and are summarized in Table 21-1.

Nasal Cannula. Nasal cannulae, which are applied easily, deliver 100 percent oxygen via two nasal prongs. The flow from each nasal prong is directed posteriorly, and the nasal passages serve as oxygen reservoirs. A rough rule of thumb for the inspired oxygen fraction (F_{IO_2}) provided using this technique is an increment of 3 percent per liter per minute of oxygen flow.[5] The oxygen can be humidified prior to delivery through the small-bore tubing of the device although care must be taken that water droplets do not accumulate in the tubing and occlude the flow of oxygen. Although these cannulae can be used at flow rates up to 7 to 8 L/min, patient comfort generally dictates a limit on flow of 4 to 6 L/min. Complications related to the use of cannulae, especially at high flow rates, include drying of the mucus membrane with subsequent pain and epistaxis. These cannulae, when properly applied, will provide supplemental oxygen continuously while allowing the patient freedom to eat, be suctioned, be out of bed, etc.—all without removal of the oxygen delivery device. The facial discomfort with the cannulae,

Table 21-1
Oxygen Delivery Devices

Device	Applications	Approximate Attainable FiO_2	Gas Flow Rate to Device	Comments
Nasal cannula	General use: adult and pediatric	≤ 0.40	1–6 L/min *	$FiO_2 \simeq 0.40$ at 6 L/min recommended maximum
Nasal catheter	Not recommended			See text
Simple mask	General use: adult and pediatric	≤ 0.60	6–12 L/min *	Uses small-bore delivery tubing; provides less humidity than aerosol mask
Aerosol mask	General use: adult and pediatric	≤ 0.60	6–12 L/min **	Uses large-bore delivery tubing
Face shield	General use: adult and pediatric	≤ 0.40	6–12 L/min **	Uses large-bore delivery tubing
Partial rebreathing mask	Limited use: adult and pediatric	≤ 0.80	Sufficient to maintain reservoir bag inflation (*)	Higher FiO_2s *and humidity* available with modification of aerosol face mask (see text)
Non-rebreathing mask	Limited use: adult and pediatric	≤ 1.00	Sufficient to maintain reservoir bag inflation *	Higher FiO_2's *and humidity* available with modification of aerosol face mask (see text)
Venturi mask	Limited use: adult and pediatric	0.24, 0.28, 0.30, 0.35, 0.40	2–8 L/min *	High total gas flow results from lower FiO_2 settings
Tracheostomy collar	General use: adult and pediatric	≤ 0.60	6–12 L/min **	Preferred oxygen/humidification source for tracheostomies
T-tube	Not recommended			See text
Hood	Limited Use: neonatal	≤ 1.00	4–8 L/min **	Delivered temperature and humidity are very important
Tent	Limited use: pediatric	≤ 0.50	10–20 L/min **	Flow requirements dependent upon size of tent; FiO_2 should be monitored continually
Incubator	General use: neonatal	≤ 0.40	5–12 L/min **	FiO_2 should be monitored continually
Mask for closed system	Limited use: adult	≤ 1.00	Sufficient to maintain reservoir bag inflation **	Application and observation as if the patient were intubated (see text)

Limited use and *not recommended* are explained in Comments or in the text. Attainable FiO_2 is an approximate maximum under ideal conditions, including appropriate maintenance of the device on the patient. Gas flow rate to the device may be oxygen (*) or an air-oxygen mixture obtained with oxygen driving a Venturi device (**).

in general, is less than with face masks and face shields.

Nasal Catheter. The nasal catheter is a device placed within one nasal passage, its distal end residing in the nasopharynx. Proper insertion and placement of the device requires visualization of the pharynx. The proximal end of the catheter must be secured outside the anterior naris with tape or other device. These two reasons, along with the fact that this technique requires a moderately large-bore catheter in the nasal passage, make this method for oxygen supplementation less desirable than the nasal cannula.

Face Masks. Oxygen masks are available commercially in several forms. All but the last to be discussed are applied in such a manner that they can be removed readily by the patient.

Simple Mask. This mask is supplied with small-bore delivery tubing. Gas flow is unidirectional within the tubing, and washout of the patient's exhalate is dependent upon fresh gas flow. Washout of the exhalate occurs through side ports in the body of the mask. This mask is suitable only for use with nonheated, bubble-type humidifiers, since aerosol particles or high humidity can produce water rain-out in the small-diameter tubing, thereby blocking oxygen flow to the mask.

Aerosol Mask. In this mask gas flow is unidirectional within the large-bore delivery tubing, and washout of the patient's exhalate through mask side ports is dependent upon fresh gas flow. The larger-diameter delivery tubing permits use of heated humidifiers and aerosol generators with the mask and therefore makes it more suitable for the recently extubated patient than the simple mask. Maximum FIO_2 attainable with this mask is limited by room air entrainment through the side ports of the mask. Higher delivered FIO_2s can be achieved with side-port reservoirs ("tusks") placed in the side port holes (see Fig. 21-8). Use of good facial mask fit, higher delivered gas flows (driving oxygen flow rate equal to or exceeding 20 L/min), and side port reservoirs will permit delivery

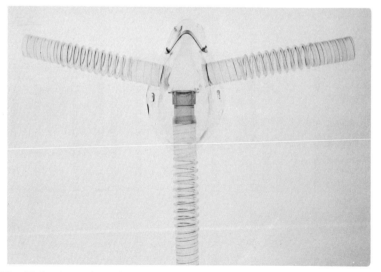

Fig. 21-8 Aerosol mask with reservoirs. This modification of an aerosol mask with "tusk" reservoirs in the exhalation ports provides an additional 100-ml reservoir for increasing FIO_2 as well as humidity. Modification merely requires use of 10-cm sections of disposable breathing circuit tubing (2 cm diameter).

not only of higher FIO_2s but also of higher humidity.

Face Shield. This variation of the simple mask, which supplies oxygen in the vicinity of the face, permits suctioning, mouth care, etc., without removal of the supplemental oxygen source from the patient. It is bulkier and heavier than the face mask and therefore is not as useful for the mobile patient.

Partial Rebreathing Mask. With this mask the patient's fresh gas source is both from a gas reservoir and directly from the fresh gas flow. Since the fresh gas flow is directed both into the reservoir bag and into the volume under the mask itself without the use of valves, exhalate can reenter the reservoir or can be washed out through the side ports in the mask. The amount of exhalate entering the reservoir bag will be dependent upon fresh gas flow, which must be adjusted so that the patient does not rebreathe exhaled carbon dioxide.

Non-rebreathing Mask. This mask is similar to the partial rebreathing mask in construction with the addition of a valve between the body of the mask and the fresh gas flowing into the reservoir bag, so that all the exhalate is directed out through the side ports in the body of the mask and cannot enter the reservoir bag. This type of mask may have one-way, flap valves on the exhalation ports to prevent room air entrainment. Fresh gas flow, therefore, must always be adjusted so that the reservoir bag never collapses.

Tracheostomy Collar. This is a device with large-bore delivery tubing for application above tracheostomy tubes, tracheostomy buttons, and laryngectomy tubes. The device is not connected directly to the tube and therefore its manner of operation is similar to that of the aerosol mask. Unless the application of distending airway pressure is required, no oxygen delivery device should be connected directly to a tracheostomy tube, since traction from the connection may lead to tracheal damage.

T-tube. This device is connected directly to an endotracheal tube or tracheostomy tube. Even though a distal reservoir ("tail") may be utilized to provide higher FIO_2s, the system is open to ambient pressure and thereby promotes loss of lung volume (decreased FRC). Therefore, the simple T-tube system is not recommended for either short-term or long-term use. Maintenance of supplemental oxygen concentrations and appropriate levels of distending airway pressure can be achieved with the breathing circuit shown in Figure 21-9.

Venturi Mask. This is a combination of mask and air entrainment mechanism which, depending upon the setting of the mechanism, will provide different delivered concentrations of oxygen. The device operates on the Venturi principle, which is illustrated in Figure 21-1. The masks operate at relatively low driving flows of pure oxygen. The total gas flow in this device or in any device operating on the Venturi principle can be calculated as shown in Figure 21-10.

Hoods, tents, and incubators are devices which surround the head or body of the patient, generally an infant or small child. The oxygen concentration provided within any one of these devices is a function of oxygen concentration delivered, tightness of all fittings and seals for the device, frequency and duration of entries into the device, and gas flowrate into the device. Since large leaks associated with any of these devices may lower the desired oxygen concentration, fresh gas flow rate will have to be increased accordingly. Each time the device is opened to the room, the desired oxygen concentration will not be reached again until the diluting gases are washed out. These devices, therefore, are not optimum for oxygen delivery if they must be entered frequently for patient care. However, they do provide supplemental oxygen in their contained atmosphere without noxious devices being applied directly to pediatric patients. Another undesirable and potentially dangerous feature of these devices can be excessive noise. Care must be

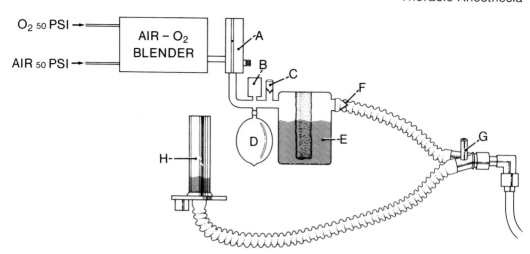

Fig. 21-9 Breathing circuit for distending airway pressure. This circuit, which is similar to the patient circuit component of the intermittent mandatory ventilation circuit (see Fig. 21-20), is used for patients receiving distending airway pressure therapy via endotracheal tube, tracheostomy tube, or tight-fitting mask. The sources for fresh gas flow are oxygen and air (each at 50 psi), which are blended to give the desired FIO_2. Other components of the circuit are as follows: (A) High-flow flowmeter. (B) Pressure relief value for preventing pressure buildup in the circuit to more than 5 mmHg above the selected expiratory airway pressure level; this should be a threshold resistor valve set approximately 5 mmHg above the selected expiratory airway pressure level. (C) Air entry valve; this is another safety feature for the circuit which provides a fresh gas source (room air) for the inspiratory limb of the circuit if the high-pressure fresh gas sources fail. (D) Reservoir bag; a 3-L reservoir bag is selected generally (see text for modifications). (E) Humidifier; a wick humidifier, which is the most efficient type for this application, is shown placed distal to the preceding three circuit components in order that humidity not interfere with their function. (F) One-way valve; this is located distal to the humidifier so that the potential compressible gas volume of the humidifier is excluded from the actual compressible gas volume of the respiratory limb (note that this also pertains to the other, preceding circuit components). (G) Port for connecting airway pressure monitoring system. (H) Exhalation–distending-airway-pressure valve; this valve serves to prevent room air entrainment via the expiratory limb during the patient's inspiration and also to provide the desired expiratory level of airway pressure (an Emerson Exhalation PEEP Valve is illustrated).

taken to ensure that the oxygen delivery system, including humidifier (as well as all other devices applied onto or near the incubator, tent, or hood) do not generate excessive noise levels which can result in subsequent hearing impairment in infants and small children.

Masks for Closed Systems. These masks permit FIO_2s up to 1.0 and the application of low levels of distending airway pressure. They fit occlusively, so that there is no gas leakage or room air entrainment, but need to be used so that patient comfort is optimum. An occlusive seal can be achieved with masks having a compliant, air-filled rim (Vital Signs Facemask, Vital Signs, Inc., Fig. 21-11) or a J-shaped lip (Bird CPAP Mask, Bird/3M Corporation, Fig. 21-12). The mask can be applied by using a mask strap, and it will exert minimum pressure on the face of the patient. The mask and the breathing circuit cannot be removed readily by the patient, who must therefore be in an environment where he is under close observation at all times, just as if he were intubated. The mask should be clear so that vomitus may be seen easily. The rim of the mask should be lifted periodically to observe the patient's face, especially the bridge of the nose, for

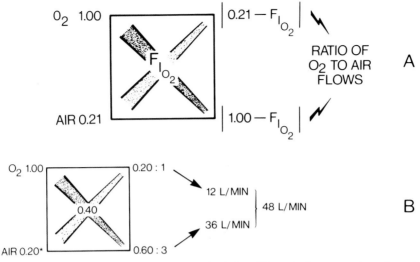

Fig. 21-10 Simplified air entrainment calculation. The entrainment ratio and total gas flow for any device operating upon the venturi principle can be calculated easily. (A) Oxygen, which is 100 percent pure, is depicted in the upper left-hand corner of the box, and air, which is 21 percent oxygen, is depicted in the lower left-hand corner. The $F_{I}O_2$ selected for the system is entered into the box, and oxygen and air are *absolutely* subtracted diagonally across the box providing $(0.21 - F_{I}O_2)$ in the upper right-hand corner and $(1 - F_{I}O_2)$ in the lower right-hand corner. This is the ratio of flows of oxygen (upper) to air (lower). (B) A mathematical example for $F_{I}O_2 = 0.40$ illustrates the principle: the oxygen/air ratio is 1:3; if oxygen is set at 12 L/min on the flowmeter, then the flow rate for the entrained air is 36 L/min, giving a resultant system flow of 48 L/min. (*For ease of subtraction in this example, air is shown as 20 percent oxygen.)

any pressure-related injury, although this generally is not a problem with the masks described if they have been properly applied. The fresh gas flow for delivery of air and oxygen in this type of system may emanate from a demand valve or from a flowmeter and reservoir, which must never empty completely. This circuit, although applicable for delivery of high known concentrations of oxygen, generally is reserved for application of distending airway pressure.

Distending Airway Pressure Therapy

Distending airway pressure therapy is the application of positive airway pressure to promote an increase in resting lung volume or functional residual capacity (FRC). The increase in FRC is achieved by increasing the volume of alveoli already open and by recruiting alveoli which were closed prior to the application of this therapy. In the spontaneously breathing patient, the application of distending airway pressure may be made in the inspiratory phase as well as in the expiratory phase; both the expiratory level and the inspiratory level have titratable therapeutic endpoints. In the apneic patient, the application of distending airway pressure can be made during the expiratory phase, and the mechanical ventilator increases airway pressure above the expiratory distending airway pressure level during delivery of the mechanical breath. In the spontaneously breathing patient who also is receiving mechanical ventilatory support, distending airway pressure can be applied during the pa-

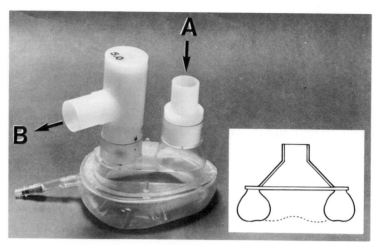

Fig. 21-11 Vital Signs face mask. Mask suitable for application of distending airway pressure therapy (see text). The air-filled rim provides a soft, cushioned seal with the patient's face. The face-mask strap may be applied by using the pegs on the front of the mask.

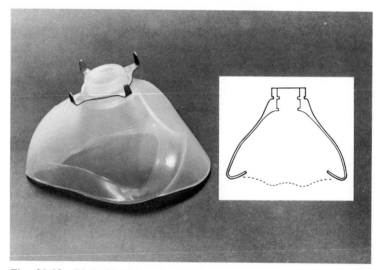

Fig. 21-12 Bird CPAP mask. Mask suitable for distending airway pressure therapy (see text). Note J-shape of lips on mask (insert). Mask straps can be attached by using strap ring on front of mask.

tient's inspiration and expiration; the delivery of a mechanical breath increases airway pressure above the expiratory airway pressure level.

Varied nomenclature has been applied to this therapy over the years. One form of nomenclature is based on the airway pressures generated by the therapy and another on the type of breathing circuit involved with generation of the positive airway pressure. The simplest approach to take, and the one in which the most information is transmitted concerning this form of therapy, is that in which the *actual airway pressure* is

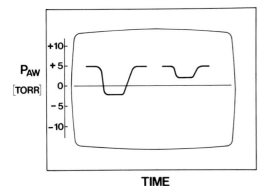

Fig. 21-13 Airway pressure monitoring. Two different airway pressures (Paw) are shown as they might appear in a calibrated oscilloscopic display of airway pressure. Time is shown on the X axis, a function of oscilloscopic sweep speed. Airway pressure is shown on the Y axis over the range -10 to $+10$. Note the difference that would be seen with the Paw = $+5/(-2)$ versus Paw = $+5/(+2)$.

indicated and no differing forms of nomenclature are utilized. The use of the term *distending airway pressure* is not an attempt to add yet another name for this therapeutic modality, but it is an effort to direct consideration toward use and quantitation of the therapy and away from acronymic confusion.

A better understanding of the therapy and its quantitation can be achieved by considering several examples. By convention, pressure during spontaneous breathing will be indicated as *expiratory/inspiratory* and its units may be either cm H_2O or mmHg.* For example, a spontaneously breathing patient with an airway pressure of 5 / (-2) is depicted in the left-hand side of Figure 21-13. If the inspiratory airway pressure level were increased to $+2$ mmHg without any change in the expiratory pressure level, the airway pressure now would appear as in the right-

hand depiction in Figure 21-13. Note that these examples appear as they would in an oscilloscopic display. Since both the inspiratory pressure level and the expiratory pressure level are titratable, it is important that the airway pressure be monitored routinely.

CIRCUIT FOR DISTENDING AIRWAY PRESSURE THERAPY

The breathing circuit for providing distending airway pressure therapy has several essential components. This circuit may or may not be a part of the circuit attached to a mechanical ventilator, since support of ventilation and support of oxygenation are separate functions.

A circuit which is independent of a mechanical ventilator is that shown in Figure 21-9. This circuit would be used for the application of all levels of distending airway pressure, ranging from low maintenance pressures (e.g., Paw = 4/0 mmHg) to very high therapeutic pressures (e.g., 32/26 mmHg).

Before each circuit component is considered separately, it should be noted that the expiratory (maximum) and inspiratory (minimum) levels of airway pressure basically are functions of the expiratory valve and the fresh gas flow rate, respectively. Although different equipment is available for delivering each, provision of distending airway pressure therapy consists merely of the selection and variation of these two system variables.

Fresh Gas Source. The fresh gas source for the circuit can be either a high-flow source and reservoir bag or a demand valve. When a fresh gas source and reservoir bag are used, the flowmeter through which the fresh gas source is provided must have the capability for metering high flow rates (which may be greater than 60 L/min). The reservoir bag must be compliant enough to provide net movement of several hundred

---

* Since airway pressure is monitored routinely on the pressure monitoring systems which are also used for vascular pressure monitoring, *mmHg* has become the conventional dimension. *mmHg* can be converted readily into mmHg × 1.36 = cm H_2O.

milliliters of gas but not so complaint as to become markedly distended at higher airway pressures; generally a 3L anesthesia bag is selected. (For higher levels of distending airway pressure, where the less compliant anesthesia bags are too small for tidal excursion of adult patients, the 3L bag can be encased within a pliable netting, e.g., women's hosiery.) With the reservoir bag in the circuit, the fresh gas flow rate is adjusted to attain the desired inspiratory level of the distending airway pressure therapy. When a demand valve is used in this circuit, the demand flow rate must be adjusted to provide the desired inspiratory pressure level for the distending airway pressure therapy.

Humidifier. Since this form of therapy is generally attendant on the maintenance of an artificial airway, the natural air conditioning system of the patient is bypassed and adequate humidification is of paramount importance. The location of the humidifier in relation to the one-way valve of the inspiratory limb also is important. If the gaseous volume within the humidifier is large, it is desirable to locate the humidifier proximal to a one-way valve in the inspiratory limb. The one-way valve must not become partially or completely dysfunctional because of the collection of condensate; to avoid such problems, another valve may have to be placed between the fresh gas source or reservoir and the humidifier. Heated wick humidifiers provide the most efficient humidification for these high-flow applications.[2]

Connection to Patient. The distending airway pressure circuit may be applied to the patient's airway via mask or via endotracheal or tracheostomy tube. The use of a mask for safe and efficient application of distending airway pressure therapy has been reported in adults and in infants.[6-9] The use of a mask does have several limitations: (1) The patient must be conscious and alert and should be able to remove the device if vomiting occurs; (2) There must be no serious facial injuries;

(3) The applied distending airway pressure should not exceed 10 to 12 cm H_2O (7 to 9 mmHg), which is less than the opening pressure of the esophagus; and (4) The duration of the distending airway pressure therapy should not exceed approximately 72 hours. Application of distending airway pressure therapy by mask may not necessitate placement of a nasogastric tube, although if one is used, it can be passed through a small sealed opening made in the mask. Distending airway pressure therapy is more commonly provided by applying the circuit described to the patient's airways via an endotracheal tube.

Expiratory Valve. For the patient receiving distending airway pressure therapy, the expiratory level of the airway pressure is determined by selection of either an expiratory valve with a fixed pressure setting or a variable valve requiring pressure adjustment. The expiratory valve which delivers the distending airway pressure should function as a *threshold resistor* and not as a flow resistor. That is, the valve should open at the desired level of expiratory airway pressure and maintain that pressure regardless of the flow rate through the valve (Fig. 21-14). If a valve has flow-resistive characteristics, then high gas flows generated within the circuit (e.g., by an attempted cough by the patient) may produce back pressure significant enough to cause pulmonary barotrauma. Also, when a flow-resistor type of valve is used, expiratory gas flow may be retarded so that mean airway pressure becomes elevated, resulting in impedance to venous return and decrease in cardiac output and systemic arterial blood pressure[10] (Fig. 21-15A and B).

This valve not only provides the expiratory pressure level but also may serve as a one-way valve in the expiratory limb, preventing entrainment of room air into the circuit. If this circuit and therefore this valve are part of a mechanical ventilator system, then the valve also may serve the function of stopping gas flow from the expiratory limb

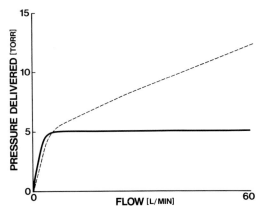

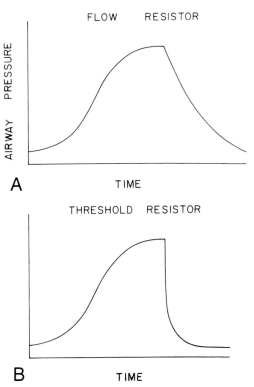

Fig. 21-14 Resistances with threshold resistor versus flow resistor. The performance of a threshold resistor (——) and a flow resistor (– – – –) are illustrated for a flow range of 0 to 60 L/min. Once the threshold resistor valve has reached its preset pressure, the delivered pressure (airway pressure) does not rise. The flow resistor valve will produce a continuing pressure increase over the entire flow range.

Fig. 21-15 Threshold versus flow resistor valves. The difference between a threshold resistor (A) and flow resistor (B) is seen in the expiratory phase of the airway pressure curve. The threshold resistor permits near instantaneous return to baseline pressure level, whereas the flow resistor impedes gas flow and thereby delays return of airway pressure to baseline. These differences can be observed easily by using airway pressure monitoring techniques.

during the mechanical breath to the patient. Several commercial valves which are available for application in any breathing circuit will be considered as will an underwater seal.

Boehringer PEEP Valves (Boehringer Laboratories, Inc.) are weighted-ball systems which also can serve as one-way valves for the expiratory limb. These devices are available for several pressure levels (2.5, 5, 10, 15 cm H$_2$O) and can be stacked serially to provide higher levels, including intercalated values of expiratory airway pressure. They must be maintained in an upright position, since their function and integrity are gravity-dependent.

The *Emerson Exhalation PEEP Valve* (J. H. Emerson Co.) is a water-weighted diaphragm. It functions as a one-way valve in the expiratory limb and also can function to close the expiratory limb during mechanical ventilation when the valve is part of a mechanical ventilator circuit. These valves also must be maintained in an upright position since they are water-filled and since the integrity of their function as a one-way valve is

dependent upon seating of the diaphragm over the expiratory port in the base of the valve.

The *Siemans-Elema PEEP Valve* (Siemans-Elema AB) is a spring-loaded platen which opposes the port connected to the expiratory limb of the breathing circuit. Tension on the spring and therefore opening pressure on the expiratory limb are variably adjustable.

The *Vital Signs PEEP Valve* (Vital Signs, Inc.) also is a spring-loaded platen, although the physical configuration of the springs is different from that in the Siemans-

Elema valve. The pressure applied by each valve is preset, and several different valves with different pressures are available (5, 7.5, 10, and 12.5 cm H_2O).

Underwater seal is the oldest means for applying distending airway pressure therapy. A rigid extension of the expiratory limb is placed beneath water, with the depth of placement determining the pressure generated within the expiratory circuit. The diameter of this extension should equal the diameter of the expiratory limb itself since this will prevent flow-resistive pressure generation.

SUPPORT OF VENTILATION

The purpose of ventilation is the maintenance of the body's acid-base homeostasis by the excretion of carbon dioxide. This is accomplished in the spontaneously breathing individual by the titration of alveolar ventilation against several feedback variables, including carbon dioxide tension, hydrogen ion concentration, and arterial oxygen tension. Ventilation must be supported mechanically when a patient cannot maintain sufficient alveolar ventilation to eliminate the carbon dioxide being presented each minute to the lungs by the pulmonary arterial circulation.

Many patients who need ventilatory support also have metabolic acid-base disturbances, predominantly metabolic alkalosis.[11] Since to make these patients eucapnic with the mechanical ventilatory support would exacerbate their metabolic alkalosis and prolong weaning from mechanical ventilation, the support of mechanical ventilation is directed primarily at assisting the body in defense of the arterial pH. Carbon dioxide tension is used as a secondary determinant unless some overriding disease process dictates otherwise (e.g., increased intracranial pressure with a need to maintain hypocapnia).

An arterial pH within a normal range (7.35 to 7.40) is maintained by mechanical ventilatory support of carbon dioxide elimination, since arterial carbon dioxide tension is proportional to alveolar carbon dioxide tension which in turn is related to alveolar ventilation:

$$PaCO_2 \propto PACO_2 \propto \dot{V}CO_2/\dot{V}A.$$

The amount of alveolar ventilation needed is determined by the amount of carbon dioxide being produced and presented to the lungs each minute. A practical approach to mechanical ventilatory support in defense of arterial pH is presented below; this section will develop the background reasons for the amount of support predicated on carbon dioxide production. If carbon dioxide production equals 200 ml/min, then to make the patient eucapnic ($PaCO_2 = PACO_2 = 40$ mmHg) would require the following level of alveolar ventilation:

$$\dot{V}A = \dot{V}CO_2/FACO_2$$
$$\dot{V}A = (200 \text{ ml/min})/(40 \text{ mmHg}/713 \text{ mmHg})$$
$$\dot{V}A = 3,565 \text{ ml/min}$$

Since the alveolar space of the lungs is in series with the conducting airways, a volume greater than the alveolar ventilatory volume must be provided to eliminate carbon dioxide. This is the volume of the conducting airways, or the anatomical dead space [$\dot{V}D(anat)$], which is approximately 2.2 ml/kg. Dead space ventilation [$\dot{V}D(anat)$] in a 70-kg individual with a respiratory rate of 8 breaths per minute would be:

$$\dot{V}D = 2.2 \text{ ml/kg} \times 70 \text{ kg} \times 8/\text{min}$$
$$\dot{V}D = 1,232 \text{ ml/min}$$

The total volume of gases moved in and out of the lungs in one minute, i.e., the minute ventilation ($\dot{V}E$), is the sum of the alveolar ventilation and the dead space ventilation:

$$\dot{V}E = \dot{V}A + \dot{V}D$$
$$\dot{V}E = 3,565 \text{ ml/min} + 1,232 \text{ ml/min}$$
$$\dot{V}E = 4,797 \text{ ml/min}$$

Mechanical ventilatory support is basically the provision of the minute ventilation based upon a knowledge of the patient's measured or estimated dead space and an estimation of the need for the level of support of the alveolar ventilation. In practice, this entails selection of a delivered tidal volume of 12 to 15 ml/kg at a mechanical frequency sufficient to support carbon dioxide excretion in defense of arterial pH.

The volume delivered by a mechanical breath is a result of the pressure difference generated between the airway* of the patient and the alveoli, since gas flow in a tubular system is the result of a pressure difference. The flow of gases into the lungs is opposed by the resistance of the patient's airways and endotracheal or tracheostomy tube and the compliance, or stiffness, of the patient's lungs. Increased resistance, either in the airways or in some portion of the mechanical system, will oppose delivery of the intended gas volume. Likewise, decreased compliance (increased stiffness) will oppose delivery of the mechanical breath. Since various pathophysiological processes of pulmonary disease, as well as mechanical components of the ventilator system, may produce increased resistance and/or decreased compliance, the resultant effect which this will have upon delivered tidal volume should be appreciated for each mechanical ventilatory system (Fig. 21-16).

Mechanical Ventilators

More than 100 mechanical ventilators are available commercially in the world today.[12] When this total is combined with the number of commercially available breathing circuits and individually constructed breathing circuits, some of which are described in the literature, there are several hundred conceivable systems which could be utilized to provide mechanical ventilation. Since it would not be reasonable to undertake detailed consideration of all of these, an over-

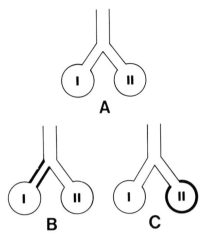

Fig. 21-16 Impedance of lung compartments. In example (A), compartments I and II are shown with equal resistance and compliances; gas flow would be distributed evenly between the two compartments. In example (B), the resistance of compartment I exceeds that of compartment II; gas flow within a finite time period would be less into compartment I than into compartment II, although over an infinite inspiratory time, gases would be evenly distributed, since the compliances of I and II are equal. In example (C), the compliance of compartment II is decreased; gas distribution will be uneven no matter what the duration of inspiration, compartment I receiving proportionately more gas than compartment II.

view of mechanical ventilators will be provided.

Mechanical ventilators can be classified into negative-pressure and positive-pressure devices. Within each category, characterization and classification of different ventilators can be made, depending upon several of their mechanical or operational features.

NEGATIVE-PRESSURE VENTILATORS

There are two types of negative-pressure ventilators available, the iron lung and the cuirass. The iron lung, which was one of the earliest forms of mechnical ventilatory support available, was described in 1929 by Drinker and McKhann and by Drinker and Shaw.[13,14] Although their early model of a ventilator is not used for routine postopera-

---

Airway indicates the point of connection of the patient to the breathing circuit.

tive care, the two types of currently available negative-pressure ventilators will be described.

Iron Lung. This large, rigid box encloses the body of the patient except for the head. Ventilation of the patient occurs when an electrically driven motor powering a bellows generates negative pressure within the box surrounding the patient. Since part of this negative pressure around the patient's chest is transmitted through the chest wall into the distal airways, a pressure gradient is produced between the patient's mouth (atmospheric pressure) and the lung parenchyma so that gas flows into the lungs. The amount of negative pressure generated within the iron lung is the primary mechanical determinant of the patient's tidal volume and is a function of the extent of the bellows' movement, which is controlled by the position of the drive arm on the drive shaft. The rate of ventilation is a function of the rotational speed and gear reduction in the drive assembly, which are controlled by a variable potentiometer. The advantages of this type of ventilatory support include the patient's continuing ability to speak and eat, as well as the lack of need to artificially maintain the airway in the awake patient who can protect his airway. Its disadvantages include the inaccessibility of the patient for nursing care and the need to pass all forms of tubing and monitor wiring required by the patient into the iron lung through specially sealed ports.

Cuirass Ventilator. Another form of negative-pressure mechanical ventilator is the cuirass, or chest shell, ventilator. This unit surrounds only the trunk of the patient, leaving the head, neck, and extremities free and accessible. The anterior and lateral portions of the shell are rigid and the remainder of the trunk is sealed into the ventilator with a plastic wrap. A negative pressure is produced within this shell by a negative pressure–generating device, which is at-

tached via a noncompliant hose. This type of mechanical ventilatory support has advantages similar to those of the iron lung, as well as improved access for patient care. Its disadvantages include the continued limited access to the trunk of the patient, the difficulty in attaining a satisfactory seal in some patients, and the relative immobility to which the patient must be subjected to be ventilated by the unit. A triggering mechanism has been described for the cuirass ventilator which permits *assisted* negative-pressure ventilation (U-Cyclit, J.H. Emerson Co.).

POSITIVE-PRESSURE VENTILATORS

The usual function of a positive-pressure ventilator is to move a volume of gas into a patient's lungs and then to permit passive expulsion of the exhalate by the patient. Since gas flow in any system of tubes occurs in response to a difference in pressure, the tidal volume delivery will occur when the pressure at the patient's airway exceeds the pressure in the alveoli. Gas flow during the inspiratory phase will be opposed by the resistance of the airways and by the resistance of components of the ventilator system, as well as by the compliance of the lung-thorax unit. Expiratory gas flow occurs when the alveolar pressure exceeds the pressure at the airway. Gas flow out of the lungs is a function of the lung-thorax compliance and is opposed by airway resistance and resistance of components of the expiratory limb of the ventilator system. To promote understanding of how this volume of gas is generated and driven into the lungs, including the frequency with which this is done, several characteristics of positive-pressure ventilators will be considered. These characteristics are also the basis of *classification* of positive-pressure ventilators and include their power source, mechanism for volume delivery, cycling mechanisms, modes of ventilation, breathing circuits, and safety and other technical features.

Power Source. The power provided for the delivery of volume by a positive-pressure mechanical ventilator is either electric or pneumatic. Pneumatic sources may have their flows directly or indirectly converted into the volume provided. Electric power generally is translated into delivered volume, with an electric motor driving a direct volume-displacement device or powering a gas compressor. In the latter case, the primary power source is electric, while the actual power utilized as the mechanism for volume delivery is pneumatic.

Mechanism for Volume Delivery. That characteristic of mechanical ventilators which describes the mechanism for volume delivery generally is considered in terms of pressure or flow generation.[12,15] A mechanical ventilator is described as a flow generator or pressure generator, depending upon which characteristic of volume delivery remains constant or relatively constant throughout the inspiratory phase. The *flow generator* maintains a constant flow rate (Fig. 21-17) or constant flow pattern (Fig. 21-18) during the

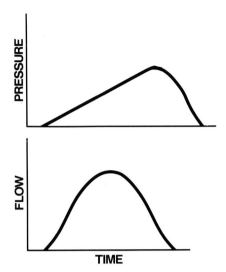

Fig. 21-18 Variable-flow generator. A mechanical ventilator functioning as a variable-flow generator will have a constant flow pattern into the patient's airways, e.g., sine wave illustrated here. Pressure will rise in a curvilinear manner until the end of inspiration.

inspiratory phase while airway pressure changes. Changes in lung or thoracic compliance or in airway resistance will have less effect on delivery of respiratory gases with ventilators that are flow generators than with ventilators that are pressure generators.[16] Ventilators that function as *pressure generators* maintain a constant amount of pressure or a constant pressure pattern during the inspiratory phase. Flow rate is variable, decaying exponentially during inspiration with a true pressure generator (Fig. 21-19). It should be noted that few ventilators function as pure pressure or pure flow generators. It also should be appreciated that this distinction does *not* correspond to the *cycling* or *limiting* mechanisms by which ventilators are classified (see below).

Cycling Mechanisms. Consideration of cycling mechanisms includes cycling from expiration to inspiration (i.e., beginning of the mechanical breath) and cycling from inspiration to expiration (i.e., ending the mechanical breath).

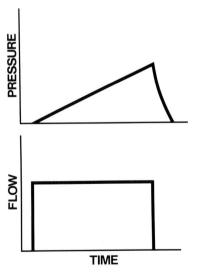

Fig. 21-17 Constant-flow generator. A mechanical ventilator that performs as a constant-flow generator will produce a constant gas flow rate into the patient's airways while airway pressure will rise linearly until the end of inspiration.

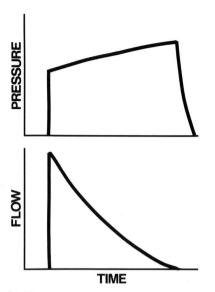

Fig. 21-19 Constant-pressure generator. A mechanical ventilator which functions as a constant-pressure generator will produce a rapidly rising, then constant, pressure upon the patient's airways, while flow decreases exponentially until the end of inspiration.

Cycling the ventilator for the cessation of the inspiratory phase (beginning of the expiratory phase) may be controlled by the time, volume, pressure, flow, or a combination of these. When ventilators are classified by a cycling mechanism, the changeover from inspiration to expiration is the cycling mechanism referred to. If the ventilator is *time-cycled,* the duration of the inspiratory phase is determined by a timing mechanism and is independent of the volume delivered, the inspiratory pressure attained, the inspiratory flow characteristics, and the patient's pulmonary condition. Time cycling may be accomplished with electronic, electromechanical, pneumatic, or fluidic techniques.

For the *volume-cycled* ventilator, the volume delivered is the independent variable, and the inspiratory phase ends when this volume has been attained. It should be noted that this volume is the volume *delivered* by the system and may not be the volume *received* by the patient. The duration of inspiration, inspiratory gas flow pattern, and

peak inspiratory pressure are variables dependent upon the patient's pulmonary condition or other system variables. Mechanisms for volume cycling would include a full excursion of a preset volume displacement device, integration of flow, and detection of an electrical signal which has characteristics proportional to the volume displaced. The last two mechanisms provide feedback to interrupt or redirect volume delivery.

With *pressure-cycled* ventilators, the inspiratory phase ends when a preset pressure is reached. Dependent variables are the absolute inspiratory time, delivered volume, and inspiratory gas flow; the normal or disease characteristics of the patient's lungs will be the primary determinant for these variables.

For the *flow-cycled* ventilator the inspiratory phase ends when the delivered gas flow has reached a preset level. Dependent variables include delivered volume and absolute time of the inspiratory phase. The mechanism used is the inspiratory valve (Bennett valve) developed for this type of cycling change from the inspiratory to the expiratory position when a predetermined low flow rate is reached (approximately 1 L/min).[12]

Some ventilators have the capacity for selection of different cycling modes; other ventilators have a built-in primary cycling mechanism and different secondary, or backup, cycling mechanisms. These ventilators are said to have combination cycling mechanisms, although many of them will have designated a primary cycling type.

Cessation of the expiratory phase (beginning of the inspiratory phase) may be initiated automatically or by the patient. Automatic cycling, or primary ventilator control, generally is accomplished with a timing mechanism. This form of cycling is independent of the pressure, expiratory volume, and expiratory gas flow rate or pattern. The time-cycling mechanisms are the same as those that end the inspiratory phase.

Inspiration may be cycled by the patient ("patient-triggered"), which provides a negative-pressure cycling mechanism in which the inspiratory phase begins when a preset negative pressure is attained. Most ventilators with this form of cycling have a variable sensitivity control, which can be adjusted to meet the needs of different inspiratory efforts by the patient. This also describes a mode of ventilation, assist mode ventilation (see below).

Modes of Ventilation. Modes of ventilation fall into one of three categories or combinations thereof: control mode ventilation (CMV), assist mode ventilation (AMV), and intermittent mandatory ventilation (IMV). CMV is the oldest form of mechanical ventilatory support and encompasses the function of the negative-pressure ventilators, as well as of the earlier models of positive-pressure ventilators. AMV was developed as an option for CMV ventilators and utilized the same circuits with modifications to detect the patient's inspiratory effort and alter subsequent cycling. IMV is a newer form of ventilation, requiring a circuit different from those for CMV and AMV.

Control mode ventilation provides mechanical breaths with equal time intervals between each. A circuit exclusively for CMV has no provision for delivery of gas volume when a patient attempts spontaneous breathing—the effort will only generate negative pressure within all or part of the breathing circuit, depending upon how the circuit's valves are arranged. These patient efforts, while not contributing to effective alveolar ventilation, can markedly increase the patient's work of breathing. True CMV is only suitable for the apneic patient, and a circuit exclusively for CMV is not recommended for general use in an intensive care unit, since ventilators and circuits which provide IMV can perform this function as well (see below).

Ventilators operating as *assist mode ventilators* will sense patient effort to inspire and will follow quickly with a mechanical breath. The detection of the patient's inspiratory effort can be made via electronic, magnetic, or pneumatic transduction, the last being the most common method. AMV circuits have no means for providing volume during a patient's spontaneous ventilatory effort other than positive-pressure delivery of gas. Since no beneficial effects of ventilatory support with AMV have been found when compared with CMV and since ventilators and circuits exclusively for CMV are not recommended, circuits designed exclusively for assist mode ventilation are not recommended either.[17]

Assist-control mode ventilation is a combination mode wherein the ventilator will provide assisted breaths in response to patient effort and also will provide a set rate of mechanical breaths to the patient each minute. Again, since this circuit has no provision for supporting the patient's spontaneous ventilatory effort with other than positive-pressure gas delivery, it is not a recommended means of support.

Intermittent mandatory ventilation is a means of ventilatory support wherein the patient may breathe spontaneously in an unimpeded, unassisted manner *and* receive a set number of mechanical breaths per minute in support of alveolar ventilation.[18] The patient may breathe at the rate and depth he selects through normal physiologic mechanisms and will receive that number of mechanical breaths selected for the IMV rate. This rate may be zero, at which point the patient could be on the IMV circuit of a mechanical ventilator or on a spontaneous breathing circuit independent of a mechanical ventilator (see section on Circuit for Distending Airway Pressure Therapy).

Figure 21-20 is a schematized presentation of an IMV circuit (e.g., modified Emerson Post-op Ventilator, Emerson IMV ventilator). The ventilator circuit can be considered as having two component circuits, one serving the mechanical ventilator and one serving the patient's spontaneous breathing. Each component of the circuit has a fresh gas source, a reservoir bag, and one-way valving to provide unidirectional gas flow. It is most efficacious to use a blender to

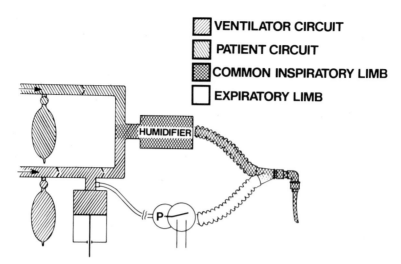

Fig. 21-20 Intermittent mandatory ventilation circuit. This simplified schematic representation of an IMV circuit shows the patient circuit component and the ventilator circuit component. Depending upon the actual ventilator employed, the fresh gas sources may be at 50 psi or less; the circuit illustrated has a premixed air-oxygen source (arrows) for each circuit subcomponent. The patient circuit (top) has its own reservoir as well as a one-way valve providing unidirectionality of flow. The ventilator circuit (bottom) also has a reservoir bag and one-way valve, as well as a means for volume generation, which is illustrated with a piston in this example. The one-way valve distal to the piston prevents any gas flow from the inspiratory limb or the patient circuit subcomponent. Both circuits enter a common humidifier, which serves the inspiratory limb. The expiratory limb ends in a combination valve, which serves to prevent room air entrainment (one-way valve function), provide the desired expiratory pressure level for distending airway pressure therapy, and occlude the expiratory limb during mechanical inspiration. The last function is accomplished by the charging line, which is shown between the piston of the ventilator circuit and the expiratory valve (attachment P).

provide the FIO_2 setting prior to flow metering the fresh gas into either circuit. Although separate humidifiers could be used for the ventilator circuit and for the patient circuit, it is more common to combine the two circuits prior to their entry into a humidifier, which then serves the inspiratory limb of the breathing circuit. The humidifier that serves the breathing circuit must be capable of efficiently warming and humidifying a high continuous gas flow; this would be a wick-type humidifier.[2]

The gas source for the ventilator circuit must have a flow rate sufficient to accommo-date the tidal volume (minute volume) needs of the patient as set for the ventilator. In this example, it would be a flow rate sufficient to prevent collapse of the reservoir bag. The flowmeter for the ventilator circuit can have a low maximum flow rate capability (15 L/min). The gas source for the patient circuit must have a flow rate capability sufficient to maintain inspiratory airway pressure at the desired level. Adequacy of the flow rate is assessed by continuously monitoring airway pressure, i.e., inspiratory level, and adjusting the flow rate to the patient circuit accordingly. The flowmeter for the patient circuit must have a high maximum flow rate capability (75 L/min; e.g., the High Flow Oxygen Flow Meter, Timeter Instrument Corporation, Lancaster, Pennsylvania). The inspiratory flow rate for the ventilator circuit has to be adjusted only when a change is made in set tidal volume or mechanical frequency. The gas flow rate into the patient circuit has to be adjusted to accommodate the patient's inspiratory needs while maintaining the desired level of inspiratory airway pressure. Expiratory gas flow proceeds via the expiratory limb through the exhalation valve and the valve for providing distending airway pressure; these two valve functions may be combined into one valve serving both purposes.

In order to provide distending airway pressure therapy and mechanical ventilatory support concomitantly, it is necessary to have a ventilator and breathing circuit capable of meeting the needs for both forms of support. It is *not* satisfactory to use a ventilator or a breathing circuit in which the demand valve or flow rate control is used simultaneously for both the ventilator circuit and the patient circuit. Since the flow rate control or demand valve may be an integral part of either the inspiratory timing or the mechanism controlling tidal volume, this will lead to undesired changes in mechanical ventilatory parameters when the flow rate for the patient's spontaneous circuit is changed, or vice versa. *Flow rate controls for the fresh gas sources must be separate for the patient circuit and the ventilator circuit.* Since utilization of one flow source for both the patient circuit and the ventilator circuit is a common design feature for many ventilators (exceptions being the Emerson IMV Ventilator and the Modified Emerson Post-op Ventilator), it is necessary to provide a spontaneous breathing circuit for the patient which is separate from the ventilator circuit. This is accomplished easily by adapting a circuit as described above to a mechanical ventilator. The ventilator circuit now serves mechanical ventilatory needs, and the externally applied circuit provides

distending airway pressure during the patient's spontaneous breathing.

Two modifications of the originally described IMV technique have been proposed in order that the delivery of the mechanical breaths may be in phase with the patient's inspiratory effort. Although no exacting convention exists for their nomenclature, they are known as synchronized intermittent mandatory ventilation (SIMV) and intermittent demand ventilation (IDV). Each of these two modifications of IMV delivers the positive-pressure mechanical breath immediately after a patient's spontaneous inspiratory effort occurs. SIMV provides a set number of mechanical breaths each minute, and each of these breaths is synchronized with patient effort, if present. Mechanical ventilatory support is provided if the patient is apneic—at the rate set for the SIMV. IDV provides synchronized mechanical breaths at a preset ratio to the number of spontaneous breaths which the patient is taking. That is, if IDV is set for 1 mechanical breath for every 6 patient breaths and the patient is breathing 18 times per minute, he will receive 3 mechanical breaths each minute. However, if he becomes apneic, there will be no mechanical breaths provided, and alveolar ventilation will be zero. The difference between SIMV and IDV, however, is moot, for there is no proven efficacy for a synchronized form of IMV.[19]

Mechanical Dead Space. Mechanical dead space results from two sources within the breathing circuit: (1) the common physical volume through which both inspiratory and expiratory gases flow; and (2) the volume amount lost with each mechanical breath owing to gas compression and system expansion that occurs during positive-pressure ventilation. The gas compression–system compliance dead space can be calculated easily. This form of dead space is compensated for readily in breathing circuits for adult patients by increasing delivered ventilation. However, in breathing circuits for neonates and children, this form of dead space is decreased by using less compliant breathing circuit components, especially tubing.

Elbow Connectors. Use of an elbow with an occlusively-sealing port provides a means for suctioning and for the introduction of a fiberoptic bronchoscope without completely disconnecting the circuit from the patient. This will prevent deleterious pressure losses within the circuit during the application of distending airway pressure therapy.

MECHANICAL VENTILATORY PATTERNS

The mechanical ventilatory cycle, as shown in Figure 21-21A, is divided into the inspiratory phase and the expiratory phase. The inspiratory phase is that period during which positive airway pressure is generated and inspiratory gas flow is occurring; it ends as airway pressure begins to become more negative and gas flow begins in the opposite direction. The expiratory phase occurs over the remainder of the ventilatory cycle, including that time during which gas flow moves out of the patient and that time during which there is no net gas flow, the expiratory pause. If an inspiratory hold (see below) is employed, it is part of the inspiratory phase even though no gas is flowing into the patient's lungs (Figure 21-21B).

Several aspects of the mechanical ventilatory pattern are important when considered in view of normalcy or disease of patients' lungs. The fundamental pulmonary features are lung and thoracic compliances and airway resistance. In many pathophysiological lung conditions, the regional differences in compliance and resistance, producing areas with different time constants, will be equally as important a consideration as the absolute abnormality in either compliance or resistance. The aspects of the mechanical ventilatory pattern to be considered include inspiratory pattern and flow rate, inspiratory time, inspiratory hold, expiratory pressure pattern, expiratory time, and inspiratory/expiratory time relationship.

Since few mechanical ventilators function as pure flow or pure pressure generators, and since inspiratory flow and pressure patterns are dependent upon the patient's compliance and resistance, consideration of a mechanical ventilator based on the concept of a constant-flow or a constant-pressure generator is more theoretical than practical. However, the type of flow pattern actually produced may have important effects depending upon the presence or absence of lung pathology and, if present, the type of pathophysiology. The inspiratory phase of the mechanical ventilator must occur over a finite time. If there is no regional resistive impedance to inspiratory gas flow, the distribution of inspiratory gases will be even. If, however, one or more compartments has increased resistance, inspiratory gases will be distributed unevenly, more going to the compartment with the lower resistance (Fig. 21-16B). An improvement in distribution with this type of pathophysiology can be achieved potentially by several means. Lower inspiratory flow rate will allow more time for even gas distribution in the face of high resistive compartments.[20] Lower inspiratory flow rates will require a longer inspiratory time to attain the desired delivered tidal volume, and this time generally should be maintained at one second or longer.[21] Since the expiratory phase should not be shortened so that the inspiratory phase may be longer, the total ventilatory time must be increased. That is, respiratory rate may have to be decreased, a factor that in and of itself has been shown to improve gas distribution in obstructive airways pathology.[22]

The different rates and patterns of inspiratory gas flow—accelerating, decelerating, or constant—have different theoretical advantages. With obstructive pathophysiology present in some compartments, decelerating or constant inspiratory gas flows may improve distribution.[20,23] However, the effi-

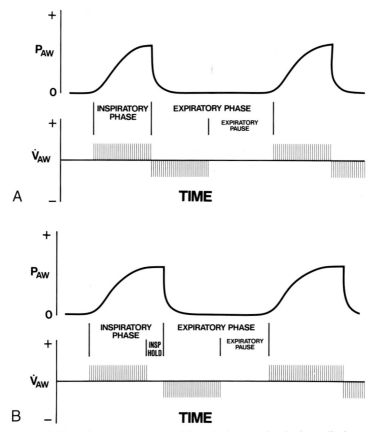

Fig. 21-21 Airway pressure and flow during mechanical ventilation (A) Relationship between airway pressure and flow in the airways is depicted for positive-pressure ventilation. Note that the expiratory pause is part of the expiratory phase; the I/E ratio is the ratio of time for the inspiratory *phase* and the expiratory *phase*. (B) Airway pressure and flow are shown with an end-inspiratory pause (note the no-flow condition); the inspiratory phase then includes the end-inspiratory pause and the I/E ratio still is the ratio of time for the inspiratory *phase* and the expiratory *phase*.

ciency of this pattern may depend upon the presence or absence of turbulence, with accelerating flow being more advantageous if inspiratory gas flow is turbulent.[20] No one inspiratory flow pattern is ideal, and in the design or selection of mechanical ventilatory patterns the waveform is not as important as other features which lead to effective alveolar ventilation.[24,25] The use of excessively high flow rates *is* detrimental, leading to increasing dead space production and decreased efficiency of alveolar ventilation.[21,24,26]

The provision of an end-inspiratory pause (inspiratory hold, inspiratory plateau) may improve gas distribution, and this may be better than increasing inspiratory time alone or decreasing inspiratory flow rate alone.[20,23,25,27] The pause generally is on the order of 0.6 to 1.2 seconds, and its application may be of benefit with several types of inspiratory flow patterns.[27,28] The use of inspiratory hold increases mean airway pressure overall, and in so doing may have adverse effects upon cardiovascular function, since increasing mean airway pressure with different ventilatory patterns is known to decrease cardiac output.[10] Inspiratory hold also has been shown to decrease arterial blood pressure, decrease ventricular stroke work, and increase pulmonary vascular resistance.[29] As with many other aspects of support of breathing, the beneficial potential of inspiratory hold must be balanced against its potentially detrimental cardiovascular effects. With the advent and appropriate utilization of distending airway pressure therapy, inspiratory hold no longer is used routinely.

The relative timing of inspiration and expiration is important, but the factors to be considered should be inspiratory and expiratory time rather than inspiratory/expiratory (I:E) ratio alone. Even in patients with normal lungs, the distribution of the tidal volume will require a finite period of time, which should be a minimum of one second.[21] Expiration must occur over a finite period of time also. The phase of the ventilatory period allotted to expiration includes that time during which expiratory gas flow is occurring and that time during which no gas flow is occurring, the expiratory pause (Fig. 21-21). Increases or decreases in mechanical ventilatory rate may change the time relationship for the expiratory pause, shortening it with increasing mechanical frequency and lengthening it with decreasing mechanical frequency. The mechanical frequency or changes in inspiratory: expiratory timing should not be executed in such a way that the period for the patient's expiratory gas flow is compromised.

Airway pressure during the expiratory phase of the ventilatory cycle may return to zero, i.e., to equilibrium with atmospheric pressure, or it may return to some preset expiratory pressure level that is being used to promote an increase in the resting lung volume (FRC). A complete consideration of this therapeutic modality is presented in the section on Distending Airway Pressure Therapy.

In the past, a negative pressure has been applied to the airways during the expiratory phase with the intention of "assisting" the patient's expiratory gas flow. However, this has been shown to increase physiologic dead space and decrease lung compliance.[21,30] Therefore, negative airway pressure should not be used during the expiratory phase. Negative pressure is employed within the circuit of some ventilators as a part of their function (e.g., Babybird Ventilator, Bird/3M Corporation); this should not be confused with negative pressure being generated within the breathing circuit.

SELECTION OF A MECHANICAL VENTILATOR

Table 21-2 summarizes the characteristics of 14 mechanical ventilators used in the United States for long-term ventilation support. Their selection should be based upon the ventilatory support needs of the patient population. Routine postoperative care will exclude negative-pressure ventilators, and the only diversity in types of positive-pressure ventilators may be the selection of devices suitable for ventilation of neonates and small children. Since there is great disparity in the efficiency of humidifiers and since there are many different types of devices for the generation of distending airway pressure therapy, consideration of mechanical ventilators should be limited to the ventilator device itself, perhaps only including the mechanism for control of inspired oxygen concentration if it is an integral part of the ventilator circuit. Selection of humidifiers, nebulizers, valves for distending airway pressure therapy, instruments for measuring airway pressure, and alarms for airway pressure and oxygen concentration should be selected separately, and the inclusion or exclusion of these items on the basic ventilator should not influence selection and purchase of the ventilator itself.

Selection of the mechanical ventilator should be based upon economy, efficiency, safety, and service. The durability of the ventilator is important since it will be used by many individuals, even though they may all be skilled professionals. Economy must be considered in view not only of initial purchase price but also of subsequent maintenance, in terms of both maintenance costs and downtime losses from service. The ventilator should be selected also on the basis of availability of parts and service. Whether the service is in-house or by maintenance agreement or repair order, it is imperative that trained individuals be readily available and have all necessary parts readily available as well. From the point of view of preventive maintenance and service, simplicity of design is a key factor.

Safety features associated with mechanical ventilators obviously are important, although deficits in ventilator system components can be eliminated with the addition of needed devices or instrumentation. The ventilator circuit or the breathing circuit should be supplied with a maximum pressure relief ("pop-off") valve or flow diversion mechanism so that excessively high pressures do not build up in the breathing circuit and patient's airways. A high-pressure alarm also may be included in the circuit for detection and notification of this problem. The breathing circuit or ventilator circuit should be supplied with an alarm device that detects circuit disconnection, which would result in no ventilatory support for the patient. These devices generally are low-pressure alarms with time delays.

Direct airway pressure monitoring serves as an integral safety feature for mechanical ventilatory support. If the airway pressure trace is continuously displayed, it will provide an ever-present visual monitor for mechanical ventilation or malfunction thereof (Fig. 21-22).

The ventilator circuit also should undergo regular frequent monitoring of inspired oxygen concentration. This may be accomplished by a continuous in-line monitor with alarms or by intermittent oxygen analysis with a device inserted into the circuit. The former approach to oxygen monitoring is more desirable.

ROUTINE APPLICATION AND WEANING OF SUPPORT

In the routine postoperative patient, several aspects of support of breathing should be provided. For support of ventilation, these include tidal volume and mechanical frequency, and for support of oxygenation, FIO_2 and distending airway pressure.

For support of ventilation, tidal volume should be delivered at 12 to 15 ml/kg. The exception to this is the postoperative pneumonectomy or lobectomy patient, in whom tidal volume should be set at 8 to 12 ml/kg. To provide support of ventilation so that initially apneic patients are eucapnic and have a normal arterial pH, mechanical frequency then is set at 7 to 8 breaths per minute.[31] For the initial support of oxygenation, FIO_2 is set at 0.80, and distending airway pressure is provided at 4/0.

Routine weaning then begins initially with FIO_2. If good oxygenation has been obtained at $FIO_2 = 0.80$, FIO_2 then may be decreased to 0.40. If oxygenation has not been completely satisfactory at the initial setting, the change in FIO_2 should be decremental, the first step lowering it perhaps to 0.60. For routine application and weaning of parameters in support of oxygenation, the distending airway pressure of 4/0 remains unchanged.

In weaning the support of ventilation, tidal volume remains unchanged throughout the weaning process. Weaning of mechanical frequency begins after muscle relaxants and their reversal, narcotics and their reversal, and patient temperature have been assessed. Weaning proceeds with decrements of 1 to 2 breaths per minute as long as arterial pH remains above an acceptable level. Since arterial PCO_2 is a secondary determinant of adequacy of ventilation, no changes are made for slight variations in arterial carbon dioxide tension. Weaning proceeds until a mechanical frequency of 0, 1, or 2 breaths per

Table 21-2
Mechanical Ventilators

Ventilator	Patient Applications	Power Source 1° (2°)	Cycling Mechanism I → E	Volume Generation	IMV Capability	Fresh Gas Sources O₂	Fresh Gas Sources Air	Comments
Bennett MA1, MA2	A, P	El (Pn)	V (P)	F	Yes	40–60 psi	Ambient (MA1) 40–60 psi or Internal air compressor (MA2)	Electronic compressor produces gas drive for bellows which deliver tidal volume.
Biomed MVP-10	N, P	Pn	T, V, P	F	Yes	45–55 psi	45–55 psi	Fluidic control
Bird Babybird Ventilator	N	Pn	T	F	Yes	50 psi	50 psi	Gas flow produces pressure changes that activate spring-loaded valves.
Bird IMV Bird	A, P	Pn	T	P	Yes	50 psi	50 psi	Control of gas flow with spring-loaded valves
Bourns Adult Volume Ventilator Bear 1	A, P	El, Pn	V (T*)	F, P**	Yes	32–100 psi	32–100 psi Internal air compressor	Electronic control of solenoid valves modulates flow.
Bourns Infant Pressure Ventilator BP200	N	El, Pn	T	F, P***	Yes	30–75 psi	15–75 psi	Solenoid valve controls gas flow, which is modulated by needle valves.

Ventilator	Patient applications	Power source	Cycling mechanism		Inspiratory hold			Volume generation
Bourns Infant Volume Ventilator LS 104-150	N	El	V∝T	F, P***	Yes	50 psi	Ambient	Volume displacement by a piston
Emerson IMV Ventilator	A, P	El	V∝T	F	Yes	Flowmeter	Flowmeter	Volume displacement by a piston
Emerson Post-op Ventilator (modified)	A, P	El	V∝T	F	Yes	Flowmeter	Flowmeter	Volume displacement by a piston
Healthdyne Ventilator 105	N, P	El, Pn	T	F	Yes	45–65 psi	45–65 psi	Fluidic control
Monaghan Volume Ventilator 225	A	Pn	V, P, T	F	yes	50 psi	50 psi	Fluidic control of gases which compress bellows
Ohio CCV1, CCV2	A, P	El, Pn	V (T*)	P, F****	Yes	50 psi	Internal air compressor	Solenoid valve controls gas flow which compresses bellows.
Sechrist Infant Ventilator IV-100	N, P	El	T	F	Yes	45–55 psi	45–55 psi	Fluidic control of gas flow
Siemans-Elema 900 Servo Ventilator	A, P, N	El	T	F	Yes	3–100 psi	3–100 psi	Servo flow control of gases from bellows source

Patient applications: A = adult, P = pediatric, N = neonatal. Power sources: Pn = pneumatic, El = electric. Cycling mechanism: T = time, V = volume, P = pressure. Volume generation: F = flow, P = pressure. *If *Inspiratory hold* is employed. **F or P dependent upon lung-thorax conditions, airway pressure, and ventilator waveform control setting. ***F under normal conditions; P if pressure limit is reached during inspiratory phase. ****F early in inspiratory phase; zero flow at end of inspiratory phase if inspiratory hold is employed.

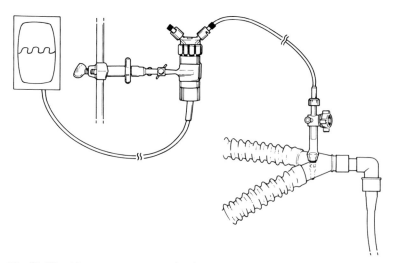

Fig. 21-22 Airway pressure monitoring system. An airway pressure monitoring system can be constructed by utilizing a circuit Y-connector with one port attached to pressure tubing, which leads to a pressure transducer. Display of the airway pressure is upon a calibrated oscilloscope. A stopcock is provided in-line for zeroing of the system. Note that the breathing circuit and pressure tubing are lower than the transducer to help prevent entry of condensate into the pressure monitoring system. The system should be air-filled and fluid-free.

minute is reached. Clinical assessment is then made of the level of consciousness and adequacy of airway protective function in the patient prior to extubation. Since a decrement in mechanical frequency from two to one breath per minute represents a 50 percent reduction in support and a decrement from one to zero represents termination of mechanical ventilatory support, an adequate clinical assessment is very important if the patient is to be extubated before a rate of zero is reached.

SPECIAL TECHNIQUES

Mechanical Ventilation with Interrupted Airways Disease

Interrupted airways disease occurs when a conducting airway or airways at the exchange level of the lung become open to the tissues surrounding it, thus permitting gas flow without the lungs through an abnormal pathway. The underlying pathophysiology with interrupted airways disease is that of bronchopleural fistula. This may result from traumatic interruption (gunshot or stab wound), surgical interruption (wedge resection, lobectomy, pneumonectomy), or pulmonary infection with subsequent airways interruption. The patient already has been or will soon be treated with a chest tube placed in the affected side, with application of negative pressure through a chest-bottle system in an attempt to aspirate the leaking air and maximally expand the affected lung. The problem of hypoventilation generally occurs when the patient is undergoing positive-pressure mechanical ventilation, which is not effective in supporting partially or completely the elimination of carbon dioxide. This is due to the loss of part of the tidal volume through the bronchopleural fistula, which is now being evacuated through the chest-bottle system. In many cases, an attempt to improve alveolar ventilation by increasing either mechanical frequency or tidal volume results in worsening of the patient's overall ventilatory status, producing a rise in $PaCO_2$ and a fall in pH. The attempt to increase minute ventilation by increasing mechanical rate or tidal volume leads not only to increasing gas loss through the fistula but also to increasing alveolar dead space as a result of the greater mean pressures being generated throughout the remaining good portion of the patient's lungs.

The underlying problem is one of gas flow, and therefore gas loss, across the bronchopleural fistula. Increasing negative pressure in the chest-bottle system will exacerbate the problem, just as does increasing ventilatory rate or volume; since this, too, increases flow across the fistula.

The goal in treatment of the bronchopleural fistula is to reduce the flow across the fistula, thereby promoting its closure. In the non-pneumonectomy patient, who has lung remaining on the affected side, an additional goal is to maximally expand the lung and eliminate the gaseous volume in the pleural space. Since either increasing negative pressure within the chest-tube system or increasing positive pressure via mechanical ventilation only worsens the situation, an effort must be made to reduce one or both of these pressures. Even though it may appear contradictory to the supportive goal in the patient, a reduction in mechanical ventilatory rate or tidal volume should be tried initially. If this fails, several additional supportive techniques are available.

Since this is generally a unilateral lung problem, selective bronchial intubation and differential treatment of the lungs may permit diminution or ablation of flow across the bronchopleural fistula on the affected side while promoting adequate support of ventilation on the unaffected side. This can be accomplished in adult patients with an endobronchial tube appropriate for long-term airway management (Broncho-Cath, National Catheter Company). For the patient who requires continued support of

ventilation after the selective bronchial intubation, dual ventilatory circuits may have to be employed. This is accomplished more easily by using separate ventilators with separate circuits than by attempting to use a split, or dual, breathing circuit with one mechanical ventilator. If it is necessary to ventilate both lungs synchronously, an adaptation of the electrical timing system for two mechanical ventilators in simultaneous use is available (J.H. Emerson Co.). Once the side with the bronchopleural fistula has been isolated by selective bronchial intubation, it may be necessary to utilize only the unaffected side for the partial or complete support of ventilation needed for the patient.

If selective bronchial intubation is not possible in the patient with bronchopleural fistula, a technique can be employed whereby gas flow through the fistula is diminished or stopped during the mechanical ventilator's inspiratory cycle. This technique employs the interruption of the vacuum-breaker bottle's aspiration of the water-seal bottle in the chest-bottle system during the positive-pressure phase of mechanical inspiration, which can be accomplished by inserting an expiratory valve (Emerson Exhalation Valve, J.H. Emerson Co.) in-line between the two bottles and activating the valve with a line teed from the charging line which activates the expiratory valve of the breathing circuit (Fig. 21-23). Therefore, when the expiratory valve is closed as the mechanical inspiratory phase begins, the vacuum applied to the chest-tube system will be interrupted and a no-flow system will be established temporarily. Since no gas flow from the pleural space is being promoted during this phase, the delivered tidal volume will enter and be distributed throughout the patient's lungs. Since the resistance in the bronchopleural fistula compartment is now increased above its previous near-zero value, gas distribution will occur depending upon relative compartmental resistances. Some leak through the fistula into the pleural space may occur, resulting in a small reduction in

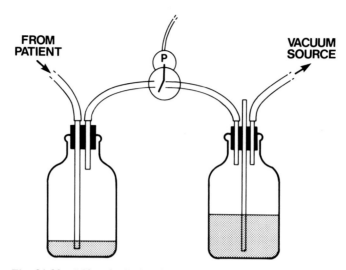

FROM PATIENT

VACUUM SOURCE

Fig. 21-23 "Charging" the chest bottle system. To stop aspiration from the pleural space during mechanical inspiration, a valve is interposed between the underwater-seal bottle and the vacuum-breaker bottle in a two-bottle system. The line that activates closure of the expiratory valve of the breathing circuit is teed to activate the valve which stops flow between the two bottles. Pressure in the vacuum-breaker bottle remains at the level preset by the depth of the vacuum-breaker straw; pressure in the water-seal bottle may increase during the mechanical breath. During the expiratory phase of mechanical ventilation, flow will resume within the system and will evacuate in a conventional manner any gas which has accumulated in the pleural space.

lung size (i.e., increase in pleural air space), but this gas will be evacuated during the expiratory phase of mechanical ventilation when once again the vacuum aspiration of the chest-tube system is applied to the pleural space.

Technical considerations with this form of therapy for interrupted airways disease include the use of a two-bottle chest-tube system, wherein gas flow through the bronchopleural fistula is diminished or stopped by interrupting the vacuum aspiration during the inspiratory phase of mechanical ventilation. Placement of the valve for this interruption must be made with a view to providing chest tube drainage as well as minimizing potential for infection. Therefore, the valve should be placed between the water-seal bottle and the vacuum-breaker bottle, not between the patient and the water-seal bottle. The valve's actuation must be timed with the closure of the expiratory valve of the breathing circuit. Therefore the length of tubing which is teed from the charging line of the ventilator must provide pressure transmission for simultaneous closure of each valve. The use of self-contained single-unit chest-bottle systems (e.g., Pleur-evac, Deknatel) is not appropriate for this form of therapy. Since there is a continued potential for increasing the gas volume within the pleural space during this form of therapy, more frequent radiographic monitoring of the patient may be required.

High-frequency positive-pressure ventilation is applicable uniquely to the treatment of the patient with interrupted airways disease.

High-Frequency Positive-Pressure Ventilation

Rhythmical movement of gases into and out of the lungs has been appreciated for centuries, and throughout this time support of breathing has been directed at emulating the cyclical movement of the respiratory gases. Quantitation of this movement, including measurement of the conducting airways' volume (anatomic dead space), was achieved at about the turn of this century.[32]

Then, in 1909, Meltzer and Auer described a non-rhythmical means of supporting respiration in which they utilized a continuous fresh gas flow delivered to the airways at a pressure of approximately 15 to 20 mmHg.[33] They studied the respiratory and cardiovascular function of their dog model over several hours, inferring good oxygenation from color and satisfactory ventilation from cardiovascular stability. They recognized specific problems associated with establishment and maintenance of the airways for these studies and utilized three different techniques: (1) tracheostomy tube through a large stoma, with gas inflow via the tracheostomy tube and gas outflow via the stoma; (2) side-by-side tubes through tracheal incisions; and (3) a catheter through an oral endotracheal tube. The conclusions from their study were anticipatory of developments of today in that they believed this non-rhythmical support could provide adequate respiration and, what is more important, could provide a means for performing cardiovascular studies without the respiratory variation overlay. In fact, almost 60 years later, other non-cyclical forms of support of ventilation were developed in conjunction with cardiovascular studies. To eliminate respiratory variation in carotid sinus blood pressure studies in dogs, Sjostrand and co-workers developed and utilized high-frequency positive-pressure ventilation (HFPPV).[34] For measuring transmyocardial pressure transmission, Lunkenheimer and co-workers developed a high-frequency oscillatory technique, which also effectively ventilated dogs.[35] The ventilatory frequencies in these early studies were 60 to 100 per minute (Sjostrand et al) and 23 to 40 Hz (Lunkenheimer et al).[34,35] In both studies, the dogs' airways were maintained with oral endotracheal tubes, an intraluminal catheter being inserted for provision of HFPPV in Sjostrand's series and the high-frequency oscillator being applied at the proximal end of the endotracheal tube in Lunkenheimer's series. Work at the same time by Heijman and coworkers introduced the first human applications of HFPPV.[36] This study was conducted in normal surgical patients in whom they reported good ventilation and oxygenation as well as cardiovascular stability during the application of HFPPV.

This technique should not be confused with the technique of *apneic oxygenation*, which has been studied by several groups, including Frumin and co-workers, who in 1959 reported adequate oxygenation for periods up to 55 minutes with the provision of a low fresh-gas flow and no rhythmical support of ventilation.[37] However, in their eight patients the carbon dioxide tensions rose as high as 250 mmHg with ventricular ectopy progressing to ventricular tachycardia in two of their eight patients—obviously not a suitable form of long-term ventilatory support.

PRINCIPLES OF HFPPV

The basic difference between HFPPV and conventional mechanical ventilation is in the means by which respiratory gases are transferred in the conducting airways. During spontaneous respiration and during conventional mechanical support of ventilation, transfer of respiratory gases through the conducting airways is accomplished by bulk flow of the gases into and out of the lungs. The carbon dioxide that is presented via the pulmonary arterial circulation to the gas compartment of the gas exchange unit is transferred from whole blood into the gas phase by diffusion. The transfer of respiratory gases within the gas exchange portion of the lung also occurs by molecular diffusion, which terminates at about the level of the terminal bronchiole, or seventeenth airway generation. Convective movement, or bulk flow, then is responsible for the transfer of carbon dioxide out and oxygen into the lungs through the conducting airways.

In the technique of HFPPV, molecular diffusion is still the primary process responsible for transfer of respiratory gases at the exchange level in the lung parenchyma. However, i) is *augmented diffusion* that is primarily responsible for transfer of these gases through the conducting airways. This was described originally in soils by Scotter and co-workers when they were able to enhance the diffusivity of oxygen 4½- to 50-fold with the application of a 5cc volume above the soil at a 1 Hz frequency.[38] Application of this principle of augmented diffusion has been described for airways by Fredberg, Slutsky et al and by Lehr et al.[39-41]

TECHNIQUES OF HFPPV

Two general considerations are relevant for any high-frequency ventilatory technique: (1) *airway management,* including gas flow patterns, and (2) the *system* for the delivery of the high-frequency positive-pressure ventilation. For airway management and gas flow patterns, essentially two types of systems exist, open and closed. With the open system, there is control over only the gas inflow, not the gas outflow. With the closed system, there is control over both gas inflow and outflow. For example, with the closed system the potential for the application and control of distending airway pressure exists, whereas it may not with the open system.

One example of an *open system* is the percutaneous placement of a transtracheal catheter, e.g., 14 gauge Angiocaths, for elective or emergent airway management for ap-

plication of HFPPV.[42] A similar open system is one in which a catheter is placed via the nose or mouth with its distal end residing in the trachea above the carina. Inflow is intraluminal* and outflow is extraluminal with this technique, which has been utilized by Erickson and Sjostrand in the development of laryngoscopic HFPPV.[43] They report satisfactory ventilation and oxygenation with 60 breaths per minute utilizing this technique, which allows a virtually unobstructed view by the endoscopist. Another open system would be that utilizing an uncuffed endotracheal tube or endotracheal tube without cuff inflation.[44,45]

When open systems are utilized, the gas outflow pathway is not established mechanically and therefore depends upon natural airway patency for adequate gas egress. Outflow can be compromised by head and neck position, cross-sectional area of the endotracheal tube exceeding an acceptable maximum cross-sectional area of the trachea, secretions in the airways, airway edema, or other airway pathology. When an endotracheal tube is utilized for provision of HFPPV in an open system, its cross-sectional area in relation to the overall cross-sectional area of the trachea may become a limiting factor for gas outflow. Aspiration is a potential problem with open systems and may occur during HFPPV, depending upon the type and position of the gas inflow pathway.[46] Although it has been reported not to occur during the actual administration of HFPPV with certain techniques, it has been shown to occur immediately after cessation of the HFPPV.[47,48]

For long-term ventilatory support, a better system would be one which guarantees airway protection and guarantees patency for gas outflow—the *closed system.* With a closed system the pathways for inflow and outflow are established physically by an artificial airway device. The two paths may exist

---

* *Lumen* in this section refers to artificial airway device, e.g., endotracheal tube lumen or tracheostomy tube lumen.

simultaneously within part of the system, providing bidirectionality of gas flow within the system, depending upon phase of ventilation. A closed system has been utilized by Sjostrand and co-workers in much of their later HFPPV work, in which they have placed a catheter within a short segment of an endotracheal tube for delivery of the HFPPV.[49] Another double-lumen technique is the use of endobronchial tubes in which the side-by-side lumens provide separate inflow and outflow tracts. The endobronchial tube may or may not be cut off beyond the end of its first lumen, but both distal ports of the tube must reside within the trachea proper. However, it should be noted that the preformed shape of many of these endobronchial tubes may force the proximal lumen against the tracheal wall, thereby partially or completely preventing gas outflow. A quadruple-lumen endotracheal tube has been designed specifically for the provision of HFPPV (Hi-Lo Jet Tracheal Tube, National Catheter Co.).

The different variables related to the provision of high-frequency positive-pressure ventilation are outlined in Table 21-3. Gas inflow and gas outflow have been discussed above. Each of the other variables will be discussed below.

Ventilators for high-frequency positive-pressure ventilation basically include four types, as shown in Table 21-4, which also lists references to representative studies or case reports. The volume displacement pump can be a piston within a cylinder which is driven by an electric motor. Systems have been described with displacement volumes of 1 to 100 ml and frequencies of 1 to 100 Hz.[44] One of the first volume-displacement high-frequency positive-pressure ventilators was the airways vibrator developed and patented by John H. Emerson in 1959.

Flow interruption can be achieved with magnetic valves and with slotted ball bearings. The electromagnetic valve is available as AGA Bronchovent (AGA Medical AB, Lidingo, Sweden), described by Sjostrand

Table 21-3
Variables Related to Provision of High-Frequency Positive-Pressure Ventilation

Volume-frequency source
Fresh gas flow
Inspiratory and expiratory timing
System compliance
Gas inflow pathway (inspirate)
Gas outflow pathway (expirate)
Patient

and co-workers.[50] The slotted ball-bearing device (J.H. Emerson Co.) is a flow interrupter whose frequency is determined by the speed of an electric motor attached to the ball bearing.

Several fluidic ventilators have been utilized in HFPPV technique; the rates attained have been between 60 and 900 per minute.[42,51] Fluidic ventilators are suited uniquely to HFPPV owing to their rapid response times and their lack of moving parts for delivery of gases—very important considerations for ventilatory rates that can exceed 15 Hz. The application of fluidic technology has been described by Klain and Smith and by Smith et al.[52,53]

Another volume-frequency source for HFPPV can be provided by high-fidelity speakers. This technique can produce a wide range of frequencies and variable volume displacement.

The frequency range in which HFPPV is accomplished is shown in Table 21-5, along with the conventional mechanical ventilatory range of 1 to 20 (0.02 to 0.3 Hz).

Humidification is available with some HFPPV techniques but not with others. When available, it varies from actual humidification of all or part of the fresh gas flow to aerosolization of a drip irrigant in the inflow pathway. Efficiency of humidification with HFPPV technology has not been studied extensively, although the deleterious effects of using dry gases with HFPPV have been reported.[54]

The timing of gas inflow and outflow can be of critical importance with the

Table 21-4
Volume-Frequency Sources for HFPPV

Devices	References
Volume displacement pumps	35, 44
Flow interruption devices	
Electromagnetic valves	34, 36, 43, 45, 49, 50, 55, 57, 58, 60, 64, 69, 70
Slotted ball bearings	67, 68
Fluidic ventilators	42, 51, 53, 56
High-fidelity speakers	40

HFPPV technique. This has been recorded in different studies as inspiration: expiration (I:E) ratio or as inspiratory time. The capability of varying the I:E ratio is available on some ventilators but not on others. When this has been studied as an independent variable in HFPPV technique, an inspiratory time equal to 22 to 32 percent of the ventilatory cycle has been found to be most efficacious.[36,49]

In Table 21-6, the various forms of airway management, including applicable breathing circuit components, are listed under the classifications of open and closed systems, with selected references.

PHYSIOLOGICAL EFFECTS OF HFPPV

Different neural effects in terms of control of breathing have been reported by different groups of investigators. Apnea has been produced in several models, sometimes immediately upon application of the HFPPV, with spontaneous ventilation re-

turning immediately following its discontinuation.[34,55] Others have reported that patients or animal models have continued spontaneous ventilatory activity during application of HFPPV[35,53,56] Although reports have differed among groups utilizing different techniques for provision of HFPPV, not enough data are available to ascertain whether the apnea is related to some aspect of the HFPPV technique or to the frequency or to some other etiology. Continued spontaneous ventilatory activity has several advantages for improving cardiovascular function but has disadvantages in terms of a quiet operative field for thoracic surgery, neurosurgery, etc. Therefore, several groups have used muscle relaxants during HFPPV for animal studies and for patient applications.[35,36,40,42-44,53-60]

The cardiovascular effects of HFPPV are the result of the lower airway pressures produced with this technique of ventilatory support and, in some series, also of the production of apnea associated with the tech-

Table 21-5
Frequency Range for HFPPV*

Designation	Hertz	Minute^{-1}	Selected References*
Conventional mechanical ventilation	0.02–0.3	1–20	49, 57, 70
Low-frequency HFPPV	1–2.5	60–150	34, 36, 42–45, 49–60, 64, 69, 70
Medium-frequency HFPPV	2.5–6	150–360	40, 53, 56
High-frequency HFPPV	6–16	360–960	35, 40, 44, 53
Ultra-high frequency HFPPV	> 16	> 960	35, 40

* Frequencies are given in rates *per minute* and *per second* (*Hertz*). Suggested designations are for ranges extant in current literature. Breakpoint of 2.5 Hz represents upper limit of range currently accepted for clinical (nonresearch) applications by FDA. Selected references are provided for each range.

Table 21-6
Airway Management for HFPPV

System	References
Open Systems	
Percutaneous transtracheal catheter	42, 53, 56
Nasotracheal catheter (for laryngoscopy)	43, 50
Endotracheal tube without cuff or without cuff inflation	44, 45
Bronchoscope (fiberoptic), inflow via suction port	62
Closed Systems	
Endotracheal tube with cuff inflated	36, 57
Tracheostomy with cuff inflated	40, 64
Endotracheal or tracheostomy tube with circumferential ligation of tube in trachea	45, 69, 70
Catheter in endotracheal tube lumen	34, 49
Endobronchial tube, both lumens in trachea	
Endobronchial tube, selective lung ventilation	59
* Bronchoscope (rigid) with side arm attachment	50, 58, 60
** Uncuffed endotracheal tubes in infants and children	55

* Listed as *closed system* even without tight airway seal because outflow path is established.
** Listed as *closed system* even without use of endotracheal tube cuff because outflow path is intraluminal and because cuffed endotracheal tubes are not used routinely in this age group of patients.

nique. A lower mean airway pressure with HFPPV results in a lower pleural pressure, which can result in increased venous return and thereby in improved cardiac output. For patients who do not become apneic during HFPPV, the continued contribution of the intrathoracic pump mechanism to venous return also will add to increased venous return and increased cardiac output.

Respiratory effects related to HFPPV compared with conventional CMV include lesser mean and peak airway pressures and more negative pleural pressures.[57] The lower peak and mean airway pressures may reduce the incidence of pulmonary barotrauma with HFPPV compared with control mode ventilation, although no series has yet been reported.

Improvement in pulmonary oxygenating ability has been shown with HFPPV as against CMV, including a reduced shunt fraction and a reduced alveolar-arterial PO_2 difference.[61] Given the potential increase in cardiac output and the potential for improved pulmonary oxygenating ability, oxygen transport certainly may be enhanced, as has been reported by Eriksson and co-workers.[57]

APPLICATIONS FOR HFPPV

Since the recent introduction of HFPPV, several patient series have been reported. These have included the use of HFPPV in elective adult surgical patients and in infants and children undergoing surgery.[36,55] Use of HFPPV in patients with normal lungs has proved to be an advantageous means of support for bronchoscopy and for laryngoscopy.[43,50,58] HFPPV has been applied to fiberoptic bronchoscopy as well as to rigid bronchoscopy.[62]

One group of patients with acute restrictive lung disease undergoing therapeutic HFPPV has been a small series of premature infants with infant respiratory distress syndrome.[63] Although there have been case reports of HFPPV in adults with adult respiratory distress syndrome, there have been no large series yet reported with ARDS.[64,65] In fact, there is evidence that HFPPV alone will not provide adequate therapy for ARDS without the concomitant application of distending airway pressure therapy.[65,66]

Many of the case reports of the application of HFPPV in acute lung injury have been related to interrupted airways disease—

traumatic, surgical, or related to infection.[67,68] The low peak and mean airway pressures, along with the ability to provide support for carbon dioxide elimination without convective gas movement, makes HFPPV an improved technique in interrupted airways disease.

Extracorporeal Membrane Oxygenation

Development of means for artificial support of heart and lung functions was directed primarily at needs related to openheart surgery prior to the early 1960s.[71] The use of extracorporeal membrane oxygenation (ECMO) for support of patients acutely ill with respiratory failure began in the late 1960s, and as of April 1975, 217 patients had been provided with this form of support; survival rate at that time was 10 percent.[72]

The most comprehensive study of the pathophysiology and treatment of ARDS was undertaken under the auspices of the National Heart, Lung, and Blood Institute of the National Institutes of Health. Beginning with their task force study in 1971, through the completion of the study in 1977, nine different medical centers compiled data on more than 500 patients, including 90 who were entered into the actual ECMO study— 42 ECMO patients and 48 conventional therapy patients. The following discussion represents the general results and conclusions drawn from this controlled study.[73]

Study of the application of ECMO was undertaken because it was felt that this would "rest the lung" while supporting other organs during lung reparation. This form of support could avoid administration of high inspired oxygen concentrations while still providing satisfactory tissue and organ oxygenation as well as removal of carbon dioxide. Use of ECMO technique and reduction of conventional ventilatory support in these patients provided potential for reducing pulmonary barotrauma. ECMO support should

have resulted in decreased pulmonary arterial pressures and flow and, theoretically, in an enhanced resorption of lung water, thereby reducing pulmonary edema.

The technique for those patients randomized to ECMO support was one of veno-arterial perfusion using membrane oxygenators. The flow, which was generated by roller pumps, was equal to or greater than 1,000 ml/min. Blood takeoff was from the right atrium, inferior vena cava, or superior vena cava via internal jugular or femoral venous cannulae. Blood return could be either central or peripheral via femoral or axillary arteries. During the study central return was found to be more favorable when utilizing the right axillary approach or longer catheters placed retrograde in the central circulation via the femoral artery. Heat was provided to maintain the patients under euthermic conditions. Hematocrits were maintained between 35 and 45 volumes percent, and anticoagulation was achieved with a heparin infusion.

Control patients underwent maximum support for their respiratory failure and full monitoring, as did the ECMO patients, with similar physiologic end-points and therapy. The ECMO patients had a minimum level of conventional ventilator support as well.

The ECMO patients averaged 6 days on bypass and a total of 8 days of therapy; the control patients averaged 7 days of conventional therapy. Of the 90 patients who entered the study and were randomized to either the ECMO or the control group, there were no differences related to type or duration of acute lung disease, sex, or age.

The results in terms of mortality are shown in Table 21-7. Of the 90 patients, 28 did not survive long enough to undergo a minimum duration of either form of therapy. Those who did survive entry plus a minimum of 8 hours of therapy of either form are shown as the "trimmed" group. There is no difference in survival between the two groups of patients.

Several problems related to the applica-

Table 21-7
Survival statistics: ECMO Study, National Heart, Lung, and Blood Institute, 1974–1977[73]

	Initial Group*		"Trimmed" Group*	
	N	Survival	N	Survival
ECMO	42	4 (10%)	32	3 (9%)
Control	48	4 (8%)	30	4 (13%)

* *Initial group* represents all patients entered into the study (N = 90); *"trimmed" group* represents those patients actually undergoing assigned therapy for a minimum of 8 hours (N = 62). There is no statistically significant difference between control and survival in either group.

tion of ECMO support occurred during the 3 years of the study. Increased requirements for blood transfusion were evident in the ECMO group, which had a three- to five-fold greater requirement than the control group. The ECMO group's daily blood needs ranged from 1,200 to 3,800 ml. Hemorrhage was a problem which was found to be greatly influenced by ECMO support, as a result of diminution of platelet counts. White blood cell count was found also to be decreased compared with the control group. Mechanical failures in ECMO support occurred in 38 percent of ECMO patients, although no deaths occurred nor was termination of ECMO required because of any one of these failures. Several difficulties were found in making conventional measurements when compared with the control group, including determination of intrapulmonary shunt fraction and measurement of cardiac output by the thermodilution technique.

Many conclusions were drawn from the results of this controlled study, three of which are applicable to the use of ECMO support today:

1. Compared with the control group of conventional respiratory care, ECMO did not improve survival, the predominant cause of death still being progressive respiratory failure.

2. ECMO did not affect the progress of disease (or lung pathology in those patients who died) any differently than conventional respiratory care.

3. Although ECMO is an effective means of short-term life support, its clinical application for the treatment of acute respiratory distress syndrome is not appropriate or economically justified.

Since the conduct and completion of the ECMO study, several advances have been made in concepts related to application of respiratory care in the critically ill patient which, if employed in a controlled study today, might provide even better morbidity and mortality statistics for the control group versus the ECMO group. These advances include an appreciation that the underlying pathophysiology of ARDS is primarily an oxygenation disability and *not one of ventilatory failure*. Therefore, simultaneous application of support of ventilation with support of oxygenation (i.e., mechanical ventilation and distending airway pressure) is unnecessary and in many cases may actually result in worse cardiovascular function and increased pulmonary barotrauma. The use of distending airway pressure therapy has been studied extensively, and it is now known that this is a therapeutic modality that should be titrated against physiological endpoints and not applied at empirically selected levels. These advances in conventional support and the very high costs of ECMO support—for both equipment and personnel—in the light of no proven efficacy in terms of reduced morbidity or mortality with ECMO have precluded its becoming a clinical tool in use today for support of breathing.

REFERENCES

1. Dery R: Determination of the alveolar humidity and temperature in the dog. Can Anaesth Soc J 18:145-151, 1977
2. Poulton TJ, Downs JB: Humidification of

rapidly flowing gas. Crit Care Med 9:59-63, 1981

3. Bates DV, Fish BR, Hatch TF et al: Deposition and retention models for internal dosimetry of the human respiratory tract. Health Phys 12:173-207, 1966

4. Beeckmans JM: The deposition of aerosols in the respiratory tract. Can J Physiol Pharmacol 43:157-172, 1965

5. Oberlin DC, Nishimura TG: Tracheal oxygen concentrations using nasal prongs. Anesthesiology 53:S384, 1980

6. Smith RA, Kirby RR, Gooding JM, et al: Continuous positive airway pressure (CPAP) by face mask. Crit Care Med 8:483-485, 1980

7. Greenbaum DM, Millen JE, Eross B et al: Continuous positive airway pressure without tracheal intubation in spontaneously breathing patients. Chest 69:615-620, 1976

8. Hoff BH, Flemming DC, Sasse F: Use of positive airway pressure without endotracheal intubation. Crit Care Med 7:559-562, 1979

9. Buck JB, McCormack WC: A nasal mask for premature infants. J Pediatr 66:123-125, 1965

10. Cournand A, Motley HL, Werko L, et al: Physiological studies of the effects of intermittent positive pressure breathing on cardiac output in man. Am J Physiol 152:162-174, 1948

11. Hodgkin JE, Soeprono FF, Chan DM: Incidence of metabolic alkalemia in hospitalized patients. Crit Care Med 8:725-728, 1980

12. Mushin WW, Rendell-Baker L, Thompson PW et al: Automatic ventilation of the lungs. Blackwell Scientific Publications, Oxford, 1980

13. Drinker P, McKhann C: The use of a new apparatus for the prolonged administration of artificial respiration. JAMA 92:1658-1660, 1929

14. Drinker P, Shaw LA: An apparatus for the prolonged administration of artificial respiration. J Clin Invest 7:229-247, 1929

15. Hunter AR: The classification of respirators. Anaesthesia 16:213-234, 1961

16. Mapleson WW: The effect of changes of lung characteristics on the functioning of automatic ventilators. Anaesthesia 17:300-314, 1962

17. Downs JB, Douglas ME, Ruiz BC, et al: Comparison of assisted and controlled mechanical ventilation in anesthetized swine. Crit Care Med 7:5-8, 1979

18. Downs JB, Klein EF, Desautels D et al: Intermittent mandatory ventilation: a new approach to weaning patients from mechanical ventilators. Chest 64:331-335, 1973

19. Heenan TJ, Downs JB, Douglas ME et al: Intermittent mandatory ventilation: is synchronization important? Chest 77:598-602, 1980

20. Lyager S: Influence of flow pattern on the distribution of respiratory air during intermittent positive-pressure ventilation. Acta Anaesthesiol Scand 12:191-211, 1968

21. Watson WE: Observations on physiological deadspace during intermittent positive pressure respiration. Br J Anaesth 34:502-508, 1962

22. Sabar EF, Norlander O, Osborn JJ, et al: Gas distribution studies in experimental unilateral bronchial constriction using an accelerating-flow, volume-controlled respirator. Surgery 58:713-719, 1965

23. Jansson L, Jonson B: A theoretical study on flow patterns of ventilators. Scand J Respir Dis 53:237-246, 1972

24. Bergman N: Effects of varying respiratory waveforms on gas exchange. Anesthesiology 28:390-395, 1967

25. Dammann JF, McAslan TC: Optimal flow pattern for mechanical ventilation of the lungs. Crit Care Med 5:128-136, 1977

26. Fairley HB, Blenkarn GD: Effect on pulmonary gas exchange of variations in inspiratory flow rate during intermittent positive pressure ventilation. Br J Anaesth 38:320-328, 1966

27. Fuleihan SF, Wilson RS, Pontoppidan H: Effect of mechanical ventilation with end-inspiratory pause on blood-gas exchange. Anesth Analg (Cleve) 55:122-130, 1976

28. Dammann JF, McAslan TC, Maffeo CJ: Optimal flow pattern for mechanical ventilation of the lungs: 2. The effect of a sine versus square wave flow pattern with and without an end-inspiratory pause on patients. Crit Care Med 6:293-310, 1978

29. Nordstrom L: Haemodynamic effects of intermittent positive-pressure ventilation with and without an end-inspiratory pause. Acta Anaesthesiol Scand 16:suppl. 47, 29-56, 1972

30. Watson WE: Some observations of dynamic lung compliance during intermittent positive pressure respiration. Br J Anaesth 34:153-157, 1962

31. Downs JB, Marston AW: A new transport

ventilator: an evaluation. Crit Care Med 5:112-114, 1977

32. Haldane JS, Priestley JG: The regulation of the lung-ventilation. J Physiol 32:225-266, 1905

33. Meltzer SJ, Auer J: Continuous respiration without respiratory movements. J Exp Med 2:622-625, 1909

34. Sjostrand U, Jonzon A, Sedin G, et al: High frequency positive pressure ventilation (discussion). Opusc Med 18:74-75, 1973

35. Lunkenheimer PP, Rafflenbeul W, Keller H et al: Application of transtracheal pressure oscillations as a modification of "diffusion respiration." Br J Anaesth 44:627, 1972

36. Heijman K, Heijman L, Jonzon A et al: High frequency positive pressure ventilation during anaesthesia and routine surgery in man. Acta Anesthesiol Scand 16:176-187, 1972

37. Frumin MJ, Epstein RM, Cohen G: Apneic oxygenation in man. Anesthesiology 20:789-798, 1959

38. Scotter DR, Thurtell GW, Taats PAC: Dispersion resulting from sinusoidal gas flow in porous materials. Soil Sci 104, 306-309, 1967

39. Fredberg JJ: Augmented diffusion in the airways can support pulmonary gas exchange. J Appl Physiol: Respir Environ Exercise Physiol 49(2):232-238, 1980

40. Slutsky AS, Drazen JM, Ingram RH Jr et al: Effective pulmonary ventilation with small-volume oscillations at high frequency. Science 209, 609-611, 1980

41. Lehr J, Barkyoumb J, Drazen JM: Gas transport during high frequency ventilation (HFV). Fed Proc 40:384, 1981

42. Smith RB, Cutaia F, Hoff BH et al: Long-term transtracheal high frequency ventilation in dogs. Crit Care Med 9:311-314, 1981

43. Eriksson I, Sjostrand U: A clinical evaluation of high-frequency positive-pressure ventilation (HFPPV) in laryngoscopy under general anaesthesia. Acta Anaesthesiol Scand (suppl 64):101-110, 1977

44. Bohn DJ, Miyasaka K, Marchak BE et al: Ventilation by high-frequency oscillation. J Appl Physiol: Respir Environ Exercise Physiol 48(4):710-716, 1980

45. Jonzon A, Sedin G, Sjostrand U: High-frequency positive-pressure ventilation (HFPPV) applied for small lung ventilation and compared with spontaneous respiration and continuous positive airway pressure (CPAP). Acta Anaesthesiol Scand, suppl, 53:23-26, 1973

46. Szele G, Keenan RL: Does percutaneous transtracheal high frequency ventilation prevent aspiration? A word of caution! Crit Care Med 9:163, 1981

47. Keszler H, Klain M, Nordin U: High frequency jet ventilation prevents aspiration during cardiopulmonary resuscitation. Crit Care Med 9:161, 1981

48. Klain M, Keszler H, Nordin U: Aspiration: a danger during high frequency ventilation? Crit Care Med 9:163, 1981

49. Jonzon A, Oberg PA, Sedin G, et al: High-frequency positive-pressure ventilation by endotracheal insufflation. Acta Anaesthesiol Scand, suppl, 43:1-43, 1971

50. Borg U, Eriksson I, Sjostrand U: High-frequency positive-pressure ventilation (HFPPV): a review based upon its use during bronchoscopy and for laryngoscopy and microlaryngeal surgery under general anesthesia. Anesth Analg (Cleve) 59:594-603, 1980

51. Carlon GC, Howland WS, Klain M et al: High frequency positive ventilation for ventilatory support in patients with bronchopleural fistulas. Crit Care Med 7:128, 1979

52. Klain M, Smith RB: Fluidic technology. Anaesthesia 31:750-757, 1976

53. Smith RB, Klain M, Babinski M: Limits of high frequency percutaneous transtracheal jet ventilation using a fluidic logic controlled ventilator. Can Anaesth Soc J 27:351-356, 1980

54. Nordin U, Keszler H, Klain M: How does high frequency jet ventilation affect the mucociliary transport? Crit Care Med 9:160, 1981

55. Heijman L, Nilsson L-G, Sjostrand U: High-frequency positive-pressure ventilation (HFPPV) in neonates and infants during neuroleptal analgesia and routine plastic surgery, and in postoperative management. Acta Anaesthesiol Scand, suppl, 64:111-121, 1977

56. Klain M, Smith RB: High frequency percutaneous transtracheal jet ventilation. Crit Care Med 5, 280-287, 1977

57. Eriksson I, Jonzon A, Sedin G, et al: The influence of the ventilatory pattern on ventilation, circulation and oxygen transport during continuous positive-pressure ventilation. Acta Anaesthesiol Scand, suppl, 64:149-163, 1977

58. Borg U, Eriksson I, Lyttkens L et al: High-

frequency positive-pressure ventilation (HFPPV) applied in bronchoscopy under general anaesthesia. Acta Anaesthesiol Scand, suppl, 64:69-81, 1977

59. Benjaminsson E, Klain M: Intraoperative dual-mode independent lung ventilation of a patient with bronchopleural fistula. Anesth Analg (Cleve) 60:118-119, 1981

60. Eriksson I, Sjostrand U: Experimental and clinical evaluation of high-frequency positive-pressure ventilation (HFPPV) and the pneumatic valve principle in bronchoscopy under general anaesthesia. Acta Anaesthesiol Scand, suppl, 64:83-100, 1977

61. Malina JR, Nordstrom SG, Sjostrand UH, et al: Clinical evaluation of high-frequency positive-pressure ventilation (HFPPV) in patients scheduled for open-chest surgery. Anesth Analg (Cleve) 60:324-300, 1981

62. Ramanathan S, Sinha K, Arismendy J et al: Bronchofiberscopic high frequency ventilation. Anesthesiology 55:A352, 1981

63. Bland RD, Kim MH, Light MJ, et al: High-frequency mechanical ventilation of low-birth-weight infants with respiratory failure from hyaline membrane disease: 92% survival. Pediatr Res 2:531, 1977

64. Bjerager K, Sjostrand U, Wattwil M: Long-term treatment of two patients with respiratory insufficiency with IPPB/PEEP and HFPPV/PEEP. Acta Anaesthesiol Scand, suppl, 64:55-68, 1977

65. Gallagher TJ, Banner MJ: High frequency positive pressure ventilation for oleic acid induced lung injury, Crit Care Med 8:232, 1980

66. Schuster DP, Klain M: High frequency ventilation during acute lung injury. Anesthesiology 55:A70, 1981

67. Hoff B, Smith RB, Wilson E et al: High frequency ventilation (HFV) during bronchopleural fistula. Anesthesiology 55:A71, 1981

68. Kuwik R, Glass DD, Coombs DW: Evaluation of high frequency positive pressure ventilation for experimental bronchopleural fistula. Crit Care Med 9:164, 1981

69. Borg U, Lyttkens L, Nilsson L-G, et al: Physiologic evaluation of the HFPPV pneumatic valve principle and PEEP. Acta Anaesthesiol Scand, suppl, 64:37-53, 1977

70. Jonzon A: Phrenic and vagal nerve activities during spontaneous respiration and positive-pressure ventilation. Acta Anaesthesiol Scand, suppl, 64:29-35, 1977

71. Peirce EC II: Extracorporeal circulation for open-heart surgery. Charles C Thomas, Springfield, Ill, 1969

72. Gille JP: World census of long-term perfusion for respiratory support. In: Artificial Lungs for Acute Respiratory Failure, 525-530, 1976

73. Extracorporeal support for respiratory insufficiency. A collaborative study. National Heart, Lung, and Blood Institute: U.S. Dept. Heath, Education & Welfare, 1979

Index